NEUROPSYCHIATRIC DISORDERS
AND INFECTION

Dedication

To my father, S. Mehdi Fatemi, whose quest for truth has been a guiding force, and to my family, S. Ali Fatemi MD, Naheed Fatemi, Parvin Fatemi, S. Mohammad Fatemi, Neelufaar Fatemi, Maryam Jalali-Mousavi, and last but not least, my mother, Fatemeh Parsa Moghaddam, whose love and support have enabled me to complete this work.

NEUROPSYCHIATRIC DISORDERS AND INFECTION

Edited by

S HOSSEIN FATEMI MD PhD
*Associate Professor of Psychiatry, Cell Biology, and Neuroanatomy
Department of Psychiatry
University of Minnesota School of Medicine
Minneapolis, Minnesota
USA*

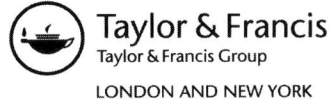

Taylor & Francis Group

LONDON AND NEW YORK

© 2005 Taylor & Francis, an imprint of the Taylor & Francis Group

First published in the United Kingdom in 2005 by
Taylor & Francis, an imprint of the Taylor & Francis Group, 2 Park Square, Milton Park, Abingdon, Oxfordshire, OX14 4RN

Tel.: +44 (0)207 017 6000
Fax.: +44 (0)207 017 6699
E-mail: info.medicine@tandf.co.uk
Website: http://www.tandf.co.uk/medicine

All rights reserved. No part of this publication may be reproduced, stored in a retrieval system, or transmitted, in any form or by any means, electronic, mechanical, photocopying, recording, or otherwise, without the prior permission of the publisher or in accordance with the provisions of the Copyright, Designs and Patents Act 1988 or under the terms of any licence permitting limited copying issued by the Copyright Licensing Agency, 90 Tottenham Court Road, London W1P 0LP.

Although every effort has been made to ensure that all owners of copyright material have been acknowledged in this publication, we would be glad to acknowledge in subsequent reprints or editions any omissions brought to our attention.

Although every effort has been made to ensure that drug doses and other information are presented accurately in this publication, the ultimate responsibility rests with the prescribing physician. Neither the publishers nor the authors can be held responsible for errors or for any consequences arising from the use of information contained herein. For detailed prescribing information or instructions on the use of any product or procedure discussed herein, please consult the prescribing information or instructional material issued by the manufacturer.

A CIP record for this book is available from the British Library.

Library of Congress Cataloging-in-Publication Data

Data available on application

ISBN 1 84184 520 5

Distributed in North and South America by
Taylor & Francis
2000 NW Corporate Blvd
Boca Raton, FL 33431, USA

Within Continental USA
Tel: 800 272 7737; Fax: 800 374 3401
Outside Continental USA
Tel: 561 994 0555; Fax: 561 361 6018
E-mail: orders@crcpress.com

Distributed in the rest of the world by
Thomson Publishing Services
Cheriton House
North Way
Andover, Hampshire SP10 5BE, UK
Tel.: +44 (0)1264 332424
E-mail: salesorder.tandf@thomsonpublishingservices.co.uk

Composition by Expo Holdings, Malaysia

Printed and bound in Great Britain by CPI Bath

Cover image: electron microscopy images of Cystic L-forms of *B. burgdorferi* courtesy of Øystein Brorson and Sverre-Henning Brorson and spirochaetal and L-forms of *B. burgdorferi* reproduced from Mursic et al. *Infection* 1996;24:218–26.

Contents

Contributors ix

Foreword xiii

Preface xv

Acknowledgements xvi

SECTION I   SCHIZOPHRENIA

Epidemiology

1. Have recent studies of the seasonality of birth in schizophrenia added to our knowledge of the disease?
   Masayoshi Kawai, Nori Takei, and Robin M Murray 1

2. Exposure to prenatal infections and psychiatric nosology: A focus on schizophrenia phenotypes
   Gerald Stöber 11

3. Epidemiological correlation of sporadic schizophrenia to Lyme borreliosis
   Markus Fritzsche 18

4. Enteroviruses and schizophrenia
   Jaana Suvisaari 31

Immunology and serology

5. The role of the immune system in the pathophysiology of schizophrenia
   Yong-Ku Kim and Michael Maes 37

6. Serologic studies of prenatal infection and schizophrenia
   Alan S Brown 43

Virology and bacteriology

7. Neurosyphilis, HIV, and psychosis
   Christian G Kohler and Courtney Johnson 51

8. Streptococcal infections and psychoses? A preliminary inquiry
   Daniel R Hanson 59

Animal models

9. Prenatal human influenza viral infection, brain development, and schizophrenia
   S Hossein Fatemi 66

10. Maternal infection causes abnormal behavior in the offspring
    Paul H Patterson 83

11. Maternal influenza A/WSN/33 virus infection in mice and persistence of viral RNA in the brains of exposed offspring
    Fredrik Aronsson and Håkan Karlsson 91

12. Maternal infection, cytokines, and risk for schizophrenia
    John H Gilmore and L Fredrik Jarskog 96

SECTION II MOOD DISORDERS

Immunology

13. Immunology and psychiatry: The role of stress as an immunomodulator in affective disorders
    Brian E Leonard 107

14. Bipolar disorder: Role of infection and immunity
    Dunja Hinze-Selch and Silja Knolle-Veentjer 112

Virology

15. Role of Borna disease virus in neuropsychiatric disorders
    Oliver Planz and Lothar Stitz 123

SECTION III PANDAS, OCD, TICS, AND TOURETTE'S SYNDROME

Epidemiology

16. Infectious trigger in obsessive compulsive and tic disorders
    Tanya K Murphy, Deborah M Herbstman, and Paula J Edge 135

17. Post-streptococcal neuropsychiatric disease: Sydenham's chorea and beyond
    Russell C Dale and Andrew J Church 154

Immunology

18. Exploring the pathophysiology of PANDAS: Streptococcus, Sydenham's, and superantigens
    Kyle A Williams, Jon E Grant, Patrick Schlievert, and Suck-Won Kim 162

SECTION IV AUTISM

Immunology

19. Antibodies against CNS antigens in autism: Possible cross-reaction with dietary proteins and infectious agent antigens
    Aristo Vojdani and Edwin L Cooper 171

20. Immunological issues in patients with autism spectrum disorders
    Harumi Jyonouchi 187

Virology

21. The gut–brain axis in childhood developmental disorders: Viruses and vaccines
    Andrew J Wakefield, Paul Ashwood, and Iain Collins 198

Animal models

22. An animal model of neurodevelopmental damage: Neonatal Borna disease virus infection
    Mikhail V Pletnikov, Steven A Rubin, Timothy H Moran, Michael W Vogel, and Kathryn M Carbone 207

SECTION V   MR AND CEREBRAL PALSY

Immunology

23. Inflammatory perinatal brain damage: Observations, experiments, explanations
    Dorothee B Bartels and Olaf Dammann 216

Virology

24. Mumps virus and CNS disease
    Steven A Rubin and Mikhail Pletnikov 222

SECTION VI   DEMENTIAS

Virology and bacteriology

25. *Chlamydia pneumoniae* as a potential etiologic agent in sporadic Alzheimer's disease
    Hérve C Gérard, Kristin L Wildt, Ute Dreses-Werringloer, Judith A Whittum-Hudson, and Alan P Hudson 229

26. Psychiatric and neurological complications of HIV infection and AIDS
    Diane M P Lawrence, Lynnae Schwartz, and Eugene O Major 239

SECTION VII   ANOREXIA AND BULIMIA

Immunology

27. Autoimmune component in anorexia and bulimia nervosa
    Serguëi O Fetissov 253

SECTION VIII   PERSONALITY DISORDERS

Epidemiology

28. Infectious etiology of adult schizotypal personality: A paradigm and the evidence
    Ricardo A Machón, Matti O Huttunen, and Sarnoff A Mednick 263

Index 271

Contributors

Fredrik Aronsson PhD
Department of Neuroscience
Karolinska Institutet
Stockholm, Sweden

Paul Ashwood PhD
Department of Rheumatology, Allergy and
Clinical Immunology
University of California at Davis
Davis, CA, USA

Dorothee B. Bartels PhD
Perinatal Infectious Disease Epidemiology Unit
Hannover Medical School
Hannover, Germany

Alan S. Brown MD
Department of Psychiatry
College of Physicians and Surgeons of
Columbia University
New York State Psychiatric Institute
New York, NY, USA

Kathryn M. Carbone MD
Center for Biologics Research and Evaluation
US Food and Drug Administration
Bethesda, MD, USA
and
Johns Hopkins University School of Medicine
Baltimore, MD, USA

Andrew C. Church BSc
Department of Neuroinflammation
Institute of Neurology
London, UK

Iain Collins BSc
Visceral, Ltd.
London, UK

Edwin L. Cooper PhD, ScD
Laboratory of Comparative Neuroimmunology
Department of Neurobiology
David Geffen School of Medicine at UCLA
Los Angeles, CA, USA

Russell C. Dale MRCP, MBChB, MSc
Neurosciences Unit
Institute of Child Health
London, UK

Olaf Dammann MD
Perinatal Infectious Disease Epidemiology Unit
Hannover Medical School
Hannover, Germany

Ute Dreses-Werringloer PhD
Department of Immunology and Microbiology
Wayne State University School of Medicine
Detroit, MI, USA

Paula J. Edge AA
Department of Psychiatry
University of Florida
Gainsville, FL, USA

S. Hossein Fatemi MD, PhD
Department of Psychiatry
University of Minnesota School of Medicine
Minneapolis, MN, USA

Sergueï O. Fetissov MD, PhD
Department of Neuroscience
Karolinska Institutet
Stockholm, Sweden

Markus Fritzsche MD
Clinic for Internal Medicine
Adliswil, Switzerland

Hérve C. Gérard PhD
Department of Immunology and Microbiology
Wayne State University School of Medicine
Detroit, MI, USA

John H. Gilmore MD
Department of Psychiatry
University of North Carolina School of Medicine
Chapel Hill, NC, USA

Jon E. Grant JD, MD
Department of Psychiatry and Human Behavior
Brown University School of Medicine
Providence, RI, USA

Daniel R. Hanson MD, PhD
Department of Psychiatry
Veterans Administration Medical Center
Minneapolis, MN, USA

Deborah M. Herbstman BS
Blackband Laboratory McKnight Brain Institute
University of Florida
Gainsville, FL, USA

Dunja Hinze-Selch MD
Department of Psychiatry and Psychotherapy
Christian-Albrechts University
Kiel, Germany

Alan P. Hudson PhD
Department of Immunology and Microbiology
Wayne State University School of Medicine
Detroit, MI, USA

Matti O. Huttunen MD, PhD
Department of Psychiatry
University of Helsinki
Helsinki, Finland
and
Department of Mental Health and Alcohol Research
National Public Health Institute
Helsinki, Finland

L. Fredrik Jarskog MD
University of North Carolina School of Medicine
Chapel Hill, NC, USA

Courtney Johnson BS
Department of Psychiatry
University of Pennsylvania
Philadelphia, PA, USA

Harumi Jyonouchi MD
Department of Pediatrics
New Jersey Medical School
Newark, NJ, USA

Håkan Karlsson PhD
Department of Neuroscience
Karolinska Institutet
Stockholm, Sweden

Masayoshi Kawai MD
Department of Psychiatry and Neurology
Hamamatsu University School of Medicine
Shizuoka, Japan

Suck-Won Kim MD
Department of Psychiatry
University of Minnesota
Minneapolis, MN, USA

Yong-Ku Kim MD, PhD
Department of Psychiatry
Korea University College of Medicine
Seoul, Korea

Christian G. Kohler MD
Department of Psychiatry
University of Pennsylvania
Philadelphia, PA, USA

Silja Knolle-Veentjer MA
Department of Psychiatry and Psychotherapy
Christian-Albrechts University
Kiel, Germany

Diane M. P. Lawrence PhD
Laboratory of Molecular Medicine and Neuroscience
National Institute of Neurological Disorders
and Stroke
Bethesda, MD, USA

Brian E. Leonard PhD, DSc, MRIA
Department of Pharmacology
National University of Ireland
Galway, Ireland
and
Brain and Behavior Research Institute
University of Maastricht
Maastricht, The Netherlands

Ricardo A. Machón PhD
Department of Psychology
Loyola Marymount University
Los Angeles, CA, USA

Michael Maes MD, PhD
Department of Psychiatry and Neuropsychology
Maastricht University
Maastricht, The Netherlands

Eugene O. Major MD, PhD
Laboratory of Molecular Medicine and Neuroscience
National Institute of Neurological Disorders
and Stroke
Bethesda, MD, USA

Sarnoff A. Mednick MD, PhD
Social Science Research Institute
University of Southern California
Los Angeles, CA, USA

Timothy H. Moran PhD
Johns Hopkins University School of Medicine
Baltimore, MD, USA

Tanya K. Murphy MD
Department of Psychiatry
University of Florida
Gainsville, FL, USA

Robin M. Murray MD, DSc, FRCP, FRCPsych
Department of Psychological Medicine
Institute of Psychiatry
London, UK

Paul H. Patterson PhD
Biology Division
California Institute of Technology
Pasadena, CA, USA

Oliver Planz PhD
Institute for Immunology
Federal Research Center for Virus Diseases of Animals
Tübingen, Germany

Mikhail Pletnikov MD, PhD
Johns Hopkins University School of Medicine
Baltimore, MD, USA

Steven A. Rubin MS
Center for Biologics Evaluation and Research
US Food and Drug Administration
Bethesda, MD, USA

Patrick Schlievert PhD
Deparment of Microbiology
University of Minnesota Medical School
Minneapolis, MN, USA

Lynnae Schwartz MD
Laboratory of Molecular Medicine and Neuroscience
National Institute of Neurological Disorders
and Stroke
Bethesda, MD, USA

Lothar Stitz VetMD
Institute for Immunology
Federal Research Center for Virus Diseases of Animals
Tübingen, Germany

Gerald Stöber MD
Department of Psychiatry and Psychotherapy
University of Würzburg
Würzburg, Germany

Jaana Suvisaari MD, PhD
Department of Mental Health and
Alcohol Research
National Public Health Institute
Helsinki, Finland
and
Department of Psychiatry
Hospital District of Helsinki and Uusimaa
Helsinki, Finland

Nori Takei MD, PhD, MSc
Department of Psychiatry and Neurology
Hamamatsu University School of Medicine
Shizuoka, Japan
and
Institute of Psychiatry
London, UK

Michael W. Vogel PhD
Maryland Psychiatric Research Center
University of Maryland
Baltimore, MD, USA

Aristo Vojdani PhD, MT, MSc
Immunosciences Lab, Inc
Beverly Hills, CA, USA
and
Laboratory of Comparative Neuroimmunology
Department of Neurobiology
David Geffen School of Medicine at UCLA
Los Angeles, CA, USA

Andrew J. Wakefield MB, BS, FRCS, FRCPath
Thoughtful House Center for Children
Austin Surgical Hospital
Austin, TX, USA

Judith Whittum-Hudson PhD
Department of Immunology and Microbiology
Wayne State University School of Medicine
Detroit, MI, USA

Kristin L. Wildt BA
Department of Immunology and Microbiology
Wayne State University School of Medicine
Detroit, MI, USA

Kyle A. Williams BA
Howard Hughes Medical School Fellow
Department of Microbiology
University of Minnesota Medical School
Minneapolis, MN, USA

Foreword

The idea that infectious agents may cause severe psychiatric disorders is not new. An editorial in an 1896 edition of *Scientific American* described the work of two physicians who had taken cerebrospinal fluid from mentally ill patients and injected it into rabbits. The rabbits thereupon become sick, although, as the editorial added, "it is not alleged that they [the rabbits] were insane." The editorial, entitled "Is Insanity Due to a Microbe?," suggested that "certain forms of insanity" could be due to infectious agents "similar to typhoid, diphtheria and cholera."[1]

This research approach to severe psychiatric disorders continued to be pursued until the late 1920s, when the infectious theory was displaced, like many other existing theories, by emerging psychoanalytic theories. The decline of the infectious hypothesis in psychiatry continued for the next half century, despite the fact that infectious research was contributing prominently to many other areas of medicine.

This book marks the full re-emergence of the infectious theory in psychiatry. As the chapters make clear, the theory holds great promise and is here to stay. Especially promising is the fact that the infectious theory is fully compatible with genetic, neurotransmitter, and neurodevelopmental theories. As polio and tuberculosis clearly illustrate, there are genes predisposing to viruses and bacteria. Many infectious agents have been shown to act directly on neurotransmitters, including dopamine, serotonin, and GABA. In addition, infectious agents in the developing brain, both *in utero* and in childhood, could well account for neurodevelopmental abnormalities.

Dr Fatemi is to be congratulated for bringing together much of the current research in this exciting approach to understanding severe psychiatric disorders. Combined with emerging work on polymorphisms, splice variants, and other genetic research that is likely to explain how infectious agents and genes interact to cause psychiatric disorders, this research is the psychiatric wave of the future.

E. Fuller Torrey MD
The Stanley Medical Research Institute
Bethesda, MD, USA

---

[1] Is insanity due to a microbe? *Scientific American* 1896;75:303.

Preface

Recent immunologic, epidemiologic, microbiologic and neuropsychiatric studies point to infectious etiologies of several important neuropsychiatric disorders e.g. schizophrenia, autism, obsessive-compulsive disorder, depression, and Tourettes disease. Additionally, several infectious diseases including human influenza virus, HIV, syphilis, and Lyme disease are associated with neuropsychiatric symptoms following transmission of infectious agents to the central nervous system of the adult individuals. An accumulation of experimental evidence also points to potential for peri-, pre-, and postnatal infections as causes for several neurodevelopmental disorders such as schizophrenia, autism, cerebral palsy, and mental retardation.

The main objective for editing this book is the near absence of a comparable book in the published literature which would cover all potential infections and immunological substrates for various neuropsychiatric disorders.

This comprehensive and integrative book examines the role that infectious agents play in the etiology of various neuropsychiatric disorders, including schizophrenia, autism, mood disorders, and obsessive-compulsive disorder. Recent advances in technology and methodology now afford a meaningful examination of the infectious etiologies of neuropsychiatric disorders. Drawing on the contributions of an international panel of experts, this work provides an unprecedented analysis of this emerging field by examining evidence from epidemiologic, serologic and animal models.

This book is the first serious attempt at enumerating experimental and clinical data regarding the infectious etiologies of several important neuropsychiatric disorders such as schizophrenia, autism, mood disorders, and obsessive-compulsive disorder. Features which make this book unique are the expertise of the authors of this book; additionally, presented data are products of years of laboratory and/or clinical studies which have been published in refereed journals.

The book is divided into eight main sections encompassing various neuropsychiatric disorders such as schizophrenia, mood disorder, PANDAS, OCD, Tics and Tourettes' disease, autism, MR, cerebral palsy, dementias, anorexia and bulimia, and personality disorders. Each section is composed of epidemiological, clinical, and experimental data pertaining to each disease entity. As evident from the list of contributors, highly eminent scientists from various laboratories and scientific centers throughout the world have provided the most up to date information about infectious causes for various neuropsychiatric disorders.

It is finally hoped that this book serves as a foundation for provision of knowledge related to immunologic and infectious etiologies for neuropsychiatric disorders for all interested clinicians and neuroscientists.

SHF

Acknowledgements

Many have helped to make the publication of this book possible including Drs. R. Machon, J. Gilmore, R. Derakshan, and K. Lieb. I am especially indebted to Ms. Teri Jane Reutiman, Ms. Anne Vandenberg Snow, and Mr. Joel Stary, for help with various aspects of editing this book. I am grateful to Ms. Janet Holland and Ms. Laurie Iversen for clerical assistance. I am also grateful to the publishers and authors who have generously given approval for reproduction of tables and figures, as well as Mr. Peter Stevenson, Ms. Caroline Milton, and Ms. Amanda May of Martin Dunitz and Parthenon Publishing/Taylor and Francis Medical Books for an excellent job in publishing the book.

SHF

1

Have recent studies of the seasonality of birth in schizophrenia added to our knowledge of the disease?

Masayoshi Kawai, Nori Takei, and Robin M Murray

INTRODUCTION

Tramer first described a winter–spring excess of schizophrenic births in 1929.[1] Since then, numerous studies from many countries have attempted to replicate the season-of-birth effect in patients with schizophrenia. Most of these studies found seasonality of birth in schizophrenic patients, predominantly in the months from December to May, with a peak in January and February. As for the magnitude of the birth excess, it ranges from 5–15%. In contrast, a smaller number of studies focused on months showing a deficit in schizophrenic births; that is, the months when individuals who develop schizophrenia are less likely to be born. The deficit period is in the summer and fall months, and the magnitude of this deficit in births has been reported to be greater than that of the excess births.[2–5]

Some have claimed the season-of-birth effect to be an artifact produced by factors such as age incidence and age prevalence effects.[6] Like other earlier studies,[2,4,5,7–14] two recent studies[15,16] have been conducted to correct for such effects. Both of these studies clearly showed a winter–spring birth excess in schizophrenic patients even after allowing for these effects. Therefore, consensus has been reached among researchers that the winter–spring seasonal birth excess for schizophrenia is not an artifact, but a genuine phenomenon.

Recently, using national case register data from the civil registration system in Denmark (2,669 cases of schizophrenia), researchers examined the extent to which the season-of-birth effect contributes to the risk of developing schizophrenia.[17] They computed the population attributable risk, an estimate of the fraction of the total number of cases of schizophrenia in the population attributable to a specific factor, and demonstrated that it is about 11% for season of birth. In other words, schizophrenia in one out of every 10 patients can be attributed to exposure to winter–spring birth.

Provided that seasonal variation of schizophrenic births is genuine, the question to be posed is: What factors are related to this phenomenon? In an overview of the literature on seasonality of birth in schizophrenia, Torrey and colleagues identified 86 separate studies published in and before 1996, and summarized the relationships between the seasonal birth excess and clinical variables of schizophrenia in order of strength and certainty.[18] The variables that have strong relations to the seasonality effect are place of birth and a negative family history. Those with a moderate relationship are lesser severity of illness and neurophysiological variables such as skin conductance response. Three of four studies that examined the relationship between seasonality of birth and skin conductance reported that winter-born schizophrenics had lower electrodermal activity than those patients born in other seasons.[19–21] On the other hand, factors with no relation to the seasonality effect include gender, social class, ethnicity, pregnancy and birth complications, clinical subtypes, and neurological, neuropsychological, or neuroimaging measures.

Other environmental factors investigated in relation to the seasonality of birth include meteorological indices, such as the amount of daytime light and temperature. The meteorological element that is related to these indices is latitude, which naturally affects the amount of daytime light and temperature in varying seasons. Some studies reported that a latitude gradient is associated with the seasonality birth excess in schizophrenia,[3,22] but another study did not.[23] Hare and colleagues found that the schizophrenia birth rate is consistently higher in colder years.[24] However, other studies found no association between winter temperatures and winter birth excess.[11,25,26]

Since Torrey and colleagues thoroughly and extensively reviewed studies published in and before 1996 that examined seasonality of schizophrenic births,[18] this chapter will focus mainly on recently published studies that deal with relevant issues. Seasonal variables that may underlie the season-of-birth effect in schizophrenia are also discussed. Finally, we will point to promising directions for future research into the seasonality of birth in schizophrenia.

CLIMATE FACTORS

A marked seasonal variation in temperature is noted in those countries, particularly in the northern hemisphere, where the winter–spring birth effect has consistently been reported.[18,27] Accordingly, a study conducted in Reunion, a tropical island in the southern hemisphere, found no seasonal fluctuation in births in patients with schizophrenia compared to the general population.[28] These findings suggest that seasonal variation in temperature or other factors that have similar seasonal fluctuations, which occur in particular in the northern hemisphere and only take place a certain distance from the equator, may be related to the seasonality effect in schizophrenia. To elucidate this further, some new studies have been conducted in the southern hemisphere. An investigation into seasonal variation in the frequencies of births among patients with a diagnosis of schizophrenia ($n = 9,655$) in equatorial Singapore found that monthly variation in births was evident for both patients and controls, and that the pattern was very similar in both groups.[29] It was concluded that no excess of seasonal births for those later developing schizophrenia is apparent in an equatorial region, where 'seasons' are virtually absent. A meta-analysis of 12 studies from the southern hemisphere, to investigate the pattern of schizophrenic births in the southern hemisphere as a whole, was unable to detect any significant season-of-birth effects.[30] These negative findings could be due to the possibility that the countries where these studies were conducted are a relatively short distance from the equator, compared to those in the northern hemisphere. In other words, seasonal factors that are pertinent to the season-of-birth effect in schizophrenia may have less fluctuation and, thus, less influence as an etiological contributor in the southern hemisphere than in the northern hemisphere. This may explain why data from the southern hemisphere have been inconsistent.[18]

Meteorological factors other than temperature have been recently investigated – the length of sunshine and rainfall. Recent research examined the links between the duration of sunshine and the pattern of schizophrenic births.[31] Researchers undertook an ecological analysis of long-term trends in the length of perinatal exposure to sunshine and schizophrenia birth rates based on mental health registers in two different countries (Queensland, Australia $n = 6,630$; the Netherlands $n = 24,474$). Both the Dutch and Australian data showed an association between decreasing long-term trends in sunshine duration around the time of birth and rising schizophrenia birth rates for males, but not for females.

Another study examined the monthly distribution of births in a sample ($n = 2,459$) of schizophrenia patients in northeastern Brazil to assess the relationship between schizophrenia births and rainfall in a tropical area.[32] This region lacks any meaningful seasonal variation in temperature, but has a marked seasonal variation in rainfall. The study found a relationship between rainfall and the number of schizophrenia births three months later, thus raising the possibility that seasonally varying rainfall rather than temperature in the tropical regions might be associated with the risk of schizophrenia.

Sunshine-related components, including direct sunshine hours in daytime, may serve as a potential risk factor for schizophrenia since it is feasible that they may mediate susceptibility to viral infections, hormonal changes, or some nutritional deficiency that in turn directly or indirectly has an effect on brain development. The relationship of rainfall to the seasonality of birth in schizophrenia described above may be accounted for by the length of sunshine rather than the amount of rainfall itself.

PREGNANCY AND BIRTH COMPLICATIONS, AND LOW BIRTHWEIGHT

Pregnancy and birth complications (PBCs) have been shown in many, but not all, studies to be increased in individuals who later develop schizophrenia.[33] Four previous studies investigated the relationship between PBCs and seasonality of birth in schizophrenia.[34–37] In Denmark, researchers found that PBCs had occurred more often in patients born in the winter than in other seasons.[34] A Swedish study used another approach – a matched-pair, case-control method – and reported that obstetric complications increased risk for schizophrenia by 80% in persons born during the winter months.[35] In contrast, the remaining two studies reported quite opposite findings. In England it was reported that a history of PBCs was more common in patients born in the summer or autumn than in the winter or spring.[36] In America it was also found that PBCs were significantly more common in patients born during May–November than December–April.[37] In short, the results have been contradictory.

Low birthweight has been confirmed as a risk factor for schizophrenia in a recent meta-analytic review.[33] And a study examining the relationship between low birthweight and season of birth in patients with schizophrenia – comparing the birthweight of 450 schizophrenic patients born in 1971–1978 with that of controls matched for sex, place of birth, date of birth, maternal age, maternal parity, and social class – reported that schizophrenics born in the second quarter of the year (April–June) had a significantly lower birthweight than the controls, and that this was not attributable to differences in the duration of gestation.[38]

INFECTIONS

An excess of winter–spring births in schizophrenia could be related to exposure to infections during the peri- and/or prenatal period, which occur seasonally, such as influenza and measles.[11,39] There are many studies supporting relationships between seasonal fluctuations in occurrence of infectious diseases and the number of schizophrenia births.[40–45]

A recent study examined the relationship between prenatal exposure to poliovirus infection and later development of schizophrenia.[46] Patients with schizophrenia (n = 13,559) born between 1951 and 1969 were identified from the Finnish Hospital Discharge Register. The investigators calculated the relative risk of prenatal exposure to poliomyelitis (at four months, five months, and six months before birth as risk periods) associated with schizophrenia. They reported an association between exposure to poliomyelitis epidemics at five months before birth (mid gestation) and later development of schizophrenia.

Another large-scale study examined the relationship between pre- and perinatal exposure to two infections (influenza and measles) and the fluctuation of schizophrenic births.[47] The study utilized a Georgia Medicaid database (n = 746,615; 11,736 persons with schizophrenia) to investigate the relationship. The authors first determined the risk exposure timing using a statistical modeling technique and defined three months prior to birth as the risk period. Although there was a relationship between winter births and schizophrenia, the prevalence of influenza or measles in the population three months prior to birth had no effect on the rate of schizophrenia.

It is also possible that the seasonal variation in infant mortality may influence the seasonal birth rate in schizophrenia. On this basis, researchers in Finland examined the seasonal variation of births in relation to epidemics of infections that occurred during the birth period.[48] They utilized the Finish National Population Register to investigate the seasonal variation among schizophrenia patients born between 1950 and 1969 (n = 16,687) who had developed the disorder before 1992. They divided the year of birth into four groups and calculated the odds ratio for patients with schizophrenia being born in a given month compared with the general population born in the same period in Finland and alive at the time of the study. They found that the odds of being born between November and April were high among patients born in the quinquennial period 1955–1959. Severe, widespread epidemics of poliomyelitis occurred in Finland in 1954 and 1956, and epidemics of influenza occurred in 1953, 1955, and 1957. The authors interpreted their results as indicating that the prominent seasonal variation among patients born between 1955 and 1959 was attributable, in part, to epidemics of the two infections, poliomyelitis and influenza, that occurred in the same period.

VITAMIN D

Seasonal variations in the serum level of vitamin D have been postulated to be associated with the seasonality of schizophrenia births.[49] Vitamin D is an important regulator of brain development in the second and third trimesters of pregnancy,[50] and low vitamin D levels in the serum have frequently been reported in regions with less sunlight.[51,52]

The relationship between population exposure to sunlight, as a proxy measure of vitamin D, and the monthly rate of schizophrenic births was examined in two large data sets – schizophrenic patients born in England or Wales between 1921 and 1960 (n = 22,000), and those born in Scotland between 1932 and 1960 (n = 8,000). No convincing evidence in support of the relationship was found in either cohort.[53]

SUBTYPES AND CLINICAL SYMPTOMS

Many attempts have been made to correlate winter birth with clinical variables such as age of onset, prognosis, specific diagnostic subtype, and symptomatology.

Age of onset

Six studies have examined the birth patterns of individuals with childhood-onset (that is, extremely early onset) schizophrenia. Of these, the largest study investigated 2,106 individuals with childhood-onset schizophrenia in a New York psychiatric hospital.[54] Patients with childhood-onset schizophrenia had an excess of births in both winter (December–March) and summer (June–August). Another study reported that 208 individuals with 'childhood psychosis' had an excess of births in the last quarter, especially December, compared to 1,040 non-psychotic controls.[55] The other four studies are too small to be meaningful.[56–59]

In Denmark, researchers used data from the Danish Civil Registration System, and identified persons who were born between 1950 and 1993.[60] There was no interaction between season of birth and age at onset in 10,246 who developed schizophrenia during the follow up period (1970–1998).

Prognosis

Studies examining the relationship between season of birth and outcome features of schizophrenia have yielded inconsistent results. Two found that winter-born patients showed a shorter duration of first hospital admission.[8,22] In contrast, another found winter birth excesses only among schizophrenics who had never married, a group that is thought to be more likely to have severe, process schizophrenia with poor premorbid history.[11] Other studies found no relationship between season of birth and a variety of clinical variables including marital status, total duration of hospitalization, and number of readmissions as well as age of onset which is, in this context, regarded as an index of prognostic variables (earlier onset corresponding to poorer outcome).[61–63]

Subtypes and symptomatology

Three early studies compared the birth seasons between paranoid and non-paranoid schizophrenics and found no significant differences between these two subtypes.[3,61,62] A much smaller study found that patients with positive syndrome schizophrenia tended to be born in non-winter months, whereas equal numbers of negative syndrome patients were born in winter and non-winter months.[64]

Summer birth has been reported as a risk factor for the deficit syndrome,[65,66] a supposed subtype of schizophrenia characterized by primary and enduring negative symptoms.[67] However, the number of subjects with deficit schizophrenia in these studies has been small. Only 26 individuals with deficit schizophrenia were included in the first study (1998), and 46 in the second (2000). More recently, researchers re-examined the relationship between deficit schizophrenia and summer birth with a large sample, using data from an epidemiological study of incident cases of psychosis in Dumfries and Galloway, Scotland (65 deficit schizophrenics and 277 non-deficit schizophrenics).[68] They found that the deficit schizophrenia group had an excess of summer births, compared to both the non-deficit schizophrenia group and all births in the regions. In contrast, a study in France found no significant difference in the pattern of month of birth or season of birth between deficit ($n = 53$) and non-deficit ($n = 158$) patients.[69]

An examination of the interaction of gender and negative symptoms with respect to seasonality of births ($n = 204$) found that female patients born in the winter and early spring had higher scores on the PANSS negative scale and anergia factor, whereas male patients born in non-winter seasons had higher scores on the PANSS anergia factor.[70]

Another recent study investigated the pattern of season of birth in Kraepelinian schizophrenia, defined on the basis of a longitudinal criterion: at least five years of continuous and complete dependence on others to maintain the basic necessities of life, including food, clothing, and shelter.[71] Among Kraepelinian patients ($n = 31$) with negative and disorganized features, there was an excess number of births in the month of July compared with 279 non-Kraepelinian schizophrenic patients. However, the sample size of this study is limited.

Thus, we can conclude that the results on clinical subtypes and symptomatology remain contradictory.

OTHER CLINICAL VARIABLES

Family history

A family history of schizophrenia is the strongest and best documented risk factor for the disease.[72] Torrey and colleagues reviewed 17 studies that examined the relationship between seasonality and a family history of the illness.[18] Based on their overview, there is some evidence that family-history-negative schizophrenic patients are more likely to be born in winter months. This was supported by 10 of the 17 studies. For instance, two studies with large samples reported that individuals with schizophrenia who did not have a family history of the disease were more likely to show a winter birth excess.[73,74]

Inaccuracy of assessment for family histories, including false negative and false positive family history, may have obscured the relationship. To resolve this problem, a direct interview method was used to examine relatives and found that the proportional excess of births in winter months among family-history-negative schizophrenics was highly significant.[75] This result provides additional evidence for the relationship between a negative family history of illness and the seasonality birth effect in schizophrenia.

Place of birth

Recent studies have established that being born or raised in a city is a risk factor for the later development of schizophrenia.[18,76,77] A comparison of the place and season of birth of individuals with schizophrenia with those of individuals with affective psychosis, personality disorders, and neurotic disorders in England and Wales revealed that city birth did not increase the risk of schizophrenia among those born in summer, but was associated with a 19% increase among the autumn-born and a 21% increase among the winter-born. Similarly, in Ireland it was reported that urban-born patients were more likely to be born in the winter than urban-born healthy controls.[78]

Data from a survey in metropolitan France was used to investigate the association between season of birth and place of birth in a sample of 4,139 schizophrenic patients.[79] Researchers found a 20% excess of winter births among patients born in highly densely populated areas compared to those born in other areas.

Another study in the Netherlands followed up all live births recorded in any of 646 Dutch municipalities through the psychiatric case register, and investigated the place and season of birth for 42,115 individuals with schizophrenia.[80] However, no significant interaction was found between Randstad (the most densely populated area) exposure at birth and winter birth.

Gender

Three previous studies reported the winter–spring birth excess in schizophrenia to be more pronounced among men,[74,81,82] whereas four studies found it to be more marked in female patients.[7,22,83,84] Another small southern hemisphere study reported markedly different seasonal birth excesses for men (in winter) and women (in spring).[84] However, many other studies examining male–female differences in the seasonal birth pattern found little or nothing.[8,14,22,61,62,86–91] For instance, a large recent study used a large population-based sample (10,264 cases of schizophrenia), and found no interaction between season of birth and gender.[60]

Social class

It has been reported that the winter birth excess is restricted to those schizophrenic patients from the lower socio-economic classes.[92] However, other studies failed to confirm these findings.[61,87,93]

Ethnicity

Only two studies of seasonal births by ethnicity have been reported. One showed that black individuals with schizophrenia were more likely to be winter-born than white patients.[94] The other found no difference in seasonal birth pattern between white and black patients.[62]

Minor physical anomalies

The association between birth season and minor physical anomalies in patients with schizophrenia has been investigated; no relationship was found between the two.[95]

NEUROANATOMICAL AND NEUROPHYSIOLOGICAL FEATURES

Nine studies have examined the relationship between birth seasonality and neuroanatomical measures on computed tomography (CT) or magnetic resonance imaging (MRI). A CT-based investigation calculated the lateral ventricle to brain ratio (VBR) in 155 individuals with schizophrenia and found that schizophrenic patients born between December and April had greater VBR than those born between May and November.[96] This finding has been reproduced by four other studies.[97–100] On the contrary, researchers who studied 88 affected individuals with a negative family history for schizophrenia with CT reported that those born in the summer and autumn had significantly larger VBRs than those born in winter and spring.[36] The remaining three studies found no association between seasonality of birth and VBR in individuals with schizophrenia using either CT[101,102] or MRI techniques.[63] No studies using recently available MRI techniques, such as region of interest (ROI) analysis and voxel-based morphometric analysis, have been reported so far in this research field.

Neurophysiological studies of schizophrenic patients have also been conducted in relation to birth seasonality. One investigated the association between season of birth and electroencephalogram (EEG) power measures in schizophrenia.[103] This study examined the resting EEGs of 28 winter-born and 81 non-winter-born schizophrenic patients, and 97 normal subjects. They found that non-winter-born, but not winter-born, schizophrenia patients had augmented low-frequency power and diminished alpha band power compared to normal subjects.

PROCREATIONAL HABITS

The 'parental procreational habits' hypothesis posits that the seasonal conception pattern of parents of schizophrenic patients differs from that of the general population. The late spring to early summer peak of births in the general population is thought to be caused by family planning, since summer is the most convenient time to care for a small baby in a cold climate in the northern countries.[104] This hypothesis predicts that the birth rate of the unaffected siblings of patients with schizophrenia should also be higher in the winter and spring.[18] Seasonal variation in births among siblings of patients with schizophrenia has been investigated in six studies, the largest of which involved 2,639 siblings.[9] Two studies found a similar seasonal variation in births among siblings and patients that differed from the variation among the general population,[105,106] but the other four, including the largest study, found no difference in seasonality of births between siblings and the general population.[9,107–109]

The most recent study investigated the seasonal variation of births in a nationwide, epidemiologically representative Finnish sample of patients with schizophrenia (n = 15,389) born from 1950 to 1969 and their unaffected siblings (37,819) born in the same time period.[48] Both patients and siblings had slightly higher odds of being born during the winter and/or spring months than the general population. However, no significant difference in the seasonal variation of births was found between siblings and the general population.

GENETICS

Five studies have consistently shown a higher frequency of HLA-DR1 in patients with schizophrenia than in the general population,[110–114] which might reflect susceptibility to infections during the pre- and/or perinatal period in individuals who go on to develop the disorder. In this regard, a significantly higher rate of births in February and March was observed in patients (n = 60) with HLA-DR1 (31.7%) than those (n = 307) without HDL-DR1 (15.6%).[115] Research into the association between season of birth and HLA-A specificities (the most frequent HLA haplotypes in the Japanese population) in Japanese patients with schizophrenia showed no significant association between HLA-A and birth season.[116]

SHIFTS OF BIRTH SEASONALITY OVER TIME

Huntington in the United States first noted that the seasonal birth pattern for individuals with schizophrenia may shift over time.[117] His 1,114 cases with schizophrenia born before 1885 had a definite October–January birth excess, whereas in the decades after 1885 there was a February–March peak.

In the latter half of the 20th century, several studies examined fluctuations in the magnitude of the seasonal variation over time in the births of individuals with schizophrenia, and shifts of seasonality have been observed in some,[26,118] but not in others.

One of the most recent studies examined data on a Scottish case register for seven decades, from 1900 through 1969.[119] For the two decades of 1900–1909 and 1910–1929, summer–autumn (June–November) births were more numerous than winter–spring (December–May) births for individuals with schizophrenia, but for each decade thereafter, winter–spring births predominated. Another study found no change over time in seasonal variation.[120]

SUMMARY

The season-of-birth phenomenon has been found in many countries, mostly in the northern hemisphere, where there is a temperate climate with clear seasonal variation in temperature. Thus, it is certain that some seasonal varying factor(s) play a role in the etiology of schizophrenia, although they may involve only a small fraction of schizophrenic patients.

The winter–spring birth excess is presumably a proxy for some other factor which remains as yet unknown. Variation in temperature or other meteorological factors such as the amount of sunshine in daytime could be important. For example, the serum level of vitamin D has been postulated to be associated with the seasonality of birth in schizophrenia. As a proxy measure of vitamin D, the amount of sunlight in daytime was examined in relation to the monthly rate of schizophrenic births, but no relationship was found.[53] This negative result may undermine the postulated relationship between vitamin D deficiency and the seasonality of birth effect in schizophrenia.

Another theory suggests that seasonally varying rainfall is a critical factor, and this has been found to be associated with the seasonality of birth in schizophrenia in Brazil where there is no marked seasonal variation in temperature.[32] On the other hand, the association between rainfall and the rate of schizophrenic births could be accounted for by a relation to the sunshine hours instead of rainfall per se, as rainfall is naturally inversely correlated to the amount of sunshine.

Low birthweight, one of the known risk factors for schizophrenia, has recently been suggested to be related to the seasonality of birth effect. Some seasonally varying factors, such as nutritional deficiencies and maternal infections, could influence intrauterine growth and, thereby, result in low birthweight in schizophrenic patients.

Many studies have reported a relationship between the seasonal birth pattern of schizophrenia and seasonal fluctuations in infections. However, the majority of these used only the numbers of live births to calculate the rate of schizophrenic births. This could be a serious limitation if the month of birth is related to mortality and, in fact, a recent report shows that there is a higher infant death rate in those born in winter.[121] If the mortality rate was lower among those otherwise destined to become schizophrenic patients who were born in winter than among the general population born in the same period, then the winter birth excess for schizophrenia would be exaggerated. Therefore, in future studies, to eliminate influence arising from varying mortality in infants or death rates in childhood/adulthood according to the month of birth, it would be optimal to utilize data such as those from computerized case register systems so as to identify individuals who are alive; then one could compare the seasonal variation of schizophrenic births with that of the rest of the living population.

Elucidating the mechanisms that underlie the seasonality effect in schizophrenia could bring about a breakthrough in our understanding of the disease. It may be the time to move to animal models. For example, it would be worth exploring in animal models whether vitamin D deficiency during gestation would produce brain abnormalities that mimic those reported in the brains of schizophrenia patients. Similarly, animal studies could be devised to test whether prenatal exposure to infections associated with a risk for schizophrenia lead to behavioral disturbances and brain abnormalities in the offspring. Indeed, such a study has recently been reported in mice.[122]

REFERENCES

1. Tramer M. Über die biologische Bedeutung des Geburtsmonates, insbesondere für die Psychoseerkrankung. Schweiz. *Arch Neurol Psychiatr* 1929; **24**: 17–24.
2. Hare EH. Season of birth in schizophrenia and neurosis. *Am J Psychiatry* 1975; **132**: 155–8.
3. Torrey EF, Torrey BB, Peterson MR. Seasonality of schizophrenic births in the United States. *Arch Gen Psychiatry* 1977; **34**: 1065–70.
4. O'Callaghan E, Gibson T, Colohan HA et al. Season of birth in schizophrenia. Evidence for confinement of an excess of winter births to patients without a family history of mental disorder. *Br J Psychiatry* 1991; **158**: 764–9.
5. Rodrigo G, Lusiardo M, Briggs G, Ulmer A. Season of birth of schizophrenics in Mississippi, USA. *Acta Psychiatr Scand* 1992; **86**: 327–31.
6. Lewis MS, Griffin PA. An explanation for the season of birth effect in schizophrenia and certain other diseases. *Psychol Bull* 1981; **98**: 589–96.
7. Pulver AE, Sawyer JW, Childs B. The association between season of birth and the risk for schizophrenia. *Am J Epidemiol* 1981; **114**: 735–49.
8. Pulver AE, Stewart W, Carpenter WT Jr, Childs B. Risk factors in schizophrenia: season birth in Maryland, USA. *Br J Psychiatry* 1983; **143**: 389–96.
9. Pulver AE, Liang KY, Wolyniec PS et al. Season of birth of siblings of schizophrenics patients. *Br J Psychiatry* 1992; **160**: 71–5.
10. Watson CG, Kucala T, Angulski G, Brunn C. Season of birth and schizophrenia: a response to the Lewis and Griffin critique. *J Abnorm Psychol* 1982; **91**: 120–5.
11. Watson CG, Kucala T, Tilleskjor C, Jacobs L. Schizophrenic birth seasonality in relation to the incidence of infectious diseases and temperature extremes. *Arch Gen Psychiatry* 1984; **41**: 85–90.
12. Shur E, Hare E. Age-prevalence and the season of birth effect in schizophrenia: a response to Lewis and Griffin. *Psychol Bull* 1983; **93**: 373–7.
13. Aschauer HN, Meszaros K, Willinger U et al. The season of birth of schizophrenics and schizoaffectives. *Psychopathology* 1994; **27**: 298–302.
14. Kim CE, Lee YS, Lim YH et al. Month of birth and schizophrenia in Korea. Sex, family history, and handedness. *Br J Psychiatry* 1994; **164**: 829–31.
15. Pallast EGM, Jongbloer PH, Straatman HM, Zielhuis GA. Excess seasonality of births among patients with schizophrenia and seasonal ovopathy. *Schizophr Bull* 1994; **20**: 269–76.

16. Tam WC, Sewell KW. Seasonality of birth in schizophrenia in Taiwan. *Schizophr Bull* 1995; **21**: 117–27.
17. Mortensen PB, Pedersen CB, Westergaard T et al. Effects of family history and place and season of birth on the risk of schizophrenia. *Engl J Med* 1999; **340**: 603–8.
18. Torrey EF, Miller J, Rawlings R, Yolken RH. Seasonality of births in schizophrenia and bipolar disorder: a review of the literature. *Schizophr Res* 1997; **7**: 1–38.
19. Ohlund LS, Ohman A, Alm T et al. Season of birth and electrodermal unresponsiveness in male schizophrenics. *Biol Psychiatry* 1990; **27**: 328–40.
20. Ohlund LS, Ohman A, Ost LG et al. Electrodermal orienting response, maternal age, and season of birth in schizophrenia. *Psychiatry Res* 1991; **36**: 223–32.
21. Katsanis J, Ficken J, Iacono WG, Beiser M. Season of birth and electrodermal activity in functional psychoses. *Biol Psychiatry* 1992; **31**: 841–55.
22. Dalèn P. *Season of Birth: A Study of Schizophrenia and Other Mental Disorders*. New York: North-Holland/American Elsevier, 1975.
23. Torrey EF, Bowler AE, Rawlings R. An influenza epidemic and the seasonality of schizophrenic births. In: *Psychiatry and Biological Factors* (Kurstak E, ed). New York: Plenum Medical Book Company, 1991: 109–16.
24. Hare E, Moran P. A relation between seasonal temperature and the birth rate of schizophrenic patients. *Acta Psychiatr Scand* 1981; **63**: 396–405.
25. Ede A, Templer DI, Brooner RK, Corgiat M. The seasonality of schizophrenic births in Alberta. *Am J Orthopsychiatry* 1985; **55**: 451–3.
26. Torrey EF, Torrey BB. A shifting seasonality of schizophrenic births. *Br J Psychiatry* 1979; **134**: 183–6.
27. Berk M, Terre-Blanche MJ, Maude C et al. Season of birth and schizophrenia: southern hemisphere data. *Aust N Z J Psychiatry* 1996; **30**: 220–2.
28. d'Amato T, Guillaud-Bataille JM, Rochet T et al. No season-of-birth effect in schizophrenic patients from a tropical island in the southern hemisphere. *Psychiatry Res* 1996; **60**: 205–10.
29. Parker G, Mahendran R, Koh ES, Machin D. Season of birth in schizophrenia: no latitude at the equator. *Br J Psychiatry* 2000; **176**: 68–71.
30. McGrath JJ, Welham JL. Season of birth and schizophrenia: a systematic review and meta-analysis of data from the southern hemisphere. *Schizophr Res* 1999; **35**: 237–42.
31. McGrath J, Selten JP, Chant D. Long-term trends in sunshine duration and its association with schizophrenia birth rates and age at first registration—data from Australia and the Netherlands. *Schizophr Res* 2002; **54**: 199–212.
32. de Messias EL, Cordeiro NF, Sampaio JJ et al. Schizophrenia and season of birth in a tropical region: relationship to rainfall. *Schizophr Res* 2001; **48**: 227–34.
33. Cannon M, Jones PB, Murray RM. Obstetric complications and schizophrenia: historical and meta-analytic review. *Am J Psychiatry* 2002; **159**: 1080–92.
34. Machon RA, Mednick SA, Schulsinger F. Seasonality, birth complications and schizophrenia in a high risk sample. *Br J Psychiatry* 1987; **151**: 122–4.
35. Cantor-Graae E, McNeil TF, Sjostrom K et al. Obstetric complications and their relationship to other etiological risk factors in schizophrenia. A case-control study. *J Nerv Ment Dis* 1994; **182**: 645–50.
36. Jones PB, Goodman R, Owen MJ et al. Neurodevelopment and the chronological curiosities of schizophrenia. In: *Developmental Neuropathology of Schizophrenia* (Mednick SA, Cannon TD, eds). New York: Plenum Press, 1992; 191–209.
37. Kinney DK, Levy DL, Yurgelun-Todd DA et al. Season of birth and obstetrical complications in schizophrenics. *J Psychiatr Res* 1994; **28**: 499–509.
38. Kendell RE, Boyd JH, Grossmith VL, Bain MB. Seasonal fluctuation in birthweight in schizophrenia. *Schizophr Res* 2002; **57**: 157–64.
39. Mednick SA, Machon RA, Huttunen MO, Bonett D. Adult schizophrenia following prenatal exposure to an influenza epidemic. *Arch Gen Psychiatry* 1988; **45**: 189–92.
40. Kendell RE, Kemp IW. Maternal influenza in the etiology of schizophrenia. *Arch Gen Psychiatry* 1989; **46**: 878–82.
41. Sham PC, O'Callaghan E, Takei N et al. Schizophrenia following pre-natal exposure to influenza epidemics between 1939 and 1960. *Br J Psychiatry* 1992; **160**: 461–6.
42. O'Callaghan E, Sham PC, Takei N et al. The relationship of schizophrenic births to 16 infectious diseases. *Br J Psychiatry* 1994; **165**: 353–6.
43. Takei N, Van Os J, Murray RM. Maternal exposure to influenza and risk of schizophrenia: a 22 year study from the Netherlands. *J Psychiatr Res* 1995; **29**: 435–45.
44. Takei N, Mortensen PB, Klaening U et al. Relationship between in utero exposure to influenza epidemics and risk of schizophrenia in Denmark. *Biol Psychiatry* 1996; **40**: 817–24.
45. Limosin F, Rouillon F, Payan C et al. Prenatal exposure to influenza as a risk factor for adult schizophrenia. *Acta Psychiatr Scand* 2003; **107**: 331–5.
46. Suvisaari JM, Haukka JK, Tanskanen AJ, Lonnqvist JK. Decline in the incidence of schizophrenia in Finnish cohorts born from 1954 to 1965. *Arch Gen Psychiatry* 1999; **56**: 733–40.
47. Battle YL, Martin BC, Dorfman JH, Miller LS. Seasonality and infectious disease in schizophrenia: the birth hypothesis revisited. *J Psychiatr Res* 1999; **33**: 501–9.
48. Suvisaari JM, Haukka JK, Lonnqvist JK. Season of birth among patients with schizophrenia and their siblings: evidence for the procreational habits hypothesis. *Am J Psychiatry* 2001; **158**: 754–7.
49. Moskovitz RA. Seasonality in schizophrenia. *Lancet* 1978; **311**: 664.
50. Altschuler EL. Low maternal vitamin D and schizophrenia in offspring. *Lancet* 2001; **358**: 1464.
51. Holick MF. Environmental factors that influence the cutaneous production of vitamin D. *Am J Clin Nutr* 1995; **61**: 638S–645S.
52. McKenna MJ. Differences in vitamin D status between countries in young adults and the elderly. *Am J Med* 1992; **93**: 69–77.
53. Kendell RE, Adams W. Exposure to sunlight, vitamin D and schizophrenia. *Schizophr Res* 2002; **54**: 193–8.
54. Sankar DVS. Demographic studies on childhood schizophrenia: preliminary report on season of birth, diagnosis, sex, IQ, and race distribution. In: *Schizophrenia: Current Concepts and Research* (Sankar DVS, ed). Hicksville, NY: PJD Publications, 1969: 450–69.
55. Fombonne E. Season of birth and childhood psychosis. *Br J Psychiatry* 1989; **155**: 655–66.
56. McNeil TF, Raff CS, Cromwell RL. A technique for comparing the relative importance of season of conception and season of birth: application to emotionally disturbed children. *Br J Psychiatry* 1971; **118**: 329–35.
57. Garralda ME, Watt AE. Seasonal variations in the child and adolescent psychoses. *J Adolesc* 1989; **12**: 315–21.
58. Atlas JA. Birth seasonality in developmentally disabled children. *Psychol Rep* 1989; **64**: 1213–4.
59. Livingston R, Adam BS, Bracha HS. Season of birth and neurodevelopmental disorders: summer birth is associated with

dyslexia. *J Am Acad Child Adolesc Psychiatry* 1993; **32**: 612–6.
60. Pedersen CB, Mortensen PB. Family history, place and season of birth as risk factors for schizophrenia in Denmark: a replication and reanalysis. *Br J Psychiatry* 2001; **179**: 46–52.
61. Kendell RE, Kemp IW. Winter-born v summer-born schizophrenics. *Br J Psychiatry* 1987; **151**: 499–505.
62. Rodrigo G, Lusiardo M, Briggs G, Ulmer A. Differences between schizophrenics born in winter and summer. *Acta Psychiatr Scand* 1991; **84**: 320–2.
63. Roy MA, Flaum M, Andreasen NC. No difference found between winter- and non-winter-born schizophrenic cases. *Schizophr Res* 1995; **17**: 241–8.
64. Opler LA, Kay SR. Birth seasonality and schizophrenia. *Arch Gen Psychiatry* 1985; **42**: 106–8.
65. Kirkpatrick B, Ram R, Amador XF et al. Summer birth and the deficit syndrome of schizophrenia. *Am J Psychiatry* 1998; **155**: 1221–6.
66. Kirkpatrick B, Castle D, Murray RM, Carpenter WT Jr. Risk factors for the deficit syndrome of schizophrenia. *Schizophr Bull* 2000; **26**: 233–42.
67. Carpenter WT Jr, Heinrichs DW, Wagman AM. Deficit and nondeficit forms of schizophrenia: the concept. *Am J Psychiatry* 1998; **145**: 578–83.
68. Kirkpatrick B, Tek C, Allardyce J et al. Summer birth and deficit schizophrenia in Dumfries and Galloway, southwestern Scotland. *Am J Psychiatry* 2002; **159**: 1382–7.
69. Dollfus S, Brazo P, Langlois S et al. Month of birth in deficit and non-deficit schizophrenic patients. *Eur Psychiatry* 1999; **14**: 349–51.
70. Troisi A, Pasini A, Spalletta G. Season of birth, gender and negative symptoms in schizophrenia. *Eur Psychiatry* 2001; **16**: 342–8.
71. Bralet MC, Loas G, Yon V, Marechal V. Clinical characteristics and risk factors for Kraepelinian subtype of schizophrenia: replication of previous findings and relation to summer birth. *Psychiatry Res* 2002; **111**: 147–54.
72. Gottesman II. *Schizophrenia Genesis. The Origins of Madness*. New York: WH Freeman, 1991.
73. Franzek E, Beckmann H. Schizophrenia and birth seasonality—contrary results in relation to genetic risk. *Fortschr Neurol Psychiatr* 1993; **61**: 22–6.
74. Chen WJ, Yeh LL, Chang CJ et al. Month of birth and schizophrenia in Taiwan: effect of gender, family history and age at onset. *Schizophr Res* 1996; **20**: 133–43.
75. Kinney DK, Jacobsen B, Jansson L et al. Winter birth and biological family history in adopted schizophrenics. *Schizophr Res* 2000; **44**: 95–103.
76. Lewis G, David A, Andreasson S, Allebeck P. Schizophrenia and city life. *Lancet* 1992; **340**: 137–40.
77. Takei N, Sham PC, O'Callaghan E et al. Schizophrenia: increased risk associated with winter and city birth—a case-control study in 12 regions within England and Wales. *J Epidemiol Community Health* 1995; **49**: 106–7.
78. O'Callaghan E, Cotter D, Colgan K et al. Confinement of winter birth excess in schizophrenia to the urban-born and its gender specificity. *Br J Psychiatry* 1995; **166**: 51–4.
79. Verdoux H, Takei N, Cassou de Saint-Mathurin R et al. Seasonality of birth in schizophrenia: the effect of regional population density. *Schizophr Res* 1997; **23**: 175–80.
80. Marcelis M, Navarro-Mateu F, Murray R et al. Urbanization and psychosis: a study of 1942–1978 birth cohorts in the Netherlands. *Psychol Med* 1998; **28**: 871–9.
81. Jones IH, Frei D. Seasonal births in schizophrenia. A southern hemisphere study using matched pairs. *Acta Psychiatr Scand* 1979; **59**: 164–72.
82. Michitsuji S, Haas S, Ohta Y et al. Seasonality of birth in schizophrenia and its heterogeneity. In: *Seasonal Effects on Reproduction, Infection and Psychoses* (Miura T, ed). The Hague: SPB Academic Publishing, 1987: 195–204.
83. Parker G, Neilson M. Mental disorder and season of birth – a southern hemisphre study. *Br J Psychiatry* 1976; **129**: 355–61.
84. García Hildebrandt JO. Estacíonalídad del nacimiento en esquizofrenicos de Lima y Callao (Peru)—un estudio en el hemisferio sur [Seasonality of births in schizophrenics from Lima and Callao (Peru) – a study in the southern hemisphere]. *Anales de Salud Mental VIII* 1992; 69–100.
85. Syme GJ, Illingworth DJ. Sex differences in birth patterns of schizophrenics. *J Clin Psychol* 1978; **34**: 633–5.
86. Torrey EF, Torrey BB. Sex differences in the seasonality of schizophrenic births. *Br J Psychiatry* 1980; **137**: 101–2.
87. Ødegård Ø. Season of birth in the general population and in patients with mental disorder in Norway. *Br J Psychiatry* 1974; **125**: 397–405.
88. Hare HE, Bulusu L, Adelstein A. Schizophrenia and season of birth. *Popul Trends* 1979; **17**: 9–11.
89. Parker G, Balza B. Season of birth and schizophrenia – an equatorial study. *Acta Psychiatr Scand* 1977; **56**: 143–6.
90. Hsieh HH, Khan MH, Atwal SS, Cheng SC. Seasons of birth and subtypes of schizophrenia. *Acta Psychiatr Scand* 1987; **75**: 373–6.
91. Goldstein JM, Santangelo SL, Simpson JC, Tsuang MT. The role of gender in identifying subtypes of schizophrenia: a latent class analytic approach. *Schizophr Bull* 1990; **16**: 263–75.
92. Barry H III, Barry H Jr. Season of birth in schizophrenics. *Arch Gen Psychiatry* 1964; **11**: 385–91.
93. Hare EH, Price JS, Slater E. Parental social class in psychiatric patients. *Br J Psychiatry* 1972; **121**: 515–24.
94. Gallagher BJ III, McFalls JA Jr, Jones BJ. Racial factors in birth seasonality among schizophrenics: a preliminary analysis. *J Abnorm Psychol* 1983; **92**: 524–7.
95. Akabaliev V, Sivkov S. Minor physical anomalies in schizophrenia. *Folia Med (Plovdiv)* 1998; **40**: 39–45.
96. Sacchetti E, Vita A, Battaglia M et al. Season of birth and cerebral ventricular enlargement in schizophrenia. In: *Etiopathogenetic Hypotheses of Schizophrenia* (Cazzullo GL, Invernizzi G, Sacchetti E, Vita A, eds). Boston: MTP Press, 1987: 93–8.
97. Zipursky RB, Schulz SC. Seasonality of birth and CT findings in schizophrenia. *Biol Psychiatry* 1987; **22**: 1288–92.
98. Degreef G, Mukherjee S, Bilder R, Schnur D. Season of birth and CT scan findings in schizophrenic patients. *Biol Psychiatry* 1988; **24**: 461–4.
99. Sacchetti E, Calzeroni A, Vita A et al. The brain damage hypothesis of the seasonality of births in schizophrenia and major affective disorders: evidence from computerised tomography. *Br J Psychiatry* 1992; **160**: 390–7.
100. d'Amato T, Rochet T, Dalèry J et al. Seasonality of birth and ventricular enlargement in chronic schizophrenia. *Psychiatry Res* 1994; **55**: 65–73.
101. Wilms G, Van Ongeval C, Baert AL et al. Ventricular enlargement, clinical correlates and treatment outcome in chronic schizophrenic inpatients. *Acta Psychiatr Scand* 1992; **85**: 306–12.
102. DeQuardo JR, Goldman M, Tandon R. VBR in schizophrenia: relationship to family history of psychosis and season of birth. *Schizophr Res* 1996; **20**: 275–85.
103. Sponheim SR, Iacono WG, Clementz BA, Beiser M. Season of birth and electroencephalogram power abnormalities in schizophrenia. *Biol Psychiatry* 1997; **41**: 1020–7.

104. Rantakallio P. The effect of a northern climate on seasonality of births and the outcome of pregnancies. *Acta Paediatr Scand Suppl* 1971; **218**: 1–67.
105. McNeil T, Kaij L, Dzierzykray-Rogalska M. Season of birth among siblings of schizophrenics. A test of the parental conception habits interpretation. *Acta Psychiatr Scand* 1976; **54**: 267–74.
106. Hare EH. The season of birth of siblings of psychiatric patients. *Br J Psychiatry* 1976; **129**: 49–54.
107. Torrey EF. The epidemiology of schizophrenia: questions needing answers. In: *Schizophrenia: Scientific Progress* (Schulz SC, Tamminga CA, eds). New York: Oxford University Press, 1989: 45–51.
108. Buch C, Simpson H. Season of birth among the sibs of schizophrenics. *Br J Psychiatry* 1978; **132**: 358–60.
109. Larson CA, Nyman GE. Birth month of schizophrenics and their sibs. *IRCS Medical Science: Anatomy and Human Biology; Psychology and Psychiatry; Social and Occupational Medicine* 1976; **4**: 56.
110. Miyanaga K, Machiyama Y, Juji T. Schizophrenic disorders and HLA-DR antigens. *Biol Psychiatry* 1984; **19**: 121–9.
111. Sasaki T, Kuwata S, Dai XY et al. HLA-DR types in Japanese schizophrenics: analysis by group-specific PCR amplification. *Schizophr Res* 1994; **14**: 9–14.
112. Sasaki T, Matsushita M, Nanko S et al. Schizophrenia and the HLA-DRB1 gene in the Japanese population. *Am J Psychiatry* 1999; **156**: 771–3.
113. Arinami T, Otsuka Y, Hamaguchi H et al. Evidence supporting an association between the DRB1 gene and schizophrenia in Japanese. *Schizophr Res* 1998; **32**: 81–6.
114. Akaho R, Matsushita I, Narita K et al. Support for an association between HLA-DR1 and schizophrenia in the Japanese population. *Am J Med Genet* 2000; **96**: 725–7.
115. Narita K, Sasaki T, Akaho R et al. Human leukocyte antigen and season of birth in Japanese patients with schizophrenia. *Am J Psychiatry* 2000; **157**: 1173–5.
116. Tochigi M, Ohashi J, Umekage T et al. Human leukocyte antigen-A specificities and its relation with season of birth in Japanese patients with schizophrenia. *Neurosci Lett* 2002; **329**; 201–4.
117. Huntington E. *Season of Birth: Its Relation to Human Abilities*. New York: Wiley, 1938.
118. Hare EH. Variations in the seasonal distribution of births of psychotic patients in England and Wales. *Br J Psychiatry* 1978; **132**: 155–8.
119. Eagles JM, Hunter D, Geddes JR. Gender-specific changes since 1900 in the season-of-birth effect in schizophrenia. *Br J Psychiatry* 1995; **167**: 469–72.
120. Procopio M, Marriott PK. Is the decline in diagnoses of schizophrenia caused by the disappearance of a seasonal aetiological agent? An epidemiological study in England and Wales. *Psychol Med* 1998; **28**: 367–73.
121. Leach CE, Blair PS, Fleming PJ et al. Epidemiology of SIDS and explained sudden infant deaths. CESDI SUDI Research Group. *Pediatrics* 1999; **104**: e43.
122. Shi L, Fatemi SH, Sidwell RW, Patterson PH. Maternal influenza infection causes marked behavioral and pharmacological changes in the offspring. *J Neurosci* 2003; **23**: 297–302.

2

Exposure to prenatal infections and psychiatric nosology: A focus on schizophrenia phenotypes

Gerald Stöber

INTRODUCTION

The neurodevelopmental model of schizophrenia pathogenesis proposes that the observed patterns of early abnormal brain development are related to and induced by genetic risk factors and/or exogenous environmental causes.[1] In accordance with the excess of schizophrenic birthrates in the winter and spring months, one attractive hypothesis suggests that viral infections during crucial periods of brain maturation are of etiological importance.[2,3] The influenza-schizophrenia theory emerged from findings on mid-gestational exposure to the 1957 influenza epidemic,[2] followed by numerous studies on schizophrenia risk among those exposed to annual peaks of infectious disease.[4] Subsequently, individual maternal viral infection was reported in schizophrenic offspring,[5–7] and altered fetal brain development was found in animal models after prenatal viral infection.[8] Based on epidemiological findings, however, the relative risk of maternal viral infection in schizophrenia seems to be low at ~1.5, indicating that prenatal infections could account only for a small proportion of schizophrenia cases.[9] Another attractive hypothesis is that the infection theory is of key importance in distinct schizophrenic phenotypes only.[5,10] Here, we present a summary of our studies on birthrate patterns and individual exposure to prenatal infections across the spectrum of schizophrenic psychoses.

PSYCHATRIC NOSOLOGY AND DIFFERENTIATED PSYCHOPATHOLOGY

Differentiated psychopathology claims to define real diseases in a psychiatric nosology and has proven to be a useful framework for investigating the spectrum of the functional psychoses with high reliability and validity.[11–14] In this system, the functional psychoses are classified into five main categories according to different cross-sectional symptomatology, which is strongly related to different types of long-term course and outcome.[12] The phasic psychoses with full recovery from each episode are represented by the monopolar affective psychoses, the bipolar affective psychoses (manic depression), and the non-affective cycloid psychoses (anxiety–happiness psychosis, confusion psychosis, motility psychosis). The psychoses with obligate psychic residual symptoms are sub-differentiated into the unsystematic schizophrenias (cataphasia, affect-laden paraphrenia, periodic catatonia) and the systematic schizophrenias (hebephrenias, systematic paraphrenias, systematic catatonias).

Cycloid psychoses show phasic, remitting episodes with polymorphic psychotic symptom patterns in between schizophrenia and affective disorders as an independent nosological entity. The psychic systems of psychomotility, affect, and thought are affected in a polymorphic bipolar course with characteristic symptom constellations.[15] In contrast to the manic depressive disease, heritability is low in cycloid psychosis as confirmed by twin and family studies.[11,12] In the unsystematic schizophrenias the symptoms again tend to be polymorphous with bipolarity, but the symptomatic pictures differ qualitatively from cycloid psychosis, and run a periodic course to psychotic residual syndromes.

One subphenotype of the unsystematic schizophrenias, periodic catatonia, has attracted some attention in recent years after successful mapping of the disease gene locus at chromosome 15q15.[13,16] Periodic catatonia is characterized by qualitatively different hyperkinetic and akinetic motor disturbances occurring during psychotic episodes, giving way to grimacing or mask-like facial expressions, iterations, and distorted stiff movements, alternating with akinetic negativism, stereotypies, or negativistic behavior. These acute psychotic episodes progress to debilitating residual states with psychomotor weakness and apathy. The periodic course and polymorphous symptomatology of periodic catatonia is distinct from the systematic catatonias.

Each of the six systematic catatonia subphenotypes has its own specific clinical presentation, but meets the general characteristics of systematic schizophrenia – chronic progressive course without remission and irreversible syndromes with sharply distinguished residual states:[12] parakinetic catatonia (parakinesia with bizarre expressive/reactive movements, erratic thought); manneristic catatonia (mannerisms within complex movements, progressive stiffness of psychomotility); proskinetic catatonia (proskinesia with abnormal tendency towards automatic movements reactive to external stimuli, impulse–automatism); negativistic catatonia (negativism with resistance or omissions, ambitendency, negativistic, aggressive excitement); speech-prompt catatonia (short-circuiting in speech, talking past the point, autism); and sluggish catatonia (sluggish verbalizations, continuous hallucinations, extinguished initiative).

In the phenotypes of unsystematic schizophrenia, the contribution of genetic factors is important, with a familial morbidity risk for first degree relatives of the index cases of ~15%, whereas in systematic schizophrenia the familial aggregation of psychoses is at ~2%, and in cycloid psychoses at ~4%, indicating that these diagnostic categories could have psychosocial and/or environmental causes in a potentially multifactorial etiological background.[12]

SEASON-OF-BIRTH EFFECT AND DIFFERENTIATED PSYCHOPATHOLOGY

In an epidemiological approach, a considerable sample of DSM-III-R schizophrenic patients demonstrated significantly distinct birthrate patterns.[17] Cycloid psychoses and systematic schizophrenias, both phenotypes with low heritability, showed a birth excess in the first half of spring, whereas the unsystematic schizophrenias (high familial pattern) even exhibited a slight decrease of births in this period compared to the general population. The sample comprised 1299 independent individuals:[12] cycloid psychosis ($n = 213$), unsystematic schizophrenia ($n = 507$), and systematic schizophrenia ($n = 579$). Patients were born between 1896 and 1965, and controls consisted of the general population registered up to December 31 1990 in West Berlin. The year was divided into eight sections, each covering a first or second half of the four seasons. A significant peak of birthrates appeared in the first half of spring in the sample compared to the control population (+2.3%; $p < .05$), which was even higher in those with cycloid psychosis (+6%; $p < .01$) or systematic schizophrenia (+5.3%; $p < .001$). Integrating the hypothesis of midgestational viral infections (fifth and sixth month of gestation), a high-risk period in the winter and spring months was defined during which – according to the Public Health Centres – a peak of acute respiratory bronchitic illnesses (without any known causative origin) repeatedly occurred in November and December. In this period of time those fetuses were in their fifth and/or sixth month of gestation, if pregnancies started later than May 1 and earlier than September 1. If the sample was classified according to the high-risk period, the effect was even more pronounced: a surplus of birthrates appeared in patients with cycloid psychosis (7.4%; $p < .05$) and systematic schizophrenias (+10.3%; $p < .001$). Conversely, those subjects with unsystematic schizophrenia (high genetic risk) showed a slight decrease of birthrates in the first half of spring (–2.7%, ns) and in the specified high-risk period (–3.7%, ns).

MATERNAL GESTATIONAL INFECTION

Contemporaneously to the epidemiological approach we started retrospective studies on individual maternal gestational infections in phenotypes of the functional psychoses.[5,18] The assessment of maternal information was based on a highly structured questionnaire.[19] All questions were asked person-to-person in an interview. Most of the interviews were carried out at the mothers' residences. Immense importance was placed on the occurrence of infectious diseases during pregnancy. The interviewer continually asked each of the mothers if she had suffered from any infectious disease during pregnancy, regularly followed by more specific questions on the kind of infectious disease of viral or bacterial origin. If any infection was recalled, the mother was questioned precisely in regard to the time of manifestation during pregnancy (month and trimester). Likewise the mother was taken through her obstetric history from prenatal and intrapartal to postnatal risk factors according to the scale of Lewis and colleagues.[20] The interviewer was not aware of the patients' diagnostic subdifferentiation and was not permitted to ask questions about the family history during the interview. This rule was applied until all mothers had been interviewed.

Prenatal infection in systematic schizophrenia

In an initial sample of 55 patients with chronic schizophrenia and 20 control cases we found evidence that individual prenatal infections are reliably recalled, are significantly increased during midgestation in chronic schizophrenia, and are associated with an increased frequency of further obstetric complications.[5,21,22] We extended these findings in a sample of 80 chronic schizophrenics and 80 physically and mentally healthy controls.[18,23] Exposure to prenatal infections occurred in 16 out of 80 individuals with chronic schizophrenia (20%) and in 10 out of 80 controls (13%). Not the frequency, but the distribution by trimester was significantly different between groups. Compared to controls, in chronic schizophrenia midgestational infections were significantly increased in trimester II compared to trimesters I and III (Figure 2.1). Eleven infections occurred in the second trimester, whereas in the control group gestational infections were equally distributed among the trimesters ($p < .02$). Regarding the monthly distribution, seven of the 16 infections (44%) were reported during the fifth month of gestation ($p < .02$). Again, this pattern was significantly different to controls ($p < .05$). The majority of infections recorded were of the respiratory tract, which accounted for 56% of all gestational infections and 64% of all midtrimester infections. No reference was made to viruses such as rubella, measles, mumps, varicella or cytomegalovirus, which are known to cause gross fetal damage.

The excess of prenatal exposure to infections was mainly restricted to systematic schizophrenia: 36% of these patients were exposed compared to 7% with unsystematic schizophrenia ($p < .01$) and to 13% of controls ($p < .01$). Focusing on the second trimester, the surplus of maternal infections in systematic schizophrenia was even more pronounced at 28% compared to unsystematic schizophrenia at 2% ($p < .001$) or controls at 4% ($p < .001$). Infections during the fifth month of gestation were exclusively reported in systematic schizophrenics. Gestational infections were consecutively followed by further obstetric complications (OCs; $p < .05$), but no specific type of OC was observed. Prenatal infections were not allocated to a specific gender in the schizophrenic offspring (males 23%, females 14%).

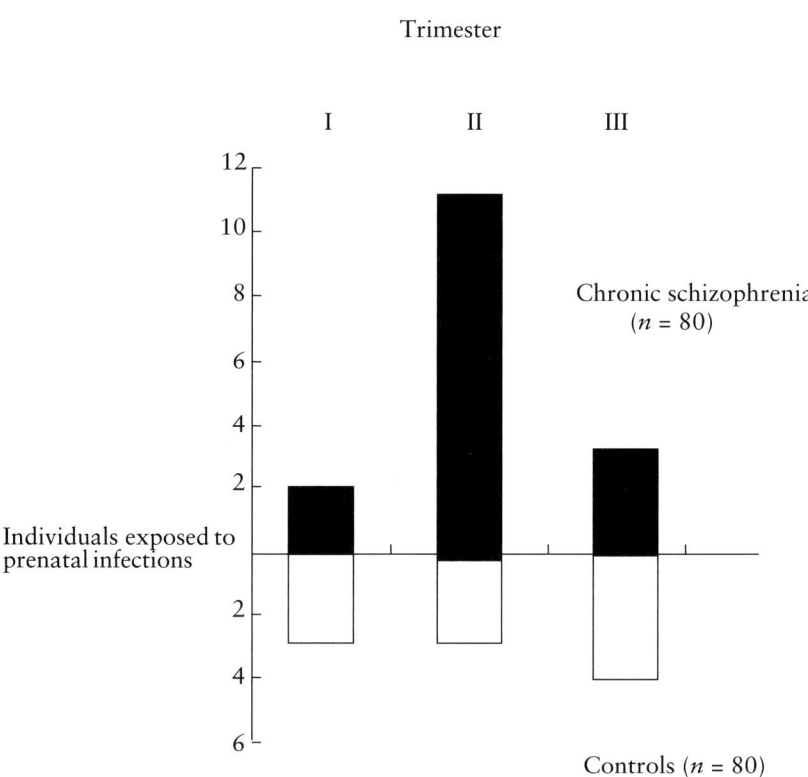

Figure 2.1 Exposure to prenatal infections in individuals with chronic DSM III-R schiophrenia and in healthy controls. In the second trimester, the incidence of midgestational infections was increased compared to the first and third trimester (11 out of 16 infections; $p < .02$), and compared to the population controls ($p < .05$).

Prenatal infections in subphenotypes of catatonia

In our last series[10] we studied individuals derived from a previous empirico-genetic family study of 139 patients with chronic catatonic DSM III-R schizophrenia, subdifferentiated according to Leonhard's classification, with intensive investigations on diagnostic reliability and stability.[24,25] In all, 83 individuals suffered from the clinical subtype periodic catatonia and 56 from systematic catatonia. To evaluate the influence of genetic predisposition, psychosocial factors, and prenatal and perinatal complications, we selected those patients whose mother was traceable and willing to participate in the study. In the systematic catatonia sample 35 mothers were alive, and 33 of them could be contacted. One mother suffered from combined systematic catatonia and was not able to give detailed information on giving birth to her children. In the periodic catatonia cases, 42 mothers were still alive and 39 could be traced. Among them, 12 had undergone previous psychiatric hospitalization; the statements of three mothers had to be excluded from evaluation due to psychotic impairment, and nine completed the interview adequately. In total we analyzed data on 36 patients with periodic catatonia (86%) and 32 with systematic catatonia (91%). For power analysis we included data from the earlier control sample ($n = 80$).

Familial transmission of periodic catatonia with unilineal transmission (documented parental cases) was evident in 16 of 36 patients (44%; nine cases of maternal transmission). This pattern contrasted with one case of an affected parent in systematic catatonia (3%; $p = .0003$). Prenatal exposure to infections was recalled in 11 of 32 cases with systematic catatonia (34%) and in three of 36 cases with periodic catatonia (8%; $p = .008$). In systematic catatonia infectious diseases included seven cases of influenza or febrile cold (64%), and one case each of tonsillitis, pyelonephritis, cystitis, and cholecystitis. In periodic catatonia one case of febrile cold and two cases of tonsillitis were reported. Exposure to second trimester infections was recalled in 10 of 32 patients with systematic catatonia compared to two cases with periodic catatonia ($p = .006$). Again, in systematic catatonia second trimester infections were significantly more frequent than first and third trimester infections, when compared to periodic catatonia ($p = .025$).

Multivariate logistic regression analyses were applied to predict the dependent variable (classification of diagnosis) with independent variables (maternal gestational infections, obstetric complications, age of onset, gender, family history, maternal age at time of birth, and maternal age at interview) as logarithmic odds-ratios. We used a forward stepwise condition with removal of terms with significant odds-ratios in subsequent analyses. Occurrence of gestational infection predicted the diagnosis of systematic catatonia at a probability of $p = .008$, and unilineal parental transmission of psychosis predicted a diagnosis of periodic catatonia at $p = .0001$ (see Table 2.1). None of the other variables, such as gender, age of onset, OCs, or maternal age, reached significant logarithmic odds-ratio. Given the prevalence of exposure to maternal infection we had a power of 72% to detect differences in the sample at a significance level of $p = .05$, which reached 89% if we added the data derived from the control sample. Regarding second trimester infections, the statistical power was 74% in the sample and 97% in the combined sample of controls and periodic catatonia cases versus the systematic catatonia sample. Thus, approximately 150 cases would be needed in each group to detect a difference at the 1% significance level with 100% power.[10]

Maternal gestational infection in cycloid psychosis

In an earlier study, first trimester respiratory infections (influenza, febrile cold) were found to be associated with cycloid psychosis, and pointed to a putatively earlier vulnerability period in these phasic, non-affective psychoses than in systematic schizophrenia.[19] The analysis compared 40 individuals with cycloid psychosis, 40 with manic depression, and 40 controls. In cycloid psychosis a non-significant surplus of infections appeared during the first trimester compared to controls and those with manic depression. Respiratory diseases (influenza, febrile cold) explained 56% of all infections and all trimester I infections in cycloid psychosis. In cycloid psychosis prenatal exposure to respiratory infections during the first trimester was observed more frequently than in controls ($p = .03$) or the combined groups of controls and patients with manic depression ($p = .03$).

DISCUSSION

The prenatal viral infection theory as a part of the neurodevelopmental concept of schizophrenia is supported by epidemiologically-based surveys on influenza and other viral/bacterial annual epidemics, and by retrospective and prospective case-control studies. Epidemiologic studies suggested that exposure to annual high risk periods of non-specific bron-

Table 2.1 Periodic catatonia and systematic catatonia: logistic regression analysis of demographic, environmental, and genetic factors

Variable	Periodic catatonia ($n = 36$)	Systematic catatonia ($n = 32$)	Score	df	p value
Gender (males/females)	21/15	25/7	3.032	1	.082
Age of onset (years ± SD)	21.1 ± 5.2	20.7 ± 7.3	.068	1	.795
Obstetric complication positive	22 (61%)	24 (75%)	1.493	1	.222
Gestational infection positive	3 (8%)	11 (34%)	7.027	1	.008
Unilineal parental transmission	16 (44%)	1 (3%)	15.426	1	.0001
Mother's age at giving birth (years ± SD)	29.7 ± 6.0	28.2 ± 7.5	.832	1	.362
Mother's age at interview (years ± SD)	63.5 ± 9.5	62.3 ± 11.6	.346	1	.556

df = degree of freedom; SD = standard deviation

chitic disease during mid-gestation are related to sporadic forms of schizophrenia, and this effect was most prominent in the phenotypes of cycloid psychosis and systematic schizophrenias.[4] In retrospective case-control studies, we found an increased incidence of midgestational infection among those who developed chronic schizophrenia later in life. Second trimester infections, in particular during the fifth month of gestation, were significantly related to the development of systematic schizophrenia with chronic nonremitting course and characteristic residual syndromes.[5,23] Respiratory infections accounted for the majority of infections (56%). In these disease phenotypes, 28% were exposed to severe midgestational infection.[18] In the subcategory of systematic catatonias we observed prenatal exposure to maternal infection in 34% of cases, and midgestational exposure in 31%. The prevalence of maternal gestational infection in the general population was found at 4%, and the risk of being exposed in systematic catatonia reached $p = .0002$ and OR = 23.33 (95% CI 11.7–273.4) compared to population controls. In systematic catatonia, exposure to prenatal infection was the main predictive diagnostic factor at a level of $p = .008$.[10]

The association of individual prenatal exposure has been confirmed in independent samples.[6,26] The DSM III-R does not classify schizophrenia based on familial/sporadic distribution,[5,6] but prenatal midgestational exposure to infections seems to be of key etiological relevance to the systematic schizophrenias, and particularly to the systematic catatonias. These phenotypes are sporadic in origin, but are the most debilitating schizophrenic diseases. In these disorders specific circumscribed functional fields seem to be affected, so that in each subtype a higher function of the nervous system is involved. After several years of illness, these sharply delimited clinical pictures of systematic schizophrenia are found to be unresponsive to pharmacological treatment, and delimited from the non-specific effects of the morbid process or environmental pathoplastic factors. The subphenotypes of systematic catatonia distinguish themselves by circumscribed qualitative psychomotor disturbances with evidence of a low intrafamilial morbidity risk for first-degree relatives.[12,25] In our studies on chronic catatonias we found exposure to maternal infection restricted to the diagnostic category of systematic catatonia, and parental transmission linked to diagnosis of periodic catatonia. These patterns put the accent on etiological heterogeneity in the spectrum of schizophrenic psychoses, and added further evidence of disparate pathophysiological mechanisms in schizophrenia subphenotypes. In periodic catatonia, familial transmission was the main predictive diagnostic factor, with $p < .001$. The phenotype of periodic catatonia is breeding true with homogeneity of psychoses. In two independent genome-wide linkage scans we mapped and replicated a major susceptibility locus on chromosome 15q15.[13,16] Perfect segregation of distinct marker haplotypes in linked pedigrees support the assumption of autosomal dominant inheritance with reduced penetrance, as indicated by a morbidity risk of first-degree relatives of ~25%.

The cycloid psychoses, phenotypes with low heritability and good long-term prognosis, were found to be associated with first trimester respiratory infections. The effect of prenatal exposure seemed to be considerably lower than in the diagnostic category of systematic schizophrenias. A first trimester effect, however, is supported by several epidemiological studies,[27,28] and these findings could point to different vulnerability periods of altered neural cell proliferation and migration in subphenotypes of the functional psychoses. Furthermore, the pattern of early gestational stress and reduced genetic determinants indicates a potentially multifactorial etiological background to the cycloid psychoses. There was no evidence for a relationship of prenatal infection with the genetically determined schizophrenia phenotypes or with manic depression and, thus, no support for the 'two-strike' hypothesis which proposes additive effects of genetic predisposition and prenatal adverse events.

In 79% of the systematic schizophrenia sample, prenatal infections were followed by further obstetric complications (OCs), which confirmed our notion that at least in the systematic schizophrenias OCs may be sequels of earlier noxious events rather than causative factors of disturbed fetal development.[21] The effect of OCs seemed to be confined to early onset cases, particularly in the non-familial psychoses,[29] but we found them non-discriminatory between periodic and systematic catatonia. Several shortcomings should be considered when interpreting the prenatal infection findings. The sample sizes in all the retrospective studies may have been too small, but the thorough clinical differentiation introduced sufficient statistical power to differentiate the diagnostic groups. Due to the retrospective nature of the study, the findings rely primarily on the validity of maternal recall. Prenatal infections were reported in a considerable number of controls, but the discriminating factor was the specific period of time when the exposure occurred. Several studies indicate that mothers show proficient ability when remembering accurately OCs and maternal gestational infections, and both sources of information, maternal interviews and maternity hospital records, showed agreement regarding OCs as well as prenatal infectious diseases.[22,30,31] The mothers did not know the differentiation of diagnosis or the hypotheses tested and, thus, it seems unlikely that a systematic bias in these regards would account for the different frequency and time periods of infections.

Recently, immense efforts have been made towards elucidating the mechanisms of prenatal infections in the developing brain, and although the pathogenic mechanisms are still under discussion, potential mechanisms include direct viral infection, altered cytokine expression, and other fetal or maternal immune response abnormalities which lead to marked cytoarchitectural, behavioral, and neurophysiological abnormalities in animal models.[5,32–34] Post-mortem investigations on the brains of schizophrenics have shown evidence for circumscribed malformations, nerve cell alterations, and cytoarchitectural deviations attributable to disruptions of neural migration in the second trimester of gestation.[1,35] These findings suggest that viral infection may result in selective destruction or imbalance of neuronal pathways in the fetal brain. An attractive hypothesis for the etiology of systematic catatonia is the involvement of developing inhibitory circuits with disinhibition of glutamatergic neurotransmission with consecutive excitotoxicity and progressive disease course. This is represented by imbalance in distributed cortical and subcortical circuits in the speech-inactive phenotype using PET imaging.[36]

CONCLUSION

The link of schizophrenia to exposure to prenatal viral infections was found to be restricted to distinct phenotypes: cycloid psychoses and systematic schizophrenias. In the systematic cases, we found evidence that systematic catatonias are the category with excess exposure to midgestational infections, and that this exposure is the main predictive diagnostic factor. In contrast to this finding, another catatonic phenotype, periodic catatonia, shows no association with prenatal infections, but was recently mapped to a major susceptibility locus on chromosome 15q15. These findings may offer a small, but significant, contribution towards a differentiated nosology of psychiatric diseases, and towards new prophylactic and therapeutic treatment strategies.

REFERENCES

1. Beckmann H. Neuropathology of the endogenous psychoses. In: *Contemporary Psychiatry, Vol. 3. Specific Psychiatric Disorders* (Henn F, Sartorius N, Helmchen H, Lauter H, eds). New York: Springer, 2001; 81–100.
2. Mednick SA, Machon RA, Huttunen MO, Bonett D. Adult schizophrenia following prenatal exposure to an influenza epidemic. *Arch Gen Psychiatry* 1988; **45**: 189–92.
3. Munk-Jorgensen P, Ewald H. Epidemiology in neurobiological research: exemplified by the influenza-schizophrenia theory. *Br J Psychiatry* 2001; **178** (Suppl. 40): 30–2.
4. Franzek E, Beckmann H. Gene-environment interaction in schizophrenia: season-of-birth effect reveals etiologically different subgroups. *Psychopathology* 1996; **29**: 14–26.
5. Stöber G, Franzek E, Beckmann H. The role of maternal infectious diseases during pregnancy in the etiology of schizophrenia in offspring. *Eur Psychiatry* 1992; **7**: 147–52.

6. Wright P, Takei N, Rifkin L, Murray RM. Maternal influenza, obstetric complications, and schizophrenia. *Am J Psychiatry* 1995; **152**: 1714–20.
7. Brown AS, Schaefer CA, Wyatt RJ et al. Maternal exposure to respiratory infections and adult schizophrenia disorders: a prospective birth cohort study. *Schizophr Bull* 2000; **26**: 287–95.
8. Patterson PH. Maternal infection: window on neuroimmune interactions in fetal brain development and mental illness. *Curr Opin Neurobiol* 2002; **12**: 115–8.
9. Takei N, Mortensen PB, Klaening U et al. Relationship between in utero exposure to influenza epidemics and risk of schizophrenia in Denmark. *Biol Psychiatry* 1996; **40**: 817–24.
10. Stöber G, Franzek E, Beckmann H, Schmidtke A. Exposure to prenatal infections, genetics, and the risk of systematic and periodic catatonia. *J Neural Transm* 2002; **109**: 921–9.
11. Franzek E, Beckmann H. *Psychoses of the Schizophrenic Spectrum in Twins*. Vienna New York: Springer, 1999.
12. Leonhard K. *The Classification of Endogenous Psychoses and their Differentiated Etiology* (2nd ed). Vienna New York: Springer, 1999.
13. Stöber G, Saar K, Rüschendorf F et al. Splitting schizophrenia: periodic catatonia susceptibility locus on chromosome 15q15. *Am J Hum Genet* 2000; **67**: 1201–7.
14. Peralta V, Cuesta MJ. Cycloid psychosis: a clinical and nosological study. *Psychol Med* 2003; **33**: 443–53.
15. Jabs BE, Pfuhlmann B, Bartsch AJ, Stöber G. Cycloid psychoses – from clinical concepts to biological foundations. *J Neural Transm* 2002; **109**: 907–19.
16. Stöber G, Seelow D, Rüschendorf F et al. Periodic catatonia: confirmation of linkage to chromosome 15 and further evidence for genetic heterogeneity. *Hum Genet* 2002; **111**: 323–30.
17. Franzek E, Beckmann H. Season-of-birth effect reveals the existence of etiologically different groups of schizophrenia. *Biol Psychiatry* 1992; **32**: 375–8.
18. Stöber G, Franzek E, Beckmann H. Schwangerschaftsinfektionen bei Müttern von chronisch Schizophrenen. Die Bedeutung einer differenzierten Nosologie. *Nervenarzt* 1994; **65**: 175–82.
19. Stöber G, Kocher I, Franzek E, Beckmann H. First-trimester maternal gestational infections and cycloid psychosis. *Acta Psychiatr Scand* 1997; **95**: 319–24.
20. Lewis SW, Owen M, Murray RM. Obstetric complications and schizophrenia: methodology and mechanisms. In: *Schizophrenia: Scientific Progress* (Schulz S, Tamminga C, eds). New York: Oxford University Press, 1989: 56–68.
21. Stöber G, Franzek E, Beckmann H. Pregnancy and birth complications in distinct schizophrenic subgroups. *Eur Psychiatry* 1993; **8**: 293–9.
22. Franzek E, Stöber G. Maternal infectious diseases during pregnancy and obstetric complications in the etiology of distinct subtypes of schizophrenia: further evidence from maternal hospital records. *Eur Psychiatry* 1995; **10**: 326–30.
23. Stöber G, Franzek E, Beckmann H. Maternal infectious illness and schizophrenia. *Am J Psychiatry* 1997; **154**: 292–3.
24. Stöber G, Franzek E, Lesch KP, Beckmann H. Periodic catatonia: a schizophrenic subtype with major gene effect and anticipation. *Eur Arch Psychiatry Clin Neurosci* 1995; **245**: 135–41.
25. Beckmann H, Franzek E, Stöber G. Genetic heterogeneity in catatonic schizophrenia: a family study. *Am J Med Genet* 1996; **67**: 289–300.
26. Mednick SA, Huttunen MO, Machón RA. Prenatal influenza infection and adult schizophrenia. *Schizophr Bull* 1994; **20**: 263–7.
27. Barr CE, Mednick SA, Munk-Jorgensen P. Exposure to influenza epidemics during gestation and adult schizophrenia. A 40-year study. *Arch Gen Psychiatry* 1990; **47**: 869–74.
28. Adams W, Kendell RE, Hare EH, Munk-Jorgensen P. Epidemiological evidence that maternal influenza contributes to the aetiology of schizophrenia. An analysis of Scottish, English, and Danish data. *Br J Psychiatry* 1993; **163**: 522–34.
29. Verdoux H, Geddes JR, Takei N et al. Obstetric complications and age at onset in schizophrenia: an international collaborative meta-analysis of individual patient data. *Am J Psychiatry* 1997; **154**: 1220–7.
30. Cantor-Graee E, Cardenal S, Ismail B, McNeil TF. Recall of obstetric events by mothers of schizophrenic patients. *Psychol Med* 1998; **28**: 1239–43.
31. Buka SL, Goldstein JM, Seidman LJ, Tsuang MT. Maternal recall of pregnancy history: accuracy and bias in schizophrenia research. *Schizophr Bull* 2000; **26**: 335–50.
32. Borrell J, Vela JM, Arévalo-Martin A et al. Prenatal immune challenge disrupts sensorimotor gating in adult rats: implications for the etiopathogenesis of schizophrenia. *Neuropsychopharmacology* 2002; **26**: 204–15.
33. Fatemi SH, Earle J, Kist D et al. Prenatal viral infections lead to pyramidal cell atrophy and macrocephaly in adulthood: implications for genesis of autism and schizophrenia. *Cell Mol Neurobiol* 2002; **22**: 25–33.
34. Shi L, Fatemi SH, Sidwell RW, Patterson PH. Maternal influenza infection causes marked behavioral and pharmacological changes in the offspring. *J Neurosci* 2003; **23**: 297–302.
35. Jakob H, Beckmann H. Prenatal development disturbances in the limbic allocortex in schizophrenia. *J Neural Transm* 1986; **65**: 303–26.
36. Lauer M, Schirrmeister H, Gerhard A et al. Disturbed neural circuits in chronic catatonic schizophrenia demonstrated by F-18-FDG-PET and F-18-DOPA-PET. *J Neural Transm* 2001; **108**: 661–70.

3

Epidemiological correlation of sporadic schizophrenia to Lyme borreliosis

Markus Fritzsche

INTRODUCTION

Following the identification of neurosyphilis, caused by the spirochaete *Treponema pallidum*, that led Kraepelin to recognize the distinctive pattern of dementia praecox as a disease entity,[1] Bleuler coined the term 'schizophrenia'.[2] Although this 'break' between reality and 'mind' is characterized by a multiplicity of signs and symptoms, it is a highly prevalent illness recognized throughout the world, and there is now international agreement on its classification. Apart from known infectious diseases, no other illness exhibits equally marked clusters by season and locality, nurturing the hope that schizophrenia could ultimately be preventable. Although Hippocrates (460 BC) recognized the importance of 'the seasons of the year and the effects they produce ... being common to all countries as well as peculiar to each locality,' psychiatrists have been slow to accept this idea.

SEASONAL CORRELATION

Systematic research into the season of psychiatric birth effects began only after the turn of the last century. Being born during winter and spring is nowadays considered one of the most robust epidemiological risk factors for developing sporadic schizophrenia later in life. The cause and exact timing of this birth excess, however, has remained elusive so far.

Since, during phylogeny, borrelia DNA has led to multiple germ-line mutations within the CB1 candidate gene for schizophrenia, a meta-analysis has been performed on all schizophrenic birth excesses published before 2003.[3–5] For statistical reasons, only birth studies compared to the normal population and encompassing no fewer than 3000 cases each have been considered. The significant numerical data were then taken together and plotted against the seasonal distributions of *Borrelia burgdorferi*-transmitting ixodes ticks worldwide.

In the United States, Europe, and Japan, seasonal correlation between the time of conception and ixodes tick activity reveals that the seasonal distribution of ixodes ticks may underlie the excess of schizophrenic births nine months later (that is, the excess in births of individuals who go on to develop schizophrenia). South of the Wallace Line, which limits the spread of *Ixodes persulcatus* ticks and *B. burgdorferi* into Australia, the seasonal trends are less significant, and in Singapore, being non-endemic for ixodes ticks and Lyme disease, schizophrenic birth excesses are absent (Figure 3.1).

In the USA, *I. scapularis* ticks exhibit a clearly defined periodicity, increasing their numbers under specific macroclimatic conditions from March to April, then in June and October. This seasonal distribution exactly mirrors the birth excess for schizophrenia nine months later, while the risk of developing schizophrenia is reduced towards a global decline in November. It should be noted that this deficit in schizophrenic births in late autumn occurs throughout the world, reflecting the lowest numbers and activity of ixodes ticks in winter-time nine months earlier. In the USA and Europe, the spring peak of tick activity with its first climax in March correlates with the rising numbers of schizophrenic births between December and January. The overall seasonal distribution of schizophrenic births across Europe, by contrast, mirrors the more complex seasonal concentration of tick populations, separated by the central European midsummer decrease in air humidity. Due to reduced tick activity, the relative decline towards a schizophrenic birth deficit in April appears earlier and more

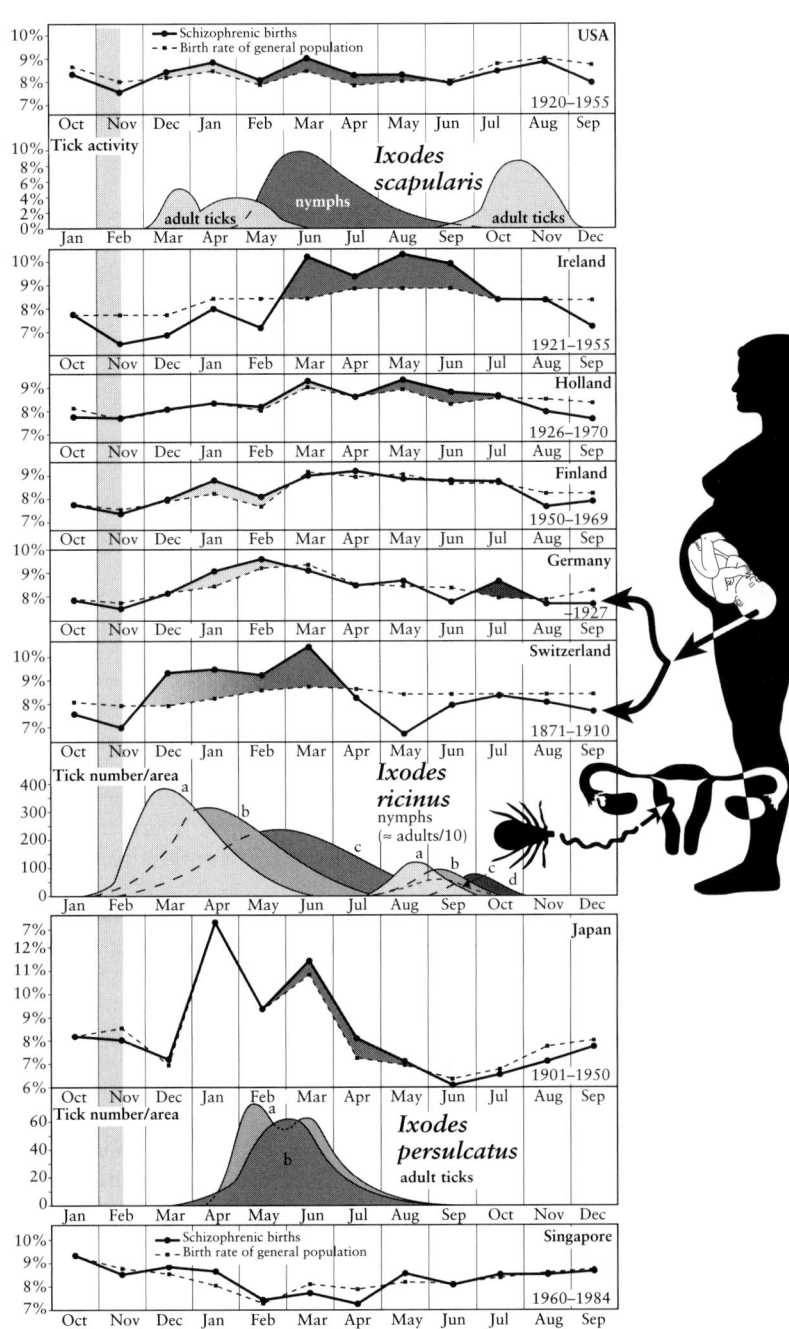

Figure 3.1 Schizophrenic birth excesses. The seasonal periodicity of the adult and juvenile stages of *I. scapularis* in the state of New York reflects the dynamics of schizophrenic births in the north-eastern United States. The same pattern of schizophrenic births applies to Europe, where the spring and autumn populations of *I. ricinus* in central Europe are affected by microclimatic conditions and a drop in humidity in midsummer (a = exposed meadow, b = dense hill vegetation or secondary deciduous woodland, c = highly sheltered habitat, d = spring-derived but autumn-feeding cohort). In northern Europe, however, there exists no late autumn cohort (d) as tick activity comes to a halt due to falling ambient temperature. The seasonal distribution of *I. persulcatus* ticks in the Far East (a = Vladivostok, b = Japan) correlates with the schizophrenic birth excess in Japan between February and March. In Singapore, by contrast, the non-significant, birth excess rates in schizophrenia are consistent with the absence of ixodes ticks and *B. burgdorferi* in that part of the world (adapted from Fritzsche).[5]

pronounced the further south we move towards Germany and Switzerland. In Ireland and the Netherlands, however, where the maritime climatic conditions remain relatively mild throughout the year, nymphal activity continues into midsummer which is immediately followed by another peak in early autumn. In Ireland, this more uniform pattern of mid-summer *I. ricinus* activity might therefore account for the somewhat delayed, but pronounced, schizophrenic birth excess in spring.[5,6]

The unimodal peak of *I. persulcatus* from April to July in Japan[7] reflects the unimodal winter–spring birth excess followed by a relative decline in May. This is also true for northern Europe, including

Scandinavia and the Karelian border between Russia and Finland, where the minimal mean temperature of seven degrees required for tick activity allows only one summer peak. The seasonal periodicity of *I. ricinus* might thus reflect the typical unimodal schizophrenic birth excess in Finland and Denmark. The harsh weather conditions in the north might also reflect the stochastic fluctuations of ticks in Scandinavia and possibly the multi-year fluctuations in schizophrenic births in Finland.[5,8]

Biological plausibility of cause and effect

Clinically, syphilis, which has long been associated with devastating congenital outcomes, resembles Lyme disease. As in humans, however, overt chronic infection of the unborn by *B. burgdorferi* is rare in mice, and placental transmission of borrelia is restricted to an exclusively narrow time window at conception. The nine-month interval between tick activity and schizophrenic birth excess, which implies an infection at conception, is therefore in line with the animal model of prenatal transuterine borrelia transmission. Without immediate detriment, *B. burgdorferi* is able to penetrate the embryonic cells of its host, which the pathogen then exploits like a virus owing to its own incomplete genome. Although counter to established views, the bacterium has thus integrated parts of its genes into our germ line, these serving as putative templates for further recombination in the course of phylogeny.[9,10]

For successful implantation into maternal tissue, and in order to suppress HLA-mediated antigen presentation, the foetal–placental unit secretes interferon gamma. This could facilitate the immune evasion and survival of intruding pathogens. Worse still, interferon gamma also upregulates the molecular machinery of genetic recombination in *B. burgdorferi*.[11] Through this cytokine-mediated mutagenesis, the simultaneous genetic expression of both embryonic and microbial DNA has arguably led to multiple germ-line mutations within our ancestral genome.[5]

Since within the cannabinoid receptor gene *CB1* (Figure 3.2), an inserted borrelia virulence factor – the flagellar basal rod protein (FBRP) – codes for intrusion into foreign tissue, it is tempting to speculate that such a mutagenic interaction with the implanting blastocyst depends on the simultaneous exposure of both borrelia and human DNA reading frames – weeks before neurons differentiate and embryonic brain development sets in. As ontogeny reflects phylogeny, the fast-switching ionotropic neuroreceptors dominate in the adult mammalian brain, whereas earlier in life and evolution the slow metabotropic neuroreceptors appear during implantation as critical elements in intercellular signaling before neurons differentiate. Intriguingly, the only metabotropic neuroreceptor gene implicated in both schizophrenia[5,10,12–14] and embryonic implantation[15] is *CB1*.

If a dysfunction of the cannabinoid system triggers schizophrenia in later life, there must also be an anatomical substrate in support of such a role (Figure 3.3). Being concentrated in the limbic lobe, including hippocampal formation and amygdala, as well as in the thalamus, basal ganglia, and cerebellum, the highest CB1 receptor densities can be found in exactly those areas that mirror the structural and functional brain abnormalities in schizophrenia.[16]

GEOGRAPHICAL CORRELATION

That exposure precedes infection is self-evident. Like other environmental causes, however, such a temporal relation is also expected to show a correlated biological gradient. In maritime Ireland and the sheltered microclimatic environment at the foot of the Swiss Alps, for example, tick abundance and the transmission of three pathogenic species of *B. burdorferi sensu lato* appear to coincide with the highest rates of schizophrenic births worldwide. Lower concentrations of ixodes ticks in the United States, by contrast, lead to relatively lower rates of infection with *B. burgdorferi sensu stricto* as well as the apparently lower rates of schizophrenic birth (Figure 3.1). Within the USA, however, the Pacific coast, New England, and the Great Lakes states have an approximately three times higher rate of schizophrenia than other states and the schizophrenic birth excesses, in particular, are more pronounced in New England and the Midwest than in the South. This trend, which has been remarkably consistent over a long period, correlates with the geographical distribution of ixodes ticks and Lyme disease in the USA.[5]

Contrary to current belief, neither the incidence nor the winter–spring birth excess of schizophrenia occurs at a constant, global rate – see Figure 3.4(a). South of the Wallace Line, which limits the spread of borrelia-carrying ixodes ticks by mammals into New Guinea and Australia as illustrated in Figure 3.4(b), schizophrenic births are less significant than in the northern hemisphere; and in Singapore, which is reportedly a non-endemic area for ixodes ticks and *B. burgdorferi*, there exists no significant schizophrenic birth excess (see also Figure 3.1).

Biological plausibility of geographical correlation

Residential development favors small tree-enclosed meadows interspersed with strips of woodland, much

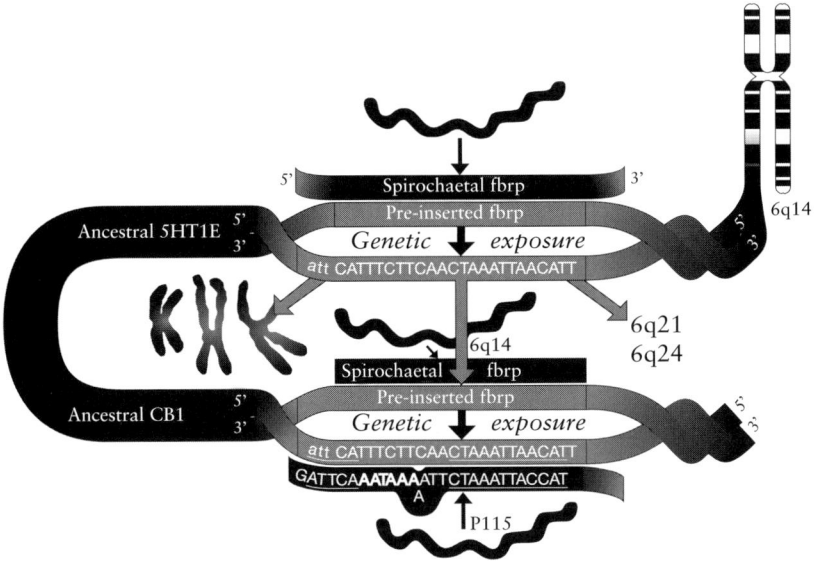

Figure 3.2 Infectious recombination between *B. burgdorferi* and human DNA. Within our germ line, infectious recombination (↓) between the spirochaetal flagellar basal rod protein (FBRP) and its pre-inserted FBRP template on ancestral *5HT1E* exposed (↓) the complementary strand on the double helix, including adjacent non-microbial nucleotides, to further genetic recombination with mammalian and borrelia DNA. Note the apparent gene shuffling from ancestral *5HT1E* onto *CB1* (⇓). Subsequent recombination with p115 (↑) introduced the second polyadenylation signal (AATAAA) into *CB1* adjacent to its 5′ methylation consensus signal (cctgG). Since the adjacent non-microbial nucleotides (indicated in lower-case letters) can still be found on *5HT1E* of the mouse and rat, but not on FBRP of *B. burgdorferi*, the spread of *B. burgdorferi* DNA originates from the ancient *5HT1E* already containing the spirochaetal insertion, and not directly from spirochaetal nucleotides (indicated in upper-case letters). If prenatal exposure to foreign DNA, which has led to these germ-line mutations on the 3′ 'hotspot' for pathology on *CB1*, re-occurs during ontogeny, epigenetic interference with foreign DNA resulting in mismatch–repair mutations or a change of its methylation status will subsequently alter the genetic expression of *CB1* in at least one of its alternative splice variants (adapted from Fritzsche).[10]

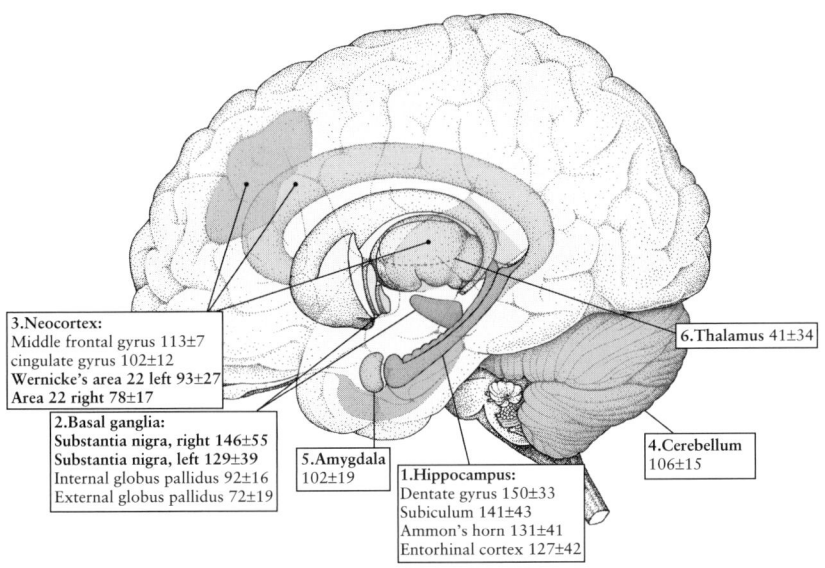

Figure 3.3 Anatomical distribution and receptor densities of CB1 in the human brain (based on Glass et al.)[17] measured in femtomoles of [^{3}H] CP55940 bound per mg of tissue. Reproduced from Fritzsche with permission.[18]

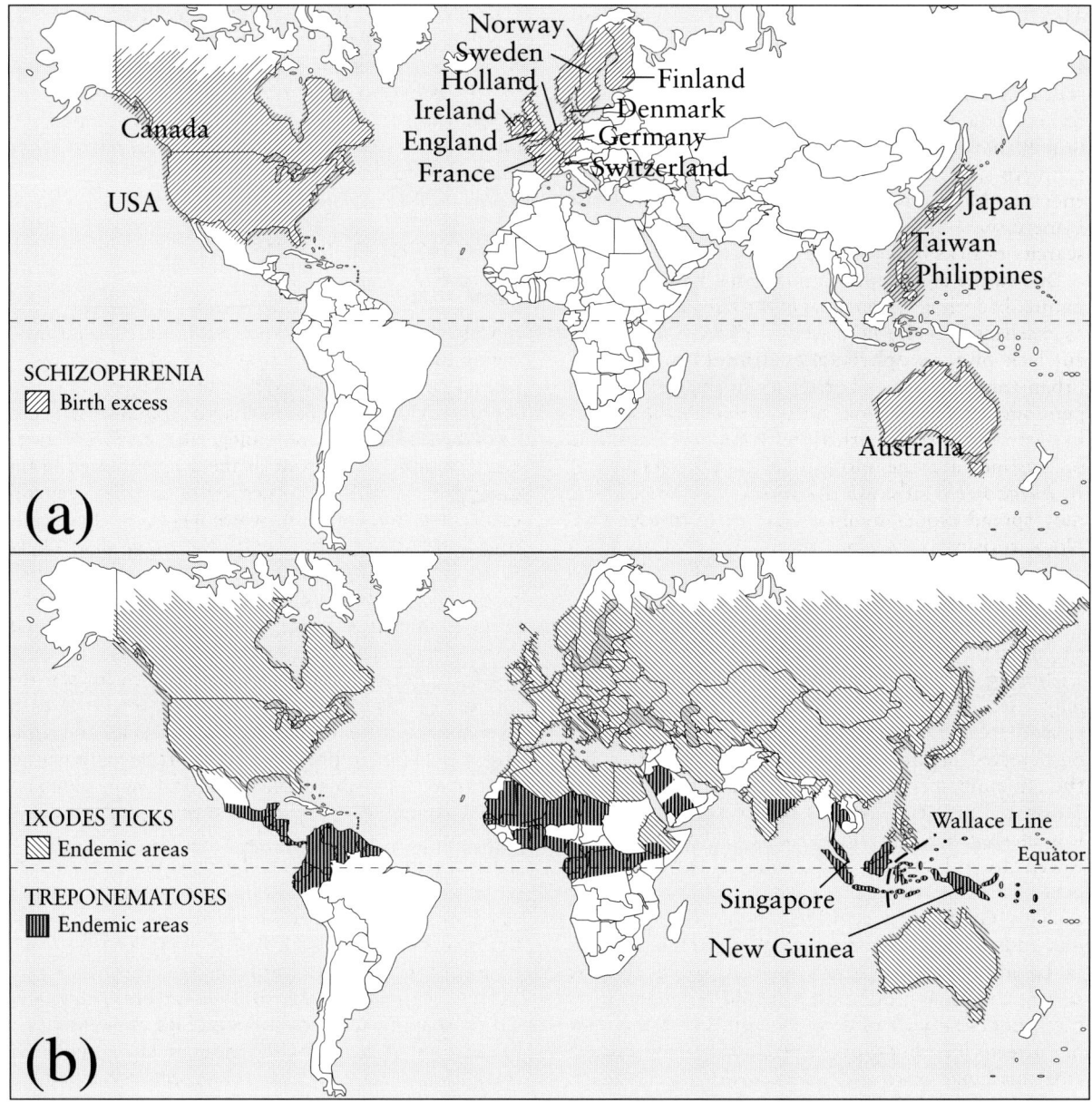

Figure 3.4 (a) Distribution of significant schizophrenic birth excesses worldwide.[3,5] (b) Global distribution of *B. burgdorferi*-transmitting ixodes ticks.[6] The genetic difference in heat shock protein expression among spirochaetes, protecting borrelia but not treponema from fluctuations in temperature, may explain the complementary distribution of endemic treponematoses versus ixodes tick activity. *B. burgdorferi* vector-borne transmission, in turn, correlates with the geographical clustering of schizophrenic birth excesses worldwide.

prized by deer, hedgehogs, mice, and cats. The widely reported correlation of schizophrenic birth excess to more densely populated urban and suburban areas[3] might thus reflect the activity of ticks, now attacking people in metropolitan areas. At first sight this phenomenon might appear counterintuitive. Yet while deer play a crucial role in the development and recent geographical dispersal of adult ticks, their spirochaetocidal antibodies exert a protective effect by clearing borrelia from the questing ticks' endolymph.

Thereby the ticks lose their infectious potential for human beings living in the countryside. This so-called zooprophylactic effect particularly applies to the southern United States, where ticks feed abundantly on lizards and skinks, and these hosts poorly maintain *B. burgdorferi* infection. Hence, compared to southern states such as Mississippi, where lizards are endemic, Michigan poses a relatively higher risk for Lyme disease and schizophrenia despite the relative scarcity of ticks in that state.[5]

Due to the continuous peridomestic parcelation of nature, hedgehogs (*Erinaceus europaeus*) also abound as excellent hosts for ixodes ticks. Worse, their apparent lack of zooprophylaxis contributes to the peri-urban transmission of borreliosis in our gardens. In peridomestic sites, various mice, *Peromyscus leucopus* in eastern North America and *Apodemus agrarius* in Europe, are the most important reservoirs of *B. burgdorferi* infection. As cats go for these mice, they spread ixodes nymphs near or in households. Not surprisingly, therefore, there is significantly often a cat in the household at the time of birth of an individual who later develops schizophrenia.[19]

Polar birds traveling from the northern hemisphere sporadically via the Antarctic introduce *I. uriae* ticks harboring *B. garinii* into Australia. These, in turn, may infect people in New South Wales and adjacent coastal areas. However, *B. burgdorferi* could neither be detected in, nor experimentally transmitted by, the endemic species *I. holocyclus*. Such maladaptation to local tick vectors might account for the low incidence of borreliosis and thus the reportedly lower rate of schizophrenia in New South Wales and other parts of Austronesia. In the remote interior of New Guinea, on an island which is reportedly non-endemic for Lyme disease, schizophrenia appears to be almost non-existent. In a neuropsychiatric survey comprising more than 10,000 Papuans from the Indonesian part of New Guinea, we found only one overtly psychotic case that had recently arrived from his home town Merauke on the western coast. In the interior of Papua New Guinea, prevalence of schizophrenia is also much lower than expected. Yet in the western coastal districts, where migratory birds are known to introduce ticks from New South Wales and Queensland, and where Rusa deer (*Cervus timorensis*) originally imported by the Dutch abound, the prevalence of schizophrenia is significantly higher.

Migratory sea birds are known to introduce *I. persulcatus* and *B. garinii* sporadically from their origin on the Eurasian mainland into pockets of northern Japan. As in Australia, however, the risk of acquiring Lyme disease is relatively low,[7] and the spirochaetes have not yet fully adapted to the local *I. ovatus*. In fact, this more widely endemic species is capable of acquiring but not transmitting *B. garinii* to its vertebrate hosts. From that perspective, the relatively recent introduction of *B. garinii* might explain the relatively recent rise of schizophrenic birth excesses occurring in Tokyo after the turn of the last century.[5,10]

GENETIC CORRELATE

About 60% of all humans are affected by gene mutations in their lifetime, 'and these variations, owing to our ignorance, are often said to arise spontaneously.'[20] The spirochaetal mutations on *CB1* corroborate Moreau de Tour's long-held hypothesis that cannabis and its pathophysiological effects on 'mental alienation' lie at the root of the schizophrenic brain disorder.[21] To tackle the question of whether prenatal exposure to foreign DNA, which has led to these multiple germ-line mutations during phylogeny, is likely to re-occur during ontogeny and expose the unborn to the risk of developing schizophrenia in later life, let us examine the functional role of the cannabinoid system from a slightly broader perspective.

CB1 is located on the candidate region for schizophrenia on *6q14*, which has been correlated to a translocation breakpoint in familial schizophrenia and a deletion responsible for neurodevelopmental abnormalities with enlarged cerebral ventricles and abnormal dermatoglyphics.[10] An early prenatal event interfering with neuronal migration, and development of dermatoglyphics and ventricles has been suggested to underlie the consistently reported pattern of cellular disarray in schizophrenic brains – a hypothesis that contrasts with the frequent reports correlating schizophrenia to third-trimester pregnancy and birth complications due to hypoxic brain damage. The seemingly contradictory findings, however, can be accounted for, as *CB1* induces both neuronal migration and hypoxic resistance to ischaemic challenge.

In the course of evolution, exposure of complementary DNA templates has furthermore led to infectious recombination with other genetic loci whose distribution is not entirely random. Rather, the chromosomal scatter presents surprising explanatory power for schizophrenic linkage studies that have remained so far unaccounted for.[10] Chromosome 6 harbours most translocations clustering across *6q14-q24* exactly within the candidate region for schizophrenia on *6q13-q25*, and one template originating from *B. burgdorferi* nucleotides even coincides with the highest lod score for schizophrenia at *6q21* (Figure 3.2).[10]

PHENOTYPIC CORRELATE

CB1 receptor knockout mice as animal models for schizophrenia

Cannabis intoxication and schizophrenia exhibit changes in the neurotransmitter profile that are surprisingly similar to those found in CB1 knockout mice.[9] The most consistent correlation is an elevated level of dynorphin A, a potent hallucinogenic kappa-opiate receptor agonist, known to induce symptoms of depersonalization as well as disturbances in the perception of time. Intriguingly, both CB1 knockout mice and schizophrenics show reduced initiation of goal-directed behavior and stereotypy. At the behavioral and molecular level, CB1 knockout mice exhibit another intriguing overlap with schizophrenia. Being triggered by a disinhibition of NMDA-mediated hippocampal long-term potentiation,[22] their long-term memories are markedly enhanced and appear to be in line with the psychotic symptoms in schizophrenia. When schizophrenic subjects are challenged with memory retrieval tasks, hippocampal baseline metabolic activity is continuously increased at a suboptimal level.[23] Such dysfunctional hippocampal hyperactivity could, according to the authors, account for the typical over-inclusive thought processes, hallucinations, and delusions in schizophrenia.[23] Unlike patients with tertiary neurosyphilis, who typically forget about their hallucinations, schizophrenics remember and their hallucinations can ultimately expand into fixed delusions.[1]

Pharmacological evidence for pathogenic involvement of CB1

Cannabinoid transmission is closely related to dopaminergic transmission, but the function of CB1 is not limited to the inhibitory i-mode of the G-protein-coupled metabotropic action, as often maintained. Depending on their mutual co-activation, CB1 and D2 rather hinge on the balance between the inhibitory and stimulatory G modes.[24] With regard to schizophrenia, this dual mode of neurotransmitter transmission is reflected at the genetic and phenotypic level. As molecular chemistry has become more sophisticated, the interaction of drugs with multiple receptor subtypes pointed to a similar binding pocket in different G-protein-coupled receptors. What was not appreciated until recently was the relatedness of these receptors at the molecular level and the sequence homology between CB1 and D2/D1 dopamine receptors. Whereas a short protein sequence of the seventh transmembrane loop essential for Gi inhibition shares similarity between CB1 and D2, a much larger portion of the CB1 peptide is similar to D1.[9]

As a pharmacological blockade of the CB1 receptor usually produces opposite and CB1 agonist-like effects, these phenotypic changes are counterintuitive. The paradoxical behavior, however, is consistent with the physiological overlap between schizophrenia and cannabis-induced psychosis.[25] It does not reflect a direct effect of CB1 receptor dysfunction, but rather appears to be related to an imbalance between CB1 and D2 co-activation (Figure 3.5).

When naloxone (Narcan®), a kappa opiate antagonist, was tested in schizophrenic patients their hallucinations disappeared promptly. After five minutes one patient reported 'complete silence within his head,' and two hours after the naloxone injection another patient with paranoid visual hallucinations noted that the phantom 'had left her for the first time in several weeks.'[26] Rather than the slow therapeutic effects of D2 antagonists, such a rapid abolishment of hallucinations indicates a more direct effect on the pathophysiological mechanism in schizophrenia.

Among the most widely replicated findings in schizophrenia are signs and symptoms of subtle morphological abnormalities in brain asymmetry, these being in line with the asymmetric distribution of CB1 receptors.[18] GABAergic modulation at strategic locations on axon initial segments, or lower-order dendrites of pyramidal cells, seems to play a pivotal role in shaping hemispheric asymmetry in the superior temporal gyrus (STG), an area that receives the strongest dopaminergic afferent within the posterior cerebral lobe. Not surprisingly, a reduction in volume of Wernicke's area (Area 22) in the left STG (see Figure 3.3) correlates with auditory hallucinations and the degree of formal schizophrenic thought disorder. As in the basal ganglia (Figure 3.5), these observations suggest that dysfunctional CB1-D2 co-activation of Gs impairs presynaptic GABAergic modulation.[18] In schizophrenia, we would furthermore expect a subsequent postsynaptic dopamine D1-mediated asymmetric activation of the Gs second messenger systems. Over the left STG of schizophrenic brains – where D1 receptors are more efficiently coupled with the adenylcyclase – this is indeed the case, suggesting enhanced responsiveness to receptor stimulation through relative preponderance of Gs over Gi in the postsynaptic membrane.[18]

Occasional consumption of tetrahydrocannabinol (THC), the psychopharmacologically most active ingredient of cannabis, appears to have few harmful effects overall. Its abuse, however, often triggers a relapse of psychotic symptoms in schizophrenic patients, and in normal but genetically vulnerable individuals, THC may increase the risk of developing schizophrenia. Conversely, eight-fold elevated levels of the endogenous CB1 agonist anandamide in the cerebrospinal

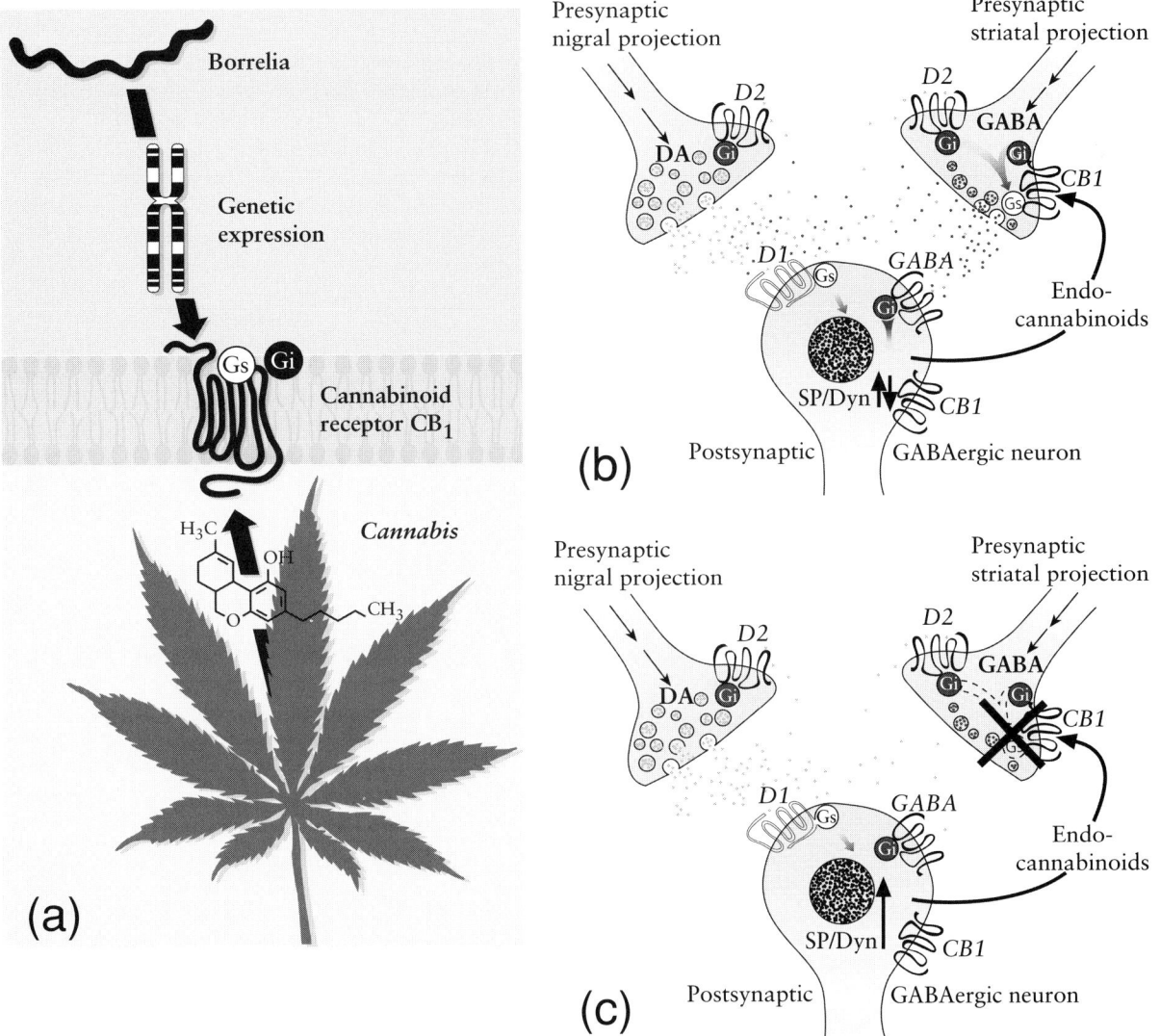

Figure 3.5 (a) Pharmacologic and genetic constraints on the mechanism of action of CB1. (b) Intact D2–CB1 receptor co-activation: it is well known that psychostimulants with dopaminergic properties produce paranoid delusions indistinguishable from schizophrenia. Owing to this functional overlap between the dopamine and the cannabinoid systems at the molecular and genetic level, the recently described retrograde messenger function of endocannabinoids entails a dual function. Balanced co-activation of both D2 and CB1 stimulates the adenylatecyclase through the third transmembrane Gs-protein-coupled loop, whereas the seventh transmembrane Gi-protein-coupled loop activation of either D2 or CB1 alone exerts an inhibitory effect on the release of GABA into the synaptic cleft. (c) Imbalanced D2–CB1 receptor co-activation: a dysbalanced activation or a genetic expression of CB1 is supposed to diminish the Gs-protein-coupled release of GABA from presynaptic striatal neurons. Reduced activation of the postsynaptic GABA receptor subsequently dysbalances the neuron in favour of the Gs-coupled D1 input which in turn increases the release of substance P (SP) and dynorphin (Dyn) in CB1 knockout mice and schizophrenia. Hence, naloxone can immediately relieve dynorphin-related psychotic effects (adapted from Fritzsche).[10]

fluid of schizopheric patients correlated with fewer psychotic symptoms in a recent study,[27] and thus appear to compensate for an altered cannabinoid receptor or second messenger system in acute paranoid schizophrenia.

Altered P300 event-related potentials, which have their electroencephalographic source within the STG, are among the most robust indices for cannabis intoxication as well as schizophrenia.[25] They do not only correlate with attention across time and goal-directed action, faculties that are typically disrupted in schizophrenia and cannabis psychosis. Altered P300 event-related potentials may also reflect genetic polymorphism of the *D2* as well as the *CB1* receptor gene.[9] If cannabis increases the risk of schizophrenia by 30%, as implied by recent epidemiological findings, then up to 13% of cases of schizophrenia could possibly be prevented if cannabis use was eliminated from the population.[28]

CORRELATION OF SPORADIC SCHIZOPHRENIA TO MULTIPLE SCLEROSIS

Since in epidemiology the concept of cause is a source of much controversy, as it is in other sciences, I would like to draw the reader's attention to the long-held concept that science 'must confine itself to the description of the correlation between observable data.'[29]

Epidemiological clusters by season and locality

Environmental constraints usually determined by probabilistic approaches are known as risk factors and these we assume – with a leap of faith – to be causative. Prevailing in the colder parts of the world, schizophrenia and multiple sclerosis (MS) exhibit a striking epidemiological overlap. In the northern USA, for example, the states with the highest rates of schizophrenia score significantly higher rates of MS than the states with the lowest schizophrenia rates in the south.[30] These biological gradients suggest a common environmental component that could be influenced. Extending the previous report from the USA, Templer and colleagues also found a high geographical correlation between MS and schizophrenia in Italy.[31] Subsequently, correlated birth patterns of MS and schizophrenia were studied: in Denmark, a significant birth excess of MS was found in early summer, but the data on schizophrenia were insignificant compared to the general population.[32] This negative result was in retrospect very unfortunate since accumulating evidence from most other studies from all around the world did yield significant schizophrenic birth excesses in winter and spring.[3]

MS prevalence parallels *B. burgdorferi* endemicity worldwide, and in America and Europe the birth excesses of those individuals who later in life develop MS not only reflect the schizophrenic birth excesses[33] but also mirror the seasonal distributions of *B. burgdorferi*-transmitting ixodes ticks at the time of birth (see Figure 3.8).

Etiological correlate

When in 1925 Adams and colleagues inoculated rhesus monkeys with material from patients with MS, spirochaetes emerged in their cerebrospinal fluid after several months.[34] In one animal, stained films showed 'several spirochaetes with rather irregular open spirals and varying from 15μ to 20μ in length and about 1μ in thickness.' In the other animal, 'on examination of the fluid from the lateral ventricle immediately after death, a single actively motile spirochaete, similar to those already noted in the first animal, was found on dark-ground examination.' In 1928, Gabriel Steiner demonstrated in the periphery of MS plaques numerous argyrophilic granules highly reminiscent of neurosyphilis and leptospirosis.[35] 'After an extremely fatiguing inspection of countless slides it was possible to find well preserved forms, which did not lie in cells and the morphological feature of which had to be specified as nothing else than the one of a spirochaete.' These findings were replicated and published by Steiner on several occasions.[36]

Yet despite living oscillating 'spirochaetes of the *Borrelia* type' independently documented in the cerebrospinal fluid of MS patients,[37] scepticism prevailed amongst neurologists, and seroepidemiological studies relating *B. burgdorferi* to MS have produced conflicting results at best. These, however, come as no surprise. When entering their hosts, spirochaetes including *B. burgdorferi* often undergo extensive antigenic and metabolic changes, which appear to prevent them from being recognized by the host's immune system. For this reason it is often difficult, if not impossible, to reach a conclusive diagnosis even with respect to clinical Lyme borreliosis.

The truth resurfaced in 2001. Cystic structures originating from spirochaetes were isolated in eight out of 10 Norwegian MS patients by means of immunofluorescence and in all 10 MS patients by transmission electron microscopy and staining after culture – see Figure 3.6(a). No such cysts could be observed in the five controls with either method, but the investigators noted a similarity between those found in the MS

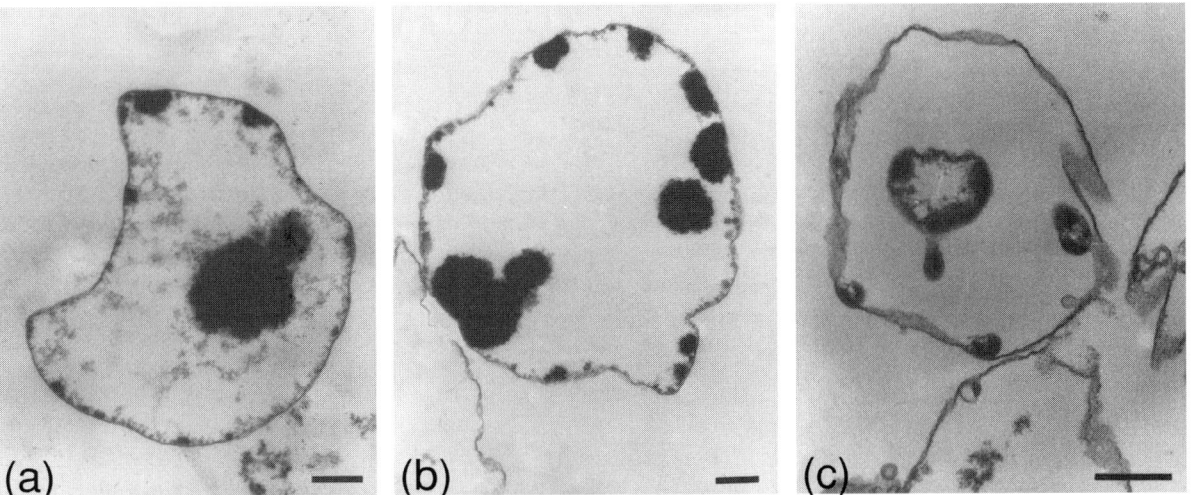

Figure 3.6 Cystic L-forms of *B. burgdorferi*. (a) Cyst collected from the cerebrospinal fluid of an MS patient, (b) from a Lyme borreliosis patient with a migrating rash, and (c) MS cysts of *B. burgdorferi* grown *in vitro*. The bar represents 500nm (EM photographs kindly presented by Øystein Brorson and Sverre-Henning Brorson).[39]

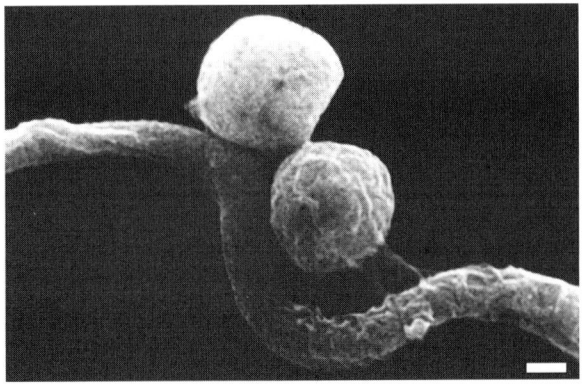

Figure 3.7 Spirochaetal and L-forms of *B. burgdorferi*. Note the two cystic structures adherent to a borrelia spirochaete. The bar represents 200nm. Reproduced with permission from Mursic et al.[40]

patients and the cystic forms characteristic of chronic *B. burgdorferi* infection – see Figure 3.6(b) and Figure 3.7. More significantly, the cysts of the MS patients exhibited positive reactions to anti-borrelia antiserum and, after culturing – see Figure 3.6(c) – curved spirochaete-like bacteria emerged and these structures could be propagated. The authors also observed that transformation of the *B. burgdorferi* to cystic forms occurred invariably and rapidly after incubation in CSF and that they could be reconverted to spirochaetes if the conditions became favorable.[38]

The MS patients in this Norwegian study in fact originated from a well-defined area where Lyme borreliosis as well as MS is endemic. Clinically, all of them had relapsing remitting MS according to Poser's criteria.[38] In spite of numerous reports citing a possible association between MS and chronic infection with *B. burgdorferi*, which in its chronic form is supposed to be an autoimmune disease triggered by these spirochaetes,[33] the same counterarguments re-emerged. In such a situation, technology plays a lesser role and the art of molecular epidemiology prevails.

Biological plausibility of the correlation

Intriguingly, the geographical gradient of MS sharply declines at 37° latitude, entirely sparing the tropical belt where human treponematoses are endemic. In more temperate climates, *B. burgdorferi s. l.* infection rates of seabird ticks match MS prevalence rates worldwide (Figure 3.8).

The inverse geographical distribution of endemic treponematoses versus MS (Figure 3.8) and schizophrenic birth excesses (Figure 3.4) can be explained by the differences in the genetic expression of heat shock proteins (HSPs), which not only protect from fluctuations in temperature, but also activate host immune defences. Molecular evidence reveals that the pathogenic spirochaetes have circumvented this immunological impasse differently. Whilst in the course of evolution treponema as an exclusively human pathogen could afford to delete the capacity

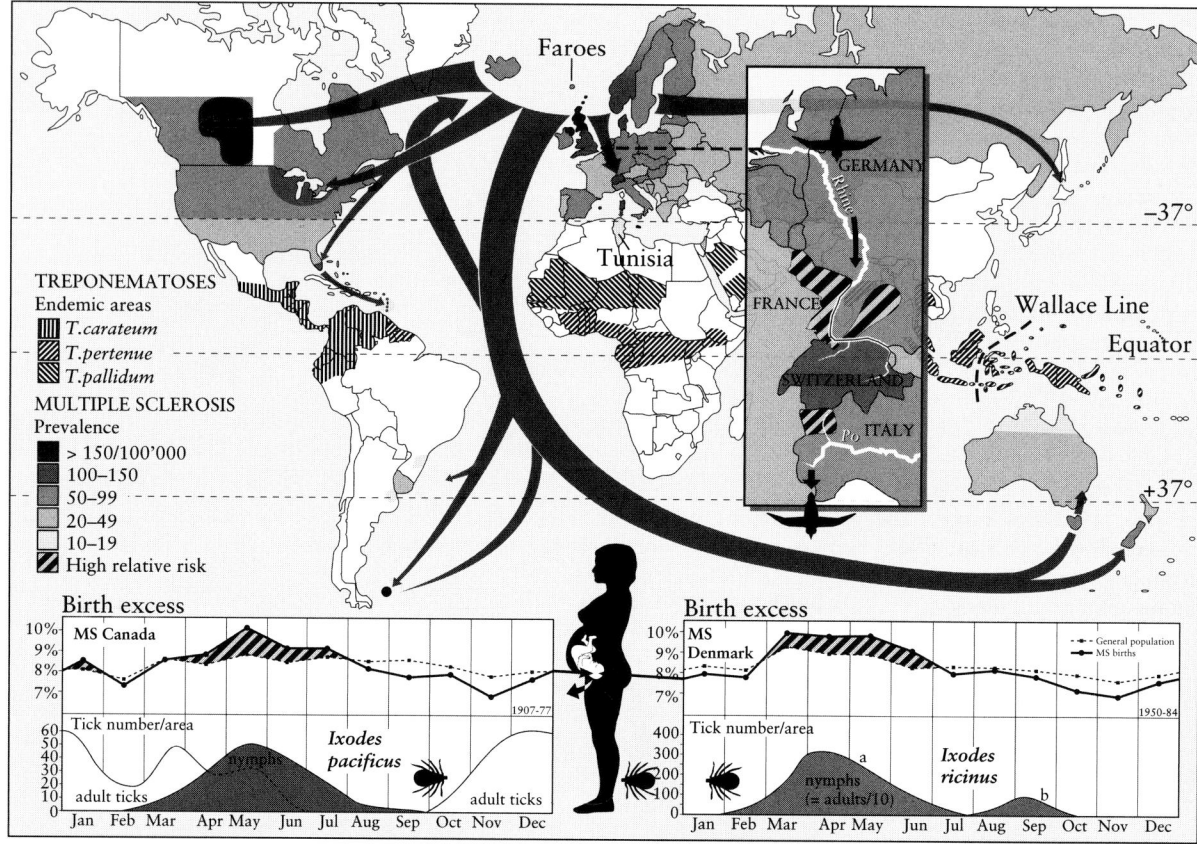

Figure 3.8 Geographical and seasonal correlation of multiple sclerosis to *B. burgdorferi*-transmitting ixodes ticks. The arrows represent the migratory routes of seabirds worldwide, if a number of species such as puffins and seagulls are taken together. In America and Europe, the birth excesses of those individuals who later in life develop MS exactly mirror the seasonal distributions of ixodes ticks at the time of birth. This seasonal correlation implies – analogous to the transmission of chronic hepatitis B infection during delivery – that one form of MS is caused by neonatal exposure to maternal *B. burgdorferi* infection. Apart from acute infections, no other disease exhibits equally marked clusters by season and locality, nurturing the hope that multiple sclerosis might ultimately be preventable (adapted from Fritzsche).[33]

of heat shock resistance and thus vector-borne transmission, *B. garinii* adapted to a broad range of changes in temperature by expressing HSPs. Rapid adaptation to preferentially 38° is critical when transmitted from the tick vector to the human brain as well as to warm-blooded seabirds with an average temperature of 38°. *Treponema pallidum* on the other hand is exquisitely sensitive to temperature, and can be eliminated by inducing fevers; this was indeed the standard treatment for tertiary neurosyphilis until penicillin became the established therapeutic choice.

The pathogen's transmission success also depends on its ability to replicate and survive within a host for long periods. One option is to remain latent inside the long-lived cells of the CNS. *In vitro* evidence suggests early invasion of the CNS by *B. burgdorferi* s. l. is by adherence of this organism to neurons. Functionally linked to a flagellar protein, Hsp-60 is thereby involved in binding to the neural cell surface for intrusion into the CNS.[41] As Hsp-60 is a major immunodominant antigen of *B. burgdorferi*, it comes as no surprise that antibodies to Hsp-60 were also detected in the synovial fluid of Lyme arthritis patients.[42]

In MS the immunologic response simply persists because the immune system is not able to remove the offending agent from the body. Worse still, hitherto hidden autoantigens can be released from damaged tissues, among which are major myelin constituents including the myelin basic protein and several members of the HSP family, thus amplifying the auto-aggressive response.

In order to become functional and virulent, intracellular pathogens sequester cytosolic HSPs in membrane-bound complexes from their human host. Subsequently, HSP autoantibodies, including anti-HSP90 cross-reacting with oligodendrocytes,[43] appear during such infections and in a subset of patients who suffer from both MS[43,44] and schizophrenia.[45–47] The expression of HSPs is thus unlikely on its own to trigger demyelinating autoimmunity, but may contribute to the amplification of local inflammatory responses in parallel with stress-producing events such as local immune responses to infectious antigens.[44]

Lyme disease is easily missed in psychiatry. The most revealing is the case report of a 19-year-old patient who presented with acute catatonic and paranoid symptoms including negativism, stereotyped movements, ideas of persecution and acoustic hallucinations. Upon isolation of *B. burgdoferi* from the CSF and the demonstration of intrathecal IgG antibodies, the patient completely recovered after antibiotic therapy.[48] This type of adult-onset encephalitis, however, whick might be explained by specific borrelia-derived excitotoxins acting on NMDA receptors in schizophrenia-like psychosis as well as in MS,[49] is rather the exception to the rule.

Although nosological criteria for MS and schizophrenia have high diagnostic reliability, affected individuals may differ substantially in their specific profile of signs and symptoms, as well as in the severity and course of their illness. What we recognise clinically as schizophrenia or MS is likely to encompass a complex set of disorders. A major task of future studies will thus be to resolve the question of heterogeneity as well as its etiologic overlap with other disease processes. The identification of flagellar borrelia DNA on human *CB1* and its functional relation to HSPs reminds us of Virchow's postulate: 'In searching for pathological systems one must clearly not construct nosological but only etiological ones.'[44]

CONCLUSION

It cannot be excluded at present that maternal infection by *B. burgdorferi* poses a risk to the unborn. The global epidemiological clustering by season and locality rather emphasizes a causal relation between sporadic schizophrenia and MS, which derives from both genetic and antigenic exposure to specific *B. burgdorferi*-mediated virulence factors at conception and birth.[5,33]

REFERENCES

1. Kraepelin E. *Psychiatrie, Ein Lehrbuch für Studierende und Aerzte. Dementia praecox*. Leipzig: Barth, 1899.
2. Bleuler E. *Handbuch der Psychiatrie. Dementia praecox oder Gruppe der Schizophrenien*. Leipzig: Deuticke, 1911.
3. Torrey EF, Miller J, Rawlings R, Yolken RH. Seasonality of births in schizophrenia and bipolar disorder: a review of the literature. *Schizophr Res* 1997; **28**: 1–38.
4. Selten JP, van der Graaf Y, Dijkgraaf M et al. Seasonality of schizophrenia and stillbirths in the Netherlands. *Schizophr Res* 2000; **44**: 105–11.
5. Fritzsche M. Seasonal correlation of sporadic schizophrenia to Lyme borreliosis. *Int J Health Geogr* 2000; **1**: 2.
6. Sonenshine DE. *Biology of Ticks*. New York: Oxford University Press, 1989.
7. Miyamoto K, Masuzawa T. Ecology of *Borrelia burgdorferi sensu lato* in Japan and East Asia. In: *Lyme Borreliosis, Epidemiology and Control* (Gray JS, Kahl O, Lane RS, Stanek G, eds). Wallingford, UK: CAB International, 2002: 201–22.
8. Fritzsche M, Schmidli J. Seasonal fluctuation in schizophrenia. *Am J Psychiatry* 2002; **159**: 499–500.
9. Fritzsche M. Are cannabinoid receptor knockout mice animal models for schizophrenia? *Med Hypotheses* 2001; **56**: 638–43.
10. Fritzsche M. Lateral gene transfer – the missing link between cannabis psychosis and schizophrenia. *Am J Med Gen* 2002; **114**: 512–5.
11. Anguita J, Thomas V, Samanta S et al. *Borrelia burgdorferi*-induced inflammation facilitates spirochaete adaptation and variable major protein-like sequence locus recombination. *J Immunol* 2001; **167**: 3383–90.
12. Dean B, Sundram S, Bradbury R et al. Studies on [3H]CP-55940 binding in the human central nervous system: regional specific changes in density of cannabinoid-1 receptors associated with schizophrenia and cannabis use. *Neuroscience* 2001; **103**: 9–15.
13. Leroy S, Griffon N, Bourdel MC et al. Schizophrenia and the cannabinoid receptor type 1 (CB1): association study using a single-base polymorphism in coding exon 1. *Am J Med Genet* 2001; **105**: 749–52.
14. Ujike H, Takaki M, Nakata K et al. *CNR1*, central cannabinoid receptor gene, associated with susceptibility to hebephrenic schizophrenia. *Mol Psychiatry* 2002; **7**: 515–8.
15. Paria BC, Song H, Wang X et al. Dysregulated cannabinoid signaling disrupts uterine receptivity for embryo implantation. *J Biol Chem* 2001; **276**: 20523–8.
16. Torrey EF. Studies of individuals with schizophrenia never treated with antipsychotic medications: a review. *Schizophr Res* 2002; **58**: 101–15.
17. Glass M, Dragunow M, Faull RL. Cannabinoid receptors in the human brain: a detailed anatomical and quantitative autoradiographic study in the fetal, neonatal and adult human brain. *Neuroscience* 1997; **77**: 299–318.
18. Fritzsche M. The origin of brain asymmetry and its psychotic reversal. *Med Hypotheses* 2003; **60**: 468–80.
19. Torrey FE, Yolken RH. Familial and genetic mechanisms in schizophrenia. *Brain Res Brain Res Rev* 2000; **31**: 113–7.
20. Darwin C. *The Descent of Man, and Selection in Relation to Sex*. London: Murray, 1871.
21. Moreau de Tours JJ. *Du Hachisch et de l'Aliénation Mentale*. Paris: Masson, 1845.
22. Bohme GA, Laville M, Ledent C et al. Enhanced long-term potentiation in mice lacking cannabinoid CB1 receptors. *Neuroscience* 2000; **95**: 5–7.

23. Heckers S, Rauch SL, Goff D et al. Impaired recruitment of the hippocampus during conscious recollection in schizophrenia. *Nat Neurosci* 1998; **1**: 318–23.
24. Glass M, Felder CC. Concurrent stimulation of cannabinoid CB1 and dopamine D2 receptors augments cAMP accumulation in striatal neurons: evidence for a Gs linkage to the CB1 receptor. *J Neurosci* 1997; **17**: 5327–33.
25. Fritzsche M. Impaired information processing triggers altered states of consciousness. *Med Hypotheses* 2002; **58**: 352–8.
26. Gunne LM, Lindstrom L, Terenius L. Naloxone-induced reversal of schizophrenic hallucinations. *J Neural Transm* 1997; **40**: 13–9.
27. Giuffrida A, Leweke FM, Gerth CW et al. Cerebrospinal anadamide levels are elevated in acute schizophrenia and are inversely correlated with psychotic symptoms. *Neuropsychopharmacology* 2004; in press.
28. Zammit S, Allebeck P, Andreasson S et al. Self reported cannabis use as a risk factor for schizophrenia in Swedish conscripts of 1969: historical cohort study. *BMJ* 2002; **325**: 1199–201.
29. Heisenberg W. Üeber den anschaulichen Inhalt der quantentheoretischen Kinematik und Mechanik. *Zeitschr Physik* 1927; **43**: 172–98.
30. Templer DI, Regier MW, Corgiat MD. Similar distribution of schizophrenia and multiple sclerosis. *J Clin Psychiatry* 1985; **46**: 73.
31. Templer DI, Cappelletty GG, Kauffman I. Schizophrenia and multiple sclerosis. Distribution in Italy. *Br J Psychiatry* 1988; **153**: 389–90.
32. Templer DI, Trent NH, Spencer DA et al. Season of birth in multiple sclerosis. *Acta Neurol Scand* 1992; **85**: 107–9.
33. Fritzsche M. Geographical and seasonal correlation of multiple sclerosis to sporadic schizophrenia. *Int J Health Geogr* 2002; **1**: 5.
34. Adams DK, Blacklock WS, Cluskiie JAW. Spirochaetes in ventricular fluid of monkeys inoculated from cases of disseminated sclerosis. *J Path Bacteriol* 1925; **28**: 117–8.
35. Steiner G. Spirochäten im menschlichen Gehirn bei multipler Sklerose. *Der Nervenarz* 1928; **8**: 457–69.
36. Steiner G. Morphology of *Spirochaeta myelophthora* in multiple sclerosis *J Neuropathol Exp Neurol* 1954; **13**: 221–9.
37. Simons HC. Spirochätenbefunde im Liquor bei multipler Sklerose. *Schweiz Med Wochenschr* 1957; **18**: 544–5.
38. Brorson O, Brorson SH, Henriksen TH et al. Association between multiple sclerosis and cystic structures in cerebrospinal fluid. *Infection* 2001; **29**: 315–9.
39. Brorson Ø, Brorson SH. 2003. Personal communication.
40. Mursic VP, Wanner G, Reinhardt S et al. Formation and cultivation of *Borrelia burgdorferi* spheroplast-L-form variants. *Infection* 1996; **24**: 218–26.
41. Kaneda K, Masuzawa T, Yasugami K et al. Glycosphingolipid-binding protein of *Borrelia burgdorferi sensu lato*. *Infect Immun* 1997; **65**: 3180–5.
42. Shanafelt MC, Hindersson P, Soderberg C et al. T cell and antibody reactivity with the *Borrelia burgdorferi* 60-kDa heat shock protein in Lyme arthritis. *J Immunol* 1991; **146**: 3985–92.
43. Cid C, Alvarez-Cermeno JC, Camafeita E et al. Antibodies reactive to heat shock protein 90 induce oligodendrocyte precursor cell death in culture. Implications for demyelination in multiple sclerosis. *FASEB J* 2004; **18**: 409–11.
44. van Noort JM, Bajramovic JJ, Plomp AC, van Stipdonk MJ. Mistaken self, a novel model that links microbial infections with myelin-directed autoimmunity in multiple sclerosis. *J Neuroimmunol* 2000; **105**: 46–57.
45. Kilidireas K, Latov N, Strauss DH et al. Antibodies to the human 60 kDa heat-shock protein in patients with schizophrenia. *Lancet* 1992; **340**: 569–72.
46. Schwarz MJ, Riedel M, Gruber R et al. Antibodies to heat shock proteins in schizophrenic patients: implications for the mechanism of the disease. *Am J Psychiatry* 1999; **156**: 1103–4.
47. Kim JJ, Lee SJ, Toh KY et al. Identification of antibodies to heat shock proteins 90 kDa and 70 kDa in patients with schizophrenia. *Schizophr Res* 2001; **52**: 127–35.
48. Pfister HW, Preac-Mursic V, Wilske B et al. Catatonic syndrome in acute severe encephalitis due to *Borrelia burgdorferi* infection. *Neurology* 1993; **43**: 433–5.
49. Halperin JJ, Heyes MP. Neuroactive kynurenines in Lyme borreliosis. *Neurology* 1992; **42**: 43–50.
50. Virchow R. *Die Einheitsbestrebungen in der Wissenschaftlichen Medizin*. Berlin: Reimer, 1849.

4

Enteroviruses and schizophrenia

Jaana Suvisaari

INTRODUCTION

There was already speculation about infections being involved in the etiology of schizophrenia back in Kraepelin and Bleuler's times:[1,2] the spirochete causing neurosyphilis had been identified, and it seemed that the involvement of infections in the etiology of schizophrenia could not be ruled out. Psychotic symptoms associated with influenza infections during the pandemic of 1918–1919 fueled these speculations. The infectious etiology theory was then forgotten until findings of abnormalities in the immune system among patients with schizophrenia, and observations that viruses were capable of causing new symptoms decades after the primary infection, revived interest.[3]

There are several hypotheses about how an infection could cause schizophrenia. It could be a direct result of an active infection which disrupts cellular and molecular functioning. Or a viral infection might act in a more subtle way, for example by mimicking CNS transmitters or receptors. Schizophrenia could also be caused by a latent virus that is periodically reactivated, or by retroviral genomic material integrated into host cell DNA. Finally, it has been suggested that it is the immune response, rather than an initial infection, that is responsible for the development of schizophrenia. The suggested timing of the infection varies from the prenatal period to the onset of schizophrenia.[4]

Enteroviruses belong to the picornaviruses, small RNA viruses, and consist of polioviruses, coxsackieviruses, echoviruses, and the newer numbered enteroviruses 68 to 71. They have a worldwide distribution, and in temperate climates, infections tend to occur particularly in the summer and fall. Most enterovirus infections beyond the neonatal period are asymptomatic. Enteroviruses enter the body usually via the upper respiratory or gastrointestinal mucosa, and submucosal lymphoid tissue is the major replication site. If viral replication is contained at this level, the infection will remain subclinical. However, the infection sometimes spreads and causes more severe illnesses.[5–7]

Enteroviruses infect the central nervous system (CNS) by hematogenous spread or by axonal transport from peripheral nerves. The best-known enteroviral CNS infection is paralytic poliomyelitis, an acute flaccid paralysis sometimes accompanied by meningitis. Paralytic poliomyelitis is caused by any of the three polio virus types; however, other enteroviruses are also capable of causing a similar paralytic illness. Enteroviruses are nowadays the most common causative agent of aseptic meningitis, a disease characterized by fever, headache, neck stiffness, photophobia, and nausea. Approximately 80–92% of aseptic meningitis cases for which the causative agent is identified are caused by enteroviruses.[7] They may also cause encephalitis, a direct infection of the brain, which may be focal, associated with seizures, or generalized, causing decreased level of consciousness.[5,6]

Besides CNS infections, enteroviruses cause myocarditis, pancreatitis, and dermatological diseases.[6,8] Evidence also strongly suggests that they are involved in the etiology of type 1 (insulin-dependent) diabetes.[9]

Enteroviruses are good candidate agents for involvement in the etiology of schizophrenia. As described, they are capable of infecting the CNS. Acute CNS infections may be accompanied by psychotic symptoms.[10] Interestingly, enteroviral meningitis occurs more commonly in males than in females,[11] and males also have a slightly higher incidence of schizophrenia than females.[12] Severe enteroviral CNS infections may cause structural changes in brain areas that are also involved in the pathogenesis of schizophrenia. For example, fetal infections leading to cerebral ventriculomegaly,[13] and bilateral lesions of the hippocampi as a sequelae of an enteroviral encephalitis,[14] have been described. Children who suffer CNS enterovirus infection during the first year of life have smaller mean head circumference, lower mean IQ, and depressed language and speech skills,[15,16] all of which have also been found among individuals who develop schizophrenia in adulthood.[17–20] Enteroviruses may persist in the body for years,[6,21] and may cause new symptoms decades after the primary infection.[22] Thus, it would be theoretically possible that a prenatal or childhood enteroviral infection could be involved in the development of schizophrenia in adulthood.

PRENATAL POLIO VIRUS INFECTION AND SCHIZOPHRENIA

It has been hypothesized that prenatal polio virus infection could contribute to the development of schizophrenia, because a decline in the incidence of schizophrenia occurred in many countries after the introduction of polio vaccination.[23,24] It has been suggested that the winter–early spring excess of schizophrenic births is caused by an infection during the second trimester of fetal development.[25] If so, polio virus epidemics, which peak in late summer and early autumn,[26] are a better candidate to explain the seasonality than the winter and spring infections usually suggested.[23] There is also a similar geographical variation in the seasonality of poliomyelitis epidemics[26] and schizophrenic births.[27] Environmental survival of polio viruses is very sensitive to both humidity and temperature.[26] In areas with high relative humidity and low variation in temperature, annual variation in the incidence of poliomyelitis was low, while it was very high in areas with large temperature and humidity variations. In the USA, seasonal variation in the incidence of poliomyelitis was highest in the New England states and lowest in the west south central states (Texas, Louisiana, Arkansas, Oklahoma). Similarly, seasonal variation of births in schizophrenia was most pronounced in New England and least pronounced in the southern USA.[27] Further support for the hypothesis comes from the latency of the effect of poliovirus. Decades after the primary infection, new symptoms – the so-called post-polio syndrome – can emerge.[22,28] Acute polio infection of the central nervous system affects, besides motor neurons and motor cortex, the hypothalamus, thalamus, cerebellum, and reticular formation in the brain stem – areas that partially correlate with those in which brain lesions have been observed in schizophrenia.[22,28,29]

Thus far, few studies have investigated the possible role of polio viruses in the etiology of schizophrenia. Three studies have compared the incidence of paralytic poliomyelitis and the number of schizophrenic births.[30–32] Two detected no association,[30,32] while the third found a significant concordance between schizophrenic births and poliomyelitis – a finding difficult to explain because poliomyelitis preceded the schizophrenic births by 18 months.[31] A fourth study found no relationship between the number of deaths caused by poliomyelitis and schizophrenic births.[33] However, death is a rare outcome of polio virus infection.

In Finland, the winter excess of schizophrenic births was exceptionally large, almost 30%, among individuals born between 1953 and 1959.[34] After this, the seasonal variation of birth in schizophrenia disappeared almost completely. When searching for an explanation for this curious phenomenon, we noticed that there were severe polio epidemics in the mid-1950s but, after that, polio was eradicated by 1965. The most severe polio epidemics were followed by a peak in the observed versus the expected number of schizophrenic births, with a latency of approximately four to five months (see Figure 4.1.). Thus, we set out to investigate whether there was any association between prenatal exposure to polio epidemics and later development of schizophrenia.[35]

We obtained the monthly reports on infectious diseases originally kept by the National Board of Health and now stored in the archives of the National Research and Development Center for Welfare and Health. These were based on the reports delivered by every Finnish physician to the National Board of Health. Each physician was required to report the cases of infectious diseases they had treated. A separate, detailed report on each case was required for some diseases, including poliomyelitis. Reports were obtained for the years 1950–1969, and included the monthly numbers of infections separately for each of the 12 provinces and for the three largest towns (Helsinki, Tampere, Turku) in Finland. In our study, we used the monthly numbers of new cases of paralytic poliomyelitis.[35]

We used a Poisson regression model with the number of schizophrenic births as the response variable and the province of birth, incidence of paralytic poliomyelitis in the province of birth at different times of gestation, birth cohort, age, sex, and month of birth as the explanatory variables. The size of population in each cell was used as weight to obtain correct estimates. Circular transformation was applied to the month of birth to analyze seasonal variation.[35]

The incidence of paralytic poliomyelitis showed very high variability, because even during epidemics there were few cases in one province or town. The high variability was first reduced by dichotomizing the incidence to an indicator variable (0 = no cases

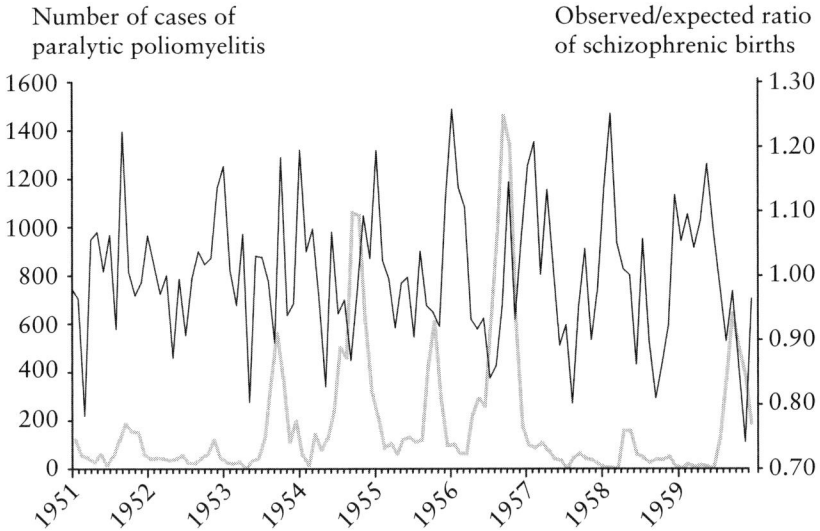

Figure 4.1 Monthly number of cases with paralytic poliomyelitis (gray line) and the observed vs. expected ratio of schizophrenic births (black line) in Finland between 1951 and 1959.

of poliomyelitis, 1 = any cases of poliomyelitis). In another analysis, a moving average with a three-month window was used before dichotomization. To investigate whether the effect would increase with the severity of exposure, the incidence of poliomyelitis was also divided into deciles; the first six deciles, in which the incidence was zero, were pooled.[35]

In the first regression model, in which the incidence of poliomyelitis was dichotomized but not smoothed, exposure to poliomyelitis epidemics five to six months before birth was associated with a significantly increased risk of later developing schizophrenia (relative risk RR 1.06, 95% confidence interval CI 1.01–1.11). When seasonality was omitted from the model, the relative risk increased slightly (RR 1.07, 95% CI 1.02–1.12).[35]

When a smoothed incidence of poliomyelitis was used, exposure to a polio epidemic five months before birth was associated with an increased risk of later developing schizophrenia (RR 1.05, 95% CI 1.00–1.11). When seasonality was omitted from the model, the effect became significant throughout the second trimester (RR 1.06–1.08 four to six months before birth). The effect did not, however, increase with the severity of exposure. The relative risk of developing schizophrenia compared with the first six deciles with no exposure was 1.13 in the seventh, 1.05 in the eight, 0.98 in the ninth, and 1.05 in the 10th decile.[35]

We observed that second trimester exposure to polio epidemics increased the risk of the later development of schizophrenia modestly but significantly. The relatively small effect of the exposure is not surprising given that genetic factors are most important in the etiology of schizophrenia and that several other possible environmental risk factors have already been identified. The timing accords with previous findings of a neurodevelopmental insult in schizophrenia during the second trimester of fetal life.[25,35]

That the effect did not increase with the severity of exposure might be because we restricted ourselves to the incidence of paralytic poliomyelitis. Paralytic symptoms develop in less than 1% of those infected with the polio virus and only after an incubation period of up to one month.[26] In addition, the case:infection ratio depends on age, level of immunity in the population, and the type of poliovirus, type 1 being the most virulent and type 2 the least.[26,35]

Neutralizing immunity against the polio virus serotype that caused the infection develops after the infection, but it does not provide neutralizing immunity to other serotypes. Polio epidemics occurred relatively frequently in the first half of the 20th century. Therefore, one reason for the rather weak association between exposure to polio epidemics during pregnancy and later development of schizophrenia could have been that most pregnant women already had immunity against the polio virus type that caused the epidemic. Results from the Finnish field trial of the polio vaccine provided some estimate of the size of the susceptible population.

The first field trial of a polio vaccine in Finland was conducted during a large polio epidemic in 1954. A large number of six- to 12-year-old children were recruited, half of whom were vaccinated while the other half served as controls. Their antibody status was measured before the vaccination, and again after the termination of the epidemic. At the baseline, 61%

of children had antibodies against type 1 virus, 44% against type 2 virus, and 62% against type 3 virus. The epidemic was caused by a type 1 virus, against which the vaccine did not protect. After the epidemic, 25% of the originally seronegative subjects had developed antibodies against the type 1 virus, regardless of whether they had received the vaccination or not. During the epidemic, the incidence of paralysis among those acquiring the infection increased from one per 250 to one per 110.[36]

According to one study, the susceptible population in the 1954 epidemic was considerable, although more than half of the six- to 12-year-old children already had antibodies against the type 1 and type 3 strains.[36] The seroconversion rate among the susceptible population was also high: the epidemic was widespread. It seems reasonable to assume that during an epidemic like this, a significant proportion of pregnant women belonged to the susceptible population, and a significant proportion of those belonging to the susceptible population also caught the infection. The findings also suggest that the virulence of the virus may change even during one epidemic.

Yet another reason for finding only a weak association between second trimester exposure to polio virus epidemic and adult schizophrenia could be that the association might be limited to one of the serotypes. Or it might be confined to one exceptionally virulent form of one of the serotypes. Thus, it would have been interesting to study the association according to the type of virus that had caused each epidemic, but unfortunately the information was not available.

We are left with many unanswered questions. An ecological study cannot prove causal association. For this, a follow-up study of pregnant women who actually had a polio virus infection during the 1950s would be needed. The type of polio virus which caused the infection should also be known. While such a study might be almost impossible to conduct, our results encourage research on other enteroviruses, which in many respects are similar to polio viruses and have become the most common viral agents causing aseptic meningitis.[5]

CHILDHOOD ENTEROVIRAL CNS INFECTIONS AND SCHIZOPHRENIA

It has been suggested that the brain abnormalities that lead to the development of schizophrenia may progress during childhood,[37] and insults on the developing brain during childhood may have an influence on the risk of developing schizophrenia in adulthood. Consistent with this hypothesis, the Northern Finland 1966 Birth Cohort study found that childhood viral central nervous system (CNS) infection was associated with almost five-fold increased odds for developing schizophrenia in adulthood.[38] In this study, two of the four individuals who had suffered childhood viral CNS infection and developed schizophrenia in adulthood had an infection caused by coxsackievirus B5 (CBV-5), an enterovirus, giving a cumulative incidence of schizophrenia of 12.5% among those with neonatal meningitis caused by CBV-5.[38] We set out to verify these findings in a sample of 320 individuals with virologically confirmed childhood CNS infection, identified from the Department of Virology at the National Public Health Institute, which had the first viral laboratory in Finland.[39]

During the 1960s and 1970s, the laboratory of the Department of Virology analyzed clinical samples sent from hospitals throughout Finland. One branch of the laboratory specialized in enteroviral infections. Samples from individuals with suspected enteroviral diseases were therefore often sent there. Results of all virological analyses from each individual patient were stored on a card which recorded the following information: name, date of birth or social security number, clinical diagnosis, often a brief description of the presenting symptoms, treating hospital, date when samples had been taken, and their type (blood, fecal, cerebrospinal fluid). From these cards, all individuals born from 1960 to 1976 who had suffered virologically confirmed CNS infection before their 15th birthday were identified. Names and birthdates of those with missing social security numbers were linked with information from the Population Register Center to obtain the social security numbers. The social security numbers were then sent to the National Hospital Discharge Register to obtain information on all hospital treatments from 1969 to 2000 for the sample. Schizophrenia was defined as a 295 diagnosis according to ICD-8 and ICD-9 diagnostic codes, used between 1969 and 1995, or an F20 diagnosis according to ICD-10 diagnostic codes, used since 1996. These include schizophrenia, schizophreniform disorder, and schizoaffective disorder. Cumulative incidence was calculated by dividing the number of individuals who developed schizophrenia by the number of individuals in the cohort. The exact 95% confidence intervals were calculated using the Bayesian method.[39,40]

The sample consisted of 370 individuals. The social security numbers for 47 of them could not be found. One had to be discarded because two different viruses had been identified and it was thus unclear which had caused the infection. Two more individuals were excluded because of missing clinical diagnoses, leaving 320 individuals in the final sample. Their clinical diagnoses were encephalitis in 28, meningitis in 256, meningoencephalitis in 17, and 'seizures' in 19 cases. The infection had been caused by adenovirus in 30 cases, by mumps in 84 cases, by enterovirus in 202 cases – including 40 caused by CBV-5 – and by other viruses in four cases. The mean age when the infection occurred was 3.80 years (SD 2.97, range 0–11.6), and the mean age at the end of the follow-up was 32.0 years (SD 4.52, range 23.3–41.0).[39]

Three individuals developed schizophrenia in adulthood. Two of them had suffered enteroviral infection (one caused by CBV-5) at the age of 42 and 25 months respectively, the clinical diagnosis being encephalitis in the former and seizures in the latter case. The age at onset of schizophrenia was 21 years in the former and 16 years in the latter case. The third individual to develop schizophrenia had adenovirus meningitis at the age of 27 months, and developed schizophrenia at the age of 23 years. In addition, there was one case with more than 30 admissions because of substance abuse and borderline personality disorder who had once received a diagnosis of psychotic disorder not otherwise specified (NOS) who we did not classify as suffering from schizophrenia. The cumulative incidence of schizophrenia was 0.94% (95% CI 0–2.72) among those with any CNS infection, and 0.99% (95% CI 0–3.53) among those with an enteroviral CNS infection. The risk of schizophrenia did not differ among those with enterovirus infection and those with other types of infection (odds ratio 1.16, 95% CI 0.10–13.0).[39]

The observed cumulative incidences were in the same range as the register-based cumulative incidence of schizophrenia of 0.74% until 1995 in Finnish birth cohorts born from 1960 to 1969, a figure we calculated using our register-based data used in the polio virus study, and the cumulative incidence of 0.91% observed in the Northern Finland 1966 Birth Cohort.[41] Thus, our data provided no support for the hypothesis that childhood viral CNS infections, or enteroviral CNS infections in particular, are associated with a markedly increased risk of developing schizophrenia. Our confidence interval overlapped with that found elsewhere,[37] suggesting that a moderate association is possible. Our sample size was still inadequate for examining whether a CNS infection caused particularly by CBV-5 would increase the risk of adult-onset schizophrenia. In our sample 40 cases had suffered a CNS infection caused by CBV-5, and one of them developed schizophrenia. A larger sample would be needed to verify the association.

There were 28 cases whose clinical diagnosis was encephalitis, and the 19 whose diagnosis was seizures probably also suffered from encephalitis. Two of these 47 cases developed schizophrenia. The possibility that the most severe viral CNS infections increase the risk of schizophrenia should be studied further with larger samples.

CONCLUSIONS

Theoretically, enteroviruses are good candidate viruses to be involved in the etiology of schizophrenia, but our data provide only weak support for the hypothesis. The results of the polio virus study suggest that maternal second trimester polio virus infection may increase risk of schizophrenia in the offspring. However, our study was an ecological study which cannot prove causality. Stronger evidence would be provided by analyzing blood samples collected during pregnancy in such cohort studies as the Collaborative Perinatal Project.[42] It would definitely be worthwhile investigating antibodies against polio virus and also against other enteroviruses in such studies. Offspring of mothers with verified prenatal polio virus infection could be followed up, but since polio virus vaccination has been used for decades in most countries, such cohorts might be very difficult to find.

We did not find any support for the hypothesis that childhood CNS infections, and enteroviral infections in particular, are involved in the etiology of schizophrenia. Although our sample was not small, the confidence intervals were rather wide, and for example a two-fold increase in the risk would be possible. Most noteworthy, individuals who have suffered CNS infections caused by coxsackie B5 virus or viral encephalitis should be studied further.

If prenatal or childhood enteroviral infections increase the risk of schizophrenia, this would be yet another reason for developing enterovirus vaccines. Fortunately, rapid diagnosis of enteroviral infections using PCR, and effective treatment for enteroviral CNS infections with pleconaril, have been developed,[7] which might reduce the risk of schizophrenia if there is association between the severity of CNS infection and risk of schizophrenia.

REFERENCES

1. Kraepelin E. *Dementia Praecox and Paraphrenia* (Barclay RM, transl). Huntington, NY: Robert E. Krieger Publishing Co Inc, 1919/1971.
2. Bleuler E. *Dementia Preacox or the Group of Schizophrenias* (Zinkin J, transl) Monograph Series of Schizophrenia No. 1. New York: International Universities Press, 1911/1950.
3. Yolken RH, Torrey EF. Viruses, schizophrenia, and bipolar disorder. *Clin Microbiol Rev* 1995; 8: 131–45.

4. Kirch DG. Infection and autoimmunity as etiologic factors in schizophrenia: a review and reappraisal. *Schizophr Bull* 1993; **19**: 355–70.
5. Muir P, van Loon AM. Enterovirus infections of the central nervous system. *Intervirology* 1997; **40**: 153–66.
6. Hovi T. Molecular epidemiology of enteroviruses with special reference to their potential role in the etiology of insulin-dependent diabetes mellitus (IDDM). A review. *Clin Diag Virol* 1998; **9**: 89–98.
7. Sawyer MH. Enterovirus infections: diagnosis and treatment. *Curr Opin Pediatr* 2001; **13**: 65–9.
8. Kim K-S, Hyfnagel G, Chapman NM, Tracy S. The group B coxsackieviruses and myocarditis. *Rev Med Virol* 2001; **11**: 355–68.
9. Hyöty H. Enterovirus infections and type 1 diabetes. *Ann Med* 2002; **34**: 138–47.
10. Wang SM, Liu CC, Chen YJ et al. Alice in Wonderland syndrome caused by coxsackievirus B1. *Ped Infec Dis J* 1996; **15**: 470–1.
11. Nigrovic LE. What's new with enteroviral infections. *Curr Opin Pediatrics* 2001; **13**: 89–94.
12. Leung A, Chue P. Sex differences in schizophrenia, a review of the literature. *Acta Psychiatr Scand* 2000; **101**: 3–38.
13. Dommergues M, Petitjean J, Aubry MC et al. Fetal enteroviral infection with cerebral ventriculomegaly and cardiomyopathy. *Fetal Diag Ther* 1994; **9**: 77–8.
14. Liow K, Spanaki MV, Boyer RS et al. Bilateral hippocampal encephalitis caused by enterovial infection. *Ped Neurol* 1999; **21**: 836–8.
15. Sells CJ, Carpenter RL, Ray CG. Sequelae of central-nervous-system enterovirus infections. *N Eng J Med* 1975; **293**: 1–4.
16. Wilfert CM, Thompson RJ, Sunder TR et al. Longitudinal assessment of children with enteroviral meningitis during the first three months of life. *Pediatrics* 1981; **67**: 811–5.
17. McNeil TF, Cantor-Graae E, Nordström LG, Rosenlund T. Head circumference in preschizophrenic and control neonates. *Br J Psychiatry* 1993; **162**: 517–23.
18. Davidson M, Reichenberg A, Rabinowitz J et al. Behavioral and intellectual markers for schizophrenia in apparently healthy male adolescents. *Am J Psychiatry* 1999; **156**: 1328–35.
19. Jones P, Rodgers B, Murray R, Marmot M. Child developmental risk factors for adult schizophrenia in the British 1946 birth cohort. *Lancet* 1994; **344**: 1398–402.
20. Cannon M, Caspi A, Moffitt TE et al. Evidence for early-childhood, pan-developmental impairment specific to schizophreniform disorder. *Arch Gen Psychiatry* 2002; **59**: 449–56.
21. Frisk G. Mechanisms of chronic enteroviral persistence in tissue. *Curr Opin Infec Diseases* 2001; **14**: 251–6.
22. Bruno RL, Cohen JM, Galski T, Frick NM. The neuroanatomy of post-polio fatigue. *Arch Physical Med Rehab* 1994; **75**: 498–504.
23. Eagles JM. Are polioviruses a cause of schizophrenia? *Br J Psychiatry* 1992; **160**: 598–600.
24. Squires RF. How a poliovirus might cause schizophrenia: a commentary on Eagles' hypothesis. *Neurochem Res* 1997; **22**: 647–56.
25. Huttunen MO, Machon RA, Mednick SA. Prenatal factors in the pathogenesis of schizophrenia. *Br J of Psychiatry* 1994; **164** (Suppl. 23): 15–9.
26. Nathanson N, Martin JR. The epidemiology of poliomyelitis: enigmas surrounding its appearance, epidemicity, and disappearance. *Am J Epidemiol* 1979; **110**: 672–92.
27. Torrey EF, Torrey BB, Peterson MR. Seasonality of schizophrenic births in the United States. *Arch Gen Psychiatry* 1977; **34**: 1065–70.
28. Dalakas MC. Pathogenetic mechanisms of post-polio syndrome: morphological, electrophysiological, virological, and immunological correlations. *Ann NY Acad Sci* 1995; **753**: 167–85.
29. Heckers S. Neuropathology of schizophrenia: cortex, thalamus, basal ganglia, and neurotransmitter-specific projection systems. *Schizophr Bull* 1997; **23**: 403–21.
30. Watson CG, Kucala T, Tilleskjor C, Jacobs L. Schizophrenic birth seasonality in relation to the incidence of infectious diseases and temperature extremes. *Arch Gen Psychiatry* 1984; **41**: 85–90.
31. Torrey EF, Rawlings R, Waldman IN. Schizophrenic births and viral diseases in two states. *Schizoph Res* 1988; **1**: 73–7.
32. Cahill M, Chant D, Welham J, McGrath J. No significant association between prenatal poliovirus epidemics and psychosis. *Aust N Z J Psychiatry* 2002; **36**: 373–5.
33. O'Callaghan E, Sham PC, Takei N. The relationship of schizophrenic births to 16 infectious diseases. *Br J Psychiatry* 1994; **165**: 353–6.
34. Suvisaari JM, Haukka JK, Tanskanen AJ, Lönnqvist JK. Decreasing seasonal variation of births in schizophrenia. *Psychol Med* 2000; **30**: 315–24.
35. Suvisaari J, Haukka J, Tanskanen A et al. An association between prenatal exposure to poliovirus infection and adult schizophrenia. *Am J Psychiatry* 1999; **156**: 1100–2.
36. Penttinen K, Pätiälä R. The paralytic/infected ratio in a susceptible population during a polio type I epidemic. *Annales Medicinae Experimentalis et Biologiae Fenniae* 1961; **39**: 195–202.
37. Woods BT. Is schizophrenia a progressive neurodevelopmental disorder? Toward a unitary pathogenetic mechanism. *Am J Psychiatry* 1998; **155**: 1661–70.
38. Rantakallio P, Jones P, Moring J, von Wendt L. Association between central nervous system infections during childhood and adult onset schizophrenia and other psychosis: a 28-year follow-up. *Int J Epidemiol* 1997; **26**: 837–43.
39. Suvisaari J, Mautemps N, Haukka J et al. Childhood central nervous system viral infections and adult schizophrenia. *Am J Psychiatry*, 2003; **160**: 1183–5.
40. Jaynes ET. Confidence intervals vs. Bayesian intervals. In: *Foundations of Probability Theory, Statistical Inference, and Statistical Theories of Science* (Harper WL, Hooker CA, eds). Dordrecht: D. Reidel, 1976: 175.
41. Isohanni M, Jones PB, Moilanen K et al. Early developmental milestones in adult schizophrenia and other psychoses. A 31-year follow-up of the Northern Finland 1966 Birth Cohort. *Schizophr Res* 2001; **52**: 1–19.
42. Buka SL, Tsuang MT, Torrey EF et al. Maternal infections and subsequent psychosis among offspring. *Arch Gen Psychiatry* 2001; **58**: 1032–7.

5

The role of the immune system in the pathophysiology of schizophrenia

Yong-Ku Kim and Michael Maes

INTRODUCTION

Schizophrenia is characterized by premorbid psychological deficits, onset of psychosis in late adolescence, and psychological deterioration in adulthood.[1] The pathophysiology of the disease involves both genes and environment.[2] The etiology of the disease is attributed to the failure of normal neuronal development due to environmental factors (such as obstetric complications or maternal viral infections) or a genetic defect manifesting itself during gestation or the perinatal period. Such defects alter the development of the CNS in some way. The resulting developmental deficit accounts for the premorbid cognitive and psychosocial dysfunction in schizophrenia.[3] The onset of psychotic symptoms in adolescence or early adulthood may be related to an excess in the normal synaptic pruning that occurs in certain brain regions, such as the prefrontal cortex.[4] Specifically, psychological stress during this period can stimulate perturbations in neuronal activity that could otherwise be endured without long-term psychological consequences.[5] The neurotransmitter alterations, including phasic and tonic dopamine transmission,[6] serotonin receptor dysfunction,[7] and NMDA receptor hypofunction,[8] can contribute to the positive, negative, and cognitive symptoms of schizophrenia that emerge during adolescence. In some schizophrenic patients, persistent, recurrent sensitization of the dopamine system over time[9] or oxidative stress by glutamate induced neurotoxicity[10] can lead to the neurodegeneration manifested by persistent morbidity, treatment resistance, and clinical deterioration. In this chapter, we describe the potential role of immunological mechanisms in the pathophysiology of schizophrenia, focusing on neurodevelopment, neurotransmitters, and neurodegeneration.

PRENATAL INFECTIONS, CYTOKINES, AND NEURODEVELOPMENT IN SCHIZOPHRENIA

Schizophrenia may be related to a defect in brain development, perhaps during the second half of gestation.[11] This view has been supported by brain imaging and post-mortem neuropathological findings indicating a failure of normal neuronal development such as neurogenesis, neuronal proliferation, neural differentiation, migration, and synaptogenesis.[12,13] Moreover, such defects predispose to a characteristic pattern of brain malfunction in early adult life and to symptoms which may respond to antidopaminergic drugs.[3] Although the reasons for the neurodevelopmental error in schizophrenia are not readily apparent, epidemiological studies suggest that environmental factors such as prenatal viral infections or birth trauma are significant risk factors for schizophrenia.[14]

During the last few decades, involvement of infections in the pathophysiology of schizophrenia has been a matter of research. Among those findings, the epidemiological studies on influenza[15,16] and rubella[17] are most interesting and reliable. Moreover, there is evidence that maternal viral infection during the second trimester is associated with later development of schizophrenia in adolescence.[18–20]

Regarding prenatal maternal influenza infection, a significant reduction in Reelin-positive cells in the cortical and hippocampal layers in mice prenatally exposed to influenza infection has been reported.[21] Reelin is the protein necessary for the normal lamination of the brain and therefore prenatal influenza infection can result in disturbed lamination of the brain. A distinct reduction of Reelin-positive cells in cortical and hippocampal layers was also demonstrated in the schizophrenic brain.[22] Other direct viral infections of the developing brain, with lymphocytic choriomeningitis virus (LCMV) and Borna disease virus (BDV), showed structural abnormalities and behavioral changes in later life in animal models. Cortical injection of LCMV leads to an acute loss of neurons in the cerebellum and delayed loss of neurons in the hippocampus, associated with altered patterns of activity in the adult hippocampus.[23] Intracerebral injection of BDV leads to neuronal death in the hippocampus, cerebellum, and neocortex, and a behavioral syndrome that includes hyperactivity, movement disorders, and abnormal social interaction.[24] These effects are correlated with major alterations in cytokine expression in various brain regions, depending on the stage of infection.[25] Cytokines induced by viral infection in pregnant women, such as IL-6, a neuropoietic cytokine, can influence developing neurons and glia. Such effects include changes in proliferation, survival, death, neurite growth, and gene expression.[26] Cytokines also regulate synaptic proteins and structural molecules in the schizophrenic brain.[27] A recent animal study demonstrated that pro-inflammatory cytokines, such as IL-1β, IL-6, and TNF-α, produce dose-dependent decreases in the number of neurons immunoreactive for MAP2, which influences dendrite morphology.[28] This finding suggests that cytokines have a role in the modulation of neuronal survival during neurodevelopment.

Regarding infection-induced immune system changes, antibodies against several neurotropic viruses have been the subject of research during recent decades. Most studies have focused on herpes viruses. Increased herpes simplex virus (HSV) antibodies in the serum and cerebrospinal fluid (CSF) of schizophrenic patients have been reported.[29,30] There was also a reported association between high HSV antibody titers and left frontal cortical atrophy in schizophrenic patients.[31] On the other hand, many researchers have failed to demonstrate the association between high HSV antibody levels and schizophrenics.[32–36] CMV antibodies were discovered in the CSF of 11% of schizophrenic patients[37] and signs of local CMV antibody production were observed in the brains of 68% of schizophrenics;[29] however, no change was observed in the serum.[33–36,38] Increased Epstein-Barr virus antibodies have been found in the serum of schizophrenics;[33] however, those infections are quite common in the general population. Antibodies in the brain or local brain region will be more closely related to psychiatric disorders than those in serum. Recent studies related to infection and schizophrenia focused on BDV, a neurotropic, single-stranded RNA virus. Three to 45% of schizophrenics had BDV serum antibodies[39–41] and a higher level was observed in patients with deficit syndrome.[40] On the other hand, some studies could not find any association between BDV infection and schizophrenia.[42,43] In experimental infections, vulnerability to BDV infection was observed in the hippocampus and retina.[44] Antibodies against toxoplasma and retroviruses have also been reported in schizophrenics, although only in a few studies.

Considering the above findings, it appears that schizophrenia is related to many viral infections and viral antibodies but no single virus is proven as a causative agent. Therefore, schizophrenia seems to be related to the humoral antibody response of the immune system rather than a single infectious agent.

CYTOKINES AND GENES IN SCHIZOPHRENIA

Genetic factors have also been implicated in the pathogenesis of schizophrenia and a multifocal, polygenetic etiology is considered most likely.[45] Since the majority of individuals exposed to neurodevelopmental insults such as infections or brain injury do not develop schizophrenia in adulthood, it is possible that a genetic vulnerability to neuronal injury contributes to the expression of schizophrenia. Interestingly, specific cytokine polymorphisms differentially modulate cytokine-mediated neuronal injury, and may represent susceptibility genes for development of schizophrenia following viral infection or brain injury during neurodevelopment.[28] The TNF-α gene is located on the short arm of chromosome 6, a locus associated with susceptibility to schizophrenia. A recent study indicated that a TNF-α polymorphism (-G308A) was significantly more frequent in schizophrenia patients compared with controls.[46] Moreover, TNF-α receptor II can modify phenotypic aspects of the disease such as brain morphology and the age of onset of the illness.[47] The number of carriers of certain alleles of IL-1β (−511; allele 1), IL-1α (−889; allele 2), and IL-1RA (allele 1) is significantly higher among schizophrenia patients than among controls.[48] Given the fact that genetic mutations could predispose a fetus to a higher risk from environmental factors such as infection or anoxia,[49] the interaction of cytokine genes and environmental factors may largely determine the risk for schizophrenia.

CYTOKINES AND NEUROTRANSMITTERS IN SCHIZOPHRENIC PSYCHOPATHOLOGY

The immune hypothesis of schizophrenia proposes that schizophrenia is accompanied by the dysregulation of cytokines in both peripheral and central nervous systems and, furthermore, that cytokine dysregulation plays a causative role in the etiology of the disease. The macrophage-T lymphocyte theory of schizophrenia proposes that chronically activated macrophages and T lymphocytes, along with excessive interleukin-2 and other cytokine secretions, are a cause of some cases of schizophrenia.[50,51] There is now increasing evidence that schizophrenia is characterized by increased nonspecific innate immunity, decreased type I helper cell cellular immunity, and a T helper 1 (Th1)–T helper 2 (Th2) imbalance with a shift to the Th2 system[52,53] or activation of the inflammatory response system.[54–56]

Abnormal brain dopamine activity has been suggested as the main neurotransmitter abnormality causing schizophrenia, but there has been much criticism and qualification of this idea.[57] Recently, another neurotransmitter, serotonin, has generated much interest in schizophrenia research. Many atypical antipsychotic drugs such as clozapine have been shown to exert potent serotonin-related activity.[58] Moreover, dopamine and serotonin play a major role in mediating the psychotic symptoms of schizophrenia.[59]

There is some evidence that a functional link exists between IL-2, central dopaminergic transmission, and positive symptoms such as delusions or hallucinations. Zalcman and his group demonstrated in mice that dopamine turnover in the prefrontal cortex is altered following an intraperitoneal injection of IL-2.[60] Also, IL-2 induces behavioral changes that are associated with alterations in central dopaminergic processes. In a recent animal study, IL-2 treatment increased climbing behavior related to an increase in dopaminergic activity, and this activity could be blocked by selective dopamine D1 and D2 receptor antagonists.[61] Furthermore, IL-2 appears to play a role in the pathogenesis of schizophrenia since levels are elevated in the CSF and plasma of neuroleptic-free patients.[62,63] Increased CSF levels of IL-2 predict the expression of psychotic symptoms.[64] Moreover, there is further evidence that plasma levels of IL-2 as well as the dopaminergic metabolite homovanillic acid are increased coincident with positive symptoms, and significantly decreased following treatment with haloperidol.[63]

Conversely, IL-6 levels are associated with both negative symptoms[63] and duration of illness.[63,65,66] These reports raise the question of whether elevated plasma IL-6 in schizophrenia might occur in response to the development of cerebral atrophy, which has been reported to be related to the duration of illness.[67] Moreover, structural brain abnormalities have been considered as pathogenic factors for production of negative symptoms.[68] Therefore, IL-6 may be associated with negative symptoms. Cytokines are known to influence central monoamine activity in a cytokine-specific manner.[61,69] In other words, IL-2 increases hypothalamic and hippocampal norepinephrine utilization and dopamine turnover in the prefrontal cortex, whereas IL-6 induces profound elevation of serotonin and mesocortical dopamine activity in the hippocampus and prefrontal cortex. IL-1, in contrast, induces a wide range of central monoamine alterations. Hence, it will be of great interest to determine which cytokines are related to specific schizophrenic symptoms and neurotransmitters.

CYTOKINE–SEROTONIN INTERACTION AND NEURODEGENERATION IN SCHIZOPHRENIA

The view that schizophrenia is a neurodegenerative disorder is supported by several pieces of clinical evidence: the progressive and deteriorating course of the disease, the long latency period, and the apparent ability of treatment to modify the course of the illness.[1] However, casting doubt on this hypothesis is the lack of progressive structural alteration and the absence of astrogliosis in the brains of schizophrenic patients; these traits would be expected for a severe and chronic neurodegenerative process.[70,71] Nonetheless, a growing number of studies support the notion of progressive cortical atrophy in schizophrenia and suggest a neurodegenerative component in the pathophysiology of schizophrenia.[72,73] Moreover, it was recently demonstrated that activated microglial cells are observed in a subset of schizophrenia patients.[74,75] Microglial activation is a key factor in defending the neural parenchyma against infectious diseases, inflammation, and neurodegeneration.[76]

Cytokines can also be mediators or inhibitors of the neurodegeneration. For example, TGF-β seems to exert primarily neuroprotective actions, while TNF-α contributes to neuronal injury and exerts protective effects.[77] Recently, the link between cytokines and serotonergic turnover has been explored. It was reported that cytokines such as IL-1β, IL-2, and IFN-γ reduce the production of 5-HT by stimulating the activity of indoleamine 2,3 dioxygenase (IDO), an enzyme which converts tryptophan, the precursor of 5-HT, to kynurenine.[78,79] The kynurenine is again metabolized into quinolinic acid and kynurenic acid.[80] Quinolinic acid is the excitotoxic NMDA receptor agonist,[81] and kynurenine is the antagonist of all three ionotropic excitatory amino acid receptors.[82] Therefore, it has been proposed that overexpression of IDO leads to the depletion of plasma tryptophan

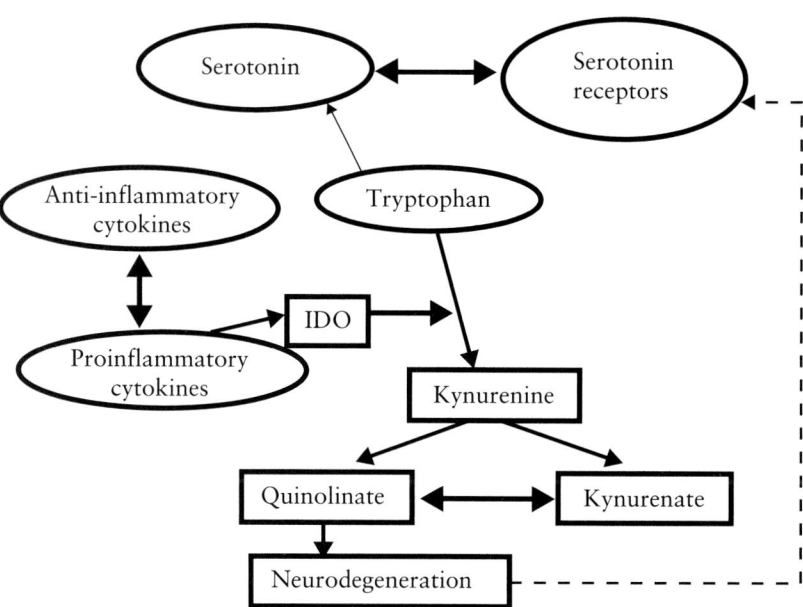

Figure 5.1 The role of cytokines in neurodegeneration in schizophrenia in relation to the serotonin degradation pathway. Cytokines activate the trpytophan degradation pathway by stimulating the activity of indoleamine 2,3 dioxygenase (IDO) enzyme which converts tryptophan to kynurenine. The balance between neurodegenerative quinolinate and neuroprotective kynurenate can lead to the neurodegeneration in schizophrenia.

and reduced synthesis of 5-HT in the brain.[83] Hence, the cytokine–serotonin interaction that leads to a challenge between neurodegenerative quinolinate and neuroprotective kynurenate in the brain may explain the neurodegeneration in schizophrenia (see Figure 5.1). In agreement with these ideas, recent studies have shown elevated levels of kynurenic acid in the CSF[84] and in the cortical brain tissue of schizophrenic patients.[85] More recently, an animal study demonstrated that an increase in endogenous kynurenic acid levels produces significant actions on the tonic afferent control of the firing pattern of rat ventral tegmental dopamine neurons. This result suggests that the elevated levels of kynurenic acid in schizophrenia may induce hyperactivity of the mesocorticolimbic dopamine system.[86] Therefore, the interactions between cytokines, the tryptophan degradation pathway, and neurodegeneration in schizophrenia need further exploration.

CONCLUSIONS

The involvement of immunological mechanisms in the pathophysiology of schizophrenia, especially in the stages of neurodevelopment, schizophrenic symptomatology, and neurodegeneration, has been an important research area. Maternal viral infections induce a failure of normal neuronal development through dysregulation of cytokines. Specific cytokine polymorphisms may represent susceptibility genes for development of schizophrenia following the insult during neurodevelopment. Cytokines also influence central monoamine activity in a cytokine-specific manner, and this activity modulates psychotic symptoms in schizophrenia. Cytokines are mediators and inhibitors of neurodegeneration. It is proposed that the interaction between cytokines and the tryptophan degradation pathway through IDO is involved in neurodegeneration in schizophrenia.

REFERENCES

1. Keshavan MS. Development, disease and degeneration in schizophrenia: a unitary pathophysiological model. *J Psychiatr Res* 1999; **33**: 513–21.
2. Bayer TA, Falkai P, Maier W. Genetic and non-genetic vulnerability factors in schizophrenia: the basis of the 'two hit' hypothesis. *J Psychiatr Res* 1999; **33**: 543–8.
3. Weinberger DR. On the plausibility of 'the neurodevelopmental hypothesis' of schizophrenia. *Neuropsychopharmacology* 1996; **14**: 1S–11S.
4. Mirnics K, Middleton FA, Lewis DA, Levitt P. Analysis of complex brain disorders with gene expression microarrays: schizophrenia as a disease of the synapse. *Trends Neurosci* 2001; **24**: 479–86.
5. Gispen-de Wied CC. Stress in schizophrenia: an integrative view. *Eur J Pharmacol* 2000; **405**: 375–84.
6. Moore H, West AR, Grace AA. The regulation of forebrain dopamine transmission: relevance to the pathophysiology and psychopathology of schizophrenia. *Biol Psychiatry* 1999; **46**: 40–55.
7. Iqbal N, van Praag HM. The role of serotonin in schizophrenia. *Eur Neuropsychopharmacol* 1995; **5**(Suppl): 11–23.
8. Olney JW, Newcomer JW, Farber NB. NMDA receptor hypofunction model of schizophrenia. *J Psychiatr Res* 1999; **33**: 523–33.

9. Duncan GE, Sheitman BB, Lieberman JA. An integrated view of pathophysiological models of schizophrenia. *Brain Res Rev* 1999; **29**: 250–64.
10. Coyle JT. The glutamatergic dysfunction hypothesis for schizophrenia. *Harv Rev Psychiatry* 1996; **3**: 241–53.
11. Weinberger DR. Implications of normal brain development for the pathogenesis of schizophrenia. *Arch Gen Psychiatry* 1987; **44**: 660–9.
12. Harrison PJ. The neuropathology of schizophrenia. A critical review of the data and their interpretation. *Brain* 1999; **122** (Pt 4): 593–624.
13. Waddington JL. Schizophrenia: developmental neuroscience and pathobiology. *Lancet* 1993; **341**: 531–6.
14. Gilmore JH, Jarskog LF. Exposure to infection and brain development: cytokines in the pathogenesis of schizophrenia. *Schizophr Res* 1997; **24**: 365–7.
15. Mednick SA, Machon RA, Huttunen MO, Bonett D. Adult schizophrenia following prenatal exposure to an influenza epidemic. *Arch Gen Psychiatry* 1988; **45**: 189–92.
16. O'Callaghan E, Sham P, Takei N et al. Schizophrenia after prenatal exposure to 1957 A2 influenza epidemic. *Lancet* 1991; **337**: 1248–50.
17. Brown AS, Cohen P, Greenwald S, Susser E. Nonaffective psychosis after prenatal exposure to rubella. *Am J Psychiatry* 2000; **157**: 438–43.
18. Torrey EF, Miller J, Rawlings R, Yolken RH. Seasonality of births in schizophrenia and bipolar disorder: a review of the literature. *Schizophr Res* 1997; **28**: 1–38.
19. Mednick SA, Huttunen MO, Machon RA. Prenatal influenza infections and adult schizophrenia. *Schizophr Bull* 1994; **20**: 263–7.
20. Kirch DG. Infection and autoimmunity as etiologic factors in schizophrenia: a review and reappraisal. *Schizophr Bull* 1993; **19**: 355–70.
21. Fatemi SH, Emamian ES, Kist D et al. Defective corticogenesis and reduction in Reelin immunoreactivity in cortex and hippocampus of prenatally infected neonatal mice. *Mol Psychiatry* 1999; **4**: 145–54.
22. Impagnatiello F, Guidotti AR, Pesold C et al. A decrease of Reelin expression as a putative vulnerability factor in schizophrenia. *Proc Natl Acad Sci USA* 1998; **95**: 15718–23.
23. Pearce BD, Valadi NM, Po CL, Miller AH. Viral infection of developing GABAergic neurons in a model of hippocampal disinhibition. *Neuroreport* 2000; **11**: 2433–8.
24. Weissenbock H, Hornig M, Hickey WF, Lipkin WI. Microglial activation and neuronal apoptosis in Bornavirus infected neonatal Lewis rats. *Brain Pathol* 2000; **10**: 260–72.
25. Plata-Salaman CR, Ilyin SE, Gayle D et al. Persistent Borna disease virus infection of neonatal rats causes brain regional changes of mRNAs for cytokines, cytokine receptor components and neuropeptides. *Brain Res Bull* 1999; **49**: 441–51.
26. Gadient RA, Patterson PH. Leukemia inhibitory factor, interleukin 6, and other cytokines using the GP130 transducing receptor: roles in inflammation and injury. *Stem Cells* 1999; **17**: 127–37.
27. Nawa H, Takahashi M, Patterson PH. Cytokine and growth factor involvement in schizophrenia – support for the developmental model. *Mol Psychiatry* 2000; **5**: 594–603.
28. Marx CE, Jarskog LF, Lauder JM et al. Cytokine effects on cortical neuron MAP-2 immunoreactivity: implications for schizophrenia. *Biol Psychiatry* 2001; **50**: 743–9.
29. Albrecht P, Torrey EF, Boone E et al. Raised cytomegalovirus-antibody level in cerebrospinal fluid of schizophrenic patients. *Lancet* 1980; **2**: 769–72.
30. Bartova L, Rajcani J, Pogady J. Herpes simplex virus antibodies in the cerebrospinal fluid of schizophrenic patients. *Acta Virol* 1987; **31**: 443–6.
31. Pandurangi AK, Pelonero AL, Nadel L, Calabrese VP. Brain structure changes in schizophrenics with high serum titers of antibodies to herpes virus. *Schizophr Res* 1994; **11**: 245–50.
32. Rimon R, Halonen P, Puhakka P et al. Immunoglobulin G antibodies to herpes simplex type 1 virus detected by radioimmunoassay in serum and cerebrospinal fluid of patients with schizophrenia. *J Clin Psychiatry* 1979; **40**: 241–3.
33. Delisi LE, Smith SB, Hamovit JR et al. Herpes simplex virus, cytomegalovirus and Epstein-Barr virus antibody titres in sera from schizophrenic patients. *Psychol Med* 1986; **16**: 757–63.
34. Toorey EF, Peterson MR, Brannon WL et al. Immunoglobulins and viral antibodies in psychiatric patients. *Br J Psychiatry* 1978; **132**: 342–8.
35. Schindler L, Leroux M, Beck J et al. Studies of cellular immunity, serum interferon titers, and natural killer cell activity in schizophrenic patients. *Acta Psychiatr Scand* 1986; **73**: 651–7.
36. Fux M, Sarov I, Ginot Y, Sarov B. Herpes simplex virus and cytomegalovirus in the serum of schizophrenic patients versus other psychosis and normal controls. *Isr J Psychiatry Relat Sci* 1992; **29**: 33–5.
37. Torrey EF, Yolken RH, Winfrey CJ. Cytomegalovirus antibody in cerebrospinal fluid of schizophrenic patients detected by enzyme immunoassay. *Science* 1982; **216**: 892–4.
38. Shrikhande S, Hirsch SR, Coleman JC et al. Cytomegalovirus and schizophrenia. A test of a viral hypothesis. *Br J Psychiatry* 1985; **146**: 503–6.
39. Iwahashi K, Watanabe M, Nakamura K et al. Clinical investigation of the relationship between Borna disease virus (BDV) infection and schizophrenia in 67 patients in Japan. *Acta Psychiatr Scand* 1997; **96**: 412–5.
40. Waltrip RW II, Buchanan RW, Carpenter WT Jr et al. Borna disease virus antibodies and the deficit syndrome of schizophrenia. *Schizophr Res* 1997; **23**: 253–7.
41. Chen CH, Chiu YL, Wei FC et al. High seroprevalence of Borna virus infection in schizophrenic patients, family members and mental health workers in Taiwan. *Mol Psychiatry* 1999; **4**: 33–8.
42. Richt JA, Alexander RC, Herzog S et al. Failure to detect Borna disease virus infection in peripheral blood leukocytes from humans with psychiatric disorders. *J Neurovirol* 1997; **3**: 174–8.
43. Kim YK, Noh KB, Han CS et al. Borna disease virus and deficit schizophrenia. *Acta Neuropsychiatrica* 2003; **15**: 262–5.
44. Taieb O, Baleyte JM, Mazet P, Fillet AM. Borna disease virus and psychiatry. *Eur Psychiatry* 2001; **16**: 3–10.
45. Prasad S, Semwal P, Deshpande S et al. Molecular genetics of schizophrenia: past, present and future. *J Biosci* 2002; **27**: 35–52.
46. Boin F, Zanardini R, Pioli R et al. Association between -G308A tumor necrosis factor alpha gene polymorphism and schizophrenia. *Mol Psychiatry* 2001; **6**: 79–82.
47. Wassink TH, Crowe RR, Andreasen NC. Tumor necrosis factor receptor-II: heritability and effect on brain morphology in schizophrenia. *Mol Psychiatry* 2000; **5**: 678–82.
48. Katila H, Hanninen K, Hurme M. Polymorphisms of the interleukin-1 gene complex in schizophrenia. *Mol Psychiatry* 1999; **4**: 179–81.
49. Jones P, Murray RM. The genetics of schizophrenia is the genetics of neurodevelopment. *Br J Psychiatry* 1991; **158**: 615–23.
50. Smith RS. Is schizophrenia caused by excessive production of interleukin-2 and interleukin-2 receptors by gastrointestinal lymphocytes? *Med Hypotheses* 1991; **34**: 225–9.
51. Smith RS, Maes M. The macrophage-T-lymphocyte theory of schizophrenia: additional evidence. *Med Hypotheses* 1995; **45**: 135–41.
52. Muller N, Riedel M, Ackenheil M, Schwarz MJ. The role of immune function in schizophrenia: an overview. *Eur Arch Psychiatry Clin Neurosci* 1999; **249** (Suppl 4): 62–8.

53. Schwarz MJ, Muller N, Riedel M, Ackenheil M. The Th2-hypothesis of schizophrenia: a strategy to identify a subgroup of schizophrenia caused by immune mechanisms. *Med Hypotheses* 2001; **56**: 483–6.
54. Maes M. Cytokines in schizophrenia. *Biol Psychiatry* 1997; **42**: 308–9.
55. Kim YK, Suh IB, Kim H et al. The plasma levels of interleukin-12 in schizophrenia., major depression, and bipolar mania: effects of psychotropic drugs. *Mol Psychiatry* 2002; **7**: 1107–14.
56. Zhang XY, Zhou DF, Zhang PY et al. Elevated interleukin-2, interleukin-6 and interleukin-8 serum levels in neuroleptic-free schizophrenia: association with psychopathology. *Schizophr Res* 2002; **57**: 247–58.
57. Davis KL, Kahn RS, Ko G, Davidson M. Dopamine in schizophrenia: a review and reconceptualization. *Am J Psychiatry* 1991; **148**: 1474–86.
58. Schmidt CJ, Sorensen SM, Kehne JH et al. The role of 5-HT2A receptors in antipsychotic activity. *Life Sci* 1995; **56**: 2209–22.
59. Lieberman JA, Koreen AR. Neurochemistry and neuroendocrinology of schizophrenia: a selective review. *Schizophr Bull* 1993; **19**: 371–429.
60. Zalcman S, Green-Johnson JM, Murray L et al. Cytokine-specific central monoamine alterations induced by interleukin-1, -2 and -6. *Brain Res* 1994; **643**: 40–9.
61. Zalcman SS. Interleukin-2-induced increases in climbing behavior: inhibition by dopamine D-1 and D-2 receptor antagonists. *Brain Res* 2002; **944**: 157–64.
62. Licinio J, Seibyl JP, Altemus M et al. Elevated CSF levels of interleukin-2 in neuroleptic-free schizophrenic patients. *Am J Psychiatry* 1993; **150**: 1408–10.
63. Kim YK, Kim L, Lee MS. Relationships between interleukins, neurotransmitters and psychopathology in drug-free male schizophrenics. *Schizophr Res* 2000; **44**: 165–75.
64. McAllister CG, van Kammen DP, Rehn TJ et al. Increases in CSF levels of interleukin-2 in schizophrenia: effects of recurrence of psychosis and medication status. *Am J Psychiatry* 1995; **152**: 1291–7.
65. Ganguli R, Yang Z, Shurin G et al. Serum interleukin-6 concentration in schizophrenia: elevation associated with duration of illness. *Psychiatry Res* 1994; **51**: 1–10.
66. Naudin J, Capo C, Giusano B et al. A differential role for interleukin-6 and tumor necrosis factor-alpha in schizophrenia? *Schizophr Res* 1997; **26**: 227–33.
67. Waddington JL. Neurodynamics of abnormalities in cerebral metabolism and structure in schizophrenia. *Schizophr Bull* 1993; **19**: 55–69.
68. Crow TJ. Molecular pathology of schizophrenia: more than one disease process. *Br Med J* 1980; **280**: 66–80.
69. Zalcman S, Murray L, Dyck DG et al. Interleukin-2 and -6 induce behavioral-activating effects in mice. *Brain Res* 1998; **811**: 111–21.
70. Arnold SE, Trojanowski JQ, Gur RE et al. Absence of neurodegeneration and neural injury in the cerebral cortex in a sample of elderly patients with schizophrenia. *Arch Gen Psychiatry* 1998; **55**: 225–32.
71. Falkai P, Honer WG, David S et al. No evidence for astrogliosis in brains of schizophrenic patients. A post-mortem study. *Neuropathol Appl Neurobiol* 1999; **25**: 48–53.
72. Knoll JL, Garver DL, Ramberg JE et al. Heterogeneity of the psychoses: is there a neurodegenerative psychosis? *Schizophr Bull* 1998; **24**: 365–79.
73. Woods BT. Is schizophrenia a progressive neurodevelopmental disorder? Toward a unitary pathogenetic mechanism. *Am J Psychiatry* 1998; **155**: 1661–70.
74. Bayer TA, Buslei R, Havas L, Falkai P. Evidence for activation of microglia in patients with psychiatric illnesses. *Neurosci Lett* 1999; **271**: 126–8.
75. Radewicz K, Garey LJ, Gentleman SM, Reynolds R. Increase in HLA-DR immunoreactive microglia in frontal and temporal cortex of chronic schizophrenics. *J Neuropathol Exp Neurol* 2000; **59**: 137–50.
76. Kreutzberg GW. Microglia: a sensor for pathological events in the CNS. *Trends Neurosci* 1996; **19**: 312–8.
77. Allan SM, Rothwell NJ. Cytokines and acute neurodegeneration. *Nat Rev Neurosci* 2001; **2**: 734–44.
78. Guillemin GJ, Kerr SJ, Pemberton LA et al. IFN-beta1b induces kynurenine pathway metabolism in human macrophages: potential implications for multiple sclerosis treatment. *J Interferon Cytokine Res* 2001; **21**: 1097–101.
79. Sakash JB, Byrne GI, Lichtman A, Libby P. Cytokines induce indoleamine 2,3-dioxygenase expression in human atheroma-associated cells: implications for persistent *Chlamydophila pneumoniae* infection. *Infect Immun* 2002; **70**: 3959–61.
80. Dang Y, Dale WE, Brown OR. Comparative effects of oxygen on indoleamine 2,3-dioxygenase and tryptophan 2,3-dioxygenase of the kynurenine pathway. *Free Radic Biol Med* 2000; **28**: 615–24.
81. Schwarcz R, Whetsell WO Jr, Mangano RM. Quinolinic acid: an endogenous metabolite that produces axon-sparing lesions in rat brain. *Science* 1983; **219**: 316–8.
82. Perkins MN, Stone TW. An iontophoretic investigation of the actions of convulsant kynurenines and their interaction with the endogenous excitant quinolinic acid. *Brain Res* 1982; **247**: 184–7.
83. Myint AM, Kim YK. Cytokine–serotonin interaction through IDO: a neurodegeneration hypothesis of depression. *Med Hypotheses* 2003; **61**: 519–25.
84. Erhardt S, Blennow K, Nordin C et al. Kynurenic acid levels are elevated in the cerebrospinal fluid of patients with schizophrenia. *Neurosci Lett* 2001; **313**: 96–8.
85. Schwarcz R, Rassoulpour A, Wu HQ et al. Increased cortical kynurenate content in schizophrenia. *Biol Psychiatry* 2001; **50**: 521–30.
86. Erhardt S, Engberg G. Increased phasic activity of dopaminergic neurones in the rat ventral tegmental area following pharmacologically elevated levels of endogenous kynurenic acid. *Acta Physiol Scand* 2002; **175**: 45–53.

6

Serologic studies of prenatal infection and schizophrenia

Alan S Brown

INTRODUCTION

Prenatal viral infection is emerging as a potentially important risk factor for schizophrenia. As early as the 1960s, a small number of investigators postulated that infection during the prenatal period may play a role in schizophrenia and other neuropsychiatric disorders.[1,2] Yet this hypothesis was not formally tested until about two decades later, fueled in part by greater attention to the neurodevelopmental hypothesis of schizophrenia,[3] and an increasing number of studies demonstrating an excess of schizophrenia births during the winter and spring.[4,5]

The neurodevelopmental hypothesis of schizophrenia

The neurodevelopmental hypothesis of schizophrenia postulates that a disruption in the programmed process of brain development increases vulnerability to schizophrenia later in life, possibly as a result of interaction with later brain developmental processes in adolescence or adulthood.[6] Evidence supporting this model in schizophrenia includes: childhood neurocognitive, behavioral, and neuromotor disturbances long before onset of the illness;[7–9] increases in minor physical anomalies;[10,11] and gross brain abnormalities in first episode patients,[12] including an increased risk of cavum septum pellucidum, a marker of disrupted development because this brain structure normally fuses *in utero*.[13] The discordance rate of schizophrenia in monozygotic twins is approximately 50%, arguing for the importance of environmental factors in its etiology.

Among these factors, infection is one of the most plausible risk factors for an *in utero* disturbance of brain development. Congenital infections including rubella, herpes simplex virus, and toxoplasmosis have long been known to damage the developing fetal brain, resulting in mental retardation, learning disabilities, congenital seizures, focal areas of calcification, and temporal lobe hypoplasia.[14]

Season of birth

It has now been well documented in several countries, and both hemispheres, that patients with schizophrenia tend to be born in the winter and early spring months, and there is a corresponding deficit in births of future schizophrenic patients in the summer and fall.[4,5] The excess of winter/spring births ranges from 5–15%. Although other factors have been implicated in this finding, infection is one of the most plausible candidates, given the fact that the incidence of many infections fluctuates significantly with season.

Urban birth

Birthrates of future schizophrenic patients also vary with place of birth. Several studies have now demonstrated a 1.5–2-fold increase in risk of schizophrenia among subjects born in cities as compared to rural areas and small towns.[5,15,16] There are, again, several potential candidates, but infection has been postulated as a likely cause because the transmission of infectious organisms occurs at a greater rate in urban compared to rural regions, due to greater crowding and, in the developing world, inadequate sanitation.

Previous studies of prenatal influenza and schizophrenia

Among the infections studied in relation to schizophrenia, most attention has focused on influenza, prompted in large part by the high annual incidence of this infection. Most of these studies were ecologic in nature; that is, influenza exposure was defined based on the dates of epidemics in the populations studied, rather than by evidence of maternal infection in individual pregnancies. Nonetheless, several of these studies yielded intriguing findings, with second trimester exposure to influenza associated with an increased risk of schizophrenia.[17,18] These associations were demonstrated in studies of individual epidemics with high morbidity, especially the 1957 A2 influenza epidemic, and also in studies that examined influenza epidemics over periods of many years.[19] These findings, however, were not replicated by some additional studies, many of which featured improved case ascertainment and larger sample sizes.[20,21] The lack of replication may have been due to inaccurate assessment of influenza infection. In these ecologic studies, it was known that an individual was *in utero* at the time of an influenza epidemic, but not whether the mother of that subject actually contracted influenza during pregnancy. In the few cohort studies conducted on influenza, no associations were found, possibly due to relatively crude assessment of exposure status – maternal reporting of influenza after delivery – and to small sample sizes.[22,23] Thus, the discrepancies between studies may have resulted in part from non-differential misclassification of influenza exposure status, which tends to bias effect sizes toward the null.

Several infectious agents, in addition to influenza, have been investigated as potential risk factors for schizophrenia.[24] These include second trimester respiratory infections other than influenza,[25] polio,[26] and herpes simplex virus.[27] These studies were limited, however, by the lack of serologic evidence that these infections actually occurred during pregnancy.

Therefore, in order definitively to address the question of a relation between prenatal influenza and schizophrenia, it is becoming increasingly apparent that new methods are necessary to document carefully the exposure in individual pregnancies. Among these methods, we initially sought to use prospective clinical documentation of infection in individual pregnancies from well-characterized birth cohorts followed into the age of risk for schizophrenia. Following on from this work, we then initiated a series of studies to improve further upon the documentation of exposure status. This was accomplished by obtaining data on exposure to infection from the analysis of serum samples collected prospectively during pregnancy in these same birth cohorts, and by relating prenatal exposure to infection to the risk of adult schizophrenia.

CLINICALLY DOCUMENTED MATERNAL RESPIRATORY INFECTION AND SCHIZOPHRENIA

In this study, we examined the relationship between maternal exposure to respiratory infections and adult schizophrenia.[25] In the Child Health and Development Study (CHDS), conducted from 1959–1966, 20,000 pregnant women were studied extensively during pregnancy. Comprehensive data were prospectively collected during pregnancy on a wide range of factors, including maternal medical illnesses, prescribed medications during pregnancy, perinatal complications, and neonatal events.

In the Prenatal Determinants of Schizophrenia (PDS) study, we completed a follow-up of the cohort for schizophrenia.[28] For this purpose, we capitalized on a key advantage of the study – the fact that all members of the CHDS were automatically enrolled in the Kaiser Foundation Health Plan (KFHP). This provided a centralized database for all subjects in the CHDS who belonged to KFHP from 1981 on. Using the KFHP database, we ascertained subjects with a history of inpatient or outpatient treatment for psychotic disorders; pharmacy records indicating a history of antipsychotic medication treatment complemented the ascertainment.

Following screening of the medical records on ascertained subjects, we conducted direct research-based interviews with these subjects; chart review diagnoses were obtained on those subjects who could not be located or who declined to be interviewed. This protocol led to the diagnosis of 71 cases of schizophrenia and other schizophrenia spectrum disorders (90% of whom had either schizophrenia or schizoaffective disorder) among the risk set of approximately 12,000 CHDS pregnancies.

Diagnostic data on most medical conditions were carefully abstracted from the charts of the mothers enrolled in KFHP during pregnancy. Most of these diagnoses were made by obstetricians or other physicians, and were based on maternal reports of symptoms and clinical examinations during prenatal visits. Along with the presence or absence of the condition, the calendar date of the condition was obtained. Inspired by previous findings on second trimester exposure to influenza and schizophrenia, we utilized the CHDS data pertaining to maternal respiratory infections. A broad category of maternal respiratory infection was used because the number of cases of clinically diagnosed maternal influenza was insufficient to provide meaningful results. The respiratory infections included: influenza, tuberculosis, bronchopneumonia, atypical pneumonia, pleurisy, empyema, viral respiratory infections, acute bronchitis, and upper respiratory infections. We tested the hypothesis that second trimester exposure to at least one of these infections was associated with an increased risk of schizophrenia.

Consistent with our hypothesis, we found that second trimester exposure to maternal respiratory infection was associated with a significantly increased risk of schizophrenia, adjusting for maternal smoking, education, and race [RR (95% CI) = 2.13 (1.05, 4.35), χ^2 = 4.36, p = .04]. First and third trimester exposure to maternal infection was not related to risk of schizophrenia. When we examined the contributions of individual maternal respiratory infections, we discovered that the overall finding was mostly accounted for by second trimester upper respiratory infection and empyema.

SEROLOGIC STUDIES

Serologic study of prenatal influenza and schizophrenia

In order to investigate the relation between prenatal exposure to influenza and schizophrenia, we have capitalized on an additional, unique resource of the PDS – maternal serum samples drawn during pregnancy. These samples were frozen immediately after the blood draws and have been archived at –20° or below since the time of the draws.

Nearly all of these cases (64 or 90%) had available prenatal serum specimens, from early pregnancy to delivery. Controls who did not have schizophrenia, a schizophrenia spectrum disorder, or a major affective disorder were matched to cases on sex, age, length of Kaiser membership, and availability of maternal sera. The control sample was representative of the source population that gave rise to the cases, due to the continuous follow-up of treated cases and KFHP records indicating precise dates of membership for both cases and controls. This latter feature minimized bias due to loss to follow-up.

These resources permitted a nested case-control design for the investigation of the prenatal influenza hypothesis of schizophrenia, using serologic measures of influenza in individual pregnancies.[29] For this purpose, we conducted influenza assays on the sera from pregnancies giving rise to schizophrenia cases (n = 64) and controls (n = 125) matched 2:1 to cases (a small number of cases had only one available matched control). Sera were assayed from the first, second, and third trimesters. Subjects with an influenza antibody titer ≥20 were considered exposed; subjects with antibody titers <20 were considered unexposed. This titer was selected as it had optimal sensitivity and specificity for the detection of influenza infection.

For influenza exposure in the first trimester, we found that the risk of schizophrenia was increased sevenfold [OR_{MH} = 7.0 (.7, 75.3), χ^2 = 3.00, p = .083]. For influenza exposure during the second trimester, there was no increase in risk of schizophrenia. There was no appreciable change in the findings after adjustment for maternal age, paternal age, maternal socioeconomic status, or maternal ethnicity.

In order to assess more carefully whether the association for the first trimester extended into the second trimester, we examined whether influenza in the first trimester (consisting of the first trimester and first half of the second trimester) was associated with an increased risk of schizophrenia. Subjects exposed to influenza during this period had a threefold increased risk of schizophrenia (OR_{MH} = 3.0, χ^2 = 3.77, p = .052).

Thus, using serologic methods we demonstrated evidence that influenza exposure during early to mid-pregnancy may be a risk factor for the later development of schizophrenia.

Prenatal rubella and schizophrenia

As noted above, prenatal exposure to rubella has long been known to be teratogenic, and this virus has particularly strong effects on the developing nervous system. Sensorineural deafness, mental retardation, learning disabilities, and cerebral palsy are all sequelae of this infection, and are most frequent when exposure occurs early in gestation.[30] In a pioneering study, Stella Chess and colleagues examined the risk of childhood psychiatric disorders in the birth cohort of the Rubella Birth Defects Evaluation Project (RBDEP).[1] This cohort was prenatally exposed to the 1964 rubella epidemic in New York City. A key advantage of this study is that the mothers in the RBDEP were not only clinically documented as having been exposed to rubella during pregnancy, but serologic documentation of infection during pregnancy was made based on IgG-specific antibody or viral isolation.

In this cohort, the researchers found an increased risk of autism, separation anxiety disorder, and impaired social relations in exposed subjects, as compared to prevalence estimates from the population.[1] Based on these findings, we reasoned that prenatal exposure to rubella might result in adult psychiatric disorders, including schizophrenia and other nonaffective psychoses.

Fortunately, this birth cohort had received additional follow-up investigations during adolescence and young adulthood for the purpose of psychiatric, psychologic, and health services research. In a follow-up study conducted in young adulthood (age 21–23) by Patricia Cohen and colleagues, a structured psychiatric interview, the Diagnostic Interview Schedule for Children (DISC), was administered via computer. This interview yielded DSM-III-R diagnoses. Two unexposed samples were used: a cohort in Albany and Saratoga counties in New York State, and the Epidemiologic Catchment Area (ECA) sample. Both of these comparison groups received similar psychiatric interviews. We hypothesized that the risk of non-affective psychosis would be greater in the exposed than in the unexposed group. (The diagnostic category 'non-affective psychosis' was used because this version of the DISC did not allow for specific diagnoses of schizophrenia and schizophrenia spectrum disorders.)

Our findings supported the hypothesis. We found that prenatal rubella exposure was associated with a markedly increased risk of non-affective psychosis.[31] The prevalence of non-affective psychosis was 15.7% (11/70) in the rubella-exposed cohort, compared to 3% (5/164) in the Albany/Saratoga cohort [RR (95% CI) = 5.2 (1.9, 14.3), $p < .001$] and 1% (13/1,346) in the ECA sample [RR (95% CI) = 16.3 (7.6, 35.0), $p < .001$]. The findings were not accounted for by deafness or differences in demographic factors.

This study led us to explore further the relation between prenatal rubella and risk of schizophrenia in this birth cohort.[32] For this purpose, we traced all of the subjects in the RBDEP cohort who had received the previous psychiatric assessment, and administered a more comprehensive and modern psychiatric interview, the Diagnostic Interview for Genetic Studies (DIGS). This permitted a more precise categorization of individual schizophrenia and spectrum disorders. As the subjects had aged 12–14 years since the previous assessment (mean age 34), nearly all of them had passed through the age of risk for schizophrenia at the time of the interview. Our follow-up rate was high: 80% of the targeted subjects were evaluated.

Using this more stringent diagnostic instrument, we found that 20.4% (11/53) of the rubella-exposed subjects met DSM-IV criteria for schizophrenia or another schizophrenia spectrum disorder. The effect was particularly strong when exposure occurred during the first two months of gestation: 11.1% of schizophrenia cases were exposed in the first month of gestation, compared to 4.5% of controls; 44% were exposed in the second gestational month, versus 22.7% of controls. These findings are consistent with an extensive literature on rubella demonstrating that the effects are strongest following first trimester exposure.[30]

The comprehensive database of the RBDEP also permitted us to investigate premorbid antecedents of schizophrenia. This was made possible by the fact that all subjects enrolled in the RBDEP were administered neurocognitive, neuromotor, and behavioral assessments during childhood and adolescence. Based on previous work, we hypothesized that rubella-exposed subjects who developed schizophrenia would have impairments in these functions, compared to subjects who remained free of the disorder.

We first examined neurocognition, which was quantified by assessments of IQ. We found that, in childhood, premorbid IQ was lower in future schizophrenia cases when compared to controls, but this effect did not reach statistical significance. However, during adolescence, the group differences widened substantially. The mean (SD) adolescent IQ for pre-schizophrenic cases was 89.5 (14.8), compared to 104.7 (15.2) in controls. This was explained by a mean 11-point decline in IQ between childhood and adolescence for pre-schizophrenic rubella-exposed cases, compared to a three-point decline in rubella-exposed controls ($p = .03$ for group × time interaction). In a further analysis, we found that 87.5% (7/8) of future schizophrenia cases evidenced an IQ decline, compared to 37% (10/27) of controls ($p = .02$). The IQ decline was clearly premorbid, as it occurred at least several years prior to illness onset.

Rubella-exposed subjects who later developed schizophrenia, as compared to rubella-exposed controls, also manifested increased neuromotor dysfunction, mannerisms, and deviant behaviors. All of the pre-schizophrenia cases, compared to 64% of the controls, had at least one of these premorbid anomalies.

These results extend the findings of previous studies which demonstrated associations between premorbid anomalies and schizophrenia,[7–9,33] in two important ways. First, these data represented the first evidence linking a specific prenatal exposure to premorbid anomalies predictive of later schizophrenia, and to the schizophrenia outcome within the same subjects. Previous studies did not have data available on prenatal insults. Second, in previous work, premorbid data such as IQ were available at only one point in time. Prospective, longitudinal data on premorbid IQ in a birth cohort with a known prenatal exposure provides evidence that a prenatal viral exposure can induce a dynamic pathogenic process long before illness onset, which ultimately becomes expressed in adulthood as schizophrenia.

Study of maternal cytokines and schizophrenia

As mentioned above, the associations between prenatal infection and schizophrenia may be explained by increases in maternal cytokines, which become activated by a broad array of infections. Cytokines represent a family of soluble, polypeptide proteins, which act as systemic mediators of the host response to infection.[34] Adverse reproductive outcomes have been linked to infection-induced cytokine elevations.[35] Based in part on this work, and on the epidemiologic findings reviewed above, Gilmore and Jarskog hypothesized that infection-induced cytokines may explain associations between *in utero* infection and schizophrenia.[36]

We aimed to determine, in the PDS cohort, whether maternal levels of four cytokines that are plausible candidates for schizophrenia – interleukin-8 (IL-8), interleukin-1-beta (IL-1β), interleukin-6 (IL-6), and tumor necrosis factor-alpha (TNF-α) – are increased in patients who developed schizophrenia.[37] We hypothesized that second trimester levels of these maternal cytokines would be increased in pregnancies giving rise to schizophrenia offspring, as compared to matched control offspring. Second trimester prenatal sera were analyzed for cytokines using the sandwich enzyme-linked immunosorbent assay (SELISA), acquired from BD Pharmingen (San Diego, CA).

We found a marked and significant increase in the mean level of serum IL-8 in the mothers of schizophrenia cases, as compared to mothers of controls ($\chi^2 = 5.41$, $p = .02$). We found no significant differences between cases and controls for IL-1-β, IL-6, or TNF-α. Adjustment for maternal ethnicity, education, and smoking did not have any appreciable effect on the results.

PATHOGENIC MECHANISMS

With regard to *in utero* exposure to rubella, it has been well documented that this virus crosses the placenta and enters the fetal brain.[38] Damage to the fetal central nervous system is believed to occur principally through two mechanisms, each of which may explain the IQ decline and the increased risk of schizophrenia. First, rubella inhibits mitosis, leading to diminished neurons and overall brain growth,[39,40] and to reduced replication of oligodendrocytes, with a subsequent deficit of myelin.[41] Second, *in utero* rubella causes a pro-inflammatory response, with production of cytokines and other immune-mediating molecules. This results in damage to the developing fetal cerebrovascular system, specifically to the endothelium, and deposits of granular material in the pericapillary area.[40,42] Consequently, ischemic damage occurs. It is also possible that other mechanisms that occur concurrent with rubella infection could play an etiologic role; for example, maternal fever, or possibly an autoimmune response could lead to fetal brain damage, theoretically predisposing to schizophrenia.[43]

The fact that the greatest risk of schizophrenia occurred following rubella exposure during the first two months of gestation is especially supportive of its biological plausibility. It has been well documented that vulnerability to teratogenic events is highest following exposure to rubella during the first trimester. This finding may also further delineate the period of brain development that is most relevant to the pathogenesis of schizophrenia. This interval consists of early embryogenic events, including cleavage and implantation, neural tube development and closure, and extensive formation of brain regions implicated in schizophrenia, such as the hippocampus, amygdala, thalamus, and cortical plate.[44]

With regard to influenza, animal models indicate that the offspring of mice infected with influenza at day nine of gestation have significantly decreased Reelin-positive Cajal-Retzius cells in the cortex and hippocampus.[45] In addition, several physiologic and pharmacologic abnormalities analogous to those found in schizophrenia have been demonstrated in mice that were prenatally exposed to influenza.[46]

Both maternal exposure to influenza and maternal respiratory infections may theoretically increase vulnerability to schizophrenia through several mechanisms. The fact that more than one infection may increase the risk of this disorder suggests the possible contribution of nonspecific factors, such as hyperthermia, which is known to cause neural tube defects in animal studies.[14] A second possibility is over-the-counter or prescribed cold or flu remedies, which may have teratogenic effects.[14]

An additional potential mechanism by which prenatal exposure to various infectious agents might increase risk of schizophrenia is through the production of pro-inflammatory cytokines, such as IL-8, which was observed to be increased during the second trimester of pre-schizophrenia cases in our study. Increased maternal IL-8 is a plausible risk factor for schizophrenia. In a previous study, maternal serum levels of IL-8 were associated with histologic chorioamnionitis among infants born at term.[35] IL-8, a chemokine,[47,48] is especially important for neutrophil attraction and activation.[47,49,50] These properties are probably important in the response of the host to pathogens.

However, our finding on IL-8 might also be explained by a non-infectious, inflammatory insult, which can elevate IL-8 levels,[51] or by reactive oxygen intermediates following tissue injury, which increase IL-8.[52]

It is worth emphasizing that these potential explanations remain speculative. Nonetheless, they do suggest future avenues of exploration (see next section).

IMPLICATIONS FOR PREVENTION AND FUTURE RESEARCH

Our findings have provided further evidence of a role for prenatal infection and inflammation in the etiology of schizophrenia. In particular, the use of serologic methods, and prospective research designs in well-characterized birth cohorts, have enabled us more definitively to document these insults in individual pregnancies, and relate them to risk of schizophrenia in the offspring. Nonetheless, these findings should be considered tentative, and will require independent replication in other cohorts before the results can be applied to clinical practice. It is not too early, however, to speculate on the implications of this work and to consider directions for future research in this area.

With regard to influenza, our results suggest that the prevention of this infection, especially in women of reproductive age, may be an effective strategy for reducing the risk of schizophrenia. However, the incorporation of these strategies to obstetric practice will require replication of the finding in independent samples.

The implications of our research on rubella are similar to those for influenza. However, in contrast to influenza, rubella vaccination is routinely administered to young children in the developed world. This has led to a dramatic reduction in the incidence of rubella in these countries. Thus, if our findings on rubella are confirmed, it is possible that this public health measure may have already prevented a sizable number of schizophrenia cases. Recent concerns that the measles/mumps/rubella vaccine could induce autism, as yet unfounded,[53] have thwarted efforts to vaccinate a substantial number of children in certain countries, with the potential threat of a recurrence of rubella. An additional problem is that immunization for rubella and other viruses is not routinely conducted in the developing world. It is our hope that studies examining previously unrecognized sequelae of rubella may facilitate further efforts by public health agencies and governments to implement vaccination programs aimed at primary prevention of this viral infection.

Our finding on IL-8 indicates that excessive activation of part of the maternal immune response may play a role in schizophrenia. Numerous factors, including many infectious agents, and non-infectious inflammatory insults, can cause increases in IL-8 during pregnancy. Genetic variation may also cause increased maternal IL-8, or genetic transmission of a functional IL-8 variant to the fetus may lead to a constitutional elevation of this cytokine, which can disrupt brain development and function throughout the lifespan. As reviewed elsewhere, increases in cytokines in adult patients have been demonstrated in many previous studies.[54] Studies of cytokine levels in the patients in our birth cohorts may allow us to test this hypothesis.

Developmental animal models

The use of developmental animal models is proving to be a promising strategy for validating the plausibility of the epidemiologic findings on prenatal risk factors for schizophrenia, and suggesting potential causal mechanisms. One key limitation of most developmental animal models, however, is that they generally do not involve the types of insults that are encountered in human experience, which restricts their generalizability. As discussed above, however, some recent animal models are attempting to utilize exposures shown to be relevant to schizophrenia in epidemiologic studies. Among other possibilities, these studies have the potential to uncover the pathogenic process by which these exposures lead to the illness, and possibly reveal new targets for pharmaceutical agents. Furthermore, this work may also lead to the identification of new risk factors or biological processes that can be further investigated in epidemiologic or other clinical studies of schizophrenia, helping to realize the potential of translational research.

Neuroimaging investigation

In order to understand better the brain regions and functions of relevance to schizophrenia that are adversely affected by *in utero* exposure to infection and cytokine elevations, we are currently conducting structural and functional neuroimaging investigations in our birth cohorts. Neuroimaging investigations conducted to date have transformed our understanding of schizophrenia. Nonetheless, etiologic heterogeneity of schizophrenia may be responsible for the marked overlap between case and control groups with regard to regional brain volumes and activation of specific brain areas. The use of subjects with homogeneous exposures of potential relevance to the etiology of schizophrenia may facilitate the isolation of specific brain regions and functions that are responsible for the syndrome of schizophrenia. Combined with animal studies, this work may also help to reveal pathogenic mechanisms that lead to the disorder.

Gene–environment interaction

As evidenced by family, twin, and adoption studies and, more recently, association and linkage studies, susceptibility genes clearly play an important role in the etiology of schizophrenia. In addition, most subjects with prenatal infection do not develop schizophrenia later in life. This indicates that if *in utero* infection plays a role in the development of schizophrenia, then it probably does so by interacting with other factors, including susceptibility genes. Therefore, studies of gene–environment interaction are warranted in future work on prenatal infectious insults and schizophrenia. The remarkable progress on the mapping of the human genome promises to shed further light on such interactions.

It seems reasonable to speculate on the types of predisposing gene that may interact with prenatal infection. One may first consider investigating genes that are being identified as increasing vulnerability for schizophrenia. It is likely that many, if not most, of these genes are not involved in infectious or inflammatory processes. Rather, they may act additively with environmental insults, including prenatal infection, to increase liability to schizophrenia. Although not strictly a gene–environment interaction, this type of model is included under this model.

A second model worth considering is the role genes may play in the causal pathway from acquiring an infection to its effects on fetal brain development. For example, certain HLA haplotypes may predispose to influenza, or result in an excessive or inappropriate inflammatory response, which leads to prenatal brain damage.

An additional mechanism worth considering with regard to gene–environment interaction is epigenetic regulation. It has been well documented that certain environmental factors exert their deleterious effects by affecting gene expression. This can occur, for example, through DNA methylation and histone modifications.[55] Conceivably, influenza or other infectious agents may increase risk for schizophrenia by perturbing the expression of susceptibility genes for schizophrenia.

Irrespective of the model or mechanism by which genetic and environmental factors interact, it is worth noting that genes may also serve a protective function. For example, genes that prevent loss of Reelin may provide resilience to an individual who is exposed *in utero* to influenza, and genes that facilitate synaptic plasticity may help to reverse a latent brain lesion induced by a viral infection.

CONCLUSION

Serologic documentation of infection during pregnancy in prospectively followed subjects from well-characterized birth cohorts has permitted a more definitive test of the hypothesis that prenatal infection plays a role in the etiology of schizophrenia. Thus far, such studies have indicated that *in utero* exposure to viral infections, including influenza, other respiratory infections, and rubella, and elevated second trimester levels of the cytokine interleukin-8, are associated with an increased risk of schizophrenia in adult offspring. Although substantial work remains, these findings hold promise for the prevention of schizophrenia. Furthermore, studies of animal models, neuroimaging, and gene–environment interactions have the potential to elucidate the role that *in utero* infection might play in the pathogenesis of schizophrenia.

REFERENCES

1. Chess S, Korn S, Fernandez P. *Psychiatric Disorders of Children with Congenital Rubella*. New York: Brunner/Mazel.
2. Torrey EF. Stalking the schizovirus. *Schizophr Bull* 1988; **14**: 223–9.
3. Murray RM, Lewis SW. Is schizophrenia a neurodevelopmental disorder? *Br Med J (Clin Res Ed)* 1987; **295**: 681–2.
4. Bradbury TN, Miller GA. Season of birth in schizophrenia: a review of evidence, methodology, and etiology. *Psychol Bull* 1985; **98**: 569–94.
5. Mortensen PB, Pedersen CB, Westergaard T et al. Effects of family history and place and season of birth on the risk of schizophrenia. *N Engl J Med* 1999; **340**: 603–8.
6. Weinberger DR. Implications of normal brain development for the pathogenesis of schizophrenia. *Arch Gen Psychiatry* 1987; **44**: 660–9.
7. Done DJ, Crow TJ, Johnstone EC, Sacker A. Childhood antecedents of schizophrenia and affective illness: social adjustment at ages 7 and 11. *Br Med J* 1994; **309**: 699–703.
8. Jones P, Rodgers B, Murray R, Marmot M. Child development risk factors for adult schizophrenia in the British 1946 birth cohort. *Lancet* 1994; **344**: 1398–402.
9. Walker EF, Savoie T, Davis D. Neuromotor precursors of schizophrenia. *Schizophr Bull* 1994; **20**: 441–51.
10. McGrath J, El Saadi O, Grim V et al. Minor physical anomalies and quantitative measures of the head and face in patients with psychosis. *Arch Gen Psychiatry* 2002; **59**: 458–64.
11. O'Callaghan E, Buckley P, Madigan C et al. The relationship of minor physical anomalies and other putative indices of developmental disturbance in schizophrenia to abnormalities of cerebral structure on magnetic resonance imaging. *Biol Psychiatry* 1995; **38**: 516–24.

12. Bogerts B, Ashtari M, Degreef G et al. Reduced temporal limbic structure volumes on magnetic resonance images in first episode schizophrenia. *Psychiatry Res* 1990; **35**: 1–13.
13. Nopoulos P, Swayze V, Flaum M et al. Cavum septi pellucidi in normals and patients with schizophrenia as detected by magnetic resonance imaging. *Biol Psychiatry* 1997; **41**: 1102–8.
14. Brown AS, Susser E. Plausibility of prenatal rubella, influenza, and other viral infections as risk factors for schizophrenia. In: *Prenatal Exposures in Schizophrenia* (Susser E, Brown AS, Gorman JM, eds). Washington DC: American Psychiatric Press Inc, 1999: 113–34.
15. Lewis G, David A, Andreasson S, Allebeck P. Schizophrenia and city life. *Lancet* 1992; **340**: 137–40.
16. Van Os J, Selten JP. Prenatal exposure to maternal stress and subsequent schizophrenia. The May 1940 invasion of the Netherlands. *Br J Psychiatry* 1998; **172**: 324–6.
17. Bagalkote H, Pang D, Jones PB. Maternal influenza and schizophrenia. *Int J Ment Health* 2001; **29**: 3–21.
18. Mednick SA, Machon RA, Huttunen MO, Bonett D. Adult schizophrenia following prenatal exposure to an influenza epidemic. *Arch Gen Psychiatry* 1988; **45**: 189–92.
19. Barr CE, Mednick SA, Munk-Jorgensen P. Exposure to influenza epidemics during gestation and adult schizophrenia. A 40-year study. *Arch Gen Psychiatry* 1990; **47**: 869–74.
20. Erlenmeyer-Kimling L, Folnegovic Z, Hrabak-Zerjavic V et al. Schizophrenia and prenatal exposure to the 1957 A2 influenza epidemic in Croatia. *Am J Psychiatry* 1994; **151**: 1496–8.
21. Susser E, Lin SP, Brown AS et al. No relation between risk of schizophrenia and prenatal exposure to influenza in Holland. *Am J Psychiatry* 1994; **151**: 922–4.
22. Cannon M, Cotter D, Coffey VP et al. Prenatal exposure to the 1957 influenza epidemic and adult schizophrenia: a follow-up study. *Br J Psychiatry* 1996; **168**: 368–71.
23. Crow TJ, Done DJ. Schizophrenia and influenza. *Lancet* 1991; **338**: 116–7.
24. Brown AS. Prenatal infection and adult schizophrenia: a review and synthesis. *Int J Ment Health* 2001; **29**: 22–37.
25. Brown AS, Schaefer CA, Wyatt RJ et al. Maternal exposure to respiratory infections and adult schizophrenia spectrum disorders: a prospective birth cohort study. *Schizophr Bull* 2000; **26**: 287–95.
26. Suvisaari J, Haukka J, Tanskanen A et al. Association between prenatal exposure to poliovirus infection and adult schizophrenia. *Am J Psychiatry* 1999; **156**: 1100–2.
27. Buka SL, Tsuang MT, Torrey EF et al. Maternal infections and subsequent psychosis among offspring. *Arch Gen Psychiatry* 2001; **58**: 1032–1.
28. Susser ES, Schaefer CA, Brown AS et al. The design of the prenatal determinants of schizophrenia study. *Schizophr Bull* 2000; **26**: 257–73.
29. Brown AS, Begg MD, Gravenstein S et al. Serologic evidence of prenatal influenza in the etiology of schizophrenia. *Arch Gen Psychiatry* 2004; **61**: 774–80.
30. South MA, Sever JL. Teratogen update: the congenital rubella syndrome. *Teratology* 1985; **31**: 297–307.
31. Brown AS, Cohen P, Greenwald S, Susser E. Nonaffective psychosis after prenatal exposure to rubella. *Am J Psychiatry* 2000; **157**: 438–43.
32. Brown AS, Cohen P, Harkavy-Friedman J et al. AE Bennett Research Award. Prenatal rubella, premorbid abnormalities, and adult schizophrenia. *Biol Psychiatry* 2001; **49**: 473–86.
33. Erlenmeyer-Kimling L, Rock D, Squires-Wheeler E et al. Early life precursors of psychiatric outcomes in adulthood in subjects at risk for schizophrenia or affective disorders. *Psychiatry Res* 1991; **39**: 239–56.
34. Weizman R, Bessler H. Cytokines: stress and immunity. In: *Cytokines: Stress and Immunity* (Plotnikoff NP, Faith RE, Murgo AJ, Good RA, eds). Boca Raton FL: CRC Press, 1999: 1–15.
35. Shimoya K, Matsuzaki N, Taniguchi T et al. Interleukin-8 level in maternal serum as a marker for screening of histological chorioamnionitis at term. *Int J Gynaecol Obstet* 1997; **57**: 153–9.
36. Gilmore JH, Jarskog LF. Exposure to infection and brain development: cytokines in the pathogenesis of schizophrenia. *Schizophr Res* 1997; **24**: 365–7.
37. Babulas V, Brown AS, Hooton J et al. Elevated maternal interleukin-8 levels and risk of schizophrenia in adult offspring. *Am J Psychiatry* 2004; **161**: 889–95.
38. Whitley RJ, Stagno S. Perinatal infections. In: *Infections of the Central Nervous System* (2nd ed, Scheld WM, Whitley RJ, Durack DT, eds). New York: Lippincott-Raven Press, 1997: 223–53.
39. Boue JG, Boue A. Effects of rubella virus infection on the division of human cells. *Am J Dis Child* 1969; **118**: 45–8.
40. Rorke LB. Nervous system lesions in the congenital rubella syndrome. *Arch Otolaryngol* 1973; **98**: 249–51.
41. Kemper TL, Lecours AR, Gates MJ, Yakovlev PI. Retardation of the myelo- and cytoarchitectonic maturation of the brain in the congenital rubella syndrome. *Res Publ Assoc Res Nerv Ment Dis* 1973; **51**: 23–62.
42. Townsend JJ. Rubella virus disease. In: *Handbook of Neurovirology* (McKendall RR, Stropp WG, eds). New York: Marcel Dekker, 1994: 603–11.
43. Clarke WL, Shaver KA, Bright GM et al. Autoimmunity in congenital rubella syndrome. *J Pediatr* 1984; **104**: 370–3.
44. O'Rahilly R, Muller F. Minireview: summary of the initial development of the human nervous system. *Teratology* 1999; **60**: 39–41.
45. Fatemi SH, Emamian ES, Kist D et al. Defective corticogenesis and reduction in Reelin immunoreactivity in cortex and hippocampus of prenatally infected neonatal mice. *Mol Psychiatry* 1999; **4**: 145–54.
46. Shi L, Fatemi SH, Sidwell RW, Patterson PH. Maternal influenza infection causes marked behavioral and pharmacological changes in the offspring. *J Neurosci* 2003; **23**: 297–302.
47. Atta UR, Harvey K, Siddiqui RA. Interleukin-8: an autocrine inflammatory mediator. *Curr Pharm Des* 1999; **5**: 241–53.
48. Mukaida N. The roles of cytokine receptors in diseases. *Rinsho Byori* 2000; **48**: 409–15.
49. Detmers PA, Lo SK, Olsen-Egbert E et al. Neutrophil-activating protein 1/interleukin 8 stimulates the binding activity of the leukocyte adhesion receptor CD11b/CD18 on human neutrophils. *J Exp Med* 1990; **171**: 1155–62.
50. Huber AR, Kunkel SL, Todd RF III, Weiss SJ. Regulation of transendothelial neutrophil migration by endogenous interleukin-8. *Science* 1991; **254**: 99–102.
51. Taub DD, Oppenheim JJ. Chemokines, inflammation and the immune system. *Ther Immunol* 1994; **1**: 229–46.
52. DeForge LE, Fantone JC, Kenney JS, Remick DG. Oxygen radical scavengers selectively inhibit interleukin-8 production in human whole blood. *J Clin Invest* 1992; **90**: 2123–9.
53. Madsen KM, Hviid A, Vestergaard M et al. A population-based study of measles, mumps, and rubella vaccination and autism. *N Engl J Med* 2002; **347**: 1477–82.
54. Gaughran F. Immunity and schizophrenia: autoimmunity, cytokines, and immune responses. *Int Rev Neurobiol* 2002; **52**: 275–302.
55. Jaenisch R, Bird A. Epigenetic regulation of gene expression: how the genome integrates intrinsic and environmental signals. *Nature Genetics* 2003; **33**: 245–54.

7

Neurosyphilis, HIV, and psychosis

Christian G Kohler and Courtney Johnson

EPIDEMIOLOGY OF SYPHILIS AND HIV

Syphilis

Globally, the World Health Organization reported 12 million new cases of syphilis among adults in 1999.[1] Southeast Asia and sub-Saharan Africa reported 4 million new cases each, Latin America and the Caribbean 3 million cases. North America, Western Europe, North Africa and the Middle East, Eastern Europe and Central Asia, and the East Asia and Pacific regions all reported between 100,000 and 370,000 new cases of syphilis. The lowest incidence was seen in Australia and New Zealand – only 10,000 new cases of syphilis.

While primary and secondary syphilis rates have greatly decreased over the past 15 years in the United States and Western Europe, there has been a striking increase in Eastern Europe. In the USA, by 2000 the rate of primary and secondary syphilis had reached its lowest point since 1941 at a rate of 2.1 per 100,000. However in 2001, a total of 6,103 cases (~2/3 in men) were reported, a 2.1% increase from the 2000 low.[2–5] Further breakdown revealed that the increase was due to a 15.4% increase in males, in particular men who have sex with men (MSM). In females, primary and secondary syphilis rates decreased by 17.7% from 2000 to 2001. Among females, the highest incidence of syphilis was in the 20–24 year age group while in males, syphilis peaked in the 35–39 year age group. In 2001, 62% of all primary and secondary syphilis cases were found in non-Hispanic blacks (a decrease from 70% in 2000). Non-Hispanics, the second largest group, accounted for 23% of total cases. By region, the South showed the highest rates of primary and secondary syphilis at 3.4 per 100,000 followed by the Midwest, the West and the Northeast (1.1 per 100,000).[2–5]

Neurosyphilis

Due to effective screening programs and early treatment with antibiotics, progression of primary and secondary syphilis to neurosyphilis is rare. However, if left untreated, 5% of individuals with syphilis will develop symptomatic neurosyphilis. Despite mandatory public health department reporting to the Centers for Disease Control (CDC), very little detailed information is available regarding the incidence of neurosyphilis. According to the CDC 2000 report, a total of 334 cases of neurosyphilis were reported with a male to female ratio of 2.5:1.[3]

Syphilis transmission

Known routes of syphilis infection are venereal transmission, blood transfusion, perinatal transmission, and intrauterine infection. Venereal transmission is by far the most common; there is a 30% chance of contracting the disease from sexual intercourse with an individual infected with early or primary syphilis.[2–5] Sexual transmission occurs when mucocutaneous syphilitic lesions are present, which are uncommon after the first year of infection.

Nontreponemal antibody tests such as the rapid plasma reagin (RPR) and Venereal Disease Research Laboratory (VDRL) tests are aimed at detection of antibody-like substances in serum and cerebrospinal fluid (CSF). These tests are used to screen for active syphilis, and monitor successful treatment and recurrence. Nontreponemal antibody tests have a false positive rate of 20–40%, typically at low titers of 1:8 or less. Titers fall and may become nonreactive after successful treatment, and also during the later stages of untreated syphilis (particularly in the CSF). Treponemal antibody tests, such as the microhemagglutination-*Treponema pallidum* (MHA-TP) or fluorescent treponemal antibody absorption (FTA-ABS) tests, are highly specific for detection of immunoglobulins directed against *Treponema pallidum*. These tests are used to confirm the presence of active syphilis; however, they remain positive after successful treatment.

HIV/AIDS

In December 2002, the United Nations AIDS Programme (UNAIDS) and the World Health Organization (WHO) estimated that there are 42 million people living with HIV/AIDS worldwide.[6] It is estimated that 5 million people were newly infected with HIV and 3.1 million people died from AIDS in 2002. Sub-Saharan Africa reported the largest incidence with 29.4 million cases of HIV/AIDS, 58% occurring in women. South and Southeast Asia accounted for 6 million cases with 36% occurring in women. Other regions reporting over 1 million cases included East Asia and Pacific, Latin America, Eastern Europe, and Central Asia. North America, Western Europe, and Australia and New Zealand estimated rates below 1 million each with the majority being MSM and injecting drug users (IDU).

In the USA, there were 816,149 AIDS cases and 467,910 AIDS deaths reported to the CDC as of December 2001. Males account for the majority of AIDS cases with 666,026 (82%). Over half of all the people living with HIV, including 70% of the men living with HIV, are MSMs, followed by IDUs at 31%. Of the total cases, 6% can be attributed to MSMs who inject drugs. Other exposure categories include heterosexual contact, blood transfusions, and hemophilia/coagulation disorders. Approximately 42% of AIDS cases reported to the CDC are white and non-Hispanic individuals, 38% are black (non-Hispanic), and 18% are Hispanic. Asian/Pacific Islanders and American Indian/Alaska Natives each accounted for less than 1% of the total.

HIV infection and transmission

HIV infection is diagnosed by tests for antibodies against HIV-1 and HIV-2 (HIV-1/2). HIV antibodies are present in at least 95% of patients within three months of infection. Although a negative antibody test result usually indicates that a person is not infected, negative antibody tests cannot exclude recent infection.

Most HIV infections in the USA are caused by HIV-1 and very few cases of HIV-2 infection have been documented. However, HIV-2 infection, which is endemic in West Africa, should be suspected in persons who have epidemiologic risk factors for HIV-2.

The CDC has outlined the modes of transmission for HIV as including blood, semen, vaginal fluid, breast milk, and other bodily fluids that contain blood. Healthcare workers may be at additional risk for HIV exposure in CSF, synovial fluid, and amniotic fluid. The most common modes of transmission are sexual contact and infected needles; only in rare cases has blood from a transfusion screened for HIV antibodies transmitted the virus. It is also possible for infected mothers to transmit the virus to their child during birth or breastfeeding.

Comorbid syphilis and HIV

Currently there are no national reporting mechanisms that capture the comorbidity of syphilis and HIV. However, individuals with syphilis appear to be at increased risk for HIV and vice versa. A recent literature review reported a median HIV seroprevalence of 15.7% in individuals infected with syphilis.[7] The median co-infection rate was 27.5% in males and 12.4% in females. In the MSM and IDU groups, co-infection rates ranged from 64–90% and 22–71% respectively. Conversely, researchers have reported FTA reactivity in 40.5% of HIV(+) and in 18.8% of HIV(–) persons, and neurosyphilis in approximately 1.5% of HIV(+) persons.[8] According to CDC data, genital ulcers caused by syphilis facilitate transmission of HIV with a two- to fivefold fold increased risk of aquiring HIV. The precise interaction between syphilis and HIV is still not fully understood, particularly at the level of the CNS. HIV positivity may be associated with delayed seroconversion and seronegative syphilis, and, due to impaired immune status, can lead to more rapid progression to neurosyphilis. In addition, individuals who are co-infected with syphilis and HIV may be more likely to fail treatment even after an initial response,[9] especially if treatment begins in the secondary stage of syphilis.

DEFINITION OF PSYCHOSIS

According to the glossary of the American Psychiatric Association, psychosis is defined as gross impairment in reality testing and characterized by hallucinations, delusions, and disorganized thinking or behavior, including some forms of aggression. Symptoms of psychosis occur in the setting of clear consciousness; if consciousness is disturbed, then the psychotic symptoms are better explained by a state of delirium. Common causes of delirium include medical conditions associated with hypoxia or metabolic disturbances, drug intoxication or withdrawal, or iatrogenic medication use. In delirium, psychotic symptoms – in particular delusions – present as fragmented and unsystematized, and are associated with impaired ability to maintain attention. Similarly, the quality of hallucinations differs in psychotic disorders and delirium. Whereas auditory hallucinations are common and visual hallucinations are rare in psychotic disorders such as schizophrenia, visual hallucinations are characteristic of delirious states. Psychotic symptoms occur in idiopathic psychiatric disorders, most commonly schizophrenia and mood disorders. Psychotic symptoms without evidence of delirium may be present in: neurological disorders such as brain tumors or vascular malformations, epilepsy, and traumatic brain injury; drugs of abuse and certain medications; autoimmune disorders, such as systemic lupus erythematodus; hypo- and hyperthyroidism; and infections – most commonly HIV and syphilis.

GENERAL CNS SYMPTOMS OF SYPHILIS

Syphilis via the pathogenic organism *Treponema pallidum* and resultant immune response has the propensity to affect almost any organ in the human body and to produce a great diversity of clinical manifestations. Neurosyphilis, specifically general paresis or dementia paralytica, was first described in the late 19th century and recognized as a common cause of dementia and psychosis. In 1913 Noguchi and Moore showed that general paresis was caused by spirochetal infection of the brain.[10] Following the detection of penicillin for treatment of all stages of syphilis in the 1940s, there was a dramatic decline in the incidence and prevalence of neurosyphilis. It has been estimated that in most cases neurosyphilis can be arrested, producing partial or complete remission of functional impairment. Between 1942 and 1965 the incidence of neurosyphilis as a cause of first admissions to psychiatric hospitals fell from 5.9/100,000 population to 0.1/100,000 and new cases became so rare that many hospitals discarded routine screening for syphilis.[11]

It is estimated that asymptomatic neurosyphilis will occur in 20–30% of untreated syphilis within two years following primary infection. Within 10 years, about one-third of patients with asymptomatic neurosyphilis will progress to symptomatic meningeal, meningovascular, or parenchymatous neurosyphilis. These different forms of neurosyphilis may occur as distinct forms but frequently overlap with other types. While meningeal and meningovascuclar syphilis present within several years after the primary genital lesion, parenchymatous neurosyphilis is typically seen more than 10 years after primary infection and may present as tabes dorsalis which involves the spinal cord and brain stem, general paresis which involves the brain, or taboparesis – a combination of both. Tabes dorsalis produces selective degeneration of the posterior columns and posterior roots of the spinal cord. Cognitive dysfunction – often to the extent of dementia – represents the hallmark of general paresis. Other common features include behavioral changes, dysarthria, optic atrophy and Argyll Robertson pupils. Untreated general paresis progresses to death within five to 10 years.

Neuroradiological findings in neurosyphilis include nonspecific brain atrophy,[12,13] white matter changes,[13] and findings more specific to neurosyphilis such as vasculitis[14,15] and syphilitic granuloma (gumma).[16–18] Neuroradiological studies have suggested that the site of brain lesions in neurosyphilis will determine the nature of behavioral symptoms. In 20 patients with newly diagnosed neurosyphilis who underwent magnetic resonance imaging (MRI) studies of the brain, psychiatric symptoms, particularly emotional withdrawal, motor slowing, and conceptual disorganization, were associated with frontal atrophy and white matter changes.[13] In the same group cognitive impairment was associated with temporoparietal brain changes.

Diagnosis of active neurosyphilis is made on account of clinical symptoms, untreated syphilis by history, and reactive nontreponemal and treponemal antibody tests.

GENERAL CNS SYMPTOMS OF HIV

Central and peripheral nervous systems of HIV-infected patients are rarely unaffected through the course of untreated disease. HIV may affect the brain as a direct consequence of the virus, transmigration of activated monocytes into the brain,[19] or via HIV-related disorders. Although less common than in the late stages of HIV infection, the nervous system may be affected as early as the stage of primary infection and seroconversion. Case reports have described examples of focal or diffuse encephalopathy, ataxia, myelopathy, and meningitis presenting within the context of HIV seroconversion. A number of HIV-related processes may lead to brain involvement in the late phase of HIV infection, including opportunistic infections and neoplasms, aseptic meningitis, AIDS dementia complex, metabolic and vascular complications of systemic disease, and toxic reactions to antiretroviral drugs.

PSYCHOSIS IN SYPHILIS

In the early part of the 20th century, psychiatric manifestations of neurosyphilis were common and accounted for 5–15% of first admissions to mental hospitals.[20] In 1935, Cheney described a large cohort of almost 4,000 patients with 'general paresis of the insane' and reported on the presence of mania (24%), schizophrenia (19%), and depression (10%).[21] Following the detection of penicillin for treatment of all stages of syphilis in the 1940s, there was a dramatic decline in the incidence and prevalence of neurosyphilis. While cognitive dysfunction – often to the extent of dementia – represents the hallmark of general paresis, behavioral changes occur in the majority of patients. Such behavioral changes include mania in up to half of people affected; less commonly seen are psychosis and depression. Several more recent reports of behavior changes in the setting of general paresis were limited to case reports and described patients with longstanding behavior changes,[22,23] probably unrelated mental illness preceding the diagnosis of neurosyphilis,[24] or patients with a past history of syphilis and more recent behavior changes.[25–27] A single case report in a middle-aged man described new onset of psychotic symptoms without evidence of active syphilis within six months of diagnosis and treatment of neurosyphilis.[28] Other reports of new onset neurosyphilis and behavioral changes described cognitive dysfunction in combination with manic and psychotic symptoms.[29–31]

In a recent case report, we described new onset psychosis in a 30-year-old, 20-week-pregnant woman without significant prior medical or psychiatric history, who experienced sudden onset of auditory hallucinations, delusions, and unstable mood over a period of two weeks.[32] Physical examination appeared unremarkable except for pregnancy and neurological abnormalities were limited to mild gait instability and apraxia. Mental status examination was remarkable for disorganized thinking and giddy affect. Routine lab studies were unremarkable, except for positive RPR (1:32) and positive MHA-TP. CSF evaluation revealed lymphocytic pleocytosis (81/ml), increased protein (97 mg/dl), and positive VDRL. Neuropsychological testing revealed marked cognitive dysfunction on measures of attention, initiation/perseveration, construction, and conceptualization. Immediately, the patient was begun on penicillin G 2.4 million units intravenously every four hours for 14 days, as recommended for the treatment of neurosyphilis. The clinical picture was consistent with general paresis, which responded to antibiotic and temporary antipsychotic treatment, producing remission of both psychosis and cognitive dysfunction.

PSYCHOSIS IN HIV INFECTION

After the initial discovery of AIDS, reports quickly emerged describing increased prevalence of anxiety and depression in persons who are HIV positive and persons with AIDS. Homosexual HIV negative men were described as being at increased risk for psychiatric disorders, in particular depression and anxiety.[33] However another study reported psychiatric disorders in homosexual men to be irrespective of HIV status and associated with previous and current lifestyle.[34] More recently, increased symptoms of anxiety and depression were found in HIV positive persons without AIDS, compared to HIV positive, but asymptomatic, and HIV negative persons.[35] This increase was unrelated to past psychiatric history and correlated with findings on quantitative EEG. The authors concluded that early brain changes, preceding the immunological and cognitive impairment of AIDS, may cause these neuropsychiatric symptoms.

Similarly, descriptions of psychosis associated with HIV infection emerged several years after recognition of the disease. Early on a distinction was made between psychogenic or reactive psychosis, thought to be a person's emotional reaction after being diagnosed with a potentially lethal disorder, and specific AIDS psychosis, thought to be a direct result of HIV effects on the brain. By the late 1980s case series reported on symptoms ranging from isolated hallucinations to catatonia in persons newly diagnosed with HIV with or without cognitive dysfunction.[36,37]

The frequency of new onset psychosis in HIV positive persons has been reported to range between .2% and 15% and may increase with progression of illness, as the highest prevalence was found in persons with AIDS.[38] Causes of psychosis in HIV positive persons include: direct viral effects on the brain; secondary infections, such as cyptococcus, herpes, and toxoplasmosis; antiretroviral drugs; recreational drugs; reactive psychotic reaction associated with the new diagnosis; and exacerbation of previous psychotic or mood disorder. Estimated frequency of HIV infection in patients with pre-existing mental illness ranges from 5–7%.[39]

Psychosis in HIV patients appears to be a poor prognosticator. Psychosis has been found to be more common in persons with AIDS than in persons who are HIV(+) without AIDS.[40] In addition, the same study found manic symptoms in almost one-third of AIDS patients being associated with more rapid disease progression and death in almost 25% of cases.[40] Following the course of psychosis in four patients, El-Mallakh proposed a window of vulnerability for psychosis in persons with HIV infection as occurring in the setting of mild to moderate brain damage from HIV.[41] Once brain damage progresses, symptoms of dementia may replace psychotic symptoms. In a comparison of 20 patients with HIV and related psychosis to 20 patients with HIV but no psychosis, delusions, followed by auditory then visual hallucinations were the most common psychotic symptoms.[42] Cognitive dysfunction was more common in the psychosis group. There were no differences with respect to MRI and CSF findings amongst the groups. Mean follow-up was 29 months, during which 11 of 20 psychotic compared to three non-psychotic patients died; however, causes of death were not described. Autopsies revealed a higher viral burden and more brain involvement in the psychosis group.

DEMENTIA IN SYPHILIS

The mechanism by which neurosyphilis produces cognitive dysfunction appears to be via diffuse effects of *Treponema pallidum* on both cortical and subcortical brain regions. Cognitive dysfunction presents as the hallmark of general paresis, but may also occur in other forms of neurosyphilis. Simple dementia without behavioral changes has been noted in about 35% of patients with general paresis.[21] Early signs include difficulties with memory, attention, and executive functioning, progressing to confabulation and apraxia, aphasia, and agnosia which indicate severe impairment of higher cortical functions. In other forms of neurosyphilis, such as the meningovascular or gummatous forms, cognitive deficits may be more localized to the area of ischemia or space occupying lesions. Untreated general paresis progresses to death within five to 10 years as patients become bedridden – hence the term 'dementia paralytica' – and suffer from malnutrition and intercurrent infections.

DEMENTIA IN HIV INFECTION

In persons with AIDS, direct HIV effects may produce a syndrome of subcortical dementia with eventual cortical involvement called AIDS dementia complex (ADC). Typically, symptoms emerge gradually with impaired concentration, motor slowing, insight, and behavioral changes, most frequently depression. Prior to antiretroviral treatment, brain related changes, most commonly leukoencephalopathy and HIV encephalitis were found in 75–90% of AIDS patients upon autopsy. ADC may be linked to alterations in the dopaminergic system,[43] as decreased levels of dopamine and substantia nigra degeneration have been found upon brain autopsy. As dopamine activates HIV in infected T-cell lymphoblasts, dopaminergic drugs, in particular cocaine, may accelerate progression to ADC. With the advent of antiviral treatment ADC has declined from 60% without treatment to 20% with dual nucleoside therapy and <10% with highly active retroviral therapy; however ADC has not declined to the same extent as other AIDS complications.[44] ADC remains a leading cause for dementia in persons under 60 years old[45] and is associated with rapid progression and death within six months.[46] In addition, cognitive dysfunction may result from HIV-related illnesses, such as opportunistic infections, brain lymphoma, and vasculitis.

CURRENT MANAGEMENT RECOMMENDATIONS

Neurosyphilis

CNS involvement may occur during any stage of syphilis. A patient who has clinical evidence of neurologic involvement with syphilis, such as cognitive dysfunction, motor or sensory deficits, ophthalmic or auditory symptoms, cranial neuropathies, and symptoms or signs of meningitis, should undergo a CSF examination.

According to current CDC recommendations,[47] patients who have neurosyphilis or syphilitic eye or ear disease should be treated with aqueous crystalline penicillin G 18–24 million units per day, administered as 3–4 million units IV every four hours or continuous infusion, for 10–14 days. If compliance with therapy can be ensured, patients may be treated with an alternative regimen of procaine penicillin 2.4 million units IM once daily plus Probenecid 500 mg orally four times a day, both for 10–14 days. Ceftriaxone may be used as an alternative treatment for patients with neurosyphilis. If CSF pleocytosis was present initially, repeat CSF examination should be performed every six months until the cell count is normal. Treatment failure and retreatment should be considered if the cell count has not decreased after six months, or if the CSF is not normal after two years.

Neurosyphilis plus HIV

CSF abnormalities are common in patients with early syphilis and in persons with HIV infection. The clinical significance of such CSF abnormalities in HIV-infected persons with primary or secondary syphilis is unknown. Most HIV-infected persons respond appropriately to standard benzathine penicillin therapy; however, some specialists recommend intensified therapy when CNS syphilis is suspected and follow-up CSF examination after initial treatment. Individuals who are co-infected with syphilis and HIV may be more likely to fail treatment even after an initial response, in particular if treatment begins in the secondary stage of syphilis.[9]

HIV

According to the current CDC report,[48] antiretroviral therapy in asymptomatic patients should be offered to individuals with low CD4 or high HIV RNA plasma levels. All patients diagnosed with advanced HIV disease (AIDS) or patients with symptomatic HIV infection without AIDS, defined as the presence of thrush or unexplained fever, should be treated. Regimens may include combinations of proteinase inhibitors (PI) with either nucleoside (NRTIs) or non-nucleoside (NNRTIs) reverse transcriptase inhibitors. Results of therapy are monitored primarily by decreased plasma HIV RNA levels. Failure of therapy at four to six months may be ascribed to non-adherence, inadequate potency of drugs, or suboptimal levels of antiretroviral agents, viral resistance, and other factors that are poorly understood.

Treatment of psychosis in syphilis and HIV

Mood and anxiety disorders are more common than psychosis in persons with syphilis or HIV infection and their treatment follows guidelines in the setting of patients with underlying medical and neurological conditions. In HIV(+) persons, there is clinical evidence that effective antiretroviral treatment will lessen psychological symptoms as the result of physical improvement,[49] and, possibly, via direct beneficial effects on mood.[50] There are special considerations regarding treatment of psychosis in persons with syphilis or HIV infection. In both conditions a psychotic disorder may present as an independent co-morbidity, most clearly if the psychiatric disorder establishes itself before the infection with syphilis or HIV. Whereas descriptions for treatment of psychotic symptoms in syphilis are limited to case studies, there are several published treatment trials in HIV(+) persons.

In syphilis with psychosis the main treatment is antibiotic therapy of the treponemal infection as indicated for the respective stage of illness, most commonly neurosyphilis. However, it is unclear whether psychotic symptoms in the setting of syphilis persist with eradication of the infection. In HIV infection, where causative treatment does not exist at the current time, treatment for psychotic symptoms is aimed at symptomatic improvement without any beneficial effect on the underlying disorder. Psychotropic and specifically antipsychotic medication should be chosen so as to produce the fewest potential adverse effects on cognition and on extrapyramidal, cardiovascular, and metabolic systems. Such side effects are common, although to differing degrees, to all antipsychotics.

Over the past 10 years, conventional atypical antipsychotics, including risperidone, olanzapine, quetiapine, ziprasidone, and most recently aripiprazole, represent the vast majority of antipsychotic medications prescribed for psychotic disorders. Each medication, while representing first line treatment for psychotic symptoms, possesses a different side effect profile. Similar to the treatment of psychosis in other medical and neurological conditions, it is recommended that antipsychotic medications should be started at doses much lower than commonly used for the treatment of acute psychotic episodes in schizophrenia. This will decrease the likelihood of emergence of antipsychotic side effects, which are more common in persons with diffuse neurological impairment, and range from extrapyramidal to anticholinergic symptoms and sedation. In HIV(+) persons, decreased dopamine and its metabolite,[43] as well as substantia nigra degeneration, have been described upon brain autopsy. This explains the increased incidence of extrapyramidal side effects associated with typical antipsychotics when used for the treatment of psychosis in patients with HIV infection.[39]

In the past 10 years, six case series have reported on beneficial effects of low dose thioridazine, haloperidol, clozapine, risperidone, and olanzapine, but not of lorazepam, on psychotic symptoms in HIV(+) persons.[51] Risperidone is known to produce a higher incidence of extrapyramidal side effects, similar to typical antipsychotics, and has recently been implicated with increased risk for stroke in elderly patients with dementia.[52] It remains to be seen whether this risk is particular to this medication or a group effect and common to all antipsychotics. In a group of 21 HIV(+) persons with psychosis, risperidone was found to be beneficial without undue side effects.[53] Olanzapine is subjectively well tolerated, but is linked with considerable weight gain in some patients and, possibly, the emergence of glucose intolerance and diabetes. Glucose intolerance and diabetes may, again, represent a risk particular to olanzapine or to the whole group of antipsychotics.[54] However, in HIV patients with psychosis, a group of patients with shortened life expectancy and risk of malnutrition, such effects may not carry the same implications as for people with schizophrenia. Quetiapine, in structure similar to clozapine, the gold standard of antipsychotic medications but restricted to people with treatment resistant schizophrenia, has a somewhat sedating but otherwise highly favorable side effect profile and has found increasing application for treatment of psychotic symptoms in the setting of disorders other than schizophrenia. Ziprasidone represents another antipsychotic medication with a favorable side effect profile; however, issues of absorption and bioavailability may produce an unpredictable reponse. More recently aripiprazole, considered to be a selective dopamine antagonist in mesolimbic pathways and dopamine agonist in mesocortical pathways, has been approved for treatment of schizophrenia, the prototypical psychotic disorder.

For grandiosity, irritability, and excitement, mood stabilizing medications such as valproic acid and carbamazepine may be beneficial. Although valproate has been shown to increase *in vitro* HIV replication,[55] this has not been replicated in HIV-infected persons who receive adequate antiretroviral treatment.[56] Carbamezepine, as a potent inducer of cytochrome 3A, may decrease antiretroviral medication levels or reach toxic levels due to inhibition of its metabolism by antiretrovirals.

Lithium, with effects on electrolyte balance, renal and thyroid function, its potential extrapyramidal side effects, and a narrow therapeutic window, remains a second line medication. In a small sample of 10 HIV(+) persons on lithium, seven patients discontinued treatment due to side effects and in some patients viral titers were increased.[57]

REFERENCES

1. World Health Organization Department of HIV/AIDS. *Global Prevalence and Incidence of Selected Curable Sexually Transmitted Infections*. 1999: http://www.who.int/docstore/hiv/grsti/005.htm
2. Centers for Disease Control and Prevention, National Center for HIV, STD and TB Prevention, Divisions of HIV/AIDS Prevention. *Basic Statistics*. 2001: http://www.cdc.gov/hiv/stats.htm
3. Centers for Disease Control and Prevention. *Primary and Secondary Syphilis: United States 2000–2001*. http://www.cdc.gov/mmwr/preview/mmwrhtml/mm5143a4.htm
4. Centers for Disease Control and Prevention, National Center for HIV, STD and TB Prevention, Division of Sexually Transmitted Diseases. *Syphilis Fact Sheet. Syphilis Elimination: History in the Making*. 2001: http://www.cdc.gov/nchstp/dstd/fact_sheets/syphilis_facts.htm
5. Centers for Disease Control and Prevention, National Center for HIV, STD and TB Prevention, Division of Sexually Transmitted Diseases. *Syphilis Surveillance Supplement*. 2001: http://www.cdc.gov/std/syphilis2001/default.htm
6. Joint United Nations Programme on HIV/AIDS (UNAIDS) and World Health Organization (WHO). *AIDS Epidemic Update*. 2002: http://www.who.int/hiv/pub/epidemiology/epi2002/en/
7. Blocker ME, Levine WC, St Louis ME. HIV prevalence in patients with syphilis, United States. *Sex Transm Dis* 2000; 27: 53–9.
8. Berger JR. Neurosyphilis in human immunodeficiency virus type 1–seropositive individuals. *Arch Neurol* 1991; 48: 700–2.
9. Gliatto MF, Caroff SN. Neurosyphilis: a history and clinical review. *Psychiatric Ann* 2001; 31: 153–61.
10. Noguchi H, Moore JW. A demonstration of treponema pallidum in the brain of general paresis. *J Exp Med* 1913; 17: 232–8.
11. Rowland LP. Neurosyphilis. In: *Meritt's Textbook of Neurology* (8th ed, Rowland LP, ed). Philadelphia: Lea & Febiger, 1989: 152–61.
12. Godt P, Stoeppler L, Wischer U, Schroeder HH. The value of computed tomography in cerebral syphilis. *Neuroradiol* 1979; 18: 197–200.
13. Russouw HG, Roberts MC, Emsley RA, Truter R. Psychiatric manifestations and magnetic resonance imaging in HIV-negative neurosyphilis. *Biol Psychiatry* 1997; 41: 467–73.
14. Holland BA, Perret LV, Mills CM. Meningiovascular syphilis: CT and MR findings. *Radiol* 1986; 158: 439–42.
15. Tien RD, Gean-Marton AD, Mark AS. MR findings in six patients. *Am J Radiol* 1992; 158: 1325–8.
16. Agrons GA, Han SS, Husson MA, Simeone F. MR imaging of cerebral gumma. *Am J Neuroradiol* 1991; 12: 80–1.
17. Kaplan JG, Sterman AB, Horoupian D et al. Luetic meningitis with gumma: clinical radiographic and neuropathologic features. *Neurol* 1981, 31: 364–7.
18. Wang AM, Barriger TK, Wesolowski DP. Intracranial gumma mimicking a tuber cinereum tumor. *Comp Med Imaging Graphics* 1991; 15: 57–60.
19. Clifford DB. AIDS dementia. *Clin North America* 2002; 86: 537–50.
20. Rosenbaum M. Similarities of psychiatric disorders of AIDS and syphilis: history repeats itself. *Bull Menninger Clinic* 1994; 58: 375–82.
21. Cheney CO. Clinical data on general paresis. *Psychiatry Quart* 1935; 9: 467–85.
22. Weaver G, Remick R. Electroconvulsive treatment of depression associated with neurosyphilis. *J Clin Psychiatry* 1982; 43: 468–9.
23. Hoffman BF. Neurosyphilis presenting as chronic mania. *J Clin Psychiatry* 1982; 43: 338–9.
24. Sivakumar K, Okocha CI. Neurosyphilis and schizophrenia. *Br J Psychiatry* 1992; 161: 251–4.
25. Hoffman BF. Neurosyphilis in a young man. *Can J Psychiatry* 1981; 26: 68–70.
26. Mapelli G, Bellelli T. Psychiatric manifestation of neurosyphilis without dementia. *Am J Psychiatry* 1981; 138: 1391–2.
27. Sirota P, Eviatar J, Spivak B. Neurosyphilis presenting as psychiatric disorders. *Br J Psychiatry* 1989; 155: 559–61.
28. Brooke D, Jamie P, Slack R et al. Neurosyphilis: a treatable psychosis. *Br J Psychiatry* 1987; 151: 556.
29. Gastal FL, Leite SS, Carnieletto GE et al. Atypical neurosyphilis: report of a case. *Arquivos de Neuro-Psiquiatria* 1995; 53: 494–7.
30. Bschorr T, Nuernbach-Ross B, Albrecht J. Organische Genese einer maniformen Psychose. *Nervenarzt* 1995; 66: 54–6.
31. Mahendran R. Clozapine in the treatment of hypomania with neurosyphilis. *J Clin Psychiatry* 2001; 62: 477–8.

32. Kohler CG, Pickholtz J, Ballas C. Neurosyphilis presenting as schizophrenia-like psychosis. *Neuropsychiatry, Neuropsychol Behav Neurol* 2000; **13**: 297–303.
33. Perkins DO, Stern RA, Golden RN et al. Mood disorders in HIV infection: prevalence and risk factors in a nonepicenter of the AIDS epidemic. *Am J Psychiatry* 1994; **151**: 233–6.
34. Gala C, Pergami A, Invernizzi G. The psychological impact of HIV infection and the 'burn-out' syndrome amongst health care workers dealing with HIV seropositive and AIDS patients. *Minerva Psichiatrica* 1993; **34**: 75–84.
35. Baldeweg T, Catalan J, Pugh K et al. Neurophysiological changes associated with psychiatric symptoms in HIV-infected individuals without AIDS. *Biol Psychiatry* 1997; **41**: 474–87.
36. Halstead S, Riccio M, Harlow P et al. Psychosis associated with HIV infection. *Br J Psychiatry* 1988; **153**: 618–23.
37. Vogel-Scibilia SE, Mulsant BH, Keshavan MS. HIV infection presenting as psychosis: a critique. *Acta Psychiatr Scand* 1988; **78**: 652–6.
38. Navia BA, Jordan BD, Price RW. The AIDS dementia complex: I. Clinical features. *Ann Neurol* 1986; **19**: 517–24.
39. Sewell DD. Schizophrenia and HIV. *Schizophr Bull* 1996; **22**: 465–73.
40. El-Mallakh RS. Mania in AIDS: clinical significance and theoretical considerations. *Int J Psychiatry Med* 1991; **21**: 383–91.
41. El-Mallakh RS. HIV-related psychosis. *J Clin Psychiatry* 1992; **53**: 293–4.
42. Sewell DD, Jeste DV, Atkinson JH et al. HIV-associated psychosis: a study of 20 cases. *Am J Psychiatry* 1994; **151**: 237–42.
43. Sardar AM, Czudek C, Reynolds GP. Dopamine deficits in the brain: the neurochemical basis of parkinsonian symptoms in AIDS. *Neuroreport* 1996; **7**: 910–2.
44. Dore GJ, Correll PK, Li Y et al. Changes to AIDS dementia complex in the era of highly active antiretroviral therapy. *AIDS* 1999; **13**: 1249–53.
45. McArthur JC, Hoover DR, Bacellar H et al. Dementia in AIDS patients: incidence and risk factors. Multicenter AIDS Cohort Study. *Neurol* 1993; **43**: 2245–52.
46. Harrison MJG, Arthur J. HIV associated dementia complex. In: *AIDS and Neurology* (Harrison MJG, McArthur J, eds). New York: Churchill Livingstone, 1995: 31–64.
47. Centers for Disease Control and Prevention. *Sexually Transmitted Diseases Treatment and Guidelines.* 2002: http://www.cdc.gov/std/treatment/
48. Centers for Disease Control and Prevention. *Guidelines for the Use of Antiretroviral Agents in HIV-infected Adults and Adolescents.* 2004: http://www.cdc.gov/hiv/treatment.htm#treatment
49. Rabkin JG, Ferrando SJ, Lin SH et al. Psychological effects of HAART: a 2-year study. *Psychosom Med* 2000; **62**: 413–22.
50. Fumaz CR, Tuldra A, Ferrer MJ et al. Quality of life, emotional status, and adherence of HIV-1-infected patients treated with efavirenz verus protease inhibitor-containing regimens. *J Acquired Immune Deficiency Syndr* 2002; **29**: 244–53.
51. Ferrando SJ, Wapenyi K. Psychopharmacological treatment of patients with HIV and AIDS. *Psychiatry Quart* 1992; **73**: 33–49.
52. Janssen Pharmaceutical Products. Letter. *Healthcare Professional* April 2003.
53. Singh AN, Golledge H, Catalan J. Treatment of HIV-related disorders with risperidone: a series of 21 cases. *J Psychosom Res* 1997; **42**: 489–93.
54. Lindenmayer JP, Czobor P, Volavka J et al. Changes in glucose and cholesterol levels in patients with schizophrenia treated with typical or atypical antipsychotics. *Am J Psychiatry* 2003; **160**: 290–6.
55. Moog C, Kuntz-Simon G, Caussin-Schwemling C, Obert C. Sodium valproate, an anticonvulsant drug, stimulates human immunodeficiency type 1 replication independently of glutathione levels. *J Gen Virol* 1996; **77**: 1003–9.
56. Maggi JD, Halman MH. The effect of divalproex sodium on viral load: a retrospective review of HIV-positive patients with manic syndromes. *Can J Psychiatry* 2001; **46**: 359–62.
57. Parenti DM, Simon GL, Scheib RG et al. Effect of lithium carbonate in HIV-infected patients with immune dysfunction. *J Acquired Immune Deficiency Syndr* 1988; **1**: 199–224.

# 8

Streptococcal infections and psychoses? A preliminary inquiry

Daniel R Hanson

INTRODUCTION

For a common disorder, schizophrenia is an uncommonly stubborn puzzle. More than 100 years have elapsed since Kraepelin and Bleuler set down the descriptive foundations for identifying the illness, yet the cause of the illness still eludes us.[1,2] When the solution to a clinical or scientific puzzle eludes us for more than a century, as with the riddle of schizophrenia, we need to try new ways of thinking about the problem.[3,4] For decades, efforts to understand schizophrenia have focused on neurons and, especially, the role of excess dopamine neurotransmission as suggested by the mechanisms of effective treatments with antipsychotic medication. This chapter presents an alternative strategy. The central hypothesis is that some psychoses are the result of damage to the microvascular system in the brain, initiated by inflammatory processes following streptococcal infections. This hypothesis adds specificity to the diathesis-stressor model.[5] It is postulated that the environmental components of the illness are infectious agents and that the inherited components are perturbations in genetically mediated inflammatory reactions to infection. Excessive and poorly regulated inflammatory reactions will damage the vascular supply to the brain resulting in pervasive but subtle disruption of metabolism. The downstream behavioral consequences result in psychoses.

THE GENETICS OF INFECTIOUS DISEASES

The concept that infectious disease may have a genetic component is, of course, not new. Many agricultural geneticists make their livings by breeding disease resistance into both plants and animals.[6,7] One of the founders of behavioral genetics, Franz Kallmann,[8] showed genetic factors influenced acquiring tuberculosis (DZ concordance = 26%, MZ concordance = 87%), an observation that was confirmed in modern times.[9,10] There appear to be genetic factors influencing susceptibility or resistance to many infections diseases.[11-21] Mechanisms for genetically mediated responses to infection occur through genetic variations in immune mediators such as cytokines[21] and HLA factors.[22,23] Let us suppose that schizophrenia develops from an infectious agent (the environmental contributor) but genetic factors influence who is susceptible to adverse outcomes from the infection. That infectious agents may be operative in schizophrenia is supported by several of lines of evidence. Summaries can be found in numerous sources.[24-30]

VASCULAR ABNORMALITIES AND PSYCHOSES

The syndrome of schizophrenia is probably etiologically heterogeneous and a multitude of CNS disorders can give rise to schizophrenic-like psychoses.[31] The idea that CNS microvascular diseases, in particular, are factors in psychotic disorders is an old idea that deserves a second look in light of new perspectives offered by developments in the genetics of inflammatory diseases. There are many examples of psychoses resulting from microvascular CNS disease including lupus and Sjogren's syndrome.[32] Neuroimaging and neurocognitive deficits in these disorders are similar to those seen in schizophrenia.[33] Psychoses associated with substance abuse are also associated with CNS vasculitis. Furthermore, infectious agents such as syphilis and rheumatic fever (RF) lead to microvascular disorders of the CNS that are associated with psychiatric symptoms including psychoses. Recently, small vessel abnormalities were found in the depressed elderly.[34] Neuroimaging studies have repeatedly found evidence of cerebral blood flow abnormalities in psychiatric syndromes.[35] CNS metabolism involves exquisitely precise regulation of cerebral blood flow[36,37] that is in part modified by dopaminergic signals.[38,39] Other lines of evidence, including genetic linkage studies, implicate microvascular abnormalities in psychoses via the close relationship between microvessel circulation and glial cell function.[40] At the same time, there is growing interest in cytokines and other inflammatory agents in psychoses,[41] as well as growing awareness that inflammatory reactions are modulated by neuropeptides.[42]

When infectious agents give rise to inflammatory vascular disease, the nature of the infectious agent may be less important than the individual's genetically influenced inflammatory response as exemplified by familial Mediterranean fever (FMF).[43,44] The gene for FMF is located on the short arm of chromosome 16 and produces pyrin (marenostrin), which functions in a negative feedback loop to suppress inflammation. Absence of pyrin leads to exaggerated inflammatory responses. Vasculitis is one of the consequences.[45] Additionally, very high rates of RF or rheumatic heart disease (RHD) are found in relatives of patients with FMF.[46] Having even one mutant gene appears to lead to immune hyperactivity to streptococcal antigens. Antibody production[47] and cytokine activity[48] in RF patients are more marked than in non-rheumatics.

PSYCHIATRIC ILLNESS AND STREPTOCOCCAL INFECTIONS

Post-streptococcal neuropsychiatric syndromes include Syndenham chorea,[49] the PANDAS/OCD syndrome, and possibly, ADHD, tics, and Tourette syndrome.[50-54] Psychotic disorders are also implicated (see below). Sydenham chorea is the best-known neuropsychiatric complication following streptococcal pharangytis. People with a history of Sydenham chorea (SC) are at high risk for developing psychotic disorders later in life, long after resolution of the chorea[55] with a relative risk for schizophrenia as high as 8.9 in a 10-year follow-up of 29 Sydenham patients.[56] There is a suggestion that the family members of Sydenham patients are also at higher risk for psychosis.[57] The association of psychoses and RF, even in the absence of chorea, was discussed in the 17th and 18th centuries starting with Sydenham himself.[58] The interest in psychoses associated with RF continued throughout the 1900s.[58-67]

Bruetsch provided extensive exploration of psychoses and RF.[61-63,69] Among 100 patients with schizophrenia 9% had rheumatic valvular disease while only 1.7% of 171 comparison patients had the disease.[69] Though schizophrenia-like psychoses were the most common psychopathology related to rheumatic brain lesions, manic depressive, involutional, and senile psychoses were also observed.[62] Bruetsch attributed the development of psychiatric symptoms to damage to cerebral arteries (see section on neuropathology below).

An analysis of 50 autopsies of people with schizophrenia found evidence of RHD in 14%, about twice the rate of RHD in a comparison sample of 200 patients from the same hospital, and led to the conclusion that 'rheumatic cerebral arteritis is a real factor in the production of schizophrenic symptoms in some patients.'[66]

Retrospective medical data from 2,658 state hospital patients with a diagnosis of schizophrenia showed that history of RF was about nine times more prevalent in these patients than in the general population.[70] Schizophrenic patients with a history of RF or RHD more often had a progressively insidious course with poor long-term outcomes. Wertheimer pursued the concept of rheumatic mental illness in a follow-up study of children with rheumatic fever. She found functional mental illness by age 25 in 6.1% of 943 children with RF or SC compared to 3.1% of 1201 non-RF/SC controls. Siblings of RF patients also had increased rates of functional psychiatric disorders.[70,71]

Another study found a high rate of histories of rheumatic chorea earlier in the lives of psychiatric patients with psychosis (schizophrenia and affective psychoses) compared to non-psychotic patients in the same psychiatric hospital (odds ratio = 13.8).[72]

NEUROPATHOLOGY OF CNS RHEUMATIC DISEASE

Vascular abnormalities in psychoses were of great interest in the 1800s[73] but have received limited attention in modern times except for ongoing imaging studies of cerebral blood flow. Neuropathological studies of Sydenham chorea and acute and chronic rheumatic fever have repeatedly found endothelial proliferation or other damage to small vessels,[59,62,66,74-78] microscopic infarcts,[58,66,67,74,79,80] hyalinization of small vessels,[74] fibrosis of the outer vascular coats,[74,81] and inflammatory cell infiltration around the small vessels.[59,77,79,81] If rheumatic cardiac valvular disease is active, then micro emboli/infarct and glial reactions are often present.[79,80] The CNS vascular lesions appear to be part of a more generalized vascular disorder seen throughout the body in RF.[82,83]

A NEW INQUIRY

The research material is derived from a collection of clinical and neuropathological data on over 2,000 patients who died at Minnesota state hospitals between 1950 and 1972 and went to a mandated autopsy. The majority of these were dementias but nearly 400 had so-called functional psychoses. The fixed CNS tissues blocks used at autopsy are available for analysis. The post mortem interval averages 7.4 hours for the entire collection.

All medical records of psychotic cases have been assembled into a detailed (anonymized) case history neuropathology data bank allowing clinical–pathological correlations. All psychiatric diagnoses have been reviewed and updated to RDC criteria by two independent clinicians (the author of this chapter and W Grove PhD, a highly experienced clinical psychologist); inter-rater reliability was high (kappa = .99).

Subjects are cases of psychoses (including schizophrenia and psychotic mood disorders) that had rheumatic fever, as proven by autopsy evidence of rheumatic heart disease. The psychoses phenotype was chosen for study because, like other psychoses with organic cause (such as the psychoses that may accompany Huntington disease), the clinical course may be schizophrenia-like or psychotic affective-like disorder. The sample contains 30 such cases of psychoses and RF.

RESULTS

RF is found in this sample of psychiatric patients at a higher rate (7%) than expected. The general population one-year prevalence ranges from 1–35/100,000. A better comparison is the pooled data from 22 autopsy studies involving over 75,000 general hospital patients between 1924 and 1974 that showed an average rate of RHD of 3.3% (references upon request). Among schizophrenic patients who came to autopsy, Bruetsch found an RHD rate of 9%[62] and Howie found a rate of 14%.[66]

The 'rheumatic psychoses' in this sample differ from other psychoses in having a later age of onset (49 vs. 37 years; $p < .000004$). They also differ in year of first psychiatric hospitalization shortly following an epidemic of RF in Minnesota with the average calendar year of onset of 1939 for non-RHD and 1948 for RHD ($p < .0007$). The temporal clustering fits with an infectious/epidemic pattern (see Figure 8.1). Additionally, the RHD cases, though presenting as rather typical psychoses, progress to an

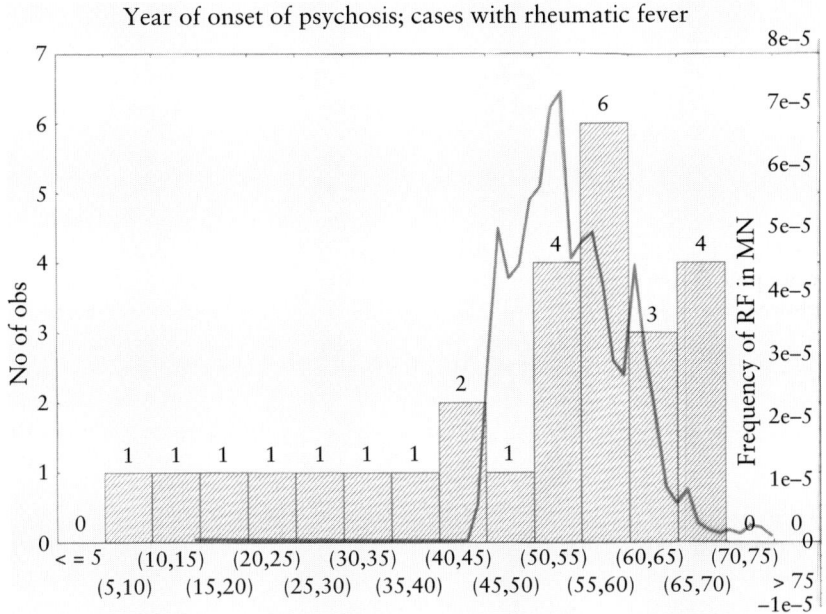

Figure 8.1 The vertical bars represent the number of cases of psychosis in people with rheumatic fever admitted to Minnesota State psychiatric hospitals for each year from 1900 to 1975 (X axis). The line plot shows the statewide incidence of rheumatic fever in Minnesota. The onset of psychiatric cases lags a few years behind the epidemic of rheumatic fever beginning during the late 1940s and ending in the early 1960s. The left vertical axis is the number of observations.

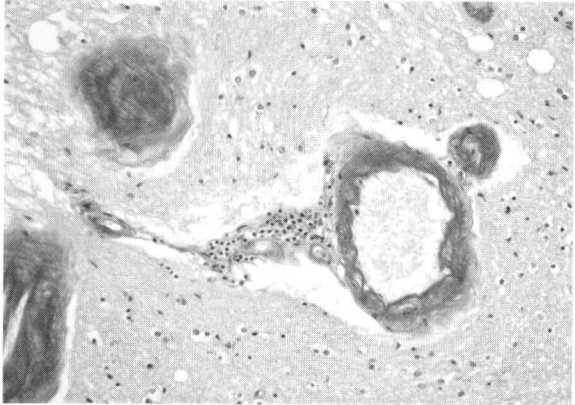

Figure 8.2 Medium-sized CNS vessel from case of RF with psychosis showing inflammatory cells in the perivascular space.

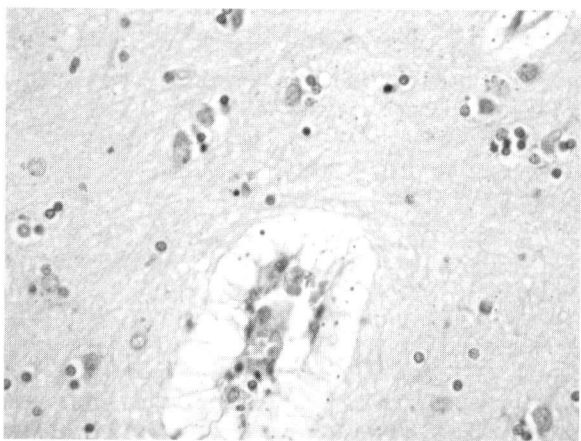

Figure 8.4 Enlarged perivascular space.

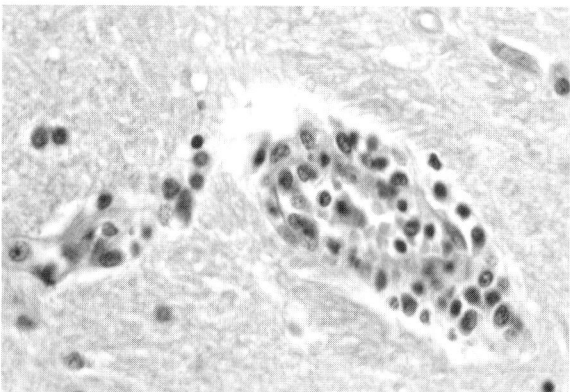

Figure 8.3 Inflammatory cells, microvascular proliferation.

organic-like (dementia praecox) state in 43% of the cases compared to only 12% of non-RHD psychotic cases in this sample (χ^2 1df, $p < .00001$). Preliminary neuropathological results indicated enlarged perivascular spaces and presence of inflammatory cells (see Figures 8.2–8.4), similar to what is reported in the literature cited above.

DISCUSSION

The ideas in this chapter are not new but bring old ideas forward into the light of new understanding of molecular genetics and inflammatory diseases. Since the late 1800s there has been evidence of inflammatory neurovascular abnormalities in psychiatric illness, initiated by infectious agents. CNS lues is the best known example. This paper expands the concept to suggest that a wide variety of infectious agents may stimulate inflammatory processes that damage the vascular supply to the brain, thus creating abnormal behaviors, in a fashion similar to the behavioral changes seen in other CNS vascular inflammatory diseases such as lupus.

This infectious–inflammatory model could explain many of the features of schizophrenia. As indicated earlier, the model incorporates both genetic and environmental components. The spontaneous fluctuations in symptoms could be the result of waxing and waning of inflammatory episodes in conjunction with other physiological and hormonal influences as seen in lupus.[84] Since the vascular system is everywhere in the brain, vascular lesions could produce the variety of symptoms seen in schizophrenia including dysfunctions of thought, emotion, memory, motor skills, and autonomic regulation. This theory also captures many of the oddities observed in schizophrenia. For example, the well-documented abnormalities of the nailfold capillary beds seen in people with schizophrenia[85] are also seen in people with inflammatory disorders such as FMF.[86] Another oddity is the negative association between schizophrenia and rheumatoid arthritis.[87] There are parallels in the post-streptococcal syndromes, where RF and acute post-streptococcal glomerulonephritis very rarely occur in the same patient.[88] It appears that different strains of streptococci may produce either heart or renal complications but not both. By analogy, individuals with vascular/CNS involvement following streptococcal infections may be systematically spared from joint involvement.

It may well be that the environmental components of psychiatric illness are acquired infections. The nature of the infection may be less important than individuals' genetically-influenced and idiosyncratic responses to infection, similar to individuals with FMF who have an exaggerated inflammatory response. Thus, the genetic components of the inherited predisposition to mental illness may lie in the immune system rather than the CNS per se. The possibility that the environmental agent may be nearly universal (who has not had a strep throat?) means that the prevalence of the etiological factor will be similar in control and experimental groups, making it easy to miss common causes in null hypothesis designs.[89] Rather than focus on infectious contributors that could be non-specific, it may be more productive to look for genotypes that respond abnormally to infection. These individuals would be the ones who are at high risk for psychiatric illness. Identification of high-risk individuals, combined with such tools as immunizations, may allow prevention of much psychiatric morbidity.

ACKNOWLEDGMENTS

This work has been approved by the Institutional Review Boards of the State of Minnesota, the University of Minnesota, and the Minneapolis VA. NARSAD and the Ramsey Hospital Foundation provided support for this project. The author thanks William Grove PhD for assistance with diagnostic re-evaluations of the psychiatric patients. Karen SantaCruz MD provided invaluable assistance with the preliminary neuropathology. Irving Gottesman PhD made many helpful suggestions in his review of the manuscript. June White RN was instrumental in preserving and organizing the collection of autopsy material. Any deficiencies in this chapter are solely those of the author.

REFERENCES

1. Kraepelin E. *Dementia Praecox and Paraphrenia*. Edinburgh: E and S Livingston, 1919.
2. Bleuler E. *Dementia Praecox or the Group of Schizophrenias*. New York: International University Press, 1950.
3. Faust D. *The Limits of Scientific Reasoning*. Minneapolis: University of Minnesota Press, 1984.
4. Wicker A. Getting out of our conceptual ruts: strategies for expanding conceptual frameworks. *Am Psychologist* 1985; **40**: 1094–103.
5. Gottesman II, Shields J. A polygeneic theory of schizophrenia. *Proc Nat Acad Sci* 1967; **58**: 199–205.
6. Richter T, Ronald P. The evolution of disease resistant genes. *Plant Molecular Biology* 2000; **42**: 195–204.
7. Mackenzie K, Bishop S. Utilizing stochastic genetic epidemiological models to quantify the impact of selection for resistance to infectious disease in domestic livestock. *Journal of Animal Science* 2001; **79**: 2057–65.
8. Kallmann FJ, Reisner D. Twin studies on the genetic variation in resistance to tuberculosis. *J Heredity* 1943; **34**: 293–301.
9. Werneck-Barroso E. Innate resistance to tuberculosis: revisiting Max Lurie genetic experiments in rabbits. *Int J Tuberculosis Lung Dis* 1999; **3**: 166–8.
10. McGue M, Gottesman II, Rao DC. The transmission of schizophrenia under a multifactorial threshold model. *Am J Human Genet* 1983; **35**: 1161–78.
11. Bion JF, Brun-Buisson C. Introduction – infection and critical illness: genetic and environmental aspects of susceptibility and resistance. *Intensive Care Med* 2000; **26** Supplement 1: S1–2.
12. Burt RA. Genetics of host response to malaria. *Int J Parasitology* 1999; **29**: 973–9.
13. Hawken RJ, Beattie CW, Schook LB. Resolving the genetics of resistance to infectious diseases. *Rev Sci Technol* 1998; **17**: 17–25.
14. Hill AV. Genetics of infectious disease resistance. *Curr Opin Genet Dev* 1996; **6**: 348–53.
15. Hill AV. Genetics and genomics of infectious disease susceptibility. *Br Med Bull* 1999; **55**: 401–13.
16. Seymour RM. Some aspects of the coevolution of virulence and resistance in contact transmission processes with ecological constraints. *IMA J Math Appl Med Biol* 1995; **12**: 83–136.
17. Kitagawa M, Aizawa S, Ikeda H, Hirokawa W. Establishment of a therapeutic model for retroviral infection using the genetic resistance mechanism of the host. *Pathol Int* 1996; **46**: 719–25.
18. Smith DA, Germolec DR. Introduction of immunology and autoimmunity. *Env Health Perspectives* 1999; **107**(Supplement 5): 661–5.
19. Cook GS, Hill AV. Genetics of susceptibility to heman infectious disease. *Nature Rev Genet* 2001; **2**: 967–77.
20. Blackwell JM. Genetics and genomics of infectious disease susceptibility. *Trends Mol Med* 2001; **7**: 521–6.
21. Knight J. Polymorphisms in tumor necrosis factor and other cytokines as risks for infectious disease and the septic shock syndrome. *Curr Infec Dis Report* 2001; **3**: 427–39.
22. Beskow AH, Gyllensten UB. Host genetic control of HPV 16 titer in carcinoma in situ of the cervix uteri. *Int J Cancer* 2000; **101**: 526–31.
23. Wang FS. Current status and prospects of studies on human genetic alleles associated with hepatitis B virus infection. *World J Gastroenterol* 2003; **9**: 641–44.
24. Munk-Jorgensen P, Ewald H. Epidemiology in neurobiological research: exemplified by the infuenza-schizophrenia story. *Br J Psychiatry* 2001; **40**: S30–2.
25. Rubenstein G. Schizophrenia, rheumatoid arthrits and natural disease resistance. *Schizophr Res* 1991; **25**: 177–81.
26. Morris JA. Schizophrenia, bacterial toxins and the genetics of redundancy. *Med Hypotheses* 1966; **46**: 362–6.
27. O'Reilly SL, Singh SM. Retroviruses and schizophrenia revisited. *Am J Med Genet* 1966; **67**: 19–26.
28. Yolken RH, Torrey EF. Viruses, schizophrenia, and bipolar disorder. *Clin Microbiol Rev* 1995; **8**: 131–45.
29. Yolken RH, Karlsson H, Yee F, Torrey EF. Endogenous retroviruses and schizophrenia. *Brain Res Rev* 2000; **31**: 193–9.
30. Torrey EF, Miller J, Rawlings R, Yolken RH. Seasonality of births in schizophrenia and bipolar disorder: a review of the research. *Schizophr Res* 1997; **28**: 1–38.
31. Davidson K, Bagley CR. Schizophrenia-like psychoses associated with organic disorders of the central nervous system: a review of the literature. In: *Current Problems in Neuropsychiatry*

(Herrington RN, ed). *British Journal of Psychiatry Special Publication No. 4*. Ashford, UK: Headly Brothers, 1969: 113–84.
32. Hess D. Cerebral lupus vasculopathy. Mechanisms and clinical relevance. *Ann New York Acad Sci* 1997; **823**: 154–68.
33. Lass P, Koseda M, Romanowicz G et al. Cerebral blood flow in Sjogren's syndrome using 99Tcm-HMPAO brain SPET. *Nuclear Med Comm* 2000; **21**: 31–5.
34. Thomas A, O'Brien J, Davis S et al. Ischemic basis for deep white matter hyperintensities in major depression. *Arch Gen Psychiatry* 2002; **59**: 785–92.
35. Honey GF, Bullmore, ET. Functional brain mapping of psychopathology. *J Neurol Neurosurgery Psychiatry* 2002; **72**: 432–9.
36. Harder D, Zhang, C, Gebremedhin, D. Astrocyte function in matching blood flow to metabolic activity. *News Physiol Sci* 2002; **17**: 27–31.
37. Yoder E. Modifications in astrocyte morphology and calcium signaling induced by brain capillary endothelial cell line. *Glia* 2002; **38**: 137–45.
38. Bacic F, Uematsu S, McCarron RM, Spatz M. Dopamine receptors linked to adenylate cyclase in human cerebromicrovascular endothelium. *J Neurochemistry* 1991; **57**: 1774–80.
39. Favard CSA, Vigny A, Nguyen-Legros J. Ultrastructural evidence for a close relationship between dopamine cell precesses and blood capillary walls in Macaca monkey and rat retina. *Brain Res* 1990; **523**: 127–33.
40. Moises HA, Zoega T, Gottesman II. The glial growth factors deficiency and synaptic destabilization hypothesis of schizophrenia. *BMC Psychiatry* 2002; **2** (www.biomedcentral.com/1471-244X/2/8).
41. Ziad K, Remick DG. Cytokines and the brain: implications for clinical psychiatry. *Am J Psychiatry* 2000; **157**: 683–94.
42. Wang H, Ochani M, Amella C et al. Nicotinic acetylcholine receptor a7 subunit is an essential regulator of inflammation. *Nature* 2003; **421**: 384–8.
43. Touitou I. The spectrum of familial mediterranean fever (FMF) mutations. *Eur J Human Genet* 2001; **9**: 473–83.
44. Scholl P. Periodic fever syndromes. *Curr Opin Pediatrics* 2000; **12**: 563–6.
45. Ozen S. Vasculopathy, Bechets syndrome and familial mediterranean fever. *Curr Opin Rheumatol* 1999; **11**: 393–8.
46. Tutar E, Akar N, Atalay S et al. Familial mediterranean fever gene (MEFV) mutations in patients with rheumatic heart disease. *Heart* 2002; **87**: 568–9.
47. Veasy LG, Hill HR. Immunologic and clinical correlations in rheumatic fever and rheumatic heart disease. *Pediatr Infect Dis J* 1997; **16**: 400–7.
48. Yegin O, Coskun M, Ertug H. Cytokines in acute rheumatic fever. *Eur J Pediatrics* 1997; **156**: 24–9.
49. Moore D. Neuropsychiatric aspects of Sydenham's chorea. *J Clin Psychiatry* 1996; **57**: 407–14.
50. Bottas A, Richer MA. Pediatric autoimmune neuropsychiatric disorders associated with streptoccal infections (PANDAS). *Pediatr Infect Dis J* 2002; **21**: 67–71.
51. Swedo S, Rapport J, Cheslow D et al. High prevalence of obsessive-compulsive symptoms in patients with Sydenham's chorea. *Am J Psychiatry* 1989; **146**: 246–9.
52. Swedo SE, Leonard HL, Kiessling LS. Speculations on antineuronal antibody-mediated neuropsychiatric disorders of childhood. *Pediatrics* 1994; **93**: 323–6.
53. Asbahr F, Negrao AB, Gentil V et al. Obsessive compulsive and related syndromes in children and adolescents with rheumatic fever with and without chorea: a prospective 6 month study. *Am J Psychiatry* 1998; **155**: 1122–4.
54. Garvey MA, Swedo SE. PANDAS: the search for environmental triggers of pediatric neuropsychiatric disorders. Lessons from rheumatic fever. *J Child Neurol* 1998; **13**: 413–23.
55. Keeler WR, Bender L. A follow-up study of children with behavior disorders and Sydenham's chorea. *Am J Psychiatry* 1952; **169**: 421–8.
56. Wilcox JA, Nasrallan H. Sydenahm's chorea and psychopathology. *Neuropsychobiol* 1988; **19**: 6–8.
57. Guttmann E. On some constitutional aspects of chorea and on its sequelae. *J Neurol Psychopathol* 1936; **17**: 16–26.
58. Van Der Horst L. Rheumatism and psychosis. *Foli Psychiatrica Neurologica et Neurochirugica Neerlandica* 1948; **1/2**: 56–64.
59. Winkelman N, Eckel JL. The brain in acute rheumatic fever. *Arch Neurol Psychiatry* 1932; **28**: 844–70.
60. Dublin W. Pathologic lesions of the brain associated with chronic rheumatic endocarditis and accompanied by psychosis. *Dis Nerv System* 1941; **2**: 390–3.
61. Bruetsch W. The histopathology of the psychoses with subacute bacterial and chronic verrucose rheumatic endocarditis. *Am J Psychiatry* 1938; **95**: 335–46.
62. Bruetsch W. Chronic rheumatic brain disease as a possible factor in the causation of some cases of dementia paraecox. *Am J Psychiatry* 1940; **97**: 276–96.
63. Bruetsch W. Rheumatic enderitis of cerebral vessels: sequelae of rheumatic fever. *Transac Am Neurol Assoc* 1942; **68**: 17–20.
64. Van Der Horst L. Rheuma und psychose. *Arxhiv fur Psychiatrie und Zierschrift Neurologie* 1949; **181**: 325–36.
65. Lewis A, Minski L. Chorea and psychosis. *Lancet* 1935; **228**: 536–8.
66. Howie D. Some pathological findings in schizophrenics. *Am J Psychiatry* 1960; **117**: 59–62.
67. Skvortsova E. Clinical neuropsychiatric changes during rheumatism. *Klinicheskaia Meditsina* 1956; **34**: 32–5.
68. Hammes E. Psychoses associated with Sydenham's chorea. *JAMA* 1922; **79**: 804–7.
69. Bruetsch W. Late cerebral sequelae of rheumatic fever. *Arch Internal Med* 1944; **73**: 972–82.
70. Wertheimer N. Rheumatic schizophrenia. *Arch Gen Psychiatry* 1961; **4**: 579–96.
71. Wertheimer N. A psychiatric follow-up of children with rheumatic fever and other chronic diseases. *J Chronic Dis* 1963; **16**: 223–37.
72. Wilcox JA, Nasrallah HA. Sydenham's chorea and psychosis. *Neuropsychobiol* 1986; **15**: 13–4.
73. Beadles C. On the degenerative lesions of the arterial system in the insane, with remarks upon the nature of the granular ependyma. *J Mental Science* 1895; **41**: 32–50.
74. Neuburger K. The brain in rheumatic fever. *Dis Nervous System* 1947; **8**: 259–62.
75. Bompiani G, Benedetti E, Cecconi D. Arteriopathie cerebrali reumatiche. *Archivo Itaaliano di Anatomi E. Istologia Pathologica* 1954; **28**: 1–35.
76. Bender L. Psychiatric, neurologic and neuropathologic studies in disseminated alterative arteriolitis. *Arch Neurol Psychiatry* 1936; **36**: 790–815.
77. Greenfield JG, Wolfson JM. The pathology of Sydenham's chorea. *Lancet* 1922; **203**: 603–6.
78. Bini L, Giovanni M. Uber den chronischen cerebralrheumatismus. *Archiv fur Psychiatrie und Zeitschrift Neurologie* 1952; **188**: 261–73.
79. Costero I. Reaccion de la microglia en el cerebro de los reumaticos. *Gaceta Medica De Mexico* 1951; **81**: 49–60.
80. Costero I. Cerebral lesions responsible for death of patients with active rheumatic fever. *Arch Neurol Psychiatry* 1949; **62**: 48–72.
81. Sachs B. The pathology of rheumatic fever. *Am Heart J* 1926; **1**: 750–72.
82. Shiokawa Y. Microcirculation in rheumatic fever. *3rd European Conference on Microcirculation* 1964; **7**: 547–51.
83. Montgomery H. Capillary fragility in rheumatic fever. *US Navy Med Bull* 1946; **46**: 1708–10.

84. Merill JT. Regulation of the vasculature: clues from lupus. *Curr Opin Rheumatol* 2002; **14**: 504–9.
85. Curtis CE, Iacono WG, Beiser M. Relationships between nailfold plexus visibility and clinical, neuropsychological, and brain structural measures in schizophrenia. *Biol Psychiatry* 1999; **46**: 102–9.
86. Dinc A, Melikoglu M, Korkmaz C et al. Nailfold capillary abnormalities in patients with familial Mediterranean fever. *Clin Exp Rheumatol* 2001; **19**(Supplement 24): S42–4.
87. Vinogradov S, Gottesman II, Moises HW, Nichol S. Negative association between schizophrenia and rheumatoid arthritis. *Schizophr Bull* 1991; **17**: 669–78.
88. Stollerman GH. Rheumatic fever. *Lancet* 1997; **349**: 935–42.
89. Hanson DR. Getting the bugs into our genetic theories of schizophrenia. In: *Behavior Genetic Principals of Development, Personality, and Psychopathology* (DiLalla L, ed). Washington DC: American Psychiatric Press, 2004: 205–16.

9

Prenatal human influenza viral infection, brain development, and schizophrenia

S Hossein Fatemi

INTRODUCTION

Schizophrenia is a debilitating disorder of brain function with genetic and environmental susceptibilities.[1] A growing body of epidemiologic evidence supports a neurodevelopmental origin for this disorder.[2] These studies link prenatal human influenza viral infection with a subsequent rise in schizophrenic births. Experimental animal data supporting this linkage are lacking. The studies described in this chapter discuss data concerning an animal model of post-viral behavioral disorder caused by prenatal exposure to human influenza virus (InfV).

The concept of schizophrenia as a neurodevelopmental disorder is based on several lines of evidence, which will be briefly discussed here. There is an association between obstetric complications and later development of schizophrenia.[3,4] The complications include periventricular hemorrhages, hypoxia, and ischemic injuries,[2] potentially causing abnormal connections in affected brains and the subsequent development of schizophrenia. Numerous published reports indicate the presence of cerebro-ventricular enlargement in schizophrenic brains, as revealed by CT and MRI imaging studies.[5] These abnormalities are present at onset of the disease, may progress with time, and distinguish affected from unaffected discordant monozygotic twins.[6–8] Moreover, gross abnormalities of various brain regions have been reported and include changes in size/volume of the hippocampus, amygdala, parahippocampal gyrus, entorhinal cortex, and temporal horns.[3] Neuropathologic reports have consistently showed abnormalities of the brain in schizophrenic subjects, including reductions in the granular layer of the dentate, disarray of pyramidal cells of the hippocampus, and decreased cell densities of prefrontal, motor cortex, and cingulate gyrus, as well as disruption and displacement of cells in the prefrontal, entorhinal, and hippocampal cortices.[9–18] Behavioral and cognitive abnormalities seen in schizophrenia can be due to pathologic involvement of various brain areas, such as the hippocampus and prefrontal cortex, causing decreased learning and memory, and inattention, respectively. Despite a large body of neuropathologic work, little or no gliosis has been observed in schizophrenic brains.[3] Because glial cells arise during the third trimester of pregnancy, their absence in schizophrenic brains has been associated with the occurrence of brain injury during the late first or mid-second trimesters of pregnancy.[19] A number of congenital and minor physical anomalies have also been reported in schizophrenic patients.[3] These include low-set ears, epicanthal eye folds, wide space between the first and second toes, and abnormal dermatoglyphics.[3,20,21] It is felt that some of these anomalies may reflect abnormal brain development *in utero*. There is also prevalence of neurologic soft signs such as slight posturing of hands and transient choreoathetoid movements in the first two years of life.[22] Moreover, pre-schizophrenic children exhibit a greater extent of social maladjustment and anxiety, and perform poorly on neuropsychologic tests.[5] Such reports conclude that developmental problems may be subtle early in life and lead to the psychosis and loss of insight observed in adolescent and young adult individuals with schizophrenia.

BRAIN DEVELOPMENT IN HUMANS

The mammalian brain develops from the embryological ectoderm as a result of a highly complex and orderly sequence of events.[5] This particular scheme of central nervous system (CNS) development exhibits several discrete stages, which include neurolation, proliferation, neurogenesis, neural migration, and cellular/regional differentiation. Human neurolation takes place during the third and fourth weeks of gestation and results in the formation of primary brain vesicles, which will give rise to cerebrum, cerebellum, and brain stem. During the proliferation phase, neurons are generated from ventricular and subventricular zones, with most neocortical areas arising from both zones, and the rostral hippocampus, subiculum, and diencephalon rising from the ventricular areas. The process of cortical neurogenesis in human beings extends from 40 days post-conception to the middle of the second trimester.[23] Aberrations occurring after day 45 in humans may lead to development of a thinner cortex, and placement of ectopic neurons, both of which have been associated with schizophrenia. Neurons that have stopped dividing will enter the migration phase of CNS development, leading to development of a laminar brain structure composed of cortical plate and subplate as early as day 54. Various genetic and environmental insults can affect migration of cells, leading to several neurodevelopmental disorders such as autism, lissencephaly, mental retardation, dyslexia, fetal alcohol syndrome, and schizophrenia. The final phase of brain development involves differentiation, which may continue into the second decade of life, and consists of synaptogenesis, dendritic and axonal growth, synaptic elimination, axonal protraction, and myelination. Indeed, the last growth spurt in brain size occurs around the age of 13–15 years.[24] This last stage of brain development coincides with the manifestations of schizophrenic signs and symptoms in susceptible individuals. Thus, abnormalities of the CNS emerging as early as the latter part of the first trimester through to relatively late postnatal life may play a role in the development of schizophrenia. This view of the pathogenesis of schizophrenia argues in favor of a neurodevelopmental origin for this disorder.

Mouse brain development progresses through four prenatal stages that exhibit various susceptibilities to prenatal insults. These stages are:

1) Cleavage and blastulation, equal to embryonic day (E) 0 to E5
2) Implantation, gastrulation, and early organogenesis, equal to E5–E10
3) Organogenesis, equal to E10–E14
4) Fetal growth and development, equal to E14–E19 or 20.[25]

These stages in mouse brain development can be roughly compared to human brain development at the first (E0–E10) and second trimesters (E10–E19/20), respectively. Mouse postnatal brain development (postnatal days 1–10) corresponds roughly to the third trimester of brain growth in humans.[2] Recent evidence points to several prenatal sensitive periods in each brain area of the mouse, when neurogenesis, gliogenesis, or neuronal migration is at its peak.[26] Thus, brain areas, such as the cerebral cortex, hippocampus, thalamus, and cerebellum, each follow specific timetables for brain growth.[26] For example, critical periods of neurogenesis for various brain areas in the mouse consist of E9 (cerebellar Purkinje cells), E11–15.5 (hippocampal pyramidal cells), E11.5–E16 (cerebral cortex), E12.5 (thalamus), E17.5–P12 (dentate gyrus), and P2–P13 (cerebellar granule cells).[27] There are additional critical periods for neurogenesis that affect specific brain cell populations. For example, neural crest-derived cells migrating to craniofacial structures are most susceptible to various insults during E8.5–E10.5 in the mouse.[28] Accordingly, retinoic acid causes deleterious effects on development of brain and craniofacial structures during the E8–E10 period.[29] Previous studies showed an increased risk of growth retardation and other morbidity/mortality in mice prenatally exposed to an H1N1 strain of influenza virus in the E8–E10 period.[30] We have also shown that administration of the same strain of virus on E9 of pregnancy results in multiple brain abnormalities in postnatal mice.[31-33] Indeed, the onset of teratogenic susceptibility begins at relatively similar temporal windows in mouse and human (E5 and E11–12 respectively).[34] However, exact extrapolation from mouse to human is not possible based on specific days of pregnancy, but can be construed qualitatively from prenatal and postnatal peaks of neurogenesis, gliogenesis, and/or neuron migration/differentiation.[26] The accumulation of various immunologic, epidemiologic, and case study data indicates that prenatal maternal exposure to human influenza infection around late first to mid-second trimester can increase the risk of births that lead to schizophrenia.[2] The critical period encompassing E8–E10 in mouse corresponds roughly to the late first trimester in man. The developing brain during this period is susceptible to multiple insults (such as retinoic acid and influenza) and mutations like a 22q11 deletion. This is a mutation in the ubiquitin fusion-degradation 1 product (UFD-1) which affects the neural-crest derived cells populating the craniofacial structures. This mutation results in mental retardation, psychosis, and dysmorphology of the face in human and mouse.[28,35]

BRAIN PROTEINS GUIDING DEVELOPMENT

Several brain proteins participate in the early growth and development of mammalian CNS. We will focus on the brain markers that help guide brain development in an orderly fashion in human and mouse. Changes in the levels of these brain markers may reflect abnormal corticogenesis. The markers include Bcl-2 (B cell lymphoma-2 gene), neuronal nitric oxide (nNOS), Reelin, synaptosome-associated protein 25 kDa (SNAP-25), polysialic-acid neural cell adhesion molecule (PSA-NCAM), and glial fibrillary acidic protein (GFAP).

Bcl-2 is a membrane-bound protein of 25 kDa that strongly inhibits programmed cell death or apoptosis.[36] Bcl-2 mRNA and protein expression are developmentally regulated in human[37] and murine brains.[38] In humans, Bcl-2 protein changes significantly with age. There is an initial rise in early gestation,[39] followed by perinatal downregulation during infancy and a subsequent gradual upregulation during adulthood.[40] Recent evidence suggests downregulation of Bcl-2 in schizophrenia.[41]

Activity of nNOS has been associated with glutamate excitotoxicity, apoptosis, growth arrest, n-nitrosylation, and glutamate release.[42] nNOS also impacts pain perception, memory, LTP processing, and synaptogenesis.[43] Several reports have implicated the abnormal translocation of NADPH-diaphorase-positive cells (which colocalize nNOS) in schizophrenic brains.[9,10]

SNAP-25 is a highly conserved, 25 kDa synaptosome-associated protein that is considered a marker of presynaptic neurons.[44] SNAP-25 is also involved in axonal growth and transport, docking and exocytosis of neurotramsmitter vesicles, and increases in response to injury.[45,46] Brain levels of SNAP-25 in schizophrenic patients are abnormal, with decrease and increase in hippocampal and cingulate cortices respectively.[47–49]

PSA-NCAM is associated with cell migration, neurite growth, and plasticity. PSA-NCAM expression in schizophrenic dentate is deficient.[50]

Reelin is a secretory glycoprotein with relative molecular mass of 388 kDa encoding a long mRNA of about 12 kilobases.[51] The amino-terminus of Reelin is 25% identical to that of F-spondin, a protein secreted by the floor plate of the developing spinal cord and thought to regulate the adhesion and extension of commissural axons, and to tenascin, another adhesion molecule.[52] Reelin mRNA is first detected in the embryonic mouse brain on days 9.5–11.5. It then increases in concentration up to early postnatal days, then declines to adult levels. The first cells expressing Reelin are the Cajal-Rezius neurons. These are transient neurons that provide precise chemical signals (in the form of extracellular Reelin) to help guide migrating neurons to the appropriate targets, and are important in normal laminar organization of the brain.[53] The reeler mutant mouse exhibits widespread morphological abnormalities in various cortical structures, including abnormal positioning of neurons and aberrant orientation of cell bodies and fibers. In the cerebral cortex of the reeler mouse, neurons destined to form the subplate zone occupy ectopic positions in superficial cortical layers. Additionally, neurons developed later, which are destined to form the cortical plate, fail to bypass previously generated neurons. Thus, an inverted pattern of cortical development takes place in the mutant mice. There is a striking similarity in migration abnormalities involving the NADPH-diaphorase-positive cells in schizophrenic brains and the reeler phenotype.[9,10] The Reelin gene is present in human beings and maps to region 22 on the long arm of chromosome 7.[51] Recent postmortem human brain studies provide evidence for reduction in Reelin mRNA and protein in schizophrenic brains.[54,55]

GFAP is a 50 kDa intermediate filament protein belonging to the type III subclass of intermediate filament proteins. GFAP is specifically found in astroglia, which are highly responsive to neurologic insults. Astrogliosis is accompanied by an increase in GFAP expression. Previous reports have demonstrated absence of gliosis in schizophrenic brains[5] and recent reports indicate reductions in GFAP in schizophrenia.[56,57] However, a few reports indicate presence of gliosis in a subpopulation of schizophrenia patients.[58,59] Finally, several reports indicate the presence of abnormalities in the expression of several other molecules in the brains of schizophrenics: decreased levels of synapsin,[60] synaptophysin,[61,62] MAP2 and MAP5,[12] and glutamic acid decarboxylase.[11] There are also reported increases in levels of SNAP-25 and syntaxin,[48,62] mRNA for NMDA-2D,[63] and GAP-43[64] in schizophrenic brains. Additionally, numerous studies have reported on abnormalities of various neurotransmitter levels and/or receptors, which is beyond the scope of this chapter.[65]

NEUROPATHOLOGIC STUDIES OF SCHIZOPHRENIA

Numerous reports have documented various neuropathologic findings in postmortem brains of patients with schizophrenia.[59] These findings consist of cortical atrophy, ventricular enlargement, reduced volume of hippocampus, amygdala, and parahippocampal gyrus, disturbed cytoarchitecture in the hippocampus, cell loss and volume reduction in the thalamus, abnormal translocation of NADPH-diaphorase-positive cells in frontal and hippocampal areas, and reduced cell size in the Purkinje cells of the cerebellum.[1,59] Collectively, these data reflect abnormal corticogenesis during the mid-gestation period in schizophrenic patients.

GENETIC FACTORS IN SCHIZOPHRENIA

Recent evidence indicates that schizophrenia is a familial disorder with a complex mode of inheritance and variable phenotypic expression. Twins studies of schizophrenia found concordance rates of 46% for MZ twins and 14% for DZ twins.[66] The lifetime expectancy of manifesting schizophrenia in relatives of schizophrenic patients varies as a function of the closeness of relationship. Among first-degree relatives, lifetime expectancies are as follows: 5.6% for a parent, 10.1% for a sibling, 16.7% for a sibling with one schizophrenic parent, and 46.3% for children with two schizophrenic parents. In second-degree and third-degree relatives, the expectancies are 3.3% and 2.4%, respectively. Furthermore, adoption studies show a lifetime prevalence of 9.4% in the adopted-away offspring of schizophrenic parents and a lifetime prevalence of 1.2% in control adoptees.[66,67] Supportive MRI studies indicate that people at high risk of developing schizophrenia – subjects with two or more first-degree or second-degree relatives affected – have structural brain abnormalities such as small amygdala–hippocampal complexes and thalami similar to those with this disorder.[68,69] These data indicate that genetic factors play a major role in development of the disease. The exact mode of transmission of schizophrenia is unknown; family studies have ruled out single dominant gene defects. A multifactorial threshold model (additive effects of numerous genes at different loci) or a mixed model (interaction between a single major gene and a number of other genes) are the most likely.

Ongoing subpair studies seem likely to identify the genetic basis for this disorder within the next several years. Linkage and association studies have produced conflicting results that point to chromosomes 6, 11, 21, and X as potential sites in the genetic transmission of schizophrenia. Candidates such as the D_2 and D_4 genes have been ruled out. Some of the candidate association sites have included the porphobilinogen deaminase gene (for porphyria), the long arm of chromosome 11, and the association between the HLA9 marker and paranoid schizophrenia. More interesting, linkage studies of the gene for the D_3 receptor, which has restricted expression in the limbic regions and has been localized to the long arm of chromosome 3, have often been positive. Recent findings and association studies point to several susceptibility loci on chromosomes 6, 8, and 22. A mutation involving the function of ubiquitin fusion-degradation 1-like product (UFD-1L), an important molecule normally expressed in neural-crest-derived embryonic tissues, leads to development of an autosomal dominant syndrome (velocardiofacial syndrome) that is associated with an increased risk of developing schizophrenia. Patients with this syndrome also exhibit congenital abnormalities involving heart, thymus, and craniofacial development.

More recently, haploinsufficiency of the UFD-1L gene product has been identified in a cohort of schizophrenic patients, giving credence to potential involvement of this protein in schizophrenia.[29,70–72] Several other genes have also been implicated in the etiology of schizophrenia including Reelin,[49,55,73,74] DISC1-2, KCNN-3, and NOTCH-4.[72]

Obviously, studies of genes that influence the genesis of schizophrenia are important; however, investigation of these genes and their products will be confounded by clinical heterogeneity of disease and the influence of environmental factors on expression of these genes. Given that over 60% of affected individuals have neither first- nor second-degree relatives with schizophrenia,[67,75] studies of environmental factors such as influenza viral infection which affect brain expression of schizophrenia-related candidate genes become more relevant.

ROLE OF ENVIRONMENTAL AGENTS IN SCHIZOPHRENIA

Several environmental factors have been associated with births that lead to schizophrenia: famine during pregnancy,[2,76] Rh factor incompatibility,[77] autoimmunity due to infectious agents,[78] and viruses.[79–81] By far, the greatest number of positive reports link schizophrenia to maternal exposure to a human influenza virus.[2,82] The mechanisms suggested for a causal relationship between maternal exposure to viruses and development of schizophrenia in the progeny include:

1) The production of a maternal antibody to the influenza virus which may cross-react with fetal neuronal proteins
2) The impact of maternal and fetal sources of cytokines on fetal neurons
3) The production of fetal anti-NCAM, anti-caudate, and subthalamic nucleus antibodies secondary to maternal *Neisseria meningitides* and group A streptococcal infections.[78]

Recent reports have also implicated borna and rubella viruses in the induction of schizophrenia.[83,84]

Prenatal viral infection and schizophrenia

There is ample evidence to indicate that the greatest risk factor for development of schizophrenia is being related to a person with schizophrenia. In some subgroups, heredity can explain up to 70% of the liability to schizophrenia.[2,75,85] However, there is also a robust collection of reports indicating that environmental factors, especially viral infections, can increase the risk for development of schizophrenia.[2,67,82,86] I will now discuss some of the literature supporting the viral etiology of schizophrenia. Emil Kraepelin referred to the potential for infections to cause causing some forms of dementia praecox (schizophrenia) during the early years of brain development.[87] Menninger described 67 cases of schizophrenia in a large cohort of patients who contracted influenza during the pandemic of 1919.[88] Later, an excess of schizophrenic patients born during late winter and spring was reported as an indicator of influenza infections being responsible for these cases.[89,90] Indeed, the majority of nearly 50 studies performed in the intervening years indicate 5–15% excess schizophrenic birth in the northern hemisphere during the months of January and March.[2,91,92] This excess winter birth has been shown not to be due to unusual patterns of conception in mothers or to a methodological artifact.[2,93] Subsequent studies showed that the risk of schizophrenia was increased by 50% in Finnish individuals whose mothers had been exposed to the 1957 A2 influenza during the second trimester of pregnancy.[90,94] Later, nine of 16 studies performed replicated a positive association between prenatal influenza exposure and schizophrenia.[20,95–108] These association studies showed that exposure during the fourth to the seventh month of gestation affords a window of opportunity for influenza virus to cause its teratogenic effects on the embryonic brain.[2] Additionally, three out of five cohort and case control studies support a positive association between schizophrenia and maternal exposure to influenza prenatally.[80,109,110] Subsequent studies have shown that other viruses may also increase the risk for development of schizophrenia in the affected progeny of exposed mothers,[2] such as rubella.[84] By far the most controversial evidence linking viral exposure to development of schizophrenia was published recently[86] with data suggestive of a possible role for retroviruses in the pathogenesis of schizophrenia.[67] Karlsson and colleagues identified nucleotide sequences homologous to retroviral polymerase genes in the cerebrospinal fluid (CSF) of 28.6% of subjects with schizophrenia of recent origin and in 5% of subjects with chronic schizophrenia.[86] In contrast, such retroviral sequences were not found in any individuals with noninflammatory neurological illnesses or in normal subjects.[67,86] The upshot of these studies and previous epidemiological reports is that schizophrenia may represent the shared phenotype of a group of disorders whose etiopathogenesis involves interaction between genetic influences and environmental risks such as viruses operating on brain maturational processes.[67] Moreover, identification of potential environmental risk factors such as influenza virus or retroviruses in general will help in targeting early interventions repressing the expression of these transcripts, thus influencing the course and outcome of schizophrenia in susceptible individuals.[67]

BEHAVIORAL ABNORMALITIES IN SCHIZOPHRENIA

We have previously alluded to the presence of certain behavioral abnormalities in schizophrenic patients that are used diagnostically to identify affected individuals. These include abnormalities of perception (hallucinations), thought (delusions, cognitive disorganization), and affect (flattening, blunting).[111,112] There are, however, more subtle behavioral and cognitive problems, which can only be detected using carefully designed behavioral tests,[113] reflecting disruption of normal cognitive operations in the schizophrenic patients.

One such behavioral deficit consists of the inability of schizophrenic patients to filter or gate most of the sensory stimuli that they receive,[114–116] leading to sensory overload and cognitive fragmentation. Similar behavioral abnormalities can be quantified accurately in humans and mice by assessment of an operational measure known as the prepulse inhibition (PPI) of startle.[116–119] Schizophrenic patients are deficient in normal inhibition of the startle reflex that occurs when the startling stimulus is preceded by a weak prestimulus.[116,120] This neural deficit originates from abnormalities within the limbic-cortico-striato-pallido-thalamic circuitry.[121] PPI deficits have also been identified in ibotenic-acid lesioned rats,[122] heterozygous reeler mutant mice,[119] hyperglycinergic rats,[118] and NCAM-180 knock out mice,[117] and are produced in rodents treated with dopamine agonists, amphetamine, and glutamate antagonist PCP.

We will now provide supportive experimental results pointing to the suitability of a potential animal model for detailed biochemical and morphometric studies of etiological environmental factors which may cause abnormal brain development – specifically, the effects of prenatal viral infection on brain development as related to schizophrenia.

MOUSE INFECTION STUDIES

On day 9 of pregnancy, 12–14 week old C57BL/6 or BALB/c mice were infected with human influenza virus A/NWS/33 (H1N1). This day precedes the timetable of proliferation, differentiation, and migration of neurons and axons in embryonic neocortex and hippocampus in mice. Neonatal brains were processed for immunocytochemistry, western blot analysis, and microarray studies. Comparison of infected and sham-infected brains showed changes in several markers as detailed below.[31–33,123–125]

nNOS immunoreactivity in neocortex and hippocampus

Two reports have implicated the abnormal translocation of NADPH-diaphorase-positive cells (which colocalize nNOS) in schizophrenic brains.[9,10] We hypothesized that prenatal viral infection would affect the expression of neuronal NOS in the hippocampus. We selected to measure nNOS by immunocytochemistry and western blot instead of histochemical estimation of NADPH-diaphorase activity, due to the fact that the latter approach underestimates counts of NOS-containing cells.[126] SDS-PAGE and western blotting of homogenized infected brains showed an increased presence of nNOS in the anterior third of affected brains on days 14 and 35, followed by a decrease on day 56.[127] Additionally, nNOS expression in the middle third of experimental brains decreased significantly by day 56 (see Figure 9.1). The early increase in nNOS (probably functionally) reflects increased potential for glutamate excitotoxicity, apoptosis, growth arrest, n-nitrosylation, and increased glutamate release.[42] There is also the likelihood that an alteration in programmed expression of nNOS impacts adversely on cellular energy production via mitochondrial damage,[128] synaptogenesis, and programmed cell death.[43] Additionally, decreased nNOS level in rostral and midbrain homogenates at day 56, in infected animals, reflects permanent alteration in the expression of this protein in the adult animal.[127] This is similar to the report of reduced NADPH-diaphorase staining in the brains of adult schizophrenic patients,[9,10] reeler mouse mutants,[119] and hypoxic guinea pigs.[129]

SNAP-25 immunoreactivity in the hippocampus

The distribution of SNAP-25 in infected neonates varied with the anatomic location of the hippocampus in a septotemporal gradient. Quantitative densito-

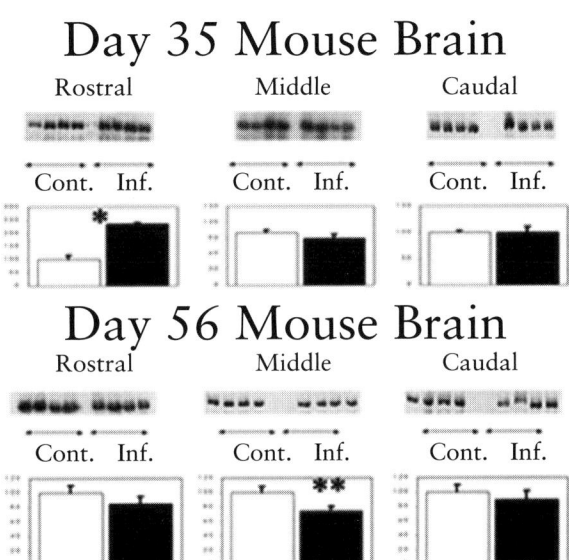

Figure 9.1 SDS-PAGE and western blotting of brain homogenates from sham (control) and prenatally-exposed P14, 35, and 56 mice. nNOS optical density is increased in rostral brain of P14 and 35 mice ($p < .005$), then decreases in P56. P56 mice also show a significant decrease in middle brain nNOS ($p < .05$).[127]

metric analysis of specific immunogold silver-enhanced SNAP-25 showed general increases in dorsal layers, except subplate, of 40–347% over control. In the experimental mid dorso-ventral hippocampus, SNAP-25 immunoreactivity (IR) increased over control in all layers, except for the hippocampal plate, but the extent of this increase was smaller than that found in the dorsal area (10–114%). Finally, in ventral levels, SNAP-25 IR was reduced in all layers except for minor increases of 9–10% in subplate and hippocampal layers (21–33% decrease against control). The region-dependent changes in expression of SNAP-25 in the hippocampi of neonates born to mothers exposed to human influenza infection during the late first trimester of pregnancy may reflect the potential for viral-induced glutamatergic excitotoxicity of the ventral hippocampus, as well as reactive synaptogenesis of dorsal and medial hippocampi in the developing brains of these neonatal mice.[32]

Reelin in neocortex and hippocampus

Prenatally-infected mouse brains from postnatal day 0 showed significant reductions in Reelin-positive cell counts in layer 1 of the neocortex and other cortical and hippocampal layers when compared to controls.[33] Although layer 1 Cajal-Retzius cells produced significantly less Reelin in infected animals, they showed normal production of calretinin and nNOS when compared to control brains (see Figure 9.2). Moreover, prenatal viral infection caused decreases in neocortical and hippocampal thickness.[33] These results implicate a potential role for prenatal viral infection in causation of neuronal migration abnormalities via reduction in Reelin production in neonatal brains. This is especially important because levels of Reelin protein are reduced in several brain areas of adult schizophrenics or in heterozygous reeler mutant mice, with both groups exhibiting defective sensorimotor gating abnormalities.[54,55,74,119] Moreover, human influenza infection in day 9 of pregnancy in our mouse model also causes significant reductions in neocortical and hippocampal Reelin protein.[33]

GFAP immunoreactivity in neocortex and hippocampus

We hypothesized that human influenza infection in E9 pregnant mice would alter the expression of glial fibrillary acidic protein (GFAP), an important marker of gliosis, neuronal migration, and reactive injury in developing brains in P0, 14, and 35 mice. Determination of cellular GFAP immunoreactivity (IR) in the cortex and hippocampus of control and experimental brains showed time-dependent increases in GFAP-positive cell counts, with further development of brains from P0 to 14 and 35 days postnatally. The GFAP-positive cells in prenatally infected brains showed hypertrophy and more stellate morphology. These results implicate a significant role for infection by human influenza virus on subsequent gliosis, which persists throughout brain development in mice from birth to adolescence.[124] These findings suggest

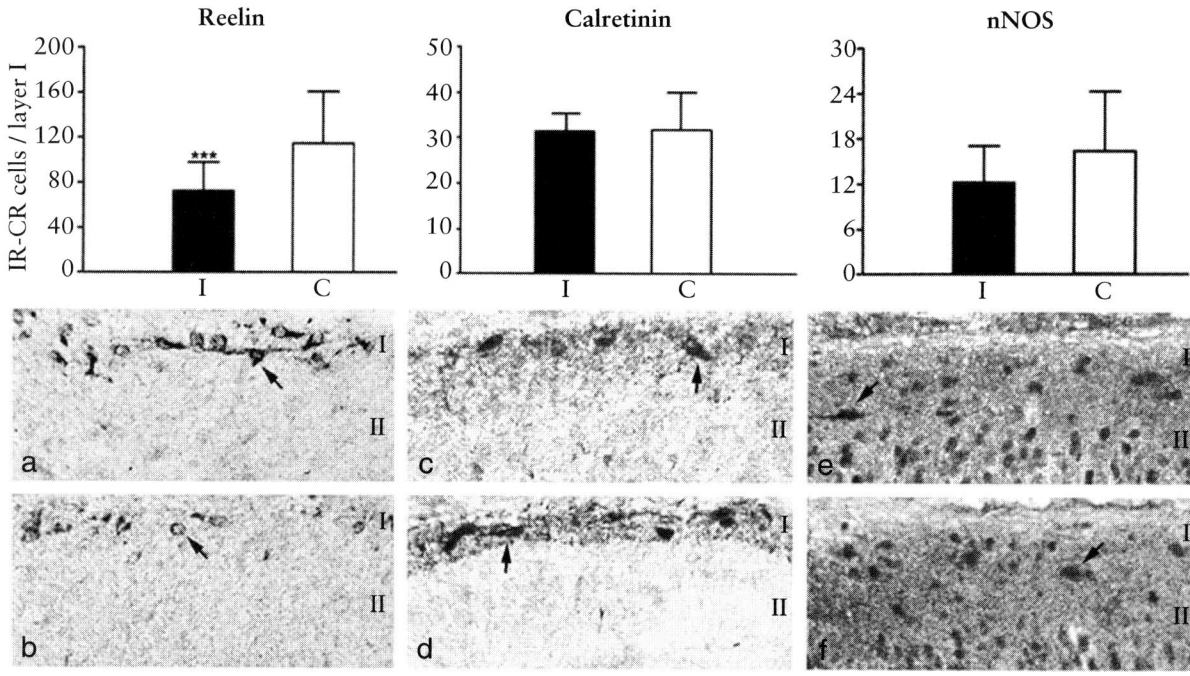

Figure 9.2 Histograms of immunoreactive Cajal-Retzius cells in cortical layer 1 of sham (upper: c; lower: a, c, e) and prenatally-exposed (upper: 1; lower: b, d, f) mouse brains. Reelin positive cells are significantly reduced in number vs unchanged calretinin and nonsignificantly reduced nNOS.[33]

that prenatal human influenza infection in mice can have deleterious effects on brain development, that persist into the prepubescent period of sexual maturation – an important developmental period which precedes manifestation of psychosis and behavioral abnormalities in schizophrenic subjects.[124]

Pyramidal cell atrophy

We investigated the role of maternal exposure to human influenza virus (H1N1) in C57BL/6 mice on day 9 of pregnancy, examining pyramidal and non-pyramidal cell density, pyramidal nuclear area, and overall brain size in day 0 neonates and 14-week-old progeny, and compared them to sham-infected cohorts. Pyramidal cell density increased significantly ($p < .0038$) by 170% in day 0 infected mice vs controls. Nonpyramidal cell density decreased by 33% in day 0 infected progeny vs controls, albeit nonsignificantly. Pyramidal cell nuclear size decreased significantly ($p < .0465$) by 29% in exposed newborn mice vs controls. Fourteen-week-old exposed mice continued to show significant increases in both pyramidal and nonpyramidal cell density values vs controls ($p < .05$). By the same token, pyramidal cell nuclear size exhibited 37–43% reduction when compared to control values; these were statistically significant vs controls ($p < .05$). Brain and ventricular area measurements in adult exposed mice also showed significant increases and decreases respectively vs controls (see Figure 9.3). Ventricular brain ratios exhibited 38–50% decreases in exposed mice vs controls. While the rate of pyramidal cell proliferation per unit area decreased from birth to adulthood in both control and exposed groups, nonpyramidal cell growth rate increased only in the exposed adult mice (see Table 9.1). These data show for the first time that exposure of pregnant mice on day 9 of pregnancy to a sublethal intranasal administration of influenza virus has both short-term and longlasting deleterious effects on developing brain structure in the progeny, as evidenced by altered pyramidal and non-pyramidal cell density values and atrophy of pyramidal cells despite a normal cell proliferation rate and final enlargement of the brain. Moreover, abnormal corticogenesis is associated with development of abnormal behavior in the exposed adult mice.[123–125]

GFAP, GAD65, and GAD67 kDa protein levels in BALB/c mice

In this study, we decided to use the same infection protocol in a different strain of pregnant mouse (BALB/c), to identify whether the same pathology would be present in the exposed neonatal and adult mice. The results indicated increased expression of GFAP protein in exposed brains across all ages vs sham-infected mice (see Figure 9.4). Levels of GFAP increased by 475% ($p < .05$), 100%, 54.5%, and 27% in 0, 14, 35, and 56-day-old exposed brains vs controls respectively (see Figure 9.5). Similarly, levels of GAD 65 kDa protein increased by 59%, 43% ($p < .05$), 24% ($p < .05$), and 16.5% in 0, 14, 35, and 56-day-old exposed brains vs controls respectively (see Figure 9.5). The level of GAD 67 kDa protein also increased by 31%, 49%, 53% ($p < .05$), and 45% ($p < .05$) in the 0, 14, 35, and 56-day-old exposed mice vs controls respectively (see Figure 9.5). The levels of β-actin varied between the two groups nonsignificantly.

We had previously shown time-dependent rises in levels of GFAP in the offspring of exposed C57BL6 mice.[124] A similar pattern of GFAP rise in BALB/c mice would connote the presence of identical mechanisms of injury in two strains of mouse secondary to viral insult *in utero*. The BALB/c exposed mice expressed 22% more GFAP during early adulthood (day 56) vs controls. This is quite striking, since in adult autistic brains, levels of GFAP are also elevated significantly in several brain sites.[123] The similarity between elevated levels of GFAP in C57Bl/6 and BALB/c mice and autistic brains may point to shared mechanisms of immune activation and injury.

GAD65 and 67 kDa proteins are important rate-limiting enzymes that modulate conversion of GABA from a pool of L-glutamate.[131] Increased GAD activity as seen here may signify greater conversion of excess glutamate (probably generated by an increased number of astrocytes), another potential marker of excitotoxicity and a parallel marker for brain injury similar to GFAP. Interestingly, the major rise in levels of GAD65/67 kDa proteins occurs beyond day 0, especially days 14–56, in the exposed brains. We had previously shown that nonpyramidal cell density increased significantly in 14-week-old adult exposed C57BL6 mice.[123] Nonpyramidal cells consist of GABAergic interneurons which localize GAD65 and 67 enzymes; this piece of evidence supports the current results indicating a parallel increase in both GAD enzymatic levels and GABAergic cells in the exposed brains.

DNA microarray studies

Preliminary results using cDNA microarray technology, spanning approximately 20,000 genes in day 0 exposed BALB/c whole brain homogenates, point to significant alterations in levels of several important gene families in response to prenatal viral insult (see Table 9.2).[132]

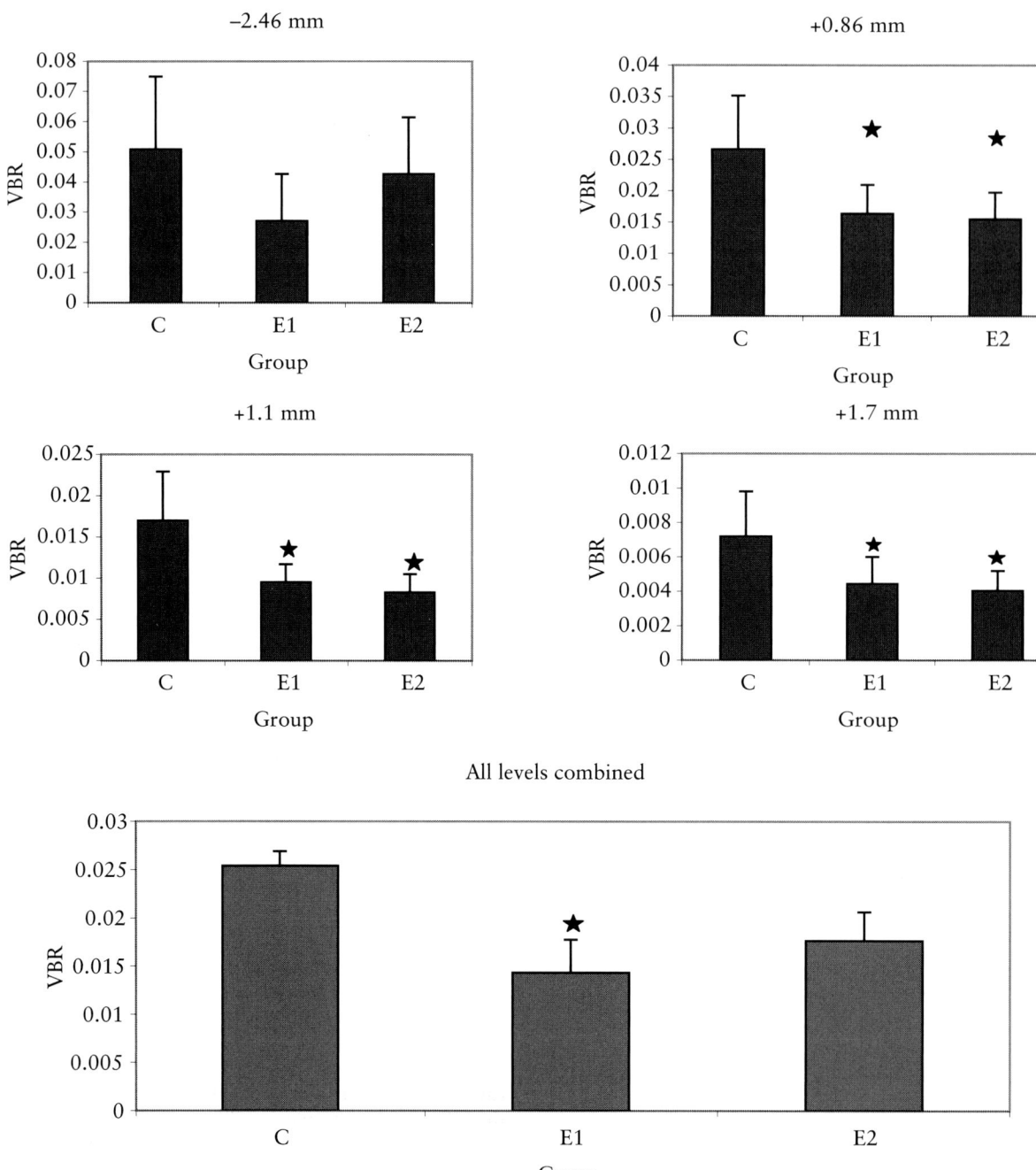

Figure 9.3 VBR measurements are shown for 14-week-old control and exposed mice at four brain levels and combined. Note the significant reductions in VBRs in the exposed brains compared to controls. E1 denotes exposed mice showing deficits in prepulse inhibition (PPI). E2 denotes exposed mice not showing deficits in PPI. Brain levels used were at −2.46, +0.86, +1.1, and +1.7 mm from bregma.[130] Asterisk (*) indicates statistical significance vs control as follows: at +0.86 mm E1 $p < .045$, E2 $p < .04$; at +1.1 mm E1 $p < .038$, E2 $p < .0166$; at +1.7 mm E1 $p < .015$, E2 $p < .0075$; at all levels combined E1 $p < .037$ (t test, unpaired).[123]

PRENATAL INFLUENZA INFECTION AND SCHIZOPHRENIA

Table 9.1 The effects of prenatal viral exposure on day 9 pregnant C57BL/6 mice progeny brain cell proliferation

	Birth		Adulthood		
	Control	Exposed	Control	Exposed PPI abnormality	no PPI abnormality
Pyramidal cell density (cells/mm^2)	4810 ± 704	8178 ± 660[1]	826 ± 118.5	1173 ± 39[3]	1075.2 ± 110.2[4]
Δ	100%	↑ 170%	100%	↑ 142%	↑ 130%
Nonpyramidal cell density (cells/mm^2)	522 ± 151	351 ± 105	329 ± 17	505 ± 62[5]	481 ± 73.5[6]
Δ	100%	↓ 33%	100%	↑ 153%	↑ 143%
Pyramidal nuclear size (mm^2)	73 ± 12.4	51.5 ± 4[2]	132 ± 28	83 ± 6.4[7]	75 ± 6.4[8]
Δ	100%	↓ 29%	100%	↓ 37%	↓ 43%

In two-tailed t tests vs control: [1]$p < .0038$; [2]$p < .0465$; [3]$p < .0085$; [4]$p < .0379$; [5]$p < .0092$; [6]$p < .0252$; [7]$p < .04$; [8]$p < .0259$.[123]

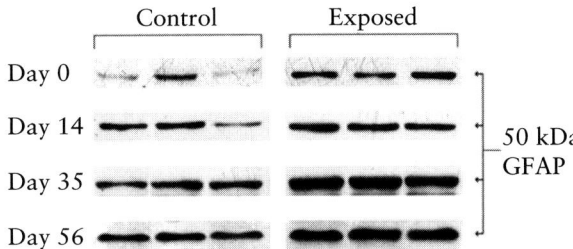

Figure 9.4 Western blot analysis of sham (control) and prenatally-exposed P0, 14, 35, and 56 mouse brains. GFAP optical density is increased in exposed brains.[133]

The dataset strongly indicates that cell structure, both intracellular and intercellular, may be disturbed as the major cytosolic chaperone system (t-complex or CCT), involved in folding many proteins that form the cytoskeleton, has altered gene expression. HSC70, which is known to function in concert with this complex, is also dysregulated. Downstream of this, the LMO4-LIM protein, which has been implicated in organization and coordination of cytoskeletal structures, also has altered gene expression. Interestingly Bicaudal D, which is also associated with cytoskeletal organization although its precise role is still not characterized, is altered. This is interesting as this and many other genes have been studied in the context of development, suggesting that this experimental dataset may well be experiencing a shift in developmental progression. Collectively, this group of gene expression changes strongly indicates that cellular integrity is compromised in this experimental system. At the intracellular level there is also evidence that cell structure and perhaps cell volume is disturbed due to altered expression of aquaporin 4 and carbonic anhydrase 3, indicating ionic homeostasis is compromised. It is also clear that the integrity and architecture of the brain and neurons is compromised in this experimental system. Two major proteins of myelin, myelin basic protein and proteolipid protein, have altered expression. Additionally there is evidence of altered neuronal function with alteration in expression of a glycine receptor and the noepinephrine transporter. Underlying these changes, there is more generic evidence of a disruption of the molecular integrity of the coordination of gene expression and protein function. Gene expression changes are evident for genes involved in transcription, translation, protein degradation, signal transduction, and post-translational modification (see Table 9.2).[132]

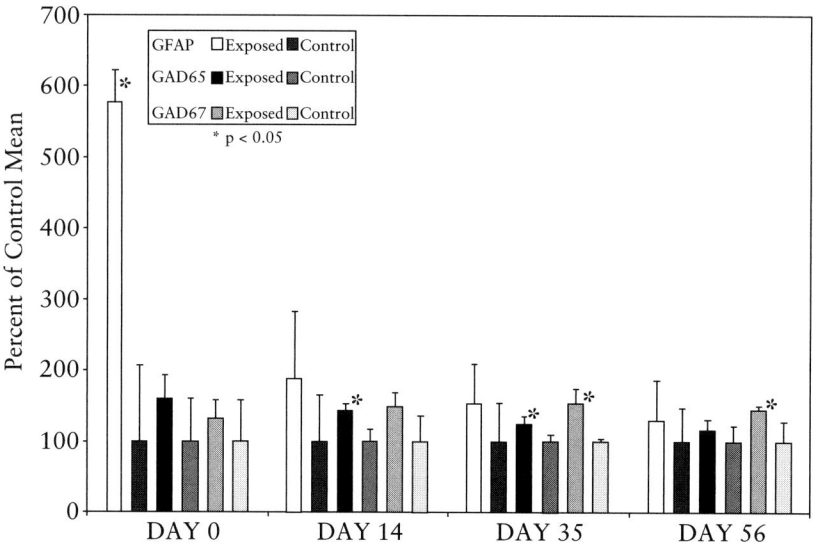

Figure 9.5 Histogram of GFAP and GAD 65 and 67 kDa proteins in P0, 14, 35, and 56 mouse brains analyzed by Western blotting. There are significant increases in GFAP in P0 exposed mice, GAD 65 in P14 and 35 exposed mice, and GAD 67 in P35 and 56 exposed mice.[133]

CONCLUSIONS

Prenatal viral infection in the mouse, on day 9 of pregnancy, causes significant deleterious effects on the growing brains of exposed offspring, leading to abnormal corticogenesis, pyramidal cell atrophy, and alterations in brain levels of Reelin, nNOS, SNAP-25, GFAP, and GAD proteins. Additionally, exposed animals exhibit reduced prepulse inhibition and other abnormal behavior in adulthood. Further preliminary study using cDNA microarray technology reveals that the viral effects are not limited to those proteins cited above, but encompass a large family of genes that affect brain development *in utero*. Experimental animal models such as this may help in gaining insights into the environmental etiologies of severe mental disorders like schizophrenia and autism.

ACKNOWLEDGMENTS

The work of this author has been generously supported by NARSAD, Stanley Medical Research Institute, March of Dimes, Minnesota Medical Foundation, Kunin Fund of St Paul Foundation, and the Jonty Foundation.

Table 9.2 Gene profile analysis in exposed mouse brains

Gene/protein	Function	Functional classification	Change
t-complex testis – 3***	Subunit of CCT-complex	Protein folding	Up
Hsc 70-interacting protein***	Heat shock protein	Protein folding	Up
LMO4***	LIM-protein	Cytoskeleton organization	Down
Bicaudal D homolog***	Cytoskeleton	Cytoskeleton organization	Down
Myelin basic protein*	Myelin stability	Axonal stability	Down
Aquaporin 4*	–	Cell integrity	Down
NET–protein synaptosomal complex***	Noepinephrine transporter	Neurotransmission	Up
Synaptosomal complex protein SC65***	–	Neurotransmission	Up
Eukaryotic translation initiation factor 2*	Translation	Protein translation	Down
UDP-galactose: N-acetyl-galactosamine-1,3-galacto-transyltransferase***	Enzyme	Post-translational modification (glycosylation)	Up
Zn-finger and BTB-domain containing protein***	Likely transcription	Gene expression	Up
SWI/SNF related protein***	Chromatin structure	Gene expression	Up
DEAD box protein*	RNA helicase	Gene expression	Down
Adipose differentiation related-protein***	–	Gene expression	Up
Mitochondrial ribosomal protein L3***	Ribosome	Gene expression	Up
Growth arrest inducible 45***	Cell cycle	Gene expression	Up
Decay accelerating factor-1***	–	Gene expression	Up
Apoptosis-associated speck-like protein***	Apoptosis	Cell death	Up

Table 9.2 Continued

Gene/protein	Function	Functional classification	Change
Protein kinase inhibitor, alpha-subunit*	Kinase	Signaling	Down
Ryanodine receptor 2***	Receptor	Signaling	Up
Insulin-like growth factor binding protein-4***	Likely receptor	Signaling	Up
Sirtuin 7 homolog***	–	Signaling	Up
RIKEN cDNA 8030469F12 gene*	Similar to protein tyrosine kinase	Signaling	Down
Cytochrome P450***	Enzyme	Stress	Up
Coagulation factor XIII, beta subunit***	Coagulation	Wound healing	Up
RNA imprinted and accumulated in nucleus*	Unknown	Unknown	Down
Zinc finger protein 93***	Unknown	Unknown	Up
RIKEN cDNA 2310009017 gene***	Unknown	Unknown	Up
RIKEN cDNA 2610036L13***	Unknown	Unknown	Down
RIKEN cDNA 2610205E22***	Unknown	Unknown	Up
Carbonic anhydrase 3**	Enzyme	Ionic homeostasis	Down
Androgen regulated protein**	Unknown	Unknown	Up
RIKEN cDNA 3732409C05 gene*	Unknown	Unknown	Down
RIKEN cDNA 3110038015 gene**	Unknown	Unknown	Down
Proteolipid protein (PLP)**	Myelin stability	Axonal stability	Down

Table 9.2 Continued			
Gene/protein	Function	Functional classification	Change
Glycine receptor, beta subunit**	Receptor	Neurotransmission	Down
AI850305 Otubain, cysteine protease in UB-pathway**	Protease	Protein degradation	Down
Transcription factor 4**	Transcription factor	Gene expression	Down
Nucleolin**	Nuclear structure	Gene expression	Down

*Gene was measured by RMA and MBEI analysis; **gene was measured by RMA analysis only; and ***gene was measured by MBEI analysis only.[132]

REFERENCES

1. Andreasen NC. A unitary model of schizophrenia. Bleuler's 'Fragmented phrene' as schizencephaly. *Arch Gen Psychiatry* 1999; **56**: 781–93.
2. Susser ES, Brown AS, Gorman JM. *Prenatal Exposures in Schizophrenia*. Washington DC: American Psychiatric Press, 1999.
3. Nasrallah HA. Neurodevelopmental pathogenesis of schizophrenia. *Psych Clin N America* 1993; **16**: 269–73.
4. Murray RM, O'Callaghan E, Castle DJ. A neurodevelopmental approach to the classification of schizophrenia. *Schiz Bull* 1992; **18**: 319–32.
5. Weinberger DR. Schizophrenia as a neurodevelopmental disorder. In: *Schizophrenia* (Hirsch SR, Weinberger DR, eds). Cambridge MA: USA Blackwell Science, 1995; 293–323.
6. Schulz SC, Killer MM, Kishore PR et al. Ventricular enlargement in teenage patients with schizophrenia spectrum disorder. *Am J Psychiatry* 1983; **140**: 1592–4.
7. Illowsky B, Juliano DM, Bigelow LB, Weinberger DR. Stability of CT scan findings in schizophrenia. *J Neurol Neurosurg Psych* 1988; **51**: 209–13.
8. Suddath RL, Christison GW, Torrey EF et al. Anatomical abnormalities in the brains of monozygotic twins discordant for schizophrenia. *N Engl J Med* 1990; **322**: 789–94.
9. Akbarian S, Bunney WE Jr, Potkin SG et al. Altered distribution of nicotinamide-adenine-dinucleotide-phosphate-diaphorase cells in frontal lobe of schizophrenics implies disturbances of cortical development. *Arch Gen Psychiatry* 1993; **50**: 169–77.
10. Akbarian S, Vinuela A, Kim JJ et al. Distorted distribution of nicotinamide-adenine-dinucleotide-phosphate-diaphorase neurons in temporal lobe of schizophrenics implies anomalous cortical development. *Arch Gen Psychiatry* 1993; **50**: 178–87.
11. Akbarian S, Kim JJ, Potkin SG et al. Gene expression for glutamic acid decarboxylase is reduced without loss of neurons in prefrontal cortex of schizophrenics. *Arch Gen Psychiatry* 1995; **52**: 258–78.
12. Arnold SE, Hyman BT, Hoesen GWV, Damasio AR. Some cytoarchitectural abnormalities of the entorhinal cortex in schizophrenia. *Arch Gen Psychiatry* 1991; **48**: 625–32.
13. Jakob H, Beckmann H. Gross and histological criteria for developmental disorders in brains of schizophrenics. *J Royal Soc Med* 1989; **82**: 466–9.
14. Selemon LD, Rajkowska G, Goldman-Rakic PS. Abnormally high neuronal density in the schizophrenic cortex: a morphometric analysis of prefrontal area 9 and occipital area 17. *Arch Gen Psychiatry* 1995; **52**: 805–18.
15. Bunney BG, Potkin SG, Bunney WE. Neuropathological studies of brain tissue in schizophrenia. *J Psychiatric Res* 1997; **31**: 159–73.
16. Benes FM, Sorensen I, Bird ED. Reduced neuronal size in posterior hippocampus of schizophrenic patients. *Schizopher Bull* 1991; **17**: 597–608.
17. Benes FM, Sorensen I, Bird ED. Reduced neuronal size in posterior hippocampus of schizophrenic patients. *Schiz Bull* 1991; **17**: 597–608.
18. Arnold SE, Ruscheinsky DD, Han LY. Further evidence of abnormal cytoarchitecture of the entorhinal cortex in schizophrenia using spatial point pattern analyses. *Biol Psychiatry* 1997; **42**: 639–47.
19. Roberts GW, Colter N, Lofthouse R et al. Gliosis in schizophrenia: a survey. *Biol Psychiatry* 1986; **21**: 1043–50.
20. Torrey EF, Bowler AE, Taylor EH, Gottesman, II. *Schizophrenia and Manic Depression Disorders: The Biological Roots of Mental Illness as Revealed by a Landmark Study of Identical Twins*. New York: Basic Books, 1994.
21. Van Oss J. Dermatoglyphic abnormalities in psychosis: a tie-in study. *Biol Psychiatry* 1997; **41**: 624–6.
22. Walker E, Lewine RJ. Prediction of adult-onset schizophrenia from childhood home movies of the patients. *Am J Psychiatry* 1990; **147**: 1052–6.
23. Rakic P. Specification of cerebral cortical areas. *Science* 1988; **241**: 170–6.
24. Epstein HT. Stages in human brain development. *Devel Brain Res* 1986; **30**: 114–9.
25. Hogan B, Beddington R, Constantini F, Lacy E. *Manipulating the Mouse Embryo. A Laboratory Manual*. Plainview NY: Cold Spring Harbor Laboratory Press, 1994.
26. Morgane PJ, Austin-LaFrance RJ, Bronzino JD et al. Malnutrition and the developing central nervous system. In: *The*

Vulnerable Brain and Environmental Risks, Volume 1: Malnutrition and Hazard Assessment (Isaacson RL, Jensen RF, eds). New York: Plenum Press, 1992; 3–44.
27. Rodier PM. Chronology of neuron development: animal studies and their clinical implications. *Develop Med Child Neurol* 1980; **22**: 525–45.
28. Yamagishi H, Garg, V, Matsuoka R et al. A molecular pathway revealing a genetic basis for human cardiac and cranio-facial defects. *Science* 1999; **283**: 1158–60.
29. Holson RR, Adams J, Ferguson SA. Gestational stage-specific effects of retinoic acid exposure in the rat. *Neurotoxicol Teratol* 1999; **21**: 393–402.
30. Molanova A, Blaskovic D. The influence of influenza infection of pregnant mice on the development of their fetuses. *Acta Virol* 1975; **19**: 259.
31. Fatemi SH, Sidwell R, Akhter P et al. Human influenza viral infection in utero increases nNOS expression in hippocampi of neonatal mice. *Synapse* 1998; **29**: 84–8.
32. Fatemi SH, Sidwell R, Kist D et al. Differential expression of synaptosome-associated protein 25 kDa (SNAP-25) in hippocampi of neonatal mice following exposure to human influenza virus in utero. *Brain Res* 1998; **800**: 1–9.
33. Fatemi SH, Emamian ES, Kist D et al. Defective corticogenesis and reduction in reelin immunoreactivity in cortex and hippocampus of prenatally infected neonatal mice. *Mol Psychiatry* 1999; **4**: 145–54.
34. Wilson JG. General principles of experimental teratology. In: *Congenital Malformations: Proceedings of the First International Conference* (Fishbein M, ed). Philadelphia: Lippincott, 1961: 191.
35. LaMantia AS. Forebrain induction, retinoic acid, and vulnerability to schizophrenia: insights from molecular and genetic analysis in developing mice. *Biol Psychiatry* 1999; **46**: 19–30.
36. Adams JM, Cory S. The Bcl-2 protein family: arbiters of cell survival. *Science* 1998; **281**: 1322–6.
37. Marshall KA, Daniel SE, Cairns N et al. Upregulation of the anti-apoptotic protein Bcl-2 may be an early event in neurodegeneration: studies on Parkinson's and incidental Lewy body disease. *Biochem Biophys Res Commun* 1997; **240**: 84–7.
38. Shimohama S, Fujimoto S, Sumida Y, Tanino H. Differential expression of rat brain bcl-2 family proteins in development and aging. *Biochem Biophys Res Commun* 1998; **252**: 92–6.
39. Chan WY, Yew IY. Apoptosis and Bcl2 oncoprotein expression in the human fetal central nervous system. *Anatom Record* 1998; **252**: 165–75.
40. Jarskog LF, Gilmore JH. Developmental expression of Bcl-2 protein in human cortex. *Brain Res Dev Brain Res* 2000; **119**: 225–30.
41. Jarskog LF, Gilmore JH, Selinger ES, Lieberman JA. Cortical bcl-2 protein expression and apoptotic regulation in schizophrenia. *Biol Psychiatry* 2000; **48**: 641–50.
42. Nicotera P, Brune B, Bagetta G. Nitric oxide: inducer or suppresser of apoptosis. *Trends Pharmacol Sci* 1997; **18**: 189–90.
43. Moore PK, Handy RLC. Selective inhibitors of neuronal nitric oxide synthase – is no NOS really good for the nervous system? *Trends Pharmacol Sci* 1997; **18**: 204–11.
44. Oyler GA, Higgins GA, Hart RA et al. The identification of a novel synaptosomal-associated protein, SNAP-25, differentially expressed by neuronal subpopulations. *J Cell Biol* 1989; **109**: 3039–52.
45. Osen-Sand A, Catsicas M, Staple JK et al. Inhibition of axonal growth by SNAP-25 antisense oligonucleotides *in vitro* and *in vivo*. *Nature* 1993; **364**: 445–8.
46. Grabs D, Bergmann M, Urban AP, Grayzl M. Rab3 proteins and SNAP-25, essential components of the exocytosis machinery in conventional synapses, are absent from ribbon synapses of the mouse retina. *Eur J Neurosci* 1996; **8**: 162–8.
47. Young CE, Arima K, Xie J et al. SNAP-25 deficit and hippocampal connectivity in schizophrenia. *Cerebral Cortex* 1998; **8**: 261–8.
48. Gabriel SM, Haroutunian V, Powchik P et al. Increased concentrations of presynaptic proteins in the cingulated cortex of subjects with schizophrenia. *Arch Gen Psychiatry* 1997; **54**: 557–66.
49. Fatemi SH, Earle JA, Stary JM et al. Altered levels of the synaptosomal protein SNAP-25 in hippocampus of subjects with mood disorders and schizophrenia. *Neuroreport* 2001; **12**: 3257–62.
50. Barbeau D, Liang JJ, Robitaille Y et al. Decreased expression of the embryonic form of the neural cell adhesion molecule in schizophrenic brains. *Proc Natl Acad Sci USA* 1995; **92**: 2785–9.
51. D'Arcangelo G, Miao GG, Chen SC et al. A protein related to extracellular matrix proteins deleted in the mouse mutant reeler. *Nature* 1995; **374**: 719–23.
52. Vrucnic N, Chiquet-Ehrismann RR. Tenascin function and regulation of expression. *Symp Soc Exp Biol* 1993; **47**: 155–62.
53. D'Arcangelo G, Nakajima K, Miyata T et al. Reelin is a secreted glycoprotein recognized by the CR-50 monoclonal antibody. *J Neurosci* 1997; **17**: 23–31.
54. Impagnatiello F, Guidotti AR, Pesold C et al. A decrease of reelin expression as a putative vulnerability factor in schizophrenia. *Proc Natl Acad Sci USA* 1998; **95**: 15718–23.
55. Fatemi SH, Earle J, McMenomy T. Reduction in reelin immunoreactivity in hippocampus of subjects with schizophrenia, bipolar disorder, and major depression. *Mol Psychiatry* 2000; **5**: 654–63.
56. Rajkowska G, Miguel-Hidalgo J, Makkos Z et al. Layer-specific reductions in GFAP-reactive astroglia in the dorsolateral prefrontal cortex in schizophrenia. *Schizophr Res* 2002; **57**: 127.
57. Fatemi SH, Laurence JA, Araghi-Niknam M et al. Glial fibrillary acidic protein is reduced in cerebellum of subjects with major depression, but not schizophrenia. *Schizophr Res* 2004; **69**: 317–23.
58. Arnold SE, Franz BR, Trojanowski JQ et al. Glial fibrillary acidic protein-immunoreactive astrocytosis in elderly patients with schizophrenia and dementia. *Acta Neuropath* 1996; **91**: 269–77.
59. Arnold SE, Trojanowski JQ. Recent advances in defining the neuropathology of schizophrenia. *Acta Neuropath* 1997; **92**: 217–31.
60. Browning MD, Dudek EM, Rapier JL et al. Significant reductions in synapsin but not synaptophysin specific activity in the brains of some schizophrenics. *Biol Psychiatry* 1993; **34**: 529–35.
61. Glantz LA, Lewis DA. Reduction of synaptophysin immunoreactivity in the prefrontal cortex of subjects with schizophrenia. *Arch Gen Psychiatry* 1997; **54**: 943–52.
62. Honer WG, Falkai P, Young C et al. Cingulate cortex synaptic terminal proteins and neural cell adhesion molecule in schizophrenia. *Neurosci* 1997; **78**: 99–110.
63. Akbarian S, Sucher NJ, Bradley D et al. Selective alterations in gene expression for NMDA receptor subunits in prefrontal cortex of schizophrenics. *J Neurosci* 1996; **16**: 19–30.
64. Perrone-Bizzozero NI, Sower AC, Bird ED et al. Levels of the growth-associated protein GAP-43 are selectively increased in association cortices in schizophrenia. *Proc Natl Acad Sci USA* 1996; **93**: 14182–7.
65. Bachus SE, Kleinman JE. The neuropathology of schizophrenia. *J Clin Psychiatry* 1996; **57**(S11): 72–83.
66. Asherson P, Mane R, McGuffin P. Genetics and schizophrenia. In: *Schizophrenia* (Hirsch SR, Weinberger DR, eds). Cambridge MA: Blackwell Scientific, 1995; 253–74.

67. Lewis DA. Retroviruses and the pathogenesis of schizophrenia. *Proc Natl Acad Sci USA* 2001; **94**: 4293–4.
68. Lawrie SM, Whalley K, Kestelman JN et al. Magnetic resonance imaging of brain in people at high risk of developing schizophrenia. *Lancet* 1999; **353**: 30–33.
69. Harrison PJ. Brains at risk of schizophrenia. *Lancet* 1999; **353**: 3–4.
70. Pasini A. Association between schizophrenia and the UFD1L promoter polymorphism-277. *Soc Neurosci* 1999; **25**: 571.
71. Riley B, Williamson R. Sane genetics for schizophrenia. *Nature Med* 2000; **6**: 253–5.
72. Mirnics K, Lewis DA. Genes and subtypes of schizophrenia. *Trends Mol Med* 2001; **7**: 169–74.
73. Fatemi SH. Reelin mutations in mouse and man: from reeler mouse to schizophrenia, mood disorders, autism and lissencephaly. *Mol Psychiatry* 2001; **6**: 129–33.
74. Guidotti A, Auta J, Davis JM et al. Decrease in reelin and glutamic acid decarboxylase67 (GAD67) expression in schizophrenia and bipolar disorder: a postmortem brain study. *Arch Gen Psychiatry* 2000; **57**: 1061–9.
75. Gottesman II, Erlenmeyer-Kimling L. Family and twin strategies as a headstart in defining prodromes and endophenotypes for hypothetical early interventions in schizophrenia. *Schizophr Res* 2001; **51**: 93–102.
76. Cannon M, Jones PB, Murray RM. Obstetric complications and schizophrenia: historical and meta-analytic review. *Am J Psychiatry* 2002; **159**: 1080–92.
77. Hollister JM, Laing P, Madnick SA. Rhesus incompatability as a risk factor for schizophrenia in male adults. *Arch Gen Psychiatry* 1996; **53**: 19–24.
78. Wright P, Murray RM. Schizophrenia: prenatal influenza and autoimmunity. *Ann Med* 1993; **25**: 497–502.
79. Franzek E, Ungvari GS (eds). *Recent Advances in Leonhardian Nosology I*. Hong Kong: Würzburg, 1997.
80. Wright P, Rakei N, Rifkin L, Muray R. Maternal influenza, obstetric complications, and schizophrenia. *Am J Psychiatry* 1995; **152**: 1714–20.
81. Takei N, Mortensen PB, Klaening U et al. Relationship between in utero exposure to influenza epidemics and risk of schizophrenia in Denmark. *Biol Psychiatry* 1996; **40**: 817–24.
82. Maher BA. The infection connection in schizophrenia. *Scientist* 2003; **17**(21): 29–33.
83. Waltrip RW, Lieberman JA, Robinson DG et al. Borna disease virus seroconversion in first episode schizophrenia. *Biol Psychiatry* 1997; **41**: 1145.
84. Brown AS, Cohen P, Susser E. Psychosis after prenatal exposure to rubella. *Biol Psychiatry* 1997; **41**: 815.
85. Gottesman II. *Schizophrenia Genesis: The Origins of Madness*. New York: Freeman, 1991.
86. Karlsson H, Bachmann S, Schroder J et al. Retroviral RNA identified in the cerebrospinal fluids and brains of individuals with schizophrenia. *Proc Natl Acad Sci USA* 2001; **98**: 4634–9.
87. Kraepelin E (ed). *Dementia Praecox and Paraphrenia*. Edinburgh: Livingstone, 1919.
88. Menninger KA. The schizophrenic syndromes as a product of acute infectious disease. *Arch Neurol Psychiatry* 1928; **20**: 464–81.
89. Hare EH, Price JS, Slater E. Schizophrenia and season of birth. *Br J Psychiatry* 1972; **120**: 125–6.
90. Machon RA, Mednick SA, Schulsinger F. The interaction of seasonality, place of birth, genetic risk and subsequent schizophrenia in a high risk sample. *Br J Psychiatry* 1983; **143**: 383–8.
91. Boyd JH, Pulver AE, Stewart W. Season of birth: schizophrenia and bipolar disorder. *Schizophr Bull* 1986; **12**: 173–86.
92. Pallast EG, Jongbloet PH, Straatman HM. Excess seasonality of births among patients with schizophrenia and seasonal ovopathy. *Schizophr Bull* 1994; **20**: 269–76.
93. Pulver AE, Liang KY, Wolyniec PS. Season of birth among siblings of schizophrenic patients. *Br J Psychiatry* 1992; **160**: 71–5.
94. Mednick SA, Machon RA, Huttunen MO. Adult schizophrenia following prenatal exposure to an influenza epidemic. *Arch Gen Psychiatry* 1988; **45**: 189–92.
95. Adams W, Kendell RE, Hare ET. Epidemiological evidence that maternal influenza contributes to the aetiology of schizophrenia: an analysis of Scottish, English, and Danish data. *Br J Psychiatry* 1993; **163**: 522–34.
96. Barr CE, Mednick SA, Munk-Jorgensen P. Exposure to influenza epidemics during gestation and adult schizophrenia: a 40-year study. *Arch Gen Psychiatry* 1990; **47**: 869–74.
97. Fahy TA, Jones PB, Sham PC. Schizophrenia in Afro-Caribbeans in the UK following prenatal exposure to the 1957 A2 influenza epidemic. *Schizophr Res* 1993; **6**: 98–9.
98. Kunugi H, Nanko S, Takei N. Schizophrenia following in utero exposure to the 1957 influenza epidemics in Japan. *Am J Psychiatry* 1995; **152**: 450–2.
99. McGrath JJ, Pemberton M, Welham JL. Schizophrenia and the influenza epidemics of 1954, 1957 and 1959: a southern hemisphere study. *Schizophr Res* 1994; **14**: 1–8.
100. O'Callaghan E, Gibson T, Colohan HA. Season of birth in schizophrenia: evidence for confinement of an excess of winter births to patients without a family history of mental disorder. *Br J Psychiatry* 1991; **158**: 764–9.
101. Sham PC, O'Callaghan E, Takei N. Schizophrenia following prenatal exposure to influenza epidemics between 1939 and 1960. *Br J Psychiatry* 1992; **160**: 461–6.
102. Takei N, Mortensen PB, Klaening U et al. Relationship between in utero exposure to influenza epidemic and risk of schizophrenia in Denmark (letter). *Schizophr Res* 1994; **11**: 95.
103. Takei N, Sham PC, O'Callaghan E. Prenatal exposure to influenza and the development of schizophrenia: is the effect confined to females? *Am J Psychiatry* 1994; **151**: 117–9.
104. Kendell RE, Kemp IW. Maternal influenza in the aetiology of schizophrenia. *Arch Gen Psychiatry* 1989; **46**: 878–82.
105. Takei N, Van Os J, Murray RM. Maternal exposure to influenza and risk of schizophrenia: a 22-year study from the Netherlands. *J Psychiatr Res* 1995; **29**: 435–45.
106. Erlenmeyer-Kimling L, Folnegovic Z, Hrabak-Zerjavic Boracic B et al. Schizophrenia and prenatal exposure to the 1957 A2 influenza epidemic in Croatia. *Am J Psychiatry* 1994; **151**: 1496–8.
107. Selten JPCJ, Sleats JPJ. Evidence against maternal influenza as a risk factor for schizophrenia. *Br J Psychiatry* 1994; **164**: 674–6.
108. Susser E, Lin SP, Brown AS. No relation between risk of schizophrenia and prenatal exposure to influenza in Holland. *Am J Psychiatry* 1994; **151**: 922–4.
109. Stober G, Franzek E, Beckmann J. The role of maternal infectious diseases during pregnancy in the aetiology of schizophrenia in offspring. *Eur Psychiatry* 1992; **7**: 147–52.
110. Mednick SA, Huttunen MO, Macon RA. Prenatal influenza infections and adult schizophrenia. *Schizophr Bull* 1994; **20**: 263–7.
111. Meltzer HY, Fatemi SH. Schizophrenia and other psychotic disorders. In: *Current Diagnosis and Treatment in Psychiatry* (Ebert MH, Loosen PT, Nurcombe B, eds). New York: McGraw-Hill, 2000: 260–77.
112. Fatemi SH. Treatment of mental disorders. In: *Psychopharmacology, An Introduction* (Spiegel R, ed). Chicester UK: John Wiley and Sons, 2003: 1–420.
113. Weiss JM, Kilts CD. Animal models of depression and schizophrenia. In: *American Psychiatric Press Textbook of*

114. Geyer MA, Braff DL. Habituation of the blink reflex in normals and schizophrenic patients. *Psychophysiol* 1982; **19**: 1–16.
115. Geyer MA, Braff DL. Startle habituation and sensorimotor gating in schizophrenia and related animal models. *Schizophr Bull* 1987; **13**: 643–68.
116. Geyer MA, Braff DL, Swerdlow NR. Startle-response measures of information processing in animals: relevance to schizophrenia. In: *Animal Models of Human Emotion and Cognition* (Haug M, ed). Washington DC: American Psychological Association, 1999.
117. Wood GK, Tomasiewicz H, Rutishauser U et al. NCAM-180 knockout mice display increased lateral ventricle size and reduced prepulse inhibition of startle. *Neuroreport* 1998; **9**: 461–6.
118. Waziri R, Baruah S. A hyperglycinergic rat model for the pathogenesis of schizophrenia: preliminary findings. *Schizophr Res* 1999; **37**: 205–15.
119. Tueting P, Costa E, Dwivedi Y et al. The phenotypic characteristics of heterozygous reeler mouse. *Neuroreport* 1999; **10**: 1329–34.
120. Braff D, Stone C, Callaway E et al. Prestimulus effects on human startle reflex in normals and schizophrenics. *Psychophysiol* 1978; **15**: 339–43.
121. Swerdlow NR, Braff DL, Barak Caine S, Geyer MA. Limbic cortico-striato-pallido-pontive substrates of sensorimotor gating in animal models and psychiatric disorders. In: *Limbic Motor Circuits and Neuropsychiatry* (Kalivas, PW, ed). Boca Raton FL: CRC Press, 1996; 311–28.
122. Lipska BK, Jaskiw GE, Weinberger DR. The effects of combined prefrontal cortical and hippocampal damage on dopamine-related behaviors in rats. *Pharmacol Biochem Behav* 1994; **48**: 1053–7.
123. Fatemi SH, Earle JA, Kanodia R et al. Prenatal viral infection leads to pyramidal cell atrophy and macrocephaly in adulthood: implications for genesis of autism and schizophrenia. *Cell Mol Neurobiol* 2002; **22**: 25–33.
124. Fatemi SH, Emamian ES, Sidwell RW et al. Human influenza viral infection in utero alters glial fibrillary acidic protein immunoreactivity in developing brains of neonatal mice. *Mol Psychiatry* 2002; **7**: 633–40.
125. Shi L, Fatemi SH, Sidwell RW, Patterson PH. Maternal influenza infection causes marked behavioral and pharmacological changes in the offspring. *J Neurosci* 2003; **23**: 297–302.
126. Doyles SA, Slater P. Localization of neuronal and endothelial nitric oxide synthase isoforms in human hippocampus. *Neuroscience* 1997; **76**: 387–95.
127. Fatemi SH, Cuadra A, El-Fakahany E, Thuras P. Prenatal viral infection causes alterations in nNOS expression in developing mouse brains. *Neuroreport* 2000; **11**: 1493–6.
128. Bolanos JP, Almeida A, Stewart V et al. Nitric oxide-mediated mitrochondrial damage in the brain: mechanisms and implications for neurodegenerative diseases. *J Neurochem* 1997; **68**: 2227–40.
129. Mallard E, Rehn A, Rees S et al. Ventriculomegaly and reduced hippocampal volume following intrauterine growth restriction: implications for the etiology of schizophrenia. *Schizophr Res* 1999; **40**: 11–21.
130. Franklin KBJ, Paxinos G. *The Mouse Brain in Stereotoxic Coordinates*. Academic Press.
131. Erlander MG, Tillakaratne NJ, Feldblum S et al. Two genes encode distinct glutamate decarboxylases. *Neuron* 1991; **7**: 91–100.
132. Fatemi SH, Pearce DA, Brooks A et al. DNA microarray studies of prenatal virally-induced brain disorder in mouse. In: *Proceedings of the Proteomics and Genomics Meeting of the Stanley Medical Research Institute*. Bethesda, MD: 2003.
133. Fatemi SH, Araghi-Niknam M, Laurence JA et al. Glial fibrillary acidic protein and glutamic acid decarboxylase 65 and 67 kDa proteins are increased in brains of neonatal BALB/c mice following viral infection *in utero*. *Schizophr Res* 2004; **69**: 121–3.

10

Maternal infection causes abnormal behavior in the offspring

Paul H Patterson

INTRODUCTION

Infection in pregnant women is relatively common. For instance, 11% of pregnant women are positive during the second and third trimesters for influenza.[1] In fact, pregnancy is known to alter the immune system's response to infection.[2,3] Although the mother may recover relatively quickly from an infection, the consequences for the fetus can be severe. Depending on the type and timing of infection, and the genotype of the mother and fetus, acute maternal infections can increase the incidence of miscarriage and stillbirth, as well as disorders in the offspring such as cerebral palsy[4–7] and mental illness[8–13] in the offspring. For instance, 'German measles' (rubella virus) or cytomegalovirus infection during the first trimester strongly increases the risk for autism in the offspring, leading one study to conclude that 'the principal nongenetic cause of autism is prenatal viral infection.'[14] In addition, respiratory infection during the second trimester can increase the risk for schizophrenia in the offspring.[11,12,15–20] Moreover, the presence of anti-influenza antibodies or increased levels of interleukin (IL)-8 during the second trimester increases the risk for schizophrenia in the offspring.[21,22]

Given this morbidity and mortality, it is important to investigate the pathophysiology of maternal infection, as well as potential avenues of prevention and therapy. Moreover, because of this connection, studies in animal models could shed light on mental retardation, autism, and schizophrenia. These models have the advantage of being based on a known risk factor for the disorders. The present article briefly reviews the effects of maternal infection on the behavior of offspring. The offspring of infected rodents can be characterized in a number of ways, including via molecular and neuropathological studies of their brains. Behavioral assays can also be useful in characterizing the mental status of these offspring. A number of relevant behavioral tests are being used in various rodent models of mental illness.[23–27] These assays include motor activity, stereotypies, and the acoustic startle response, as well as tests of latent inhibition, social interaction, learning and memory, and responses to stressful environments. Of these assays, only a few have been used thus far in testing the offspring of infected or immune-activated mothers.

MATERNAL VIRAL INFECTION

To mimic human respiratory infection, human influenza virus A/NWS/33H1N1 has been administered intranasally to BALB/c or C57BL/6 mice at day 9.5 of pregnancy (E9.5). This results in sickness behavior (lethargy, sleepiness, ruffled hair, lack of grooming) and lung edema in the mother. At the appropriate viral dose, loss of pregnancy is not severe, as long as the mice are not disturbed. Neuropathology in the offspring includes abnormal neuroblast migration patterns and layer- and region-specific changes in the expression of the presynaptic marker SNAP-25, as well as in nNOS and Reelin.[28,29] In addition, we find that hippocampal pyramidal cells display atrophy and increased density.[29] We also have preliminary evidence for highly localized abnormalities in the adult cerebellum of prenatally exposed mice, which strikingly resemble the most robust neuropathology found in autism.[30]

Spontaneous activity and sensorimotor coordination

Locomotor activity can be readily monitored using an automated photobeam crossing system (e.g., San Diego Instruments, San Diego, USA). A translucent cage is placed between photobeams and ambulatory activity of individual mice is monitored as successive interruption of two of the four beams crossing the cage over a 40-hour period. It is important to allow the mice to adapt to this environment before collecting data. Once adapted to this environment, the adult offspring of infected and sham-infected mothers display equivalent ambulation.[31]

A commonly used method of assessing sensorimotor coordination and balance is to place the animal on a rotating metal rod and measure the time it takes to fall off the rod (e.g., the Rota-rod Treadmill, UGO Basile, Comerid, Italy). This can be done at fixed rotation speeds or in an accelerating mode. The adult offspring of infected and sham-infected mothers are able to stay on the accelerating rod for similar periods of time.[31] These two tests indicate that the exposed offspring do not exhibit obvious abnormalities in motor activity or balance.

Exploratory behavior

We have also utilized a number of behavioral tests that are thought to be relevant for mental illness. The open field and novel object tests are thought, at least in part, to assess the anxiety an animal exhibits in a mildly stressful situation.[32,33] In the open field test, we quantified the time spent in the center of the box, and the number of times the mice entered the center. Quantitation reveals highly significant differences in several measures of exploratory behavior (Figure 10.1). The mice born to infected mothers spend nearly eight times less time in the center squares, most of their time being spent in corners of the box. These mice also enter the center squares nearly six times less often, and they explore their environment by rearing on their hind legs four times less often.[31] While these mice spend a great portion of the test period in the corners of the box, they do not exhibit freezing behavior; they often move around in the corner.

Novelty stress is an assay that is highly relevant for autism,[34] and autistic children display reduced exploratory behavior in novel situations.[35] Two measures of anxiety about exploring a novel object can distinguish the offspring of sham- and influenza-infected mice. Mice born to infected mothers have an almost twofold greater latency in first contacting the object, and they initiate almost threefold fewer contacts with the object (Figure 10.2).[31] Thus, under mildly stressful conditions, exposed mice display marked signs of apparent anxiety.

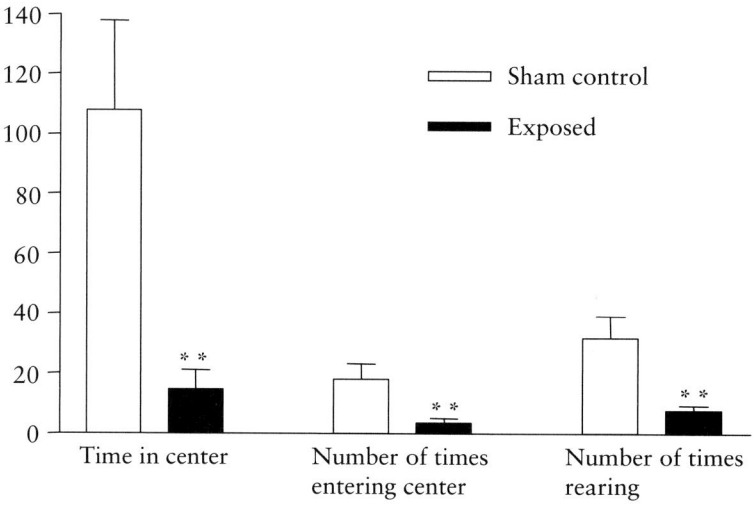

Figure 10.1 Maternal infection yields offspring that display increased apparent anxiety under mildly stressful conditions. Here, 15 control (7 males) and 23 experimental (12 males) BALB/c mice were tested in the open field for 10 minutes. Their time, in seconds, of being in the center squares of the field, and the other measures of behavior were quantified from videotapes viewed by an observer blind to the history of the mice. Data are given as mean ± SEM. A two-tailed t test was used to assess the significance of the differences between the two groups in each test (** $p < .0016$).

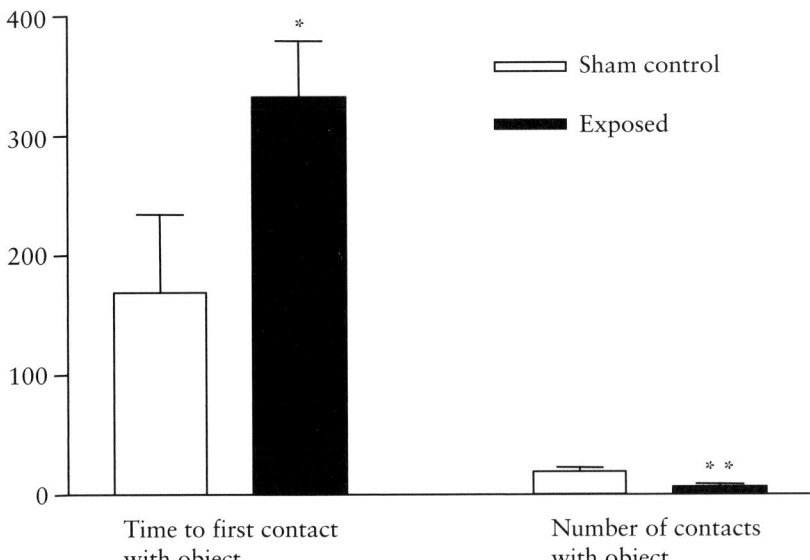

Figure 10.2 Maternal infection yields offspring that are more reluctant to interact with a novel object than controls. The same mice as in Figure 10.1 were tested for touching a novel object during a 10-minute period. Their time, in seconds, for each measure of behavior was quantified from videotapes viewed by an observer blind to the history of the mice. Data are given as mean ± SEM. A two-tailed t test was used to assess the significance of the differences between the two groups in each test (** $p < .01$; * $p < .05$).

Sensorimotor gating

Of particular interest is the acoustic startle response, which is a measure of sensorimotor gating and is used in both animals and humans.[36] Abnormal startle responses, changes in the rate of habituation, and/or the degree of pre-pulse inhibition (PPI) of the startle have been observed in several mental disorders, including schizophrenia, attention deficit disorder, Tourette syndrome, and autism.[37] Deficits in PPI have been hypothesized to be a sign of cognitive fragmentation, psychosis, and thought disorder. The large amount of work done on both humans and rodents allows direct inter-species comparisons to be made. A common paradigm is to measure the amount of startle to a loud noise (e.g., 120 dB) using a detector under the platform on which the animal sits (e.g., in an automated startle chamber, San Diego Instruments, San Diego, USA). This response is compared to a startle elicited by the same stimulus preceded by 50–100 ms by a much smaller pre-pulse (e.g., 10 dB above background noise level). The pre-pulse causes a stimulus strength-dependent inhibition of the startle. This effect is termed pre-pulse inhibition (PPI).

When the acoustic startle response is applied to adult offspring of influenza-infected mothers, we find that they display a deficit in PPI compared to mice born to sham-infected mothers. That is, similar to subjects with schizophrenia, the pre-pulse is not as effective in inhibiting the startle in the mice born to infected mothers.[31] While the difference between the exposed and control groups is quite significant ($p < .01$ for a pre-pulse of 80 dB, and $p < .05$ for a pre-pulse of 75 dB), there can be variation among the mice in the virus-exposed group (Figure 10.3). In one experiment, at a pre-pulse of 80 dB, a significant fraction of exposed mice display PPI within the range of the control mice. In this case, it appears that the exposed group may be composed of two populations – those with normal PPI and those with a deficit. In other experiments, however, all of the exposed mice display PPI values below those of the control mice; the experimental and control curves do not overlap at all in this case (data not shown).

In comparing the exposed mice with normal and abnormal PPI (Figure 10.3), we were unable to detect significant differences in weight as neonates or adults, nor was there a significant bias in gender. Moreover, offspring from individual infected mothers were found in both normal and abnormal PPI groups. Since the mice (BALB/c) are thought to be genetically identical, it is puzzling how the same infected mother could give rise to offspring with such different acoustic startle behavior. One possibility is that this difference is related to the position of the fetus in the uterus. It has been found, for instance, that there are differences in blood flow to placentae in relation to intrauterine location in pregnant rats.[38,39] There are also differences in fetal weight, cholesterol, sex steroids, and insulin-like growth factor-I, based on intrauterine position in pigs.[40,41]

The PPI assay also reveals very striking differences between the mice born to sham- and influenza-infected mothers following acute administration of

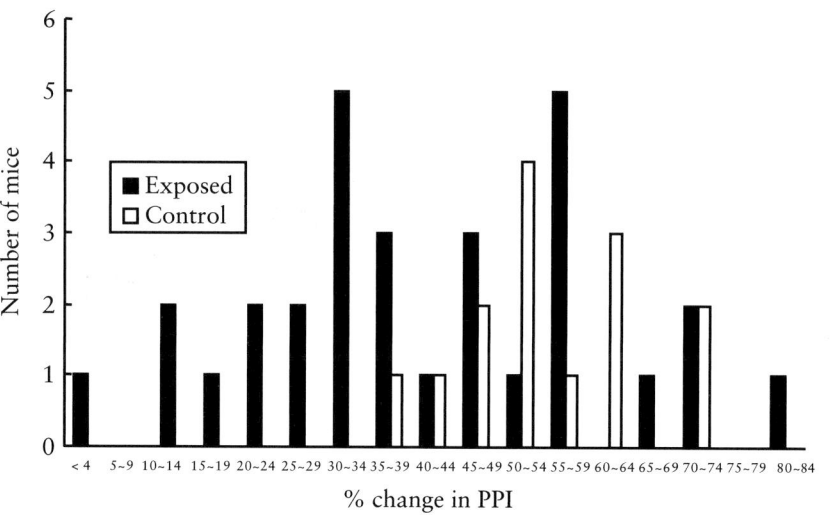

Figure 10.3 Maternal infection yields offspring with a deficit in PPI. Compared to mice born to sham-infected mothers (control; $n = 14$; 8 females), the mice born to infected mothers (exposed; $n = 29$; 15 females) display reduced PPI when analyzed as a group.[31] Nonetheless, many of the mice in this group display PPI responses in the normal range, as illustrated here.

psychoactive drugs.[31] Clozapine, a commonly used, atypical antipsychotic drug, is known to increase PPI in rodents,[42] and it does so in our control BALB/c mice after acute administration, in a dose-dependent manner. Moreover, the Balb/C mice born to infected mothers display a far greater increase in PPI than controls in response to clozapine. The same results are seen in C57BL/6 mice. In addition, very similar results are obtained with both strains of mice using chlorpromazine, a typical antipsychotic. That is, mice born to infected mothers are far more sensitive than control mice to antipsychotics.[31] This suggests an abnormality in the dopaminergic system.

There is also a striking difference in response to ketamine. This NMDA-antagonist impairs PPI and exacerbates psychotic symptoms in humans, and can be used to predict antipsychotic effects of other drugs.[42-44] As expected from the work of others, the PPI of sham-infected control mice is reduced by ketamine. In contrast, mice born to infected mothers show a very different response to ketamine.[31] Importantly, nearly identical findings were obtained with offspring of infected C57Bl/6 mice. This suggests that maternal infection may cause an abnormality in the glutamatergic system of the offspring.

These pharmacological results also indicate that exposed mice do not have an intrinsic auditory deficit, as they respond better than control mice to the pre-pulse under these circumstances. In addition, exposed mice respond very well to pre-pulse intensities only 6 dB above background noise level in the absence of drug treatment.

Social behavior

There are many assays of social behavior that would be informative. Thus far, an extremely simple test has been utilized, wherein two mice of the same sex and same experimental group, but unknown to one another, are placed in an open field box. Mice born to infected mothers contact each other 2.7 times less frequently than mice born to sham-infected mothers ($p < .01$).[31] There is also a 4.5-fold difference in latency to first contact, although this did not reach statistical significance. The large variance in the latter dataset is probably due to placing the mice near one another at the outset of the test. This was done to avoid the confound of reluctance in exploring the box that the exposed mice clearly display.

Pup–mother attachment

Behavioral tests of particular relevance to autism are those that measure the pup's bonding with, or recognition of, the mother, deficits in which are characteristic of autistic infants and toddlers. We have preliminary results indicating that pups born to influenza-infected mothers are deficient in maternal attachment. In one assay, the pup (3–21 days old) is placed in a center chamber that is bordered on one side by a chamber with the pup's own mother, and on the other side by a chamber with a lactating female unknown to the pup. We find that control pups move towards and contact their own mothers (through a small opening) 75–90% of the time, while pups born to infected mothers find the correct mother only 25–50% of the time (unpublished data). In a second assay, ultrasonic vocalizations made by pups removed from their mothers are quantified. Pups born to infected mothers make many fewer calls than control pups when removed from their mothers (unpublished data).

MATERNAL BACTERIAL INFECTION

Intraperitoneal or subcutaneous injection of lipopolysaccharide (LPS) from *E. coli* in rodents is a model of bacterial infection, and causes sickness behavior in the recipient. This is due to the induction of cytokines in the periphery as well as within the brain.[45] In hyporesponsive mouse strains such as C3H/HeN, maternal LPS injection can cause fetal death, which is due at least in part to tumor necrosis factor (TNF)α production.[46] LPS has also been injected into pregnant rats, where it leads to significant increases in cytokine levels in the placenta, as well as increased TNFα in amniotic fluid.[47,48] While little neuropathology has been reported thus far on the offspring of rats treated on alternate days with LPS during pregnancy, increased tyrosine hydroxylase immunoreactivity is seen in the nucleus accumbens and in the bed nucleus of the stria terminalis of adult exposed offspring.[49] Moreover, it is striking that such adult offspring display signs of astrocyte and microglial activation in several brain areas, as well as elevated serum IL-2 and -6 levels. This indicates an ongoing inflammatory reaction long after the fetal insult.[49] Activated astrocytes have also been observed in neonatal offspring of influenza-infected mothers.[29] The cause of this ongoing inflammation is an important question. Interestingly, while astrocyte numbers are generally not found to increase in the schizophrenic brain, the presence of reactive astrocytes has been reported in a demented subgroup of these patients.[50] Moreover, HLA-DR+ microglia are increased in the schizophrenic brains.[51,52]

Sensorimotor gating

There is one study of the behavioral consequences for the offspring of maternal LPS administration.[49] The adult offspring of rats injected with LPS subcutaneously on alternate days throughout pregnancy were assayed for PPI using an auditory stimulus preceded by either an auditory or visual pre-pulse. Such offspring display significant deficits in PPI, with the effects being greater for the auditory stimulus and the male offspring. In addition, the antipsychotic drugs haloperidol and clozapine significantly reverse this deficit. Thus, the primary features of the PPI results are quite similar in the maternal LPS and influenza infection models.

Exploratory behavior

The offspring of LPS-treated mothers have also been tested for exploratory behavior. Surprisingly, it has been reported in abstract form that LPS-exposed offspring display signs of reduced anxiety and increased exploratory behavior in the open field and elevated plus maze tests.[53] In light of the parallels between the histological and other behavioral results between maternal influenza infection and LPS administration, it will be worthwhile to examine further exploratory behavior in LPS-exposed offspring.

DOUBLE STRANDED RNA

Key aspects of microbial infection can be mimicked by injection of synthetic double stranded RNA, particularly poly(I:C). This RNA is the best candidate for the molecular trigger released by infection that induces cytokines. That is, poly(I:C) can induce flu symptoms as well as a cytokine cascade very similar to that induced by bacterial or viral infection.[54] There are, however, several differences between the cytokines induced by bacterial and viral infection, most notably the induction of interferon by viruses. While poly(I:C) induces interferon, this double stranded RNA does not perfectly mimic all of the changes induced in animals or cells by viral infection. Moreover, poly(I:C) injection does not lead to some of the antibody responses induced by viral infection.

In terms of neuropathology, it is striking that injection of poly(I:C) in pregnant rats on E15 yields adult offspring with moderate to severe neuron loss in the hippocampus and entorhinal cortex. Moreover, many of the remaining neurons exhibit a pyknotic appearance, suggesting an ongoing problem in the mature brain.[55]

Sensorimotor gating

Using poly(I:C) injection on E9.5 in pregnant mice, we found a significant PPI deficit in the adult offspring.[31] This result mimics that caused by influenza infection described above, indicating that at least part of the abnormal behavioral profile of these offspring is probably due to the cytokine cascade induced by the viral infection.

Latent inhibition

Another well-established behavioral assay that tests the ability to ignore irrelevant stimuli is that of latent inhibition (LI). In this assay, one experimental group is given repeated exposure to a stimulus without consequences, and then compared to a non-pre-exposed group in the performance of a learning task in which that stimulus is paired with negative reinforcement. Pre-exposure normally results in a weaker learning performance, which is termed LI. Schizophrenic subjects in the acute phase display abnormal LI, which can be normalized by treatment with antipsychotic drugs.[56] Injection of pregnant rats with poly(I:C) on E15 results in disrupted LI in the adult offspring, which can be corrected by antipsychotic drug treatment.[55] In addition, LI is normal in the offspring when they are tested at prepubertal ages, which is reminiscent of the long latency between developmental insult and the onset of psychotic schizophrenic symptoms.

Locomotor stimulation by amphetamine

The dopamine releaser amphetamine produces and exacerbates psychotic symptoms in high-schizotypal humans and in subsets of schizophrenia subjects. Antipsychotic drugs reverse amphetamine-induced disruption of LI.[55] Amphetamine increases locomotor activity in rodents, and prenatal immune activation by injection of poly(I:C) results in postpubertal emergence of increased sensitivity to amphetamine in this assay.[55]

PERSPECTIVES

As with human maternal infection, influenza, LPS, or poly(I:C) administration to pregnant rodents leads to marked abnormalities in the behavior of the adult offspring. Many additional behavioral tests could be applied to these offspring to characterize further their mental state, particularly assays of learning and memory as well as social interaction. Nonetheless, the results obtained thus far have generated a number of intriguing questions.

1) Would infection at different times during pregnancy yield diverse behavioral phenotypes? For instance, infection during the second trimester increases the risk for schizophrenia while infection during the first trimester increases the risk for autism.
2) Can any of the behavioral abnormalities observed in the offspring of infected mothers be linked to specific histological or molecular changes in the brains of these animals? The pharmacological results with the PPI assay suggest that there may be alterations in the dopaminergic and/or glutamatergic transmitter systems, as is seen in schizophrenia. In addition, a study of autistic children linked deficits in novel object exploration with localized pathology in the cerebellum,[35] and both of these changes are observed in the offspring of infected mice.
3) What are the signals that alter fetal brain development in maternal infection? Direct viral infection of the fetus does not appear to be necessary since activating the immune system in the absence of virus using synthetic double stranded RNA or LPS causes a PPI deficit in the offspring similar to that seen following maternal viral infection. Moreover, using highly sensitive RT-PCR methods, we were unable to detect viral RNA in the fetal brain following maternal influenza infection.[57,58] Activating the immune system elicits cytokine production and elevates corticosteroid levels, and both of these classes of signal are known to affect the development of neurons and glia.
4) Are these findings relevant to the issue of vaccination of pregnant women? Would maternal vaccination with an inactivated virus yield results for the offspring similar to those seen with viral infection? It has been recommended for many years that maternal vaccination be done routinely,[59] yet the incidence of schizophrenia in the offspring has not been assessed. Such an experiment is feasible in the animal model.

REFERENCES

1. Irving WL, James DK, Stephenson T et al. Influenza virus infection in the second and third trimesters of pregnancy: a clinical and seroepidemiological study. *Br J Obstet Gynecol* 2000; **107**: 1282–9.
2. Hanson LA. The mother-offspring dyad and the immune system. *Acta Pediatrics* 2000; **89**: 252–8.
3. Sacks G, Sargent I, Redman C. Innate immunity in pregnancy. *Immunol Today* 2000; **21**: 200–1.
4. Nelson KB, Grether JK. Cerebral palsy in low-birthweight infants: etiology and strategies for prevention. *Ment Retard Dev Dis Rev* 1997; **3**: 112–7.
5. Gilstrap LC, Ramin SM. Infection and cerebral palsy. *Semin Perinatol* 2000; **24**: 200–3.
6. Dammann O, Kuban KCK, Leviton A. Perinatal infection, fetal inflammatory response, white matter damage, and cognitive limitations in children born preterm. *Ment Retard Dev Dis Rev* 2002; **8**: 46–50.
7. Wu YW. Systematic review of chorioamnionitis and cerebral palsy. *Ment Retard Dev Dis Rev* 2002; **8**: 25–9.
8. Garvey MA, Giedd J, Swedo SE. PANDAS: the search for environmental triggers of pediatric neuropsychiatric disorders. Lessons from rheumatic fever. *J Child Neurol* 1998; **13**: 413.

9. Rodier PM, Hyman SL. Early environmental factors in autism. *Ment Retard Dev Dis Rev* 1998; **4**: 121–8.
10. Torrey EF, Yolken RH. Familial and genetic mechanisms in schizophrenia. *Brain Res Rev* 2000; **31**: 113–7.
11. Brown AS, Schaefer CA, Wyatt RJ et al. Maternal exposure to respiratory infections and adult schizophrenia spectrum disorders: a prospective birth cohort study. *Schizophr Bull* 2000; **26**: 287–95.
12. Brown AS, Susser ES. In utero infection and adult schizophrenia. *Ment Retard Dev Dis Rev* 2002; **8**: 51–7.
13. Patterson PH. Maternal infection: window on neuroimmune interactions in fetal brain development and mental illness. *Curr Opin Neurobiol* 2002; **12**: 115–8.
14. Ciaranello AL, Ciaranello RD. The neurobiology of infantile autism. *Ann Rev Neurosci* 1995; **18**: 101–28.
15. Wright P, Takei N, Rifkin L, Murray RM. Maternal influenza obstetric complications and schizophrenia. *Am J Psychiatry* 1995; **152**: 1714–20.
16. Ellenbroek BA, Cools AR. The neurodevelopment hypothesis of schizophrenia: clinical evidence and animal models. *Neurosci Res Commun* 1998; **22**: 127–36.
17. Izumoto Y, Inoue S, Yasuda N. Schizophrenia and the influenza epidemics of 1957 in Japan. *Biol Psychiatry* 1999; **46**: 119–24.
18. Tsuang M. Schizophrenia: genes and environment. *Biol Psychiatry* 2000; **47**: 210–20.
19. Pearce BD. Schizophrenia and viral infection during neurodevelopment: a focus on mechanisms. *Mol Psychiatry* 2001; **6**: 634–46.
20. Machon RA, Huttunen MO, Mednick SA et al. Adult schizotypal personality characteristics and prenatal influenza in a Finnish birth cohort. *Schizophr Res* 2002; **54**: 7–16.
21. Brown AS, Hooton J, Schaefer CA et al. Elevated maternal interleukin-8 levels and risk of schizophrenia in adult offspring. *Am J Psychiatry* 2004; **161**: 889–95.
22. Brown AS, Schaefer CA, Gravenstein S et al. Prenatal infection and immune abnormalities in adult schizophrenia. *Biol Psychiatry* 2004; **55**: 1285.
23. De Hert M, Ellenbroek B. Animal models of schizophrenia. *Neurosci Res Commun* 2000; **26**: 279–88.
24. Lipska BK, Weinberger DR. To model a psychiatric disorder in animals: schizophrenia as a reality test. *Neuropsychopharmacology* 2000; **23**: 223–39.
25. Wolterink G, Daenen EWPM, Van Ree JM. Animal models for schizophrenia. *Neurosci Res Commun* 2000; **27**: 143–54.
26. Weiss IC, Feldon J. Environmental animal models for sensorimotor gating deficiencies in schizophrenia: a review. *Psychopharmacology* 2001; **156**: 305–26.
27. Ferguson JN, Young LJ, Insel TR. The neuroendocrine basis for social recognition. *Frontiers Neuroendocrinol* 2002; **23**: 200–24.
28. Fatemi SH, Emamian ES, Kist D et al. Defective corticogenesis and reduction in reelin immunoreactivity in cortex and hippocampus of prenatally neonatal mice. *Mol Psychiatry* 1999; **4**: 145–54.
29. Fatemi SH, Earle J, Kmodia R et al. Prenatal viral infection leads to pyramidal neuron atrophy and macrocephaly in adulthood: implications for genesis of autism and schizophrenia. *Cell Mol Neurobiol* 2002; **22**: 25–33.
30. Patterson PH, Shi L. Maternal influenza virus causes a cerebellar defect resembling that in autism. *Internl Mtg for Autism Res* 2002; S334.
31. Shi L, Fatemi SH, Sidwell RW, Patterson PH. Maternal influenza infection causes marked behavioral and pharmacological changes in the offspring. *J Neurosci* 2003; **23**: 297–302.
32. File SE. Models of anxiety. *Br J Clin Practice* 1985; **38**: 15–20.
33. Weiss SM, Lightowler S, Stanhope KJ et al. Measurement of anxiety in transgenic mice. *Rev Neurosci* 2000; **11**: 59–74.
34. Tecott LH, Logue SF, Wehner JM, Kauer JA. Perturbed dentate gyrus function in serotonin 5-HT2C receptor mutant mice. *Proc Natl Acad Sci USA* 1998; **95**: 15026–31.
35. Pierce K, Courchesne E. Evidence for a cerebellar role in reduced exploration and stereotyped behavior in autism. *Biol Psychiatry* 2001; **49**: 655–64.
36. Koch M. The neurobiology of startle. *Progr Neurobiol* 1999; **59**: 107–28.
37. Geyer MA, Wilkinson LS, Humby T, Robbins TW. Isolation rearing of rats produces a deficit in prepulse inhibition of acoustic startle similar to that in schizophrenia. *Biol Psychiatry* 1993; **34**: 361–72.
38. Even MD, Laughlin MH, Krause GF, vom Saal FS. Differences in blood flow to uterine segments and placentae in relation to sex, intrauterine location and side in pregnant rats. *J Reprod Fertilization* 1994; **102**: 245–52.
39. Wentzel P, Jansson L, Eriksson UJ. Diabetes in pregnancy: uterine blood flow and embryonic development in the rat. *Pediatr Res* 1995; **38**: 598–606.
40. Wise TH, Christenson RK. Relationship of fetal position within the uterus to fetal weight, placental weight, testosterone, estrogens, and thymosin β4 concentrations at 70 and 104 days of gestation in swine. *J Animal Med Sci* 1992; **70**: 2787–93.
41. Wise TH, Roberts AJ, Christenson RK. Relationships of light and heavy fetuses to uterine position, placental weight, gestational age, and fetal cholesterol concentrations. *J Animal Med Sci* 1997; **75**: 2197–207.
42. Swerdlow NR, Bakshi V, Waikar M et al. Seroquel, clozapine and chlorpromazine restore sensorimotor gating in ketamine-treated rats. *Psychopharmacology* 1998; **140**: 75.
43. Ellison G. The N-methyl-D-aspartate antagonists phencyclidine, ketamine, dizocilpine as both behavioral and anatomical models of the dementias. *Brain Res Rev* 1995; **20**: 250–67.
44. Malhotra AK, Pinals DA, Adler CM et al. Ketamine-induced exacerbation of psychotic symptoms and cognitive impairment in neuroleptic-free schizophrenics. *Neuropsychopharmacology* 1997; **17**: 141–50.
45. Konsman JP, Parnet P, Dantzer R. Cytokine-induced sickness behaviour: mechanisms and implications. *Trends Neurosci* 2002; **25**: 154–9.
46. Silver RM, Lohner WS, Daynes RA et al. Lipopolysaccharide-induced fetal death – the role of tumor-necrosis-factor-alpha. *Biol Reprod* 1994; **50**: 1108–12.
47. Fidel PL, Romero R, Wolf N et al. Systemic and local cytokine profiles in endotoxin-induced preterm parturition in mice. *Am J Obstet Gynecol* 1994; **170**: 1467–75.
48. Urakubo A, Jarskog LF, Lieberman JA, Gilmore JH. Prenatal exposure to maternal infection alters cytokine expression in the placenta, amniotic fluid, and fetal brain. *Schizophr Res* 2001; **47**: 27–36.
49. Borrell J, Vela JM, Arevalo-Martin A et al. Prenatal immune challenge disrupts sensorimotor gating in adult rats: implications for the etiopathogenesis of schizophrenia. *Neuropsychopharmacology* 2002; **26**: 204–15.
50. Arnold SE, Franz BR, Trohanowski JQ et al. Glial fibrillary acidic protein-immunoreactive astrocytosis in elderly patients with schizophrenia and dementia. *Acta Neuropathol* 1996; **91**: 269–77.
51. Bayer TA, Buslei R, Havas L, Falkai P. Evidence for activation of microglia in patients with psychiatric illnesses. *Neurosci Lett* 1999; **271**: 126–8.
52. Radewicz K, Garey LJ, Gentleman SM, Reynolds R. Increase in HLA-DR immunoreactive microglia in frontal and temporal cortex of chronic schizophrenics. *J Neuropathol Exp Neurobiol* 2000; **59**: 137–50.
53. Golan HM, Lev V, Hallak M et al. Maternal inflammation induces behavioral alterations in offspring. *Soc Neurosci Abstract* 2002; **427**: 19.

54. Majde JA. Viral double-stranded RNA, cytokines, and the flu. *J Interferon Cytokine Res* 2000; **20**: 259–72.
55. Zuckerman L, Rehavi M, Nachman R, Weiner I. Immune activation during pregnancy in rats leads to a postpubertal emergence of disrupted latent inhibition, dopaminergic hyperfunction, and altered limbic morphology in the offspring: a novel neurodevelopmental model of schizophrenia. *Neuropsychopharmacology* 2003; **26**: 1–12.
56. Baruch I, Hemsley D, Gray JA. Differential performance of acute and chronic schizophrenics in a latent inhibition task. *J Nerv Ment Disord* 1988; **176**: 598–606.
57. Shi L, Tu N, Patterson PH. Maternal influenza infection is likely to alter fetal brain development indirectly: the virus is not detected in the fetus. *Int J Dev Neurosci* 2004; in press.
58. Aronsson F, Lannebo C, Paucar M et al. Persistence of viral RNA in the brain of offspring to mice infected with influenza A/WSN/33 virus during pregnancy. *J Neuro Virol* 2002; **8**: 353–7.
59. Glezen WP. Maternal immunization for the prevention of infections in late pregnancy and early infancy. *Infect Med* 1999; **16**: 585–95.

11

Maternal influenza A/WSN/33 virus infection in mice and persistence of viral RNA in the brains of exposed offspring

Fredrik Aronsson and Håkan Karlsson

INTRODUCTION

The development of schizophrenia has, in a number of studies, been suggested to result from disturbances in the maturation of the nervous system.[1] Although controversy still exists, there is a common belief that certain neuronal populations in the brains of patients suffering from schizophrenia have failed to develop normally due to disturbances in their migration and/or synaptogenesis. The problem with this view is the lack of an explanation for the long delay between the time of insult and the onset of symptoms. Rarely do other human diseases or even animal models exhibit this kind of latency. Therefore, a progressive component has lately been put forward as an addendum to the purely neurodevelopmental hypothesis.[2]

Epidemiological studies suggest that the development of schizophrenia may be related to exposure to infectious diseases during early life.[3] For example, maternal influenza A virus infections during the second trimester of pregnancy have in many, but not all, studies been associated with the appearance of neuropsychiatric diseases in the offspring.[4] Thus, it may be hypothesized that an infectious agent targeting the fetal brain adversely affects neuronal migration and synaptogenesis leading to the development of psychiatric symptoms in the adult individual.

Latency, in such a model, may be caused by the development of viral persistence followed by late-onset symptoms due to as of yet unknown mechanisms. Subacute sclerosing panencephalitis (SSPE) may develop years after acute measles virus infection. SSPE is caused by aberrant measles virus persisting in the CNS of individuals infected at a very young age and is an example of a viral disease exhibiting asymptomatic latency, during which the virus persists.[5] Alternatively, the infection may cause acute damage to the infected neurons leading to an imbalance in synaptic activities that progresses over time, eventually leading to the development of overt symptoms. Such a scenario may be exemplified by neonatal infection of Lewis rats with lymphocytic choriomeningitis virus, causing a loss of inhibitory GABAergic activity and resulting in progressive excitotoxic neurodegeneration in the hippocampus.[6]

In general, influenza A virus infections are limited to the respiratory epithelium, but viremia has been observed in both humans and experimental animals.[7–10] Despite the fact that transplacental transfer of influenza virus in humans has only rarely been described,[11,12] influenza poses a serious risk to the fetus during maternal infection.[13,14]

In experimental studies, only scattered reports exist of transplacental passage of influenza A virus. The A/PR/8 strain was reported to cross the placenta in mice,[15,16] and the recombinant A/PR/8-A/England/939/69 strain in ferrets[9,17] and guinea-pigs.[18] However, in a large study of A/WSN/33 infection in mice, no evidence for transplacental passage was obtained, as examined by virus cultivation.[19]

INFLUENZA A/WSN/33

The first isolated human influenza A/WS/33 virus strain[20] was inoculated into the brains of mice where the virus multiplied and produced neurological symptoms giving rise to the neurotropic influenza A/WSN/33 virus strain.[21] This strain is also pneumovirulent for mice as a result of earlier propagation in mouse lung. Intracerebral injection of the WSN/33 strain in mice resulted in specific targeting of viral antigens to the substantia nigra zona compacta and hippocampus giving rise to a lethal encephalitis.[22] When this strain was introduced into the olfactory bulbs of C57BL/6 and immunodefective TAP1 –/– (lacking functional CD8+ T-cells) mice, it selectively attacked the medial habenular and the paraventricular thalamic nuclei as well as neurons in the anterior olfactory nuclei, the piriform cortex, the ventral tegmental area, the dorsal raphe nuclei, the locus coeruleus, lateral nuclei in the hypothalamus, and the posterior mammillary nuclei in both types of mice.[23] This influenza virus infection was, however, non-lethal.

Furthermore, we previously reported that the A/WSN/33 strain causes a persistent infection at levels of the upper brainstem in TAP1 –/– mice after injection into the olfactory bulb.[24] No clonality of the persisting virus was detected in this study. The WSN/33 strain selectively infects neurons in the olfactory epithelia after intranasal inoculation and has the intrinsic capacity to spread anterogradely into the olfactory bulbs and target areas in the brain connected to these.[25] Furthermore, this spread is restricted by components of the innate immune response, interferon-α, -β, -γ, and nitric oxide, and the cellular immune response, CD8+ T-cells.

TRANSPLACENTAL PASSAGE AFTER MATERNAL INFECTION

C57BL/6 mice were inoculated intranasally with 750 or 7500 plaque forming units (PFU) of influenza A/WSN/33 virus (kindly provided by Dr S Nakajima of the Institute of Public Health, Tokyo, Japan) on day 14 of pregnancy (E14).[26] Control mice were inoculated similarly with phosphate buffered saline (PBS).

On day E17, the pregnant mice were sacrificed, the chorio-amniotic sacs containing the fetuses and placentas sampled, put on ice, and transferred to a separate laboratory. Brains, lungs, and corresponding placentas were subsequently dissected out, using new sets of tools for every fetus in order to avoid cross-contamination. For verification of maternal infection, lungs from the mothers were dissected out in a separate room. Data from two litters ($n = 17$), using a virus titer of 750 PFU for maternal inoculation, shows that influenza A virus RNA encoding matrix (M) and/or nucleoprotein (NP) could be detected in a proportion of the fetal brains and lungs. Viral RNA was also detected in some of the placentas (see Figure 11.1a). Using the higher dose of 7500 PFU for maternal inoculation of one animal gave similar

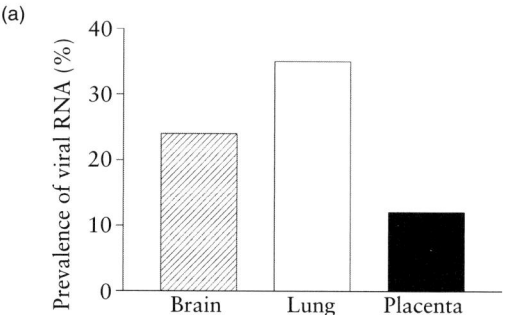

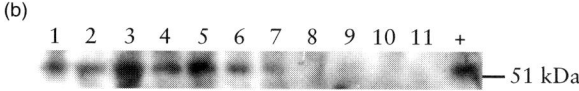

Figure 11.1 Transplacental passage of influenza A/WSN/33 virus. (a) Prevalence of viral RNA in fetal brain, lung, and corresponding placenta ($n = 17$). (b) Detection of the 56 kDa influenza A virus nucleoprotein in individual fetal brains (1–11) and a positive control (+). The tissues were sampled three days after maternal infection with 750 PFU of influenza A/WSN/33 virus. Reprinted from *Journal of Neurovirology* with permission from Taylor & Francis.

results (data not shown). Organs from fetuses whose mothers received PBS were always negative for viral RNA. Maternal infection was verified in lung tissue by RT-PCR amplification of the RNA encoding NP. mRNA encoding glyceraldehyde-3-phosphate dehydrogenase (GAPDH) was detected in all samples. In a fourth litter, the presence of viral protein in the fetal brains was investigated by Western blotting of homogenized whole brains. As seen in Figure 11.1b, viral nucleoprotein was detected in seven out of 11 brains tested.

SURVIVAL OF OFFSPRING

Mice born to mothers instilled intranasally with the higher dose of virus, 7500 PFU, showed signs of disease after three days and died within eight days of birth (Figure 11.2). This is in accordance with a previous study where a high rate of neonatal death within 10 days of birth was seen using the PR8 strain.[16] Offspring of mice infected with the lower dose of virus, 750 PFU, survived the observation period of three months. They had normal growth rates and showed no obvious signs of disease (see Figure 11.2).

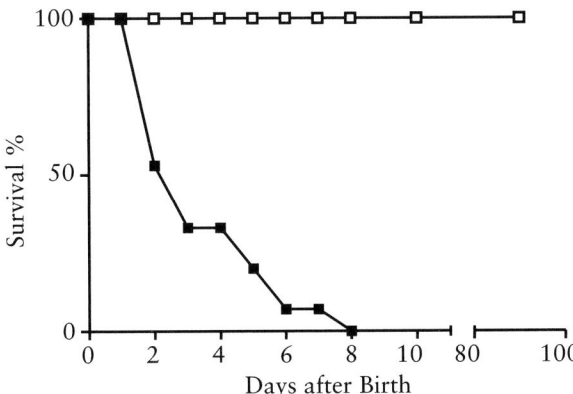

Figure 11.2 Survival of mice. Offspring to mothers exposed to 750 (□, n = 17) or 7500 (■, n = 15) PFU of influenza A/WSN/33 virus. Reprinted from *Journal of Neurovirology* with permission from Taylor & Francis.

Table 11.1 Persistence of influenza A/WSN/33 virus RNA in brains of animals exposed *in utero*

Age (days)	Virus RNA positive brains*
10	2/4
20	1/4
35	1/4
60	1/4
90	2/8

* Number of animals where viral RNA encoding M or NP was detected out of total number of animals tested at each time point of postnatal life. Reprinted from *Journal of Neurovirology* with permission from Taylor & Francis.

These mice were then sacrificed, and the brains were dissected out and subjected to further analyses.

PERSISTENCE OF VIRAL RNA

In order to examine whether viral RNA could persist in the brain of offspring of infected animals, mice were sacrificed at 10, 20, 35, 60, and 90 days of age. Their brains were analyzed for the presence of viral RNA. As seen in Table 11.1, viral RNA encoding M and/or NP could be detected in animals at all time points. Such sequences were never detected in animals born to sham-inoculated mice.

In a previous study, RNA corresponding to all viral segments was found to persist for up to 17 months in the brains of immunodefective TAP1 knockout mice after intracerebral inoculation.[24] However, no sign of persistence beyond 35 days was seen in wild-type animals,[23] which agrees with the notion that influenza A virus does not establish persistent infection in the immunocompetent host.[27,28] Hence, in the animals infected prenatally, the virus may either be tolerated or escape recognition by residing in an immunoprivileged site, such as neurons.[29–31] For a number of viral infections, the age of the host determines whether a persistent infection will be established or not. The most notable example is lymphocytic choriomeningitis (LCM) virus infections, in which the virus persists in all organs for the entire lifespan of mice infected neonatally, while the virus is rapidly cleared after infection of adult mice.[32] However, persistence of LCM virus has been reported, at very low levels, even in immunocompetent mice infected in adulthood.[33]

POSTNATAL INFECTION

Since the nervous system develops over a long period of time with synaptogenesis and myelination continuing throughout puberty in both humans and animals, it is relevant to consider the effects of postnatal infections on these parts of the developing central nervous system. We infected pups, intranasally, on days one or eight of postnatal life with 750 PFU of influenza A/WSN/33. All pups infected on day one of postnatal life died within one week. Pups infected on postnatal day eight survived for at least 90 days. Viral RNA could not be detected in the brains of these animals at this time point (unpublished data).

EFFECTS OF A MATERNAL VIRAL INFECTION ON THE OFFSPRING?

The key issue, of course, is whether the maternal influenza A/WSN/33 infection influences the development of the fetal central nervous system in ways leading to behavioral disturbances during adult life. This is still, in many ways, an open question. Researchers recently reported on marked behavioral disturbances in the offspring of mice infected in midgestation (E9.5) with 6000 PFU of the influenza A/NWS/33 strain.[34] Although the virus could not be detected in the brains of the offspring from these mothers they showed marked sickness behavior. Upon testing, these animals exhibited reduced exploratory behavior and social interactions as well as a reduction in pre-pulse inhibition to an acoustic startle. Interestingly, the induction of a maternal antiviral immune response using intra-abdominal injections of double-stranded RNA (poly I:C) resulted in similar effects on pre-pulse inhibition in the offspring. A similar study, where pregnant rats were injected with poly I:C, noted a disrupted latent inhibition which was evident in the adult, but not juvenile, offspring.[35]

CONCLUSION

Reports on the effects of congenital influenza A virus infections have previously been limited to neural tube defects in chick embryos[36–38] and fetal death with severe malformations in mice[39] after infection during early gestation. Our surviving mice showed no such gross changes in brain development. The surprising finding of virus persistence in the CNS of *in utero* infected offspring suggests that the virus has the potential to affect differentiated neuronal functions. This may become overt later in life due to reactivation of the virus, as has been shown for persisting Sindbis virus in immunocompetent BALB/c mice,[40] or by an altered vulnerability of the nervous tissue to other environmental factors. In the context of human neuropsychiatric diseases the key issues are these: to what extent are findings in mice applicable to humans, and do such events play any role in the etiology of human disease. Studies aiming to directly identify foreign (viral) nucleic acids in brain tissue or body fluids from individuals with schizophrenia or other neuropsychiatric diseases have, so far, not been successful.[41] Circumstantial evidence for a viral involvement is, however, accumulating at a steady pace, illustrated by a recent report of a significant association between serologic evidence of herpes simplex 1 infection and cognitive dysfunction in individuals with schizophrenia.[42] Additionally, the influenza–schizophrenia association was recently replicated in an epidemiological study carried out in France.[43] This study reported a significant association between maternal exposure to influenza epidemics during the fifth month of gestation and an elevated risk for the development of schizophrenia in the adult offspring.

The identification of viral agents as causative for some cases of schizophrenia according to Koch's postulates will be extremely difficult. Therefore attempts should be made to identify archival samples collected at time points preceding the onset of symptoms. Maternal sera obtained for rubella serology during early pregnancy, and blood routinely drawn from all newborn babies for screening of metabolic disorders (PKU-filters), may constitute a valuable source of information on infectious events during pregnancy and early life. Questions regarding the presence of specific antibodies and maternal seroconversion during the later part of pregnancy may be addressed in such samples. We recently reported that RNA suitable for amplification by PCR can be extracted from PKU-filters that have been stored for up to 27 years.[44] Hence, studies on gene expression in circulating white blood cells or the presence of foreign RNA may, theoretically, be performed on such archival PKU-filters.

ACKNOWLEDGMENTS

This work was supported by the Stanley Medical Research Institute, Bethesda, MD, USA.

REFERENCES

1. Raedler TJ, Knable MB, Weinberger DR. Schizophrenia as a developmental disorder of the cerebral cortex. *Curr Opin Neurobiol* 1998; **8**: 157–61.
2. Woods BT. Is schizophrenia a progressive neurodevelopmental disorder? Toward a unitary pathogenetic mechanism. *Am J Psychiatry* 1998; **155**: 1661–70.
3. Rantakallio P, Jones P, Moring J, Von Wendt L. Association between central nervous system infections during childhood and adult onset schizophrenia and other psychoses: a 28-year follow-up. *Int J Epidemiol* 1997; **26**: 837–43.
4. Munk-Jorgensen P, Ewald H. Epidemiology in neurobiological research: exemplified by the influenza–schizophrenia theory. *Br J Psychiatry* 2001; Suppl 40: S30–2.
5. Schneider-Schaulies J, Meulen V, Schneider-Schaulies S. Measles infection of the central nervous system. *J Neurovirol* 2003; **9**: 247–52.
6. Pearce BD, Steffensen SC, Paoletti AD et al. Persistent dentate granule cell hyperexcitability after neonatal infection with lymphocytic choriomeningitis virus. *J Neurosci* 1996; **16**: 220–8.
7. Ritova VV, Schastnyi EI, Ratushkina LS, Shuster IY. Investigation of the incidence of influenza A viraemia caused by virus strains circulating among children in 1968–1977. *J Hyg Epidemiol Microbiol Immunol* 1979; **23**: 35–41.
8. Reinacher M, Bonin J, Narayan O, Scholtissek C. Pathogenesis of neurovirulent influenza A virus infection in mice. Route of entry of virus into brain determines infection of different populations of cells. *Lab Invest* 1983; **49**: 686–92.
9. Rushton DI, Collie MH, Sweet C et al. The effects of maternal influenzal viraemia in late gestation on the conceptus of the pregnant ferret. *J Pathol* 1983; **140**: 181–91.
10. Mori I, Komatsu T, Takeuchi K et al. Viremia induced by influenza virus. *Microb Pathog* 1995; **19**: 237–44.
11. Yawn DH, Pyeatte JC, Joseph JM et al. Transplacental transfer of influenza virus. *JAMA* 1971; **216**: 1022–3.
12. McGregor JA, Burns JC, Levin MJ et al. Transplacental passage of influenza A/Bangkok (H3N2) mimicking amniotic fluid infection syndrome. *Am J Obstet Gynecol* 1984; **149**: 856–9.

13. Berkowitz K, LaSala A. Risk factors associated with the increasing prevalence of pneumonia during pregnancy. *Am J Obstet Gynecol* 1990; **163**: 981–5.
14. Steininger C, Holzmann H, Zwiauer KF, Popow-Kraupp T. Influenza A virus infection and cardiac arrhythmia during the neonatal period. *Scand J Infect Dis* 2002; **34**: 782–4.
15. Siem RA, Ly H, Imagawa DT, Adams JM. Influenza virus infections in pregnant mice. *J Neuropathol Exp Neurol* 1960; **19**: 125–9.
16. Takeyama T. Virological studies on experimental infection of pregnant mice with influenza virus. *Tohoku J Exp Med* 1966; **89**: 321–40.
17. Sweet C, Toms GL, Smith H. The pregnant ferret as a model for studying the congenital effects of influenza virus infection in utero: infection of foetal tissues in organ culture and in vivo. *Br J Exp Pathol* 1977; **58**: 113–23.
18. Sweet C, Collie MH, Toms GL, Smith H. The pregnant guinea-pig as a model for studying influenza virus infection in utero: infection of foetal tissues in organ culture and in vivo. *Br J Exp Pathol* 1977; **58**: 133–9.
19. Williams K, Mackenzie JS. Influenza infections during pregnancy in the mouse. *J Hyg (Lond)* 1977; **79**: 249–57.
20. Smith W, Andrewes CH, Laidlaw PP. A virus obtained from influenza patients. *Lancet* 1933; **1**: 66–8.
21. Francis T, Moore AM. A study of the neurotropic tendency in strains of the virus of epidemic influenza. *J Exp Med* 1940; **72**: 717–28.
22. Takahashi M, Yamada T, Nakajima S et al. The substantia nigra is a major target for neurovirulent influenza A virus. *J Exp Med* 1995; **181**: 2161–9.
23. Mori I, Diehl AD, Chauhan A et al. Selective targeting of habenular, thalamic midline and monoaminergic brainstem neurons by neurotropic influenza A virus in mice. *J Neurovirol* 1999; **5**: 355–62.
24. Aronsson F, Karlsson H, Ljunggren HG, Kristensson K. Persistence of the influenza A/WSN/33 virus RNA at midbrain levels of immunodefective mice. *J Neurovirol* 2001; **7**: 117–24.
25. Aronsson F, Robertson B, Ljunggren H-G, Kristensson K. Invasion and persistence of the neuroadapted influenza virus A/WSN/33 in the mouse olfactory system. *Viral Immunol* 2003; **16**: 415–23.
26. Aronsson F, Lannebo C, Paucar M et al. Persistence of viral RNA in the brain of offspring to mice infected with influenza A/WSN/33 virus during pregnancy. *J Neurovirol* 2002; **8**: 353–7.
27. Doherty PC, Topham DJ, Tripp RA. Establishment and persistence of virus-specific CD4+ and CD8+ T cell memory. *Immunol Rev* 1996; **150**: 23–44.
28. Hawke S, Stevenson PG, Freeman S, Bangham CR. Long-term persistence of activated cytotoxic T lymphocytes after viral infection of the central nervous system. *J Exp Med* 1998; **187**: 1575–82.
29. Kristensson K, Norrby E. Persistence of RNA viruses in the central nervous system. *Ann Rev Microbiol* 1986; **40**: 159–84.
30. Joly E, Mucke L, Oldstone MB. Viral persistence in neurons explained by lack of major histocompatibility class I expression. *Science* 1991; **253**: 1283–5.
31. Stevenson PG, Hawke S, Sloan DJ, Bangham CR. The immunogenicity of intracerebral virus infection depends on anatomical site. *J Virol* 1997; **71**: 145–51.
32. Lehmann-Grube F. Persistent infection of mice with lymphocytic choriomeningitis virus. In: *Virus Infections and the Developing Nervous System* (Johnson RT, Lyon G, eds). Lancaster: Kluwer Academic Publisher, 1988: 69–83.
33. Ciurea A, Klenerman P, Hunziker L et al. Persistence of lymphocytic choriomeningitis virus at very low levels in immune mice. *Proc Natl Acad Sci USA* 1999; **96**: 11964–9.
34. Shi L, Fatemi SH, Sidwell RW, Patterson PH. Maternal influenza infection causes marked behavioral and pharmacological changes in the offspring. *J Neurosci* 2003; **23**: 297–302.
35. Zuckerman L, Rehavi M, Nachman R, Weiner I. Immune activation during pregnancy in rats leads to a postpubertal emergence of disrupted latent inhibition, dopaminergic hyperfunction, and altered limbic morphology in the offspring: a novel neurodevelopmental model of schizophrenia. *Neuropsychopharmacol* 2003; **28**: 1778–89.
36. Hamburger V, Habel K. Teratogenetic and lethal effects of influenza-A and mumps viruses on early chick embryos. *Proc Soc Exp Biol NY* 1947; **66**: 608–17.
37. Robertson GG, DeBandi HO Jr, Williamson AP, Blattner RJ. Brain abnormalities in early chick embryos infected with influenza-A virus. *Anat Rec* 1967; **158**: 1–9.
38. Johnson KP, Klasnja R, Johnson RT. Neural tube defects of chick embryos: an indirect result of influenza A virus infection. *J Neuropathol Exp Neurol* 1971; **30**: 68–74.
39. Adams JM, Heath HD, Imagawa DT et al. Viral infections in the embryo. *AMA J Dis Child* 1956; **92**: 109–14.
40. Levine B, Griffin DE. Persistence of viral RNA in mouse brains after recovery from acute alphavirus encephalitis. *J Virol* 1992; **66**: 6429–35.
41. Karlsson H. Viruses and schizophrenia, connection or coincidence. *Neuroreport* 2003; **14**: 535–42.
42. Dickerson FB, Boronow JJ, Stallings C et al. Association of serum antibodies to herpes simplex virus 1 with cognitive deficits in individuals with schizophrenia. *Arch Gen Psychiatry* 2003; **60**: 466–72.
43. Limosin F, Rouillon F, Payan C et al. Prenatal exposure to influenza as a risk factor for adult schizophrenia. *Acta Psychiatr Scand* 2003; **107**: 331–5.
44. Karlsson H, Guthenberg C, von Dobeln U, Kristensson K. Extraction of RNA from dried blood on filter papers after long-term storage. *Clin Chem* 2003; **49**: 979–81.

12

Maternal infection, cytokines, and risk for schizophrenia

John H Gilmore and L Fredrik Jarskog

INTRODUCTION

The cause(s) of schizophrenia remain elusive. While there is clear evidence that risk for schizophrenia can run in families and that genes play a role in risk for schizophrenia, the search for individual genes has been disappointing. The genes that have been identified confer only a small portion of overall risk. Against this backdrop, there has been renewed interest in perinatal environmental risk factors for schizophrenia. A large population-based study found that place of birth and season of birth accounted for 41.4% of the cases of schizophrenia based on population attributable risk, clearly demonstrating the importance of perinatal environmental factors in the etiology of schizophrenia.[1] The pathological mechanisms underlying prenatal and perinatal risk factors for schizophrenia remain largely unstudied. Understanding the mechanisms through which pre- and perinatal risk factors alter brain development will ultimately inform us about the underlying cellular and circuit pathology of schizophrenia, and provide strategies for preventing or mitigating risk. This chapter will review the evidence that suggests prenatal exposure to infection increases risk for schizophrenia, and consider mechanisms through which maternal infection could impact the developing fetal brain. Finally, it will focus on the role that inflammatory cytokines, generated by the maternal immune system in response to infection, play in altering fetal brain development and increasing risk for schizophrenia.

PRENATAL EXPOSURE TO INFECTION AND SCHIZOPHRENIA

Most research on prenatal exposure to infection and schizophrenia has focused on a specific viral infection – influenza. The weight of the evidence indicates that maternal influenza infection during pregnancy is associated with a higher incidence of schizophrenia in offspring.[2,3] While the emphasis has been on influenza, other types of infection have also been implicated. These include pneumonia and diphtheria,[4] measles, varicella-zoster, and polio,[5] and bronchopneumonia.[6] More recent studies have moved beyond epidemiologic association to studies that link infections in individual mothers with schizophrenia in their children. Respiratory infections, broadly defined, in the second trimester increase risk for schizophrenia.[7] In this same cohort, serologic evidence of maternal exposure to influenza also increased risk of schizophrenia in offspring.[8] Rubella[9] and poliovirus[10] infections during pregnancy have also been linked to increased risk for schizophrenia. Finally, the offspring of mothers with elevated IgG and IgM levels, and antibodies to herpes simplex virus type 2 during pregnancy, have an increased risk for schizophrenia.[11]

These studies indicate that a variety of maternal infections during pregnancy, both viral and bacterial, are associated with increased risk for schizophrenia. There are other more indirect lines of evidence implicating maternal infection as a contributor to risk for schizophrenia. If infections in general, rather than specific types of infection, are the main association with subsequent development of schizophrenia in offspring, the methodology of prior studies that focused on individual infectious agents may not be adequate to detect the contributions of individual diseases against a broad background of infection. A more accurate picture of the association between *in utero* exposure to infection and schizophrenia may be gained by comparing periods with low versus high rates of infection of all kinds. An excess of late winter/early spring births has consistently been found in patients with schizophrenia; this excess has been attributed to infectious, nutritional, or other environmental factors such as temperature.[12]

A variety of obstetric complications are more frequent in pregnancies in which the offspring develop schizophrenia.[13,14] There is increasing evidence that prenatal infection is associated with many of the obstetric complications linked to schizophrenia, including premature birth,[15-17] fetal growth restriction,[18] the signs of birth asphyxia such as low APGAR scores and neonatal seizures,[19] and preeclampsia.[20] Therefore many of the obstetric complications associated with increased risk of schizophrenia, including low birth weight and short gestation,[21] preeclampsia,[22] and perinatal hypoxia and low APGAR scores,[22] may in fact be associated with clinical or subclinical infection. The presence of chorioamnionitis has largely been ignored as a risk factor for schizophrenia, though it is a major cause of premature birth and other perinatal complications.

Infections during pregnancy have also been associated with subsequent abnormalities of brain development. The Collaborative Perinatal Study found that urinary tract infections with fever, pneumonia, and puerperal infections during pregnancy were associated with poor outcomes, including neurological abnormalities at age one.[23] In one study, chorioamnionitis was associated with a 4.8-fold increased risk for cerebral palsy.[24] Intra-amniotic infection is associated with poor neurodevelopment in premature infants.[25] Prenatal infections also have an association with mental retardation,[26] autism,[27] lissencephaly,[28] neural tube defects,[29] and neurologic 'handicap' (cerebral palsy, mental retardation, epilepsy, or severe defects of hearing and vision) in four-year-olds.[30]

CYTOKINES: A KEY MECHANISTIC ROLE

A variety of maternal infections during pregnancy increase risk for schizophrenia and other neurodevelopmental disorders, indicating that the association between *in utero* exposure to infection and schizophrenia is a more general phenomenon related to infection, and not limited to a single etiologic viral agent such as influenza. In 1997, we proposed that proinflammatory cytokines, generated by the maternal immune system in response to infection, play a key mechanistic role in altering early brain development and increasing risk for schizophrenia.[31]

Theoretically, several factors could mediate the association between maternal exposure to infection and altered brain development increasing the risk for schizophrenia. Hypotheses about the role of *in utero* exposure to infection in the etiology of schizophrenia have focused on direct infection of the developing fetus[32] or the generation of antibodies that cross-react with neuronal antigens.[33] Studies of influenza infection during pregnancy suggest that direct infection of the fetus is a rare event. While there have been a few reports of direct fetal infection with influenza virus,[34-36] other studies have failed to detect transplacental passage of virus in humans.[37,38] A large case control study of over 1,600 pregnancies failed to detect virus-specfic IgM antibodies in fetal cord blood in any case of maternal infection, indicating no transplacental transmission of virus.[39] Support for the hypothesis that inflammatory cytokines are important in the association between prenatal exposure to infection and schizophrenia comes from studies that find production of IL-1β, IL-6, and TNF-α is increased by infection with influenza in humans and animals.[40-42]

It is well known that cytokines, including IL-1β, IL-6, and TNF-α, have a variety of effects on the central nervous system (CNS) and are expressed by glial and neuronal elements within the CNS.[43-45] Cytokines regulate normal brain development and have been implicated in abnormal brain development.[46-48] Expression of cytokine mRNA in the CNS is developmentally regulated in mouse, rat, sheep, and human brain,[49-54] an indication of the important role that cytokines play in normal neurodevelopment.

Maternally generated cytokines cross the placenta and regulate cell growth and development in the fetus; granulocyte colony-stimulating factor (G-CSF) injected into pregnant rats can stimulate fetal granulopoiesis.[55] Maternal transforming growth factor-β1 (TGF-β1) can cross the placenta and 'rescue' TGF-β1 null embryos.[56] Chorioamnionitis stimulates human fetal granulopoiesis in the second trimester, an effect presumably mediated by cytokines.[57] Levels of G-CSF are increased in the fetal circulation during chorioamnionitis; the likely source of G-CSF in the fetal circulation is the maternal circulation.[58] IL-1β, IL-6, and TNF-α all cross placenta membranes *in vitro*[59] and a recent study found that maternally administered IL-1 receptor antagonist crosses the placenta into amniotic fluid.[60] An additional source of cytokines in prenatal infection may be the placenta, as the human placenta synthesizes IL-1β, IL-6, and TNF-α in response to infection.[61-63] Finally, recent studies indicate the the fetus itself can mount an inflammatory response, especially of IL-6, in the face of maternal infection.[64,65]

IL-1β, IL-6, and TNF-α cross the blood–brain barrier in mature rodents.[66-70] In addition, IL-1β, IL-6, and TNFα each can break down the blood–brain barrier.[71,72] Finally, the blood–brain barrier is incomplete in the fetus,[73,74] making it very likely that systemically generated cytokines gain entry into the fetal brain.

CYTOKINES AND SCHIZOPHRENIA

Since we first proposed the hypothesis that cytokines play a key role in the association between maternal infection, altered brain development, and risk for schizophrenia, several studies have been published that lend support. Maternal blood levels of TNFα are elevated in pregnancies in which the offspring goes on to develop schizophrenia.[75] Studies have also found associations between schizophrenia and cytokine genes, including TNFα[76-78] and IL-1.[79] Further, associations between brain morphology in patients with schizophrenia and polymorphisms for IL-1β[80] and the TNR receptor-II[81] have been described. It is likely that genes regulating the immune response would have an effect on early brain development, especially in the setting of infection. For example, a TNFα promoter variant that increases TNFα production is associated with high rates of premature birth, an association thought to be related to exposure to infection.[82,83]

LESSONS FROM PERIVENTRICULAR LEUKOMALACIA AND CEREBRAL PALSY

A theory of cytokine mediation in the association between maternal infection and altered brain development would predict that levels of these cytokines are altered in human pregnancies complicated by infection. This is indeed the case. IL-1β, IL-6, and TNFα levels are all significantly increased in the amniotic fluid in the setting of infection, typically chorioamnionitis, in human pregnancies.[84-87] More importantly, cytokine levels in the fetal circulation, including IL-1β, IL-6, and IL-8, are increased in the setting of infection.[85,88-90]

It has been proposed that the maternal immune response to infection can have a harmful effect on brain development – an effect mediated by cytokines.[91] This hypothesis has been specifically applied to the role of TNFα in periventricular leukomalacia (PVL).[92] Intrauterine infection greatly increases the risk of PVL and cerebral palsy in premature infants and term infants,[19,93,94] and cytokines have been implicated in this association.[95] Elevated levels of IL-6 in fetal cord blood, and of IL-6 and IL-1β in amniotic fluid, are associated with white matter lesions and cerebral palsy in premature infants.[96,97] Children with cerebral palsy have high neonatal blood levels of cytokines, including IL-1β and TNFα.[98] Finally, premature infants with cerebral lesions on MRI (including germinal layer or intraventricular hemorrhage, periventricular lesions, and cystic lesions of the caudate) exhibit high levels of IL-1β, IL-6, IL-10, and TNF-α in cord blood at birth.[99] Interestingly, infants with cerebral lesions in this study also had evidence of T-cell activation, indicating that the fetus was mounting an immune response, and that this response was associated with high risk for brain damage.

Beyond elevations of cytokines in fetal blood and amniotic fluid, there is evidence that cytokines are elevated in the brain tissue of infants with white matter lesions. IL-1β, IL-6, and TNFα are highly expressed in white matter around PVL lesions, especially in astrocytes and microglial cells.[96,100,101] Both IL-1β and TNFα are toxic to developing oligodendrocytes and are thought to play a role in the development of PVL.[102] A recent study also indicates that there is increased expression of IL-1β and TNFα by cortical and subcortical neurons in the brains of infants with PVL,[103] indicating that the same inflammatory processes that lead to PVL may also alter neuron development. This study provides evidence that the inflammatory response within the developing cortex to maternal infection could lead to altered neuron development and increased risk for schizophrenia.

We reported a case of a young woman who had premature birth and evidence of PVL on neonatal ultrasound who went on to develop early-onset schizophrenia; MRI at age 14 years showed enlarged, asymmetric ventricles and periventricular white matter abnormalities.[104] This case illustrates how lessons learned from PVL can inform our understanding of the causes of schizophrenia. While gross white matter lesions are not more frequently seen in schizophrenia,[105] imaging studies reveal more subtle abnormalities of white matter volume and diffusion tensor properties in schizophrenia.[106,107] This raises the possibility that prenatal exposure to infection could alter white matter development in a way that would lead to the dysconnectivity believed to underlie schizophrenia. It has been hypothesized that abnormalities of the corticocortical and thalamocortical connections underlie the cognitive and attentional abnormalities often found in children born prematurely.[108] These same connections have been implicated in schizophrenia. Therefore, prenatal exposure to infection can cause the abnormalities of connectivity thought to underlie schizophrenia through subtle alterations of white matter development, cortical neuron development, or both.

CYTOKINES AND NEURON DEVELOPMENT

Studies of postmortem schizophrenic human brains indicate that there is loss of synapses and dendritic

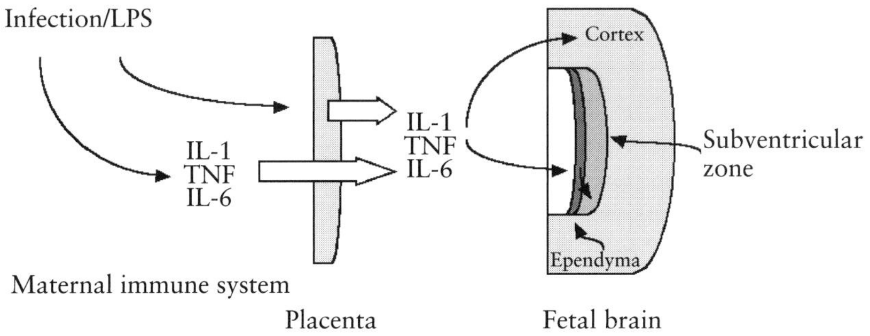

Figure 12.1 Mechanisms by which cytokines, generated by the maternal or placental immune system, can alter early brain development. Developing neurons and glia are directly exposed to cytokines in the fetal circulation through an immature blood–brain barrier. In addition, cytokine activation of the developing ependyma that lines the ventricles can potentially alter ependymal cell interactions with developing neurons and glia in the subventricular zone as well as increase CSF levels of cytokines.

spines in cortical neurons.[109,110] Cytokines regulate the neuron development that would give rise to these abnormalities. Most studies have focused on neuronal survival *in vitro* and indicate that IL-1β, IL-6, and TNF-α can each be neurotoxic to developing neurons. For example, we found that IL-1β, IL-6, and TNF-α decreased the survival of fetal serotonergic neurons and dopaminergic neurons[111] and embryonic cortical neurons.[112] IL-1β also decreases neuron survival in primary cultures of embryonic rat hippocampus.[113] TNFα is neurotoxic in primary human fetal cortical cultures, an effect mediated by glutamate.[114] TNFα also potentiates glutamate neurotoxicity in cultures of human fetal brain.[115] IL-1 and TNFα have synergistic neurotoxic effects in mixed cultures of mouse fetal cortex.[116]

Cytokine regulation of other neuron developmental processes has been less well studied. However, there is growing evidence that cytokines, including IL-1β, IL-6, and TNF-α, can regulate neuronal phenotype, as well as morphologic and functional maturation as reflected in dendritic complexity.[117–120] Recently, it has been shown that TNFα inhibits neurite outgrowth and branching in hippocampal neurons,[121] indicating that cytokine overexpression in the setting of maternal infection could cause long-lasting changes in synaptic connectivity that would increase risk for schizophrenia.

CYTOKINES REGULATE NEUROTROPHIC FACTOR EXPRESSION

Neurotrophic factors are a family of growth factors that include nerve growth factor (NGF), brain derived neurotrophic factor (BDNF), neurotrophin 3 (NT-3), and neurotrophin 4/5 (NT-4/5). These neurotrophic factors bind to tyrosine kinase receptors, with NGF binding preferentially to TrkA and BDNF and NT-4/5 binding preferentially to TrkB; NT-3's activity appears to be mediated through TrkC.[122] The neurotrophins also bind to the low affinity NGF receptor or p75^{NTR}, one of a group of structurally related cytokine receptors which can promote cell death, that includes tumor necrosis factor receptors.[123] Neurotrophic factors have been implicated in a variety of neurodevelopmental processes including programmed cell death, neuronal differentiation, and the establishment of neuronal connections.[122]

There is increasing evidence of interactions between cytokines and neurotrophic factors in the CNS. IL-1β and TNFα increase NGF expression by cortical astrocytes[124,125] and in cultures of human microglia.[126] IL-6 also induces NGF and NT-3 expression in astrocyte cultures.[127] Activated microglia in multiple sclerosis plaques express BDNF[128] and lipopolysaccharide stimulates BDNF expression in microglia in culture.[129] Whether NGF and BDNF release is an attempt to compensate for the neurotoxic effects of cytokines, or whether it may ultimately participate in the neurotoxicity of cytokines (perhaps through the p75^{NTR} receptor) is unknown at this time. Much work needs to be done to elucidate the interactions of cytokines and neurotrophic factors. Cytokine regulation of neurotrophic factor expression in the developing brain represents a potential mechanism through which early exposure to infection could alter neuron development, including the establishment and maintenance of synaptic connectivity, processes that have been implicated in schizophrenia and other neurodevelopmental disorders.

LPS: IMPACT OF SYSTEMIC INFECTION

Several animal models indicate that prenatal exposure to maternal infection can cause longlasting behavioral changes consistent with schizophrenia. Maternal infection with human influenza virus in mice, a model developed by Hossein Fatemi and described in his Chapter 9, results in abnormalities in pre-pulse inhibition.[130] Maternal exposure to poly I:C, a synthetic double-stranded RNA that stimulates a cytokine response, causes pre-pulse inhibition abnormalities[130] and disrupted latent inhibition.[131,132] Maternal exposure to *E. coli* cell wall endotoxin lipopolysaccharide (LPS) also stimulates a cytokine response and disrupts sensorimotor gating in the offspring.[133] In Fatemi's influenza model, no virus is detected in the fetal brain,[130] suggesting that it is the maternal immune response to the infection that causes the behavioral changes. In the poly I:C and LPS models also, it is the immune response to the challenge that must be the mechanism of action, as no infectious agent is present.

There has been very little systematic study of the impact of infection on the developing brain. Peripheral administration of the cell wall endotoxin LPS has been used as a model of infection in rodents. LPS stimulates cytokine expression in the CNS. For example, LPS induces IL-1β, IL-6, and TNF-α mRNA expression in the thalamus, hippocampus, striatum, hypothalamus, and pituitary.[134–136] The response of the CNS to LPS offers clues about how early exposure to infection may impact the developing brain.

In general there are two phases of response to LPS in the adult rat. The initial phase is localized to the ependyma, choroid plexus, cerebral vasculature, and the hypothalamus, followed by a more diffuse activation of the cerebral cortex. IL-1β mRNA is expressed in the choroid and blood vessels maximally at two hours and declines by four hours, while a later diffuse cortical expression, mainly in microglia, peaks at 8–12 hours and is still present 24 hours after LPS exposure.[137–141] The expression of IL-1β mRNA in microglia parallels expression of OX-42 (a marker of activated microglia) in the cortex, which is maximal 8–24 hours after LPS injection.[142] The response of IL-6 and TNFα in the brain to LPS has been less well studied. IL-6 increases in the cortex and hippocampus.[143] TNFα protein increases in the hypothalamus one hour after exposure to LPS[144] and is increased throughout the brain after higher doses of LPS.[145]

Studies in animal pregnancies indicate that LPS increases cytokine levels in the maternal circulation and amniotic fluid, and can have a significant impact on fetal brain development. LPS administered to pregnant rats and hamsters produces a variety of CNS abnormalities including enlarged ventricles, microcephaly, and neuronal necrosis.[146,147] LPS increases IL-1α, IL-6, and TNF-α in the maternal circulation and IL-1α and IL-6 in the amniotic fluid of mice,[148] and increases TNFα in the maternal circulation in sheep.[149] LPS does not enter the fetal circulation,[150] thus any effect on fetal brain development would be a result of the maternal or placental immune system response to LPS. A study in goats indicated that the fetus is minimally responsive (cortisol and prostaglandin F2α) to direct LPS exposure, providing additional support for the view that the maternal/placental immune response is critical in the impact of LPS exposure on the developing brain.[151]

Models of intrauterine infection indicate that maternal infection can increase TNF expression in the fetal brain and increase programmed cell death. Intrauterine inoculation of LPS in rabbits results in increased programmed cell death in the fetal brain.[152] Intracervical injection of LPS was found to increase programmed cell death and TNFα immunohistochemistry in the fetal brain as well.[153] Maternal exposure to systemic LPS at E18 during pregnancy in rats increases IL-1β and TNF-α mRNA in the fetal brain.[154] This same study found decreased myelin basic protein and increased GFAP protein in the cortex and hippocampus of neonatal pups after prenatal exposure to LPS.[154]

To study the regulation of cytokine expression after maternal infection, we injected E16 pregnant rats i.p. with *E. coli* LPS.[155] Placenta, amniotic fluid, and fetal brains were collected two and eight hours after LPS exposure. There was a significant treatment effect of low dose (0.5 mg/kg) LPS on placenta cytokine levels, with significant increases of IL-1β, IL-6, and TNFα over the two and eight hour time course. In amniotic fluid, there was a significant effect of treatment on IL-6 levels. Two hours after maternal administration of high dose (2.5 mg/kg) LPS, there were significant elevations of placenta IL-6 and TNFα, a significant increase of TNFα in amniotic fluid, and a small but significant decrease of TNFα in fetal brain. The observed differences between this study and the one described above[154] may be due to differences in mRNA transcription and protein translation after challenge, or may reflect a maturation of the immune responses within the fetal brain from day 16 to day 18 – or perhaps maturation of microglia cells.

We have also examined the regulation of the neurotrophic factors BDNF and NGF in the developing brain after LPS exposure.[156] We found that prenatal maternal LPS exposure significantly increased BDNF in the fetal brain and signifcantly increased NGF levels in the cortex of six-day-old pups. NGF levels were increased in the placenta and amniotic fluid of exposed rats. In the setting of infection, the neurotrophic factor expression response may represent a neuroprotective response to the toxicity of inflammatory mediators.[128] Increased BDNF in the developing cortex after exposure to maternal infection could ultimately change the number and specificity of synaptic contacts between neurons, altering connectivity in functional circuits that underlie the symptoms associated with schizophrenia and other neurodevelopmental disorders. For example, BDNF can inhibit ocular dominance formation,[157] and can inhibit dendritic growth in layer 6 of the visual cortex while stimulating dendritic growth in layer 4.[158]

Interestingly, NGF and TNFα are decreased in the fetal liver/spleen after maternal LPS exposure. The decrease in TNFα in fetal liver/spleen (and fetal brain) is unexpected and in contrast to increases of TNFα mRNA in the liver and spleen[159] and in the brain of adult rodents after LPS exposure.[160] Our finding is consistent with studies that find TNFα in fetal cord blood of human pregnancies in the setting of infection to be unchanged or decreased.[85,88] The increase in BDNF in fetal brain after maternal infection is also in contrast to the decrease of BDNF described in the adult hippocampus after systemic IL-1β administration,[161] and indicates that the fetal brain may respond to inflammatory stimuli in a different manner compared to the mature brain. It is not possible to predict the response of the fetal immune system or the fetal brain to infection based on studies in mature animals.

CONCLUSIONS

Over 40 years ago, Adams and colleagues summarized the concept of the relationship between infection during pregnancy and its effect on the fetus:

... moderate to severe infections early in pregnancy will cause abortion. However, if the infection is mild enough and abortion does not result, there are several possible courses which may follow: (a) the offspring may develop normally and be born at term with no detectable evidence of abnormalities, (b) it is conceivable that there may be mild changes which would manifest themselves later in infancy or childhood, (c) the baby may be born with congenital abnormalities of varying degree.[162]

While there is mounting evidence that maternal infection can alter fetal brain development in a way that increases the risk of schizophrenia and other neurodevelopmental disorders, little is known about how this happens. The inflammatory cytokine response of the mother, the placenta, and even the fetus itself probably plays a key role. The ultimate impact of the cytokine and neurotrophic factor response to maternal infection on fetal brain development is probably dependent both on the timing and severity of the infection in relation to critical periods of brain development, and on interactions with other environmental and genetic risk factors. In the spectrum of neurodevelopmental outcomes associated with prenatal exposure to maternal infection such as autism, cerebral palsy, and mental retardation, schizophrenia is on the less severe end, at least in terms of neuropathologic abnormalities.

Infection during pregnancy can be associated with other mechanisms that would also adversely affect fetal brain development, including stress hormones,[163–165] hypoxia,[166] reduced blood flow to the fetus,[166] malnutrition,[167] and hyperthermia.[168] Ultimately, a true mechanistic understanding of the impact of maternal infection on fetal brain development will have to integrate inflammatory, hormonal, and other potential mechanisms. Genetic determinants of the maternal and/or fetal immune response will also probably play a role in the ultimate impact of maternal infection on the developing brain.

If one assumes that schizophrenia is a disorder of synaptic connectivity, then any process or molecule that regulates dendritic growth and synaptic formation in the developing brain may contribute to risk. Given the consistent evidence for prenatal exposure to maternal infection as a risk factor for some forms of schizophrenia, the inflammatory cytokine response becomes a candidate mechanism. The study of interactions between the immune system and the developing brain is just beginning, but offers a key to understanding one of the contributing causes of schizophrenia and other neurodevelopmental disorders. This line of investigation may also offer potential targets for therapeutic strategies that may prevent or reduce the risk of abnormal brain development in the setting of infection.

REFERENCES

1. Mortensen PB, Pedersen CB, Westergaard T et al. Effects of family history and season of birth on the risk of schizophrenia. *N Engl J Med* 1999; **340**: 603–8.
2. McGrath J, Murray R. Risk factors for schizophrenia. In: *Schizophrenia* (Hirsh SR, Weinberger DR, eds). Cambridge MA: Blackwell Science, 1995: 196–9.
3. Bagalkote H, Pang D, Jones PB. Maternal influenza and schizophrenia in offspring. *Intl J Ment Health* 2001; **39**: 3–21.

4. Watson CG, Kucala T, Tilleskjor C, Jacobs L. Schizophrenic births seasonality in relation to the incidence of infectious diseases and temperature extremes. *Arch Gen Psychiatry* 1984; **41**: 85–90.
5. Torrey EF, Rawlings R, Waldman IN. Schizophrenic births and viral diseases in two states. *Schizophr Res* 1988; **1**: 73–7.
6. O'Callaghan E, Sham PC, Talei N et al. The relationship of schizophrenic births to 16 infectious diseases. *Br J Psychiatry* 1994; **165**: 353–6.
7. Brown AS, Schaefer CA, Wyatt RJ et al. Maternal exposure to respiratory infections and adult schizophrenia spectrum disorders: a prospective birth cohort study. *Schizophr Bull* 2000; **26**: 287–95.
8. Brown AS, Begg M, Gravenstein S et al. Serologic evidence for prenatal influenza in the etiology of schizophrenia. *Arch Gen Psychiatry* 2004; **61**: 774–80.
9. Brown AS, Cohen P, Greenwald S, Susser E. Nonaffective psychosis after exposure to rubella. *Am J Psychiatry* 2000; **157**: 438–43.
10. Suvisaari J, Haukka J, Tanskanen A et al. Association between prenatal exposure to poliovirus infection and adult schizophrenia. *Am J Psychiatry* 1999; **156**: 1100–2.
11. Buka SL, Tsuang MT, Torrey EF et al. Maternal infections and subsequent psychosis among offspring. *Arch Gen Psychiatry* 2001; **58**: 1032–7.
12. Torrey EF, Miller J, Rawlings R, Yolken RH. Seasonality of birth in schizophrenia and bipolar disorder: a review of the literature. *Schizophr Res* 1997; **28**: 1–38.
13. Geddes JR, Lawrie SM. Obstetric complications and schizophrenia: a meta-analysis. *Br J Psychiatry* 1995; **167**: 786–93.
14. Cannon M, Jones PB, Murray RM. Obstetric complications and schizophrenia: historical and meta-analytic review. *Am J Psychiatry* 2000; **159**: 1080–92.
15. Greci LS, Gilson GJ, Nevils R et al. Is amniotic fluid analysis the key to preterm labor? A model using interleukin-6 for predicting rapid delivery. *Am J Obstet Gynecol* 1998; **179**: 172–8.
16. Gibbs RS, Romero R, Hillie SL et al. A review of premature birth and subclinical infection. *Am J Obstet Gynecol* 1992; **166**: 1515–28.
17. Arntzen KJ, Kjollesdal AM, Halgunset J et al. TNF, IL-1, IL-6, IL-8 and soluble TNF receptors in relation to chorioamnionitis and premature labor. *J Perinat Med* 1998; **26**: 17–26.
18. Beckmann I, Meisel-Mikolajczyk F, Leszczynski P et al. Endotoxin-induced fetal growth retardation in the pregnant guinea pig. *Am J Obstet Gynecol* 1993; **168**: 714–8.
19. Grether JK, Nelson KB. Maternal infection and cerebral palsy in infants of normal birth weight. *JAMA* 1997; **278**: 207–11.
20. Hsu CD, Witter FR. Urogenital infection in preeclampsia. *Int J Gynecol Obstet* 1995; **49**: 271–5.
21. Jones PB, Rantakallio P, Hartikainen A et al. Schizophrenia as a long term outcome of pregnancy, delivery, and perinatal complications: a 28-year follow-up of the 1966 North Finland general population birth cohort. *Am J Psychiatry* 1998; **155**: 355–64.
22. Dalman C, Allebeck P, Cullberg J et al. Obstetric complications and the risk of schizophrenia: a longitudinal study of a national birth cohort. *Arch Gen Psychiatry* 1999; **56**: 234–40.
23. Niswander KR, Gordon M. *The Women and Their Pregnancies: The Collaborative Perinatal Study of the National Institute of Neurological Diseases and Stroke.* Philadelphia: WB Sanders Co, 1972.
24. Nelson KB, Ellenberg JH. Antecedents of cerebral palsy 1. Univariate analysis of risk. *Am J Dis Childhood* 1985; **139**: 1031–8.
25. Gibbs RS, Duff P. Progress in the management of clinical intraamniotic infection. *Am J Obstet Gynecol* 1991; **164**: 1317–26.
26. Rantakallio P, Von Wendt L. Risk factors for mental retardation. *Arch Disease Childhood* 1985; **60**: 946–52.
27. Ciaranello AL, Ciaranello RD. The neurobiology of autism. *Ann Rev Neurosci* 1995; **18**: 101–28.
28. Dobyns WB, Elias ER, Newlin AC et al. Causal heterogeneity in isolated lissencephaly. *Neurology* 1992; **42**: 1375–88.
29. Lynberg MC, Khoury MJ, Lu X, Cocian T. Maternal flu, fever, and the risk of neural tube defects: a population-based case-control study. *Am J Epidemiol* 1994; **140**: 244–55.
30. Holst K, Andersen E, Philip J, Henningsen I. Antenatal and perinatal conditions correlated to handicap among 4-year-old children. *Am J Perinatology* 1989; **6**: 258–67.
31. Gilmore JH, Jarskog LF. Exposure to infection and brain development: cytokines in the pathogenesis of schizophrenia. *Schizophr Res* 1997; **24**: 365–36.
32. Yolken RH, Torrey EF. Viruses, schizophrenia, and bipolar disorder. *Clin Microbiol Rev* 1995; **8**: 131–45.
33. Wright P, Gill M, Murray RM. Schizophrenia: genetics and the maternal immune response to viral infection. *Am J Med Genet (Neuropsychiatric Genet)* 1993; **48**: 40–6.
34. Ruben FL, Winkelstein A, Sabbagha RE. In utero sensitization with influenza virus in man. *Proc Soc Exp Biol Med* 1975; **149**: 881–3.
35. Ruben FL, Thompson DS. Cord blood lymphocyte in vitro responses to influenza A antigens after an epidemic of influenza A/Port Chalmers/73 (H_3N_2). *Am J Obstet Gynecol* 1981; **141**: 443–7.
36. Conover PT, Roessmann U. Malformation complex in an infant with intrauterine influenza viral infection. *Arch Pathol Lab Med* 1990; **114**: 535–8.
37. Monif GRG, Sowards DL, Eitzman DV. Serologic and immunologic evaluation of neonates following maternal influenza during the second and third trimesters of gestation. *Am J Obstet Gynecol* 1972; **114**: 239–42.
38. Ramphal R, Donnelly WH, Small PA Jr. Fatal influenza pneumonia in pregnancy: failure to demonstrate transplacental transmission of influenza virus. *Am J Obstet Gynecol* 1980; **138**: 347–8.
39. Irving WL, James DK, Stephenson T et al. Influenza virus infection in the second and third trimesters of pregnancy: a clinical and seroepidemiological study. *Br J Obstet Gynecol* 2000; **107**: 1282–9.
40. Peschke T, Bender A, Nain M, Gemsa D. Role of macrophage cytokines in influenza A virus infections. *Immunobiol* 1993; **189**: 340–55.
41. Conn CA, McClellan JL, Maassab HF et al. Cytokines and the acute phase response to influenza in mice. *Am J Physiol* 1995; **268**: R78–84.
42. Kragsbjerg P, Jones I, Vikerfors T, Holmberg H. Diagnostic value of blood cytokine concentrations in acute pneumonia. *Thorax* 1995; **50**: 1253–7.
43. Bartfai T, Schultzberg M. Cytokines in neuronal cell types. *Neurochem Int* 1993; **22**: 435–44.
44. Hopkins SJ, Rothwell NJ. Cytokines and the nervous system I: expression and recognition. *Trends Neurosci* 1995; **18**: 83–8.
45. Rothwell NJ, Hopkins SJ. Cytokines and the nervous system II: actions and mechanisms of actions. *Trends Neurosci* 1995; **18**: 130–6.
46. Merrill JE. Tumor necrosis factor alpha, interleukin 1 and related cytokines in brain development: normal and pathological. *Dev Neurosci* 1992; **14**: 1–10.
47. Mehler MF, Kessler JA. Growth factor regulation of neuronal development. *Dev Neurosci* 1994; **16**: 180–95.
48. Mehler MF, Kessler JA. Hematolymphopoetic and inflammatory cytokines in neural development. *Trends Neurosci* 1997; **20**: 357–65.

49. Burns TM, Clough JA, Klein RM et al. Developmental regulation of cytokine expression in the mouse brain. *Growth Factors* 1993; **9**: 253–8.
50. Gadient RA, Otten U. Differential expression of interleukin-6 (IL-6) and interleukin-6 receptor (IL-6R) mRNA in rat hypothalamus. *Neurosci Lett* 1993; **153**: 13–6.
51. Gadient RA, Otten U. Expression of interleukin-6 (IL-6) and interleukin-6 receptor (IL-6R) mRNAs in rat brain during postnatal development. *Brain Res* 1994; **637**: 10–4.
52. Pousset F. Developmental expression of cytokine genes in the cortex and hippocampus of the rat central nervous system. *Dev Brain Res* 1994; **81**: 143–6.
53. Mousa A, Seiger A, Kjaeldgaard A, Bakhiet M. Human first trimester forebrain cells express genes for inflammatory and anti-inflammatory cytokines. *Cytokine* 1999; **11**: 55–60.
54. Dziegielewska KM, Moller JE, Potter AM et al. Acute-phase cytokines IL-1β and TNF-α in brain development. *Cell Tissue Res* 2000; **299**: 335–45.
55. Medlock ES, Kaplan DL, Cecchini M et al. Granulocyte-stimulating factor crosses the placenta and stimulates fetal granulopoiesis. *Blood* 1993; **81**: 916–22.
56. Letterio JJ, Geiser AG, Kulkarni AB et al. Maternal rescue of transforming growth factor-β1 null mice. *Science* 1994; **264**: 36–8.
57. Stallmach T, Karolyi L. Augmentation of fetal granulopoiesis with chorioamnionitis during the second trimester of gestation. *Hum Pathol* 1994; **25**: 244–7.
58. Li Y, Ohls RK, Rosa C et al. Maternal and umbilical serum concentrations of granulocyte colony-stimulating factor and its messenger RNA during clinical chorioamnionitis. *Obstet Gynecol* 1995; **86**: 428–32.
59. Kent ASH, Sullivan MHF, Elder MG. Transfer of cytokines through human fetal membranes. *J Reprod Fertility* 1994; **100**: 81–4.
60. McDuffie RS, Dabies JK, Leslie KK et al. A randomized control trial of interleukin-1 receptor antagonist in a rabbit model of ascending infection in pregnancy. *Infec Dis Obstet Gynecol* 2001; **9**: 233–7.
61. Fortunato SJ, Menon RP, Swan KF, Menon R. Inflammatory cytokines (interleukins 1,6,8 and tumor necrosis factor-α) release from cultured fetal membranes in response to endotoxic lipopolysaccharide mirrors amniotic fluid. *Am J Obstet Gynecol* 1996; **174**: 1855–62.
62. Taniguchi T, Matsuzaki N, Kameda T et al. The enhanced production of placental interleukin-1 during labor and intrauterine infection. *Am J Obstet Gynecol* 1991; **165**: 131–7.
63. Menon R, Swan KF, Lyden TW et al. Expression of inflammatory cytokines (interleukin-1β and interleukin-6) in amniochorionic membranes. *Am J Obstet Gynecol* 1995; **172**: 493–500.
64. Gomez R, Romero R, Ghezzi F et al. The fetal inflammatory syndrome. *Am J Obstet Gynecol* 1998; **179**: 194–202.
65. Yoon BH, Romero R, Moon J et al. Differences in the fetal interleukin-6 response to microbial invasion of the amniotic cavity between term and preterm gestation. *J Maternal-Fetal Neonatal Med* 2003; **13**: 32–8.
66. Banks WA, Kastin AJ, Durham DA. Bidirectional transport of interleukin-1 alpha across the blood–brain barrier. *Brain Res Bull* 1989; **23**: 433–7.
67. Banks WA, Ortiz L, Plotkin SR, Kastin AJ. Human interleukin (IL) 1α, murine IL-1α and murine IL-1β are transported from blood to brain in the mouse by a shared saturable mechanism. *J Pharmacol Exp Therapeutics* 1991; **259**: 988–96.
68. Guiterrez EG, Banks WA, Kastin AJ. Murine tumor necrosis factor alpha is transported from blood to brain in the mouse. *J Neuroimmunol* 1993; **47**: 169–76.
69. Guiterrez EG, Banks WA, Kastin AJ. Blood-borne interleukin-1 receptor antagonist crosses the blood–brain barrier. *J Neuroimmunol* 1994; **55**: 153–60.
70. Banks WA, Kastin AJ, Guiterrez EG. Penetration of interleukin-6 across the murine blood-brain barrier. *Neurosci Lett* 1994; **179**: 53–6.
71. de Vries HE, Blom-Roosemalen MCM, van Oosten M et al. The influence of cytokines on the integrity of the blood–brain barrier in vitro. *J Immunol* 1996; **64**: 37–43.
72. Quagliarello VJ, Wispelwey B, Long WJ Jr, Scheld WM. Recombinant human interleukin-1 induces meningitis and blood-brain barrier injury in the rat. Characterization and comparison with tumor necrosis factor. *J Clin Investigation* 1991; **87**: 1360–5.
73. Adinolfi A, Beck SE, Haddad SA, Seller MJ. Permeability of the blood–cerebrospinal fluid barrier to plasma proteins during foetal and perinatal life. *Nature* 1976; **259**: 140–1.
74. Adinolfi A. The development of the human blood-CSF-brain barrier. *Dev Med Child Neurol* 1985; **27**: 532–7.
75. Buka SL, Tsuang MT, Torrey EF et al. Maternal cytokine levels during pregnancy and adult psychosis. *Brain Behav Immunity* 2001; **15**: 411–20.
76. Boin F, Zanardini R, Pioli R. Association between -G308A tumor necrosis factor alpha gene polymorphism and schizophrenia. *Mol Psychiatry* 2001; **6**: 79–82.
77. Jun T-Y, Pae C-U, Chae J-H et al. TNFB polymorphism may be associated with schizophrenia in the Korean population. *Schizophr Res* 2003; **61**: 39–45.
78. Meira-Lima IV, Pereira AC, Mota GF et al. Analysis of a polymorphism of the promoter region of the tumor necrosis factor alpha gene in schizophrenia and bipolar disorder: further support for an association with schizophrenia. *Mol Psychiatry* 2003; **8**: 718–20.
79. Katila H, Hanninen K, Hurme M. Polymorphisms of the interleukin-1 gene complex in schizophrenia. *Mol Psychiatry* 1999; **4**: 179–81.
80. Meisenzahl EM, Rujescu D, Kirner A et al. Association of an IL-1β genetic polymorphism with altered brain structure in patients with schizophrenia. *Am J Psychiatry* 2001; **158**: 1316–9.
81. Wassink TH, Crowe RR, Andreasen NC. Tumor necrosis factor receptor-II: heritability and effect on brain morphology in schizophrenia. *Mol Psychiatry* 2000; **5**: 678–82.
82. Roberts AK, Monzon-Bordonada F, Van Deerlin PG et al. Association of a polymorphism within the promoter of the tumor necrosis factor alpha gene with increased risk of preterm rupture of the fetal membranes. *Am J Obstet Gynecol* 1999; **180**: 1297–302.
83. Aidoo M, McElroy PD, Kolczak MS et al. Tumor necrosis factor-α variant 2(TNF2) is associated with preterm delivery, infant mortality, and malaria morbidity in western Kenya: Asembo Bay cohort project IX. *Genet Epidemiol* 2001; **21**: 201–11.
84. Saito S, Kasahara T, Kato Y et al. Elevation of amniotic fluid interleukin 6 (IL-6), IL-8, and granulocyte colony stimulating factor (G-CSF) in term and preterm parturition. *Cytokine* 1993; **5**: 81–8.
85. Stallmach T, Hebisch G, Joller-Jemelka HI et al. Cytokine production and visualized effects in the feto-maternal unit: quantitative and topographic data on cytokines during intrauterine disease. *Laboratory Investigation* 1995; **73**: 384–92.
86. Romero R, Brody DT, Oyarzun E et al. Infection and labor III. Interleukin-1: a signal for the onset of parturition. *Am J Obstet Gynecol* 1989; **160**: 1117–23.
87. Romero R, Manogue KR, Mitchell MD et al. Infection and labor IV. Cachectin-tumor necrosis factor in the amniotic fluid

of women with intraamniotic infection and preterm labor. *Am J Obstet Gynecol* 1989; **161**: 336–41.
88. Miller LC, Isa S, LoPreste G et al. Neonatal interleukin-1β, interleukin-6, and tumor necrosis factor: cord blood levels and cellular production. *J Pediatrics* 1990; **117**: 961–5.
89. Lencki SG, Maciulla MB, Eglinton GS. Maternal and umbilical cord serum interleukin levels in preterm labor with clinical chorioamnionitis. *Am J Obstet Gynecol* 1994; **170**: 1345–51.
90. Salafia CM, Sherer DM, Spong CY et al. Fetal but not maternal serum cytokine levels correlate with histologic acute placental inflammation. *Am J Perinatology* 1997; **14**: 419–22.
91. Adinolfi A. Infectious diseases and pregnancy, cytokines and neurological impairment: an hypothesis. *Dev Med Child Neurol* 1993; **35**: 549–58.
92. Leviton A. Preterm birth and cerebral palsy: is tumor necrosis factor the missing link? *Dev Med Child Neurol* 1993; **35**: 549–58.
93. Wu YW, Colford JM. Chorioamnionitis as a risk factor for cerebral palsy: a meta-analysis. *JAMA* 2000; **284**: 1417–24.
94. Wu YW. Systemic review of chorioamnionitis and cerebral palsy. *Ment Retard Dev Disabil Res Rev* 2002; **8**: 25–9.
95. Dammann O, Leviton A. Maternal intrauterine infection, cytokines, and brain damage in the premature infant. *Pediatr Res* 1997; **42**: 1–8.
96. Yoon BH, Romero R, Yang SH et al. Interleukin-6 concentrations in umbilical cord plasma are elevated in neonates with white matter lesions associated with periventricular leukomalacia. *Am J Obstet Gynecol* 1996; **174**: 1433–40.
97. Yoon BH, Romero R, Park JS et al. Fetal exposure to an intraamniotic inflammation and the development of cerebral palsy at the age of three years. *Am J Obstet Gynecol* 2000; **182**: 675–81.
98. Nelson KB, Dambrosia JM, Grether JK, Phillips TM. Neonatal cytokines and coagulation factors in children with cerebral palsy. *Ann Neurol* 1998; **44**: 665–75.
99. Duggan PJ, Maalouf EF, Watts TL et al. Intrauterine T-cell activation and increased proinflammatory cytokine concentrations in preterm infants with cerebral lesions. *Lancet* 2001; **358**: 1699–700.
100. Deguchi K, Mizuguchi M, Takashima S. Immunohistochemical expression of tumor necrosis factor-α in neonatal leukomalacia. *Pediatr Neurol* 1996; **14**: 13–16.
101. Kadhim H, Tabarki B, Verellen G et al. Inflammatory cytokines in the pathogenesis of periventricular leukomalacia. *Neurology* 2001; **56**: 1278–84.
102. Rezaie P, Dean A. Periventricular leukomalacia, inflammation and white matter lesions within the developing nervous system. *Neuropathology* 2002; **22**: 106–32.
103. Kadhim H, Tabarki B, De Prez C, Sebrire G. Cytokine immunoreactivity in cortical and subcortical neurons in periventricular leukomalacia: are cytokines implicated in neuronal dysfunction in cerebral palsy? *Acta Neuropathol* 2003; **105**: 209–16.
104. Gilmore JH, Castillo M, Rojas M. Early onset schizophrenia in a patient with premature birth, germinal matrix hemorrhage and periventricular leukoencephalopathy. *Schizophr Res* 2000; **44**: 158–60.
105. Rivkin P, Kraut M, Barta P et al. White matter hyperintensity volume in late-onset and early-onset schizophrenia. *Int J Geriatric Psychiatry* 2000; **15**: 1085–9.
106. Sigmundsson T, Suckling J, Maier M et al. Structural abnormalities in frontal, temporal, and limbic regions and interconnecting white matter tracts in schizophrenic patients with prominent negative symptoms. *Am J Psychiatry* 2001; **158**: 234–43.
107. Kubicki M, Westin C-F, Maier SE et al. Uncinate fasciculus findings in schizophrenia: a magnetic resonance diffusion tensor imaging study. *Am J Psychiatry* 2002; **159**: 813–20.
108. Volpe JJ. Subplate neurons – missing link in brain injury of the premature infant? *Pediatrics* 1996; **97**: 112–3.
109. Glantz LA, Lewis DA. Reduction of synaptophysin immunoreactivity in the prefrontal cortex of subjects with schizophrenia: regional and diagnostic specificity. *Arch Gen Psychiatry* 1997; **54**: 943–52.
110. Glantz LA, Lewis DA. Decreased dendritic spine density on prefrontal cortical pyramidal neurons in schizophrenia. *Arch Gen Psychiatry* 2000; **57**: 65–73.
111. Jarskog LF, Xiao H, Wilkie MB et al. Cytokine regulation of embryonic dopaminergic and serotonergic neuron survival *in vitro*. *Int J Dev Neurosci* 1997; **15**: 711–6.
112. Marx CE, Jarskog LF, Lauder JM et al. Cytokine effects on cortical neuron MAP-2 immunoreactivity: implications for schizophrenia. *Biol Psychiatry* 2001; **50**: 743–9.
113. Araujo DM, Cotman CW. Differential effects of interleukin-1b and interleukin-2 on glia and hippocampal neurons in culture. *Int J Dev Neurosci* 1995; **13**: 201–12.
114. Gelbard HA, Dzenko KA, DiLoreto D et al. Neurotoxic effects of tumor necrosis factor in primary human neuronal cultures are mediated by activation of the glutamate AMPA receptor subtype: implications for AIDS neuropathogenesis. *Dev Neurosci* 1993; **15**: 417–22.
115. Chao CC, Hu S. Tumor necrosis factor-alpha potentiates glutamate neurotoxicity in human fetal brain cultures. *Dev Neurosci* 1994; **16**: 171–9.
116. Jeohn GH, Kong LY, Wilson B, Hong J. Synergistic neurotoxic effects of combined treatments with cytokines in murine primary mixed neuron/glia cultures. *J Neuroimmunol* 1998; **85**: 1–10.
117. Mehler MF, Rozental R, Dougherty M et al. Cytokine regulation of neuronal differentiation of hippocampal progenitor cells. *Nature* 1993; **362**: 62–5.
118. Munoz-Fernandez MA, Cano E, O'Donnell CA et al. Tumor necrosis factor-α (TNF-α), interferon-γ, and interleukin-6 but not TNF-β induce differentiation of neuroblastoma cells: the role of nitric oxide. *J Neurochem* 1994; **62**: 1330–6.
119. Mehler MF, Marmur R, Gross R et al. Cytokines regulate the cellular phenotype of developing neural lineage species. *Int J Dev Neurosci* 1995; **13**: 213–40.
120. Sarder M, Abe K, Saito H, Nishiyama N. Comparative effect of IL-2 and IL-6 on morphology of cultured hippocampal neurons from fetal rat brain. *Brain Res* 1996; **715**: 9–16.
121. Neumann H, Schweigreiter R, Yamashita T et al. Tumor necrosis factor inhibits neurite outgrowth and branching of hippocampal neurons by a rho-dependent mechanism. *J Neurosci* 2002; **22**: 854–62.
122. Reichardt LF, Farinas I. Neurotrophic factors and their receptors: roles in neuronal development and function. In: *Molecular and Cellular Approaches to Neuronal Development* (Cowan WM, Jessell TM, Zipursky SL, eds). New York: Oxford University Press, 1997: 220–63.
123. Carter BD, Lewin GR. Neurotrophins live or let dies: does p75[NTR] decide? *Neuron* 1997; **18**: 187–90.
124. Gadient RA, Cron KC, Otten U. Interleukin-1β and tumor necrosis factor-a synergistically stimulate nerve growth factor (NGF) release from cultures rat astrocytes. *Neurosci Lett* 1990; **117**: 335–40.
125. Juric DM, Carman-Krzan M. Interleukin-1β, but not IL-1α, mediates nerve growth factor secretion from rat astrocytes via type I IL-1 receptor. *Int J Dev Neurosci* 2001; **19**: 675–83.
126. Heese K, Hock C, Otten U. Inflammatory signals induce neurotrophin expression in human microglia cells. *J Neurochem* 1998; **70**: 699–707.
127. Marz P, Heese K, Dimitriades-Schmutz B et al. Role of interleukin-6 and soluble IL-6 receptor in region-specific induction

128. of astrocyte differentiation and neurotrophin expression. *Glia* 1999; **26**: 191–200.
128. Stadelmann C, Kerschensteiner M, Misgeld T et al. BDNF and gp145trkB in multiple sclerosis brain lesions: neuroprotective interactions between immune and neuronal cells? *Brain* 2002; **125**: 75–85.
129. Nakajima K, Tohyama Y, Kohsaka S, Kurihara T. Ceramide activates microglia to enhance the production/secretion of brain-derived neurotrophic factor (BDNF) without induction of deleterious factors in vitro. *J Neurochem* 2002; **80**: 697–705.
130. Shi L, Fatemi SH, Sidewell RW, Patterson PH. Maternal influenza infection causes marked behavioral and pharmacological changes in the offspring. *J Neurosci* 2003; **23**: 297–302.
131. Zuckerman L, Weiner I. Post-pubertal emergence of disrupted latent inhibition following prenatal immune activation. *Psychopharmacol* 2003; **169**: 308–13.
132. Zuckerman L, Rehavi M, Weiner I. Immune activation during pregnancy in rats leads to a postpubertal emergence of disrupted latent inhibition, dopaminergic hyperfunction, and altered limbic morphology in the offspring: a novel neurodevelopmental model of schizophrenia. *Neuropsychopharmacol* 2003; **28**: 1778–89.
133. Borrell J, Vela JM, Arevalo-Martin A et al. Prenatal immune challenge disrupts sensorimotor gating in adult rats: implications for the etiopathogenesis of schizophrenia. *Neuropsychopharmacol* 2002; **26**: 204–15.
134. Gatti S, Bartfai T. Induction of tumor necrosis factor-α mRNA in the brain after peripheral endotoxin treatment: comparison with interleukin-1 family and interleukin-6. *Brain Res* 1993; **624**: 291–4.
135. Laye S, Parnet P, Goujon E, Dantzer R. Peripheral administration of lipopolysaccharide induces the expression of cytokine transcripts in the brain and pituitary of mice. *Mol Brain Res* 1994; **27**: 157–62.
136. Reinisch N, Wolkersdorfer M, Kahler C et al. Interleukin-1 receptor type I mRNA in mouse brain as affected by administration of bacterial lipopolysaccharide. *Neurosci Lett* 1994; **166**: 165–7.
137. Konsman JP, Kelly K, Dantzer R. Temporal and spacial relationships between lipopolysaccharide-induced expression of Fos, interleukin-1 beta and inducible nitric oxide synthase in rat brain. *Neurosci* 1999; **89**: 535–48.
138. Quan N, Whiteside M, Herkenham M. Time course and localization patterns of interleukin-1b messenger RNA expression in brain and pituitary after peripheral administration of lipopolysaccharide. *Neuroscience* 1998; **83**: 281–93.
139. Wong ML, Bongiorno PB, Rettori V et al. Interleukin (IL) 1β, IL-1 receptor antagonist, IL-10, and IL-13 gene expression in central nervous system and anterior pituitary during systemic inflammations: pathophysiological implications. *Proc Nat Acad Sci USA* 1997; **94**: 227–32.
140. Buttini M, Boddeke H. Peripheral lipopolysaccharide stimulation induces interleukin-1β messenger RNA in rat brain microglial cells. *Neuroscience* 1995; **65**: 523–30.
141. van Dam AM, Bauer J, Tilders FJH, Berkenbosch F. Endotoxin-induced appearance of immunoreactive interleukin-1β in ramified microglia in rat brain: a light and electron microscopic study. *Neuroscience* 1995; **65**: 815–26.
142. Buttini M, Limonta S, Boddeke HWGM. Peripheral administration of lipopolysaccharide induces activation of microglial cells in rat brain. *Neurochem Intl* 1996; **29**: 25–35.
143. Pitossi F, del Ray A, Kabiersch A, Besedovsky H. Induction of cytokine transcripts in the central nervous system and pituitary following peripheral administration of endotoxin to mice. *J Neurosci Res* 1997; **48**: 287–98.
144. Sacoccio C, Dornand J, Barbanel G. Differential regulation of brain and plasma TNFα produced after endotoxin shock. *Neuroreport* 1998; **9**: 309–13.
145. Quan N, Stern EL, Whiteside MB, Herkenham M. Induction of pro-inflammatory cytokine mRNAs in the brain after peripheral injection of subseptic doses of lipopolysaccharide in the rat. *J Neuroimmunol* 1999; **93**: 72–80.
146. Ornoy A, Altshuler G. Maternal endotoxemia, fetal anomalies, and central nervous system damage: a rat model of a human problem. *Am J Obstet Gynecol* 1976; **124**: 196–204.
147. Collins JG, Smith MA, Arnold RR, Offenbacher S. Effects of escherichia coli and porphyromonas gingivalis lipopolysaccharide on pregnancy outcome in the golden hamster. *Infect Immunity* 1994; **62**: 4652–5.
148. Fidel PL Jr, Romero R, Wolf N et al. Systemic and local cytokine profiles in endotoxin-induced preterm parturition in mice. *Am J Obstet Gynecol* 1994; **170**: 1467–75.
149. Schlafer DH, Yuh B, Foley GL et al. Effect of salmonella endotoxin administered to pregnant sheep at 133–142 days gestation on fetal oxygenation, maternal and fetal adrenocorticotropic hormone and cortisol, and maternal plasma tumor necrosis factor α concentrations. *Biol Reprod* 1994; **50**: 1297–302.
150. Goto M, Yoshioka T, Ravindranath T et al. LPS injected into the pregnant rat late in gestation does not induce fetal endotoxemia. *Res Comm Mol Path Pharm* 1994; **85**: 109–12.
151. Kijima K, Yoneyama Y, Sawa R, Araki T. Effects of fetal endotoxin administration on plasma prostoglandin F2α and cortisol levels in late-gestation fetal goats. *Fetal Diag Therapy* 1999; **14**: 240–3.
152. Debillon T, Gras-Leguen C, Verielle V et al. Intrauterine infection induces programmed cell death in rabbit periventricular white matter. *Pediatr Res* 2000; **47**: 736–42.
153. Bell MJ, Hallenbeck JM. Effects of intrauterine inflammation on developing rat brain. *J Neurosci Res* 2002; **70**: 570–9.
154. Cai Z, Pan Z-L, Pang Y et al. Cytokine induction in fetal rat brain and brain injury in neonatal rats after maternal lipopolysaccharide administration. *Pediatr Res* 2000; **47**: 64–72.
155. Urakubo A, Jarskog LF, Lieberman JA, Gilmore JH. Prenatal exposure to maternal infection alters cytokine expression in the placenta, amniotic fluid, and fetal brain. *Schizophr Res* 2001; **47**: 27–36.
156. Gilmore JH, Jarskog LF, Vadlamudi S. Maternal infection alters BDNF and NGF expression in the fetal and neonatal brain and maternal-fetal unit of the rat. *J Neuroimmunol* 2003; **138**: 49–55.
157. Cabelli RJ, Hohn A, Shatz CJ. Inhibition of ocular dominance column formation by infusion of NT-4/5 or BDNF. *Science* 1995; **267**: 1662–6.
158. McAllister AK, Katz LC, Lo DC. Opposing roles for endogenous BDNF and NT-3 in regulating cortical dendritic growth. *Neuron* 1997; **18**: 767–78.
159. Turrin NP, Gayle D, Ilyin SE et al. Pro-inflammatory and anti-inflammatory cytokine mRNA production in the periphery and brain following intraperitoneal administration of bacterial lipopolysaccharide. *Brain Res Bull* 2001; **54**: 443–53.
160. Nadeau S, Rivest S. Regulation of the gene encoding tumor necrosis factor alpha (TNF-α) in the rat brain and pituitary in response to different models of systemic immune challenge. *J Neuropathol Exp Neurol* 1999; **58**: 61–77.
161. Lapchak PA, Araujo DM, Hefti F. Systemic interleukin-1β decreases brain-derived neurotrophic factor messenger RNA expression in the rat hippocampal formation. *Neuroscience* 1993; **53**: 297–301.
162. Adams JM, Heath HD, Imagawa DT et al. Viral infections in the embryo. *Am J Dis Child* 1956; **92**: 109–14.

163. Reichlin S. Neuroendocrine-immune interactions. *N Engl J Med* 1993; **329**: 1246–53.
164. Trejo JL, Machin C, Arahuetes RM, Rua C. Influence of maternal adrenalectomy and glucocorticoid administration on the development of rat cerebral cortex. *Anat Embryol* 1995; **192**: 89–99.
165. Koenig JI, Kirkpatrick B, Lee P. Glucocorticoid hormones and early brain development in schizophrenia. *Neuropsychopharmacol* 2002; **27**: 309–18.
166. Altshuler G. Some placental considerations related to neurodevelopmental and other disorders. *J Child Neurol* 1993; **8**: 78–94.
167. Butler PD, Susser ES, Brown AS et al. Prenatal nutritional deprivation as a risk factor in schizophrenia: preclinical evidence. *Neuropsychopharmacol* 1994; **11**: 227–35.
168. Upfold JB, Smith MSR. Maternal hyperthermia as a cause of 'idiopathic' mental retardation. *Med Hypoth* 1988; **27**: 89–92.

13

Immunology and psychiatry: The role of stress as an immunomodulator in affective disorders

Brian E Leonard

INTRODUCTION

The hypothesis that emotions and mental processes are interlinked can be traced back to antiquity. However, the scientific basis of the mechanisms underlying these processes have only recently been uncovered, largely due to the research of Hans Seyle and his collaborators.[1] These investigators showed that the hypothalamus and the pituitary gland play a crucial role in controlling the release of stress hormones, particularly the glucocorticoids, which not only assist the body in adapting to external and internal stressors but also in modulating immune function. Subsequently, it was shown that the immunotransmitters, the cytokines, and related secretory products from immune cells can communicate with the endocrine and central nervous systems to modulate their functions.[2] It is now generally recognized that the endocrine-immune systems and the brain are functionally linked to provide a co-ordinated response to external and internal stressors. This network is also linked to the central and peripheral sympathetic systems thereby providing a mechanism whereby the nervous system can directly affect the activity of the immune system by activating adrenoceptors that are located on immune cells. Psychoneuroimmunology has now developed into a specialist discipline for the study of the immune-endocrine-neurotransmitter-behavioral network.[3,4]

Over the past 40 years, evidence has accumulated on the nature of the interactions between the central neurotransmitters and the immune system. The immune system is autoregulated in that most immune cells distinguish normal cells that belong to the body (self) from foreign (non-self) cells so that mounting an immune response against foreign cells does not require a major contribution from the brain. However, it is now evident that the brain plays a major role in modulating the function of the immune system and, conversely, the immune system plays a major role in the symptoms of patients suffering from major psychiatric disorders such as depression, schizophrenia, and anxiety disorders.[5,6] Thus despite the widely held view that the immune system is primarily an autoregulated system concerned with protection of the body against infectious diseases, it is now evident that there is constant 'cross-talk' between the immune-endocrine and neurotransmitter systems.

It is now generally accepted that psychological stress and psychiatric illness can compromise immune function[7,8] and that the cytokines can cause changes in behavior in man and animals. Acute infections in both animals and man are usually accompanied by a cluster of non-specific symptoms which include fever, hypersomnia, anorexia, anhedonia, amnesia, and loss of libido.[9] It is known that the release of pro-inflammatory cytokines from macrophages and monocytes (such as interleukin-1 and -6 and tumor necrosis factor) is an integral part of the host response to infection. These cytokines play a pivotal role not only in attenuating the release of the biogenic amine neurotransmitters noradrenaline, dopamine, and serotonin in the brain, but also in stimulating the hypothalamic-pituitary-adrenal (HPA) axis, thereby increasing the release of the glucocorticoids from the adrenals.[10] The pro-inflammatory cytokines are not only released from immune cells in the periphery but also from immune cells in the brain. Thus interleukin-1 (IL-1) appears to play a key role in orchestrating the cascade of inflammatory mediators from the microglia and astrocytes in addition to stimulating the release of adrenocorticotrophic hormone (ACTH) from the anterior pituitary gland.[11] Interleukin-6 (IL-6), in addition to its pro-inflammatory role in the brain, also activates the liver to produce acute phase proteins, such as anti-chymotrypsin, haptoglobulin, and protein C, the latter playing an important role in activating the complement cascade which causes the lysis of the cell walls of invading bacteria.

In man, evidence that the pro-inflammatory cytokines cause sickness behavior arose from clinical trials in which recombinant or purified cytokines were used in cancer chemotherapy or in the treatment of chronic viral infections such as hepatitis B or C. The side effects of the immunotherapy used to treat these conditions resembled symptoms seen in patients with major depression,[12] thereby leading to the suggestion that major depression was a form of sickness behavior caused by an increase in pro-inflammatory cytokines within the brain.[13]

Experimental studies in rats further demonstrated that intracerebral or systemic injections of IL-1, or the injection of lipopolysaccharide (the antigen from the cell wall of pathogenic bacteria that stimulates the release of cytokines from macrophages), caused the symptoms of sickness behavior.[13] Such symptoms could be attenuated by prior administration of the IL-1 antagonist IL-10.[14] It is now apparent, however, that the changes in behavior initiated by the pro-inflammatory cytokines also involve other mediators such as prostaglandin E2, nitric oxide, and corticotrophin releasing factor (CRF).[15] These substances contribute to the changes in central neurotransmitter function which are causally associated with the symptoms of major depression and anxiety, which is a common feature of depression.

The hypersecretion of glucocorticoids is a common feature of major depression and chronic anxiety. It would therefore be anticipated that cellular immunity would be decreased as a consequence of the anti-inflammatory effects of the glucocorticoids. While there is evidence that some aspects of cellular immunity are decreased (for example, natural killer cells and T-cell mitogenesis),[16] the activity of the pro-inflammatory secreting cells is increased under these conditions.[17] It is evident that the glucocorticoid receptors in the brain and on some types of immune cells become subsensitive following the hypersecretion of glucocorticoids.[18] This accounts not only for the failure of elevated plasma glucocorticoids to inhibit the release of ACTH (which implies a failure in the feedback inhibitory mechanism) but also the failure of the glucocorticoids to inhibit the activity of the pro-inflammatory cytokine secreting cells. Glucocorticoid receptors return to normal activity following the clinical recovery of the patient.[19] Thus depression and chronic anxiety states are often accompanied by elevated plasma acute phase proteins, elevated tissue pro-inflammatory cytokines, prostaglandin E2, and nitric oxide, which implicates activation of the immune system as an important component in the pathogenesis of these disorders. Such evidence provides a basis for the macrophage theory of depression.[6]

STRESS AND CELLULAR IMMUNITY

Acute stress is known to cause an increase in the number of lymphocytes in the blood.[20] Such changes are probably a reflection of the release of these cells from the spleen, or the cells becoming detached from the endothelial cells lining the blood vessel walls. The secretion of adrenaline in response to an acute stressor also results in an increase in the number of lymphocytes in circulation.[21] Acute stress also causes a large increase in the number of circulating NK cells, an effect which has been associated with an increased activation of beta adrenoceptors on the NK cell membrane.[22] In contrast to the effects of acute stress on cellular immunity, chronic stress, which is associated with a hypersecretion of glucocorticoids and catecholamines, decreases the number of lymphocytes in the blood; this change is associated with a reduction in the non-specific antigenic response.[20]

While it is generally assumed that stress suppresses the host defence system, leading to an increased vulnerability to infections, it is now apparent that the severity and duration of the stress can result in qualitatively different types of response. For example, social conflict in rodents causes an enhancement of phagocytic cells in the spleen.[23] Similarly, the number of lymphocytes infiltrating the skin in a delayed hypersensitivity reaction to an immunogenic challenge increases in rodents following stress.[24] Other studies have demonstrated qualitative differences between the effects of mild and severe stress on the number of B-lymphocytes producing antibodies. Severe stress causes a suppression of antibody synthesis while mild stress enhances the antigen specific immune response. Such studies serve to emphasize the complexity of the effects of glucocorticoids on immune cells and how the immune response can change depending on the severity, nature, and duration of the stress. To date most of these studies have been conducted on rodents and it is uncertain to what extent the results may be extrapolated to the effects of stress in the human.

Nevertheless, there is evidence from clinical studies that not all stressors produce identical changes in the immune and endocrine systems.[25] Furthermore, coping strategies play an important role in modifying the adverse impact of a stressor.[26]

The impact of stress on antibody synthesis depends on the temporal relationship between the antigen challenge and the time at which the stressor is applied. It has been demonstrated that a stressor will only interfere with antibody synthesis if it is applied near the time of the antigen exposure.[27] Furthermore, many immune changes are non-specific and reflect an intermediate aspect of the immune response (for example, the synthesis of interleukins or the proliferative response of the T-cell to a mitogen), rather than the end point of the immune response that destroys, for example, a virus-infected cell. It is also apparent that the immune system contains a high degree of redundancy so that changes in a specific aspect of the immune cascade are not sufficient evidence of a significant change in the overall immune process.[28] Despite these caveats, there is evidence that stressful events predispose an individual to physical illness and while such correlations are relatively small, probably accounting for about 10% of the variance,[29] they are consistent across populations and following different types of stress.

STRESS AND LIFE EVENTS

While bereavement stress has been the subject of many studies, it is now apparent that the risk of physical ill-health following marital separation or divorce is greater than that following a bereavement.[30] Similarly, the effects of chronic stress on the caregivers of patients with Alzheimer's disease have been correlated with a high incidence of depression[31] and an impairment in some aspects of immune function.[20] Even relatively short-term stress can impair different aspects of the immune response. For example, examination stress in university students has been shown to decrease the activity of NK cells;[32] surprisingly, relaxation techniques do not fully reverse the changes in cellular immunity caused by examination stress.

DEPRESSION

Evidence implicating a role for the pro-inflammatory cytokines in the etiology of depression has been provided by studies of the effects of IL-1, IL-6, TNF-α, and interferon-α (INF) on psychiatrically normal individuals being treated for a malignancy. In addition, experimental and clinical studies have implicated these cytokines as causative factors in the symptoms of major depression. These symptoms include depressed mood, anxiety, cognitive impairment, lack of motivation, loss of libido, and disturbances in short-term memory. These symptoms usually disappear once the plasma cytokine concentration returns to normal.[33] Such effects appear to be a consequence of the neurotransmitter and endocrine changes induced by the cytokines rather than the pathological condition for which the treatment has been administered.[33] The symptoms of depression also frequently occur in those recovering from various types of infection, while high incidences of depression have also been reported in patients with multiple sclerosis,[34] allergies,[35] and rheumatoid arthritis.[36] In all these situations, and in auto-immune disease, pro-inflammatory cytokines are known to be over-expressed.[37]

The initial studies linking depression with an abnormality of the immune system indicated that there was an impairment in neutrophil phagocytosis,[38] impaired mitogen stimulated lymphocyte proliferation,[39] and reduced NK cell activity in untreated depressed patients,[40] changes which largely return to normal values once the patient recovers following antidepressant treatment.

Recent research into the immune changes occurring in depressed patients has concentrated on cytokines, soluble cytokine receptors, and plasma acute phase proteins. For example, one study reported that the positive acute phase proteins were increased while the negative acute phase proteins (for example, albumin) were reduced.[41] These changes are a reflection of the actions of IL-1 and IL-6 on the liver. In addition, the complement proteins (C3, C4, and immunoglobulin M) are increased in depressed patients. Such changes are evidence of immune activation involving the pro-inflammatory cytokines (acute phase proteins) and B-cells (IgM) that are activated by the cytokines.

Further evidence of immune activation in depressed patients is provided by the studies showing that the plasma concentration of IL-1, IL-6, IFN, soluble IL-6 and IL-2 receptors, and the IL-1 receptor antagonist are raised, these changes being correlated with a rise in the plasma acute phase proteins.[42] Effective antidepressant treatments attenuated these immune changes.

In addition to the changes in the pro-inflammatory cytokines, there is evidence for an increased number of T-helper, T-memory, activated T-cells, and B-cells, which are the source of the plasma cytokines. Precisely how these changes in cytokine concentration are linked to those in central biogenic amine transmission (assumed to be responsible for the behavioral changes associated with depression) is uncertain but there is evidence that depressed patients display increased serum antibody titers to serotonin,[43] which could impair central serotonergic function. In

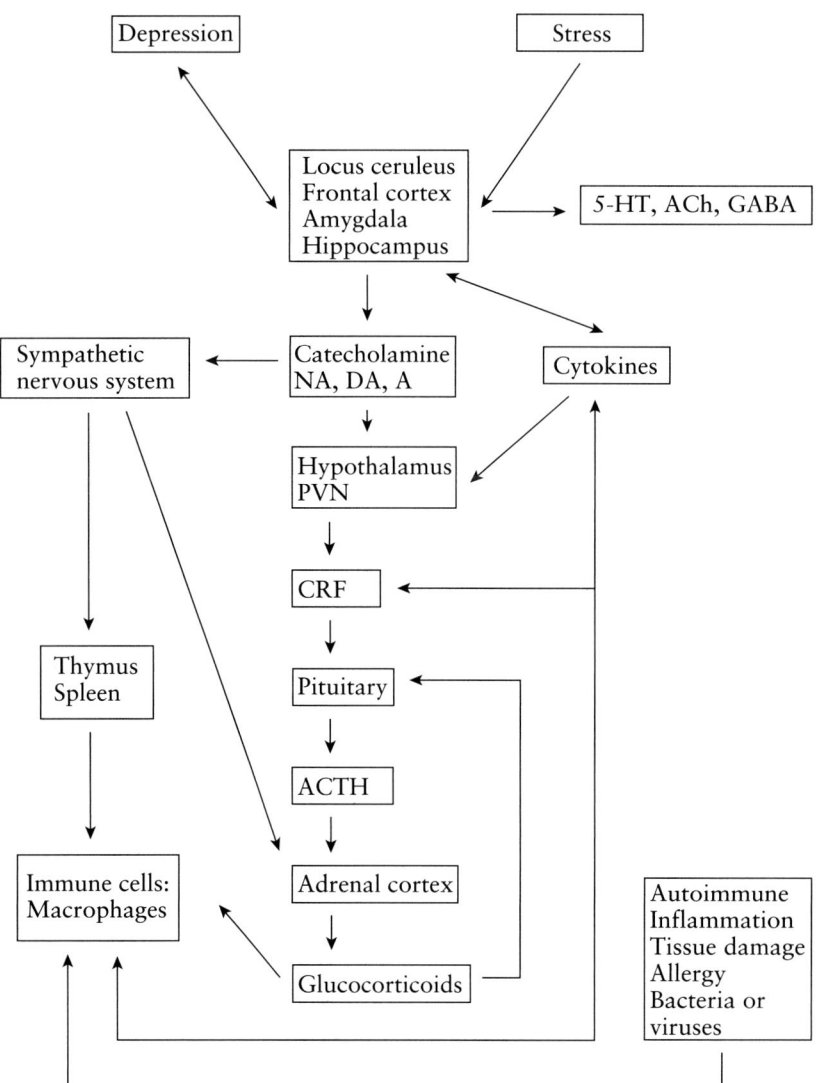

Figure 13.1 The relationship between cytokines, CRF, neurotrasmitters, glucocorticoids, and immunity in depression and stress.

addition, IL-1 is known to increase the metabolism of tryptophan to kynurenin and quinolinic acid by activating indoleamine 2,3 dioxygenase activity both in the periphery and in the brain,[44] which would further deplete brain serotonin concentrations.

Another inflammatory factor which could contribute to a central monoamine deficit is prostaglandin E2, which is raised in the plasma and cerebrospinal fluid of depressed patients.[45] This change is initiated by the activation of cyclooxygenase in the brain by IL-1, the increase in PGE2 causing a reduction in the release of brain monoamines.[46] Such findings may provide the essential link between immune activation, a deficit in monoamine neurotransmission, and the onset of symptoms of depression. Effective antidepressant treatments correct these immune and neurotransmitter changes, suggesting that the immune changes are state, rather than trait, markers of depression.[42,47]

Figure 13.1 summarizes the main interactions between the pro-inflammatory cytokines, the HPA axis, and central neurotransmission in depression.

CONCLUSION

Despite the substantial evidence for a disorder of the immune system with depression, controversy exists regarding the causal relationship between the increase in pro-inflammatory cytokines, PGE2, glucocorticoids, and the psychopathology of the disorder. Are the changes in the immune system a reflection of a stress-induced pathological state or are they responsible for the changes in central neurotransmitter function that, following a stress-related activation of the immune system, causes the behavioral changes? Only more extensive research in the field of psychoneuroimmunology will help to unravel the complex relationship between the immune-endocrine-neurotransmitter systems and the symptoms of depression.

REFERENCES

1. Seyle H. *The Stress of Life*. New York: McGraw-Hill, 1956.
2. Besedovsky HO, DelRey A. Immune-neuroendocrine interactions: facts and hypotheses. *Endocrine Rev* 1996; **17**: 64–102.
3. Ader R, Felton DL, Cohen N. *Psychoneuroimmunology* (2nd ed). San Diego: Academic Press, 1991.
4. Song C, Leonard BE. *Fundamentals of Neuropsychoimmunology*. Chichester UK: John Wiley and Sons, 2000.
5. Hickie I, Lloyd A. Are cytokines associated with neuropsychiatric syndromes in humans? *Int J Immunopharmacol* 1995; **17**: 677–83.
6. Smith RS. The macrophage theory of depression. *Med Hypothesis* 1991; **35**: 298–306.
7. Leonard BE. Brain cytokines and the psychopathology of depression. In: *Antidepressants* (Leonard BE, ed). Basle: Birkhauser Verlag, 2000: 109–22.
8. Leonard BE. The immune system, depression and the action of antidepressants. *Prog Neuropsychopharm Biol Psychiatry* 2001; **25**: 767–80.
9. Hart BL. Biological basis of the behaviour of sick animals. *Neurosci Biobehav Rev* 1988; **12**: 123–37.
10. Rivier C, Vale W, Brown M. In the rat, interleukin-1 alpha and beta stimulate adrenocorticotrophin and catecholamine release. *Endocrinol* 1989; **125**: 3096–102.
11. Turnbull AV, Rivier C. Regulation of the HPA axis by cytokines. *Brain Behav Immunol* 1995; **9**: 253–75.
12. Meyers CA, Valentine AD. Neurologic and psychiatric adverse effects of immunological therapy. *CNS Drugs* 1995; **3**: 56–68.
13. Dantzer R, Bluthe RM, Ghensi G. Molecular basis of sickness behaviour. *Ann NY Acad Sci* 1998; **856**: 132–8.
14. Bluthe RM, Casanon N, Pousset F et al. Central injection of IL-10 antagonises the behavioural effects of lipopolysaccharide in rats. *Psychoneuroimmunol* 1999; **24**: 301–11.
15. Rothwell NJ, Hopkins SJ. Cytokines and the nervous system: actions and mechanisms. *Trends Neurosci* 1995; **18**: 130–6.
16. Irwin M, Patterson T, Smith TL et al. Reduction in immune function in life stress and depression. *Biol Psychiatry* 1990; **27**: 22–30.
17. Maes M, Smith RS, Scharpe S. The monocyte and T-lymphocyte hypothesis of major depression. *Psychoneuroendocrinol* 1995; **20**: 111–6.
18. Dinan TG. Glucocorticoids and the genesis of depressive illness: a psychobiological model. *Br J Psychiatry* 1994; **164**: 365–71.
19. Cooney JM, Dinan TG. Type 2 glucocorticoid receptors mediate fast feedback inhibition of the hypothalamic-pituitary-adrenal axis in man. *Life Sci* 1996; **59**: 1981–8.
20. Kiecolt-Glaser JK, Dura JR, Speicher CE et al. Spousal caregivers of dementia victims: longitudinal changes in immunity and health. *Psychosomat Med* 1991; **53**: 345–62.
21. Samuel AJ. Primary and secondary leucocyte changes following intramuscular injections of epinephrine hydrochloride. *J Clin Invest* 1951; **30**: 941–7.
22. Benschop RJ, Rodriguezfeuerhahn M, Schlowski M. Catecholamine induced leucocytosis: early observations, current research and future directions. *Brain Behav Immunol* 1996; **10**: 77–91.
23. Lyte M, Nelson SG, Thompson ML. Innate and adaptive immune responses in a social conflict paradigm. *Clin Immunol Immunopathol* 1990; **57**: 137–47.
24. Dhabhar FS, Miller AH, McEwern BS, Spencer RI. Stress-induced changes in blood leucocyte distribution—role of adrenal steroid hormones. *J Immunol* 1996; **157**: 1638–44.
25. Mason JW. A re-evaluation of the concept of non-specificity in stress theory. *J Psychiatr Res* 1971; **8**: 123–34.
26. Mormede P, Dantzer R, Michaul B et al. Influence of stressor predictability and behavioural control on lymphocyte reactivity, antibody response and neuroendocrine activation in rats. *Physiol Behav* 1988; **43**: 577–83.
27. Fleshner M, Bellgrau D, Watkins LR et al. Stress induced reduction in the rat mixed lymphocyte reaction is due to macrophages and not to changes in T-cell phenotypes. *J Neuroimmunomodulation* 1995; **56**: 45–52.
28. Cunnick JE, Cohens S, Rabin BS, Carpenter AB. Alterations in specific antibody production due to rank and social instability. *Brain Behav Immunol* 1991; **5**: 357–69.
29. Weisse CS. Depression and immunocompetence: a review of the literature. *Psychol Bull* 1992; **111**: 475–87.
30. Kiecolt-Glaser JK, Kennedy S, Malkoff S et al. Marital quality, marital disruption and immune function. *Psychosomat Med* 1987; **49**: 13–34.
31. Crook TH, Miller NW. The challenge of Alzheimer's disease. *Am Psychol* 1985; **40**: 1245–50.
32. Kiecolt-Glaser JK, Kennedy S, Malkoff S et al. Marital discord and immunity in males. *Psychosomat Med* 1987; **50**: 213–29.
33. Meyers CA, Valentine AD. Neurological and psychiatric adverse effects of immunological therapy. *CNS Drugs* 1995; **3**: 56–68.
34. Minden SL, Schiffer RB. Affective disorders in multiple sclerosis in review and recommendations for clinical research. *Arch Neurol* 1990; **47**: 98–104.
35. Marshall PS. Allergy and depressions: a neurochemical threshold model of the relation between the illnesses. *Psychol Bull* 1993; **113**: 23–43.
36. Katz PP, Yelim EH. Prevalence and correlates of depressive symptoms among persons with rheumatoid arthritis. *J Rheumatol* 1993; **20**: 790–6.
37. Schrott LM, Crnic LS. The role of performance factors in active avoidance-conditioning deficit in autoimmune mice. *Behav Neurosci* 1996; **110**: 486–97.
38. O'Neill B, Leonard BE. Abnormal zymosan-induced neutrophil chemilumunescence as a marker of depression. *J Affect Dis* 1991; **19**: 265–72.
39. Kronfol Z, House JD. Lymphocyte mitogenesis, immunoglobulin and complement levels in depressed patients and normal controls. *Acta Psychiatr Scand* 1989; **80**: 142–7.
40. Irwin M, Daniels M, Smith TH et al. Impaired natural killer cell activity during bereavement. *Brain Behav Immunol* 1997; **1**: 98–104.
41. Song C, Dinan TG, Leonard BE. Changes in immunoglobulins, complement and acute phase protein concentrations in depressed patients and normal controls. *J Affect Dis* 1994; **30**: 283–8.
42. Sluzewska A, Rybakowski J, Bosmans E et al. Indicators of immune activation in major depression. *Psychiatry Res* 1996; **64**: 161–7.
43. Schott K, Batra A, Klein R et al. Increased serum antibody titres to serotonin in depressed patients. *Eur Psychiatry* 1992; **7**: 209–12.
44. Myint AM, Kim YK. Cytokine-serotonin interaction through IDO: a neurodegeneration hypothesis of depression. *Med Hypoth* 2003 (in press).
45. Calabrese J, Skwerer RG, Barna B. Depression, immunocompetence and prostaglandins of the E series. *Psychiatry Res* 1986; **17**: 44–7.
46. Hedqvist P. Effects of prostaglandins on autonomic neurotransmission. In: *Prostaglandins: Physiological, Pharmacological and Pathological Aspects* (Karim SMM, ed). Lancaster UK: MTP Press, 1976: 37–41.
47. McAdams C, Leonard BE. Neutrophil and monocyte phagocytosis in depressed patients. *Neuropsychopharmacol Biol Psychiatry* 1991; **17**: 971–84.

14

Bipolar disorder: Role of infection and immunity

Dunja Hinze-Selch and Silja Knolle-Veentjer

INTRODUCTION

The present chapter discusses bipolar disorder and whether infection and immunity play a role in the etiology and pathophysiology of this major psychiatric disorder, and if so, how. We will begin with a short introduction to bipolar disorder, summarizing issues of diagnosis, epidemiology, and the relevance of correct diagnosis for research. We will then briefly review the studies published to date on infections and immunity in bipolar disorder. A short section on the effect of psychotropic medication on measures of infection and immunity will follow. The major part of this chapter will introduce suggestions about how infections and peculiarities in immunity might play a role in the pathophysiology and etiology of bipolar disorder. Finally, there will be a short discussion that integrates all of these findings with respect to the etiology and pathophysiology of major psychiatric disorders.

BIPOLAR DISORDER

Diagnosis

Bipolar disorder is characterized by the presence of depressive as well as manic (bipolar I) or hypomanic (bipolar II) episodes. The *Diagnostic and Statistical Manual of Mental Disorders* (DSM-IV)[1] provides prevalence data on bipolar I and bipolar II disorder as 0.4–1.6% and 0.5%, respectively. Quite unanimously, the DSM-IV and the *International Classification of Diseases* (ICD-10)[2] require at least two episodes of different affective states for diagnosis, for example one depressive episode, as described within the -diagnosis of major depression, and at least one hypomanic, manic, or mixed episode. Manic and hypomanic episodes differ in severity, duration, and amount of manic symptoms. A mixed episode is characterized by the presence of manic and depressive episodes simultaneously. Psychotic features can be present in either episode but the diagnostic definitions vary between the ICD-10 and the DSM-IV. This is also relevant with respect to a differential diagnosis, which includes schizoaffective disorder.

Differential diagnoses

Schizophrenia lacks cycling affective symptoms and is dominated by psychotic features, making this diagnosis relatively simple to differentiate. Prevalence data for schizophrenia are given as 0.2–2.0%.[1] Schizoaffective disorder is difficult to differentiate from bipolar disorder because, as mentioned before, diagnostic criteria vary between the DSM-IV and the ICD-10. The main difference between both diagnostic systems is that the DSM-IV requires that affective and psychotic symptoms be present during the same episode but not simultaneously, whereas the ICD-10 explicitly requires that affective and well defined psychotic symptoms must be present simultaneously. Moreover, the ICD-10 defines the psychotic features that are allowed for bipolar disorder as all psychotic features that do not meet the criteria for psychotic symptoms in schizoaffective disorder, whereas the DSM-IV does not make this distinction. Thus, ICD-10 splits psychotic symptomatology to two different diagnoses whereas the DSM-IV does not.

Even if at first sight the differential diagnosis against unipolar depression (with a given prevalence of 5–25%)[1] appears simplistic, it is not. Firstly, evaluating one episode is not sufficient, as the patient's history must also be considered. Secondly, relying on history given by patients or family is difficult, particularly as recollection of previous episodes might not be very accurate.

Relevance of correct diagnosis

There is a growing body of literature on the misdiagnosis and underdiagnosis of bipolar disorder.[3] In particular, bipolar II disorder seems vastly underdiagnosed. Whereas the DSM-IV quotes 0.5% prevalence, more recent studies find up to 2% and, with slightly varied diagnostic criteria, up to 5% prevalence rates for bipolar II disorder.[4] Additionally, 30–50% of patients diagnosed with major depression meet the criteria for bipolar disorder, particularly bipolar II disorder.[5] Poor outcome and suicidality have been identified as significant consequences of this misdiagnosis.[6,7] Thus, the issue of correct diagnosis is much more than an academic exercise. Consequently, there has been considerable effort to better characterize depressive episodes clinically, and to ascertain epidemiologic features in bipolar patients in order to diagnose bipolar disorder correctly in first episode patients.

Relevance for research

As was previously discussed, diagnosing bipolar disorder early on and correctly is difficult. Thus, research on this disorder depends on the correct diagnosis. The patients securely diagnosed with bipolar disorder and investigated by researchers might be a small subgroup only, that is, those patients with clear manic or hypomanic and depressive episodes as well as with several episodes in their history. If bipolar disorder per se is to be investigated, studies should be conducted with patients experiencing either affective states, and for practical reasons this is for the most part during remission or in depressive episodes. If the question is why the affective episodes span both extremes, research needs to be done in all affective stages. If the hypothesis is that the course of the disorder is triggered once in the beginning, a study during the first episode would be needed; this is the most challenging alternative.

In summary, there are several issues hampering research on bipolar disorder: correct diagnosis, the cycling course, the difficulty of involving manic patients in systematic studies, relatively low prevalence compared to unipolar depression or schizophrenia, and the requirement of a preceding relevant course before diagnosis.

The latter issue is interesting with respect to the topic of this chapter and will be discussed later in more detail. If infectious/immunologic features are essential in triggering the symptomatic onset of an independent disorder, the chances of finding them will be extremely low in bipolar disorder because of its diagnostic peculiarities. In addition, investigating an active disorder is also more likely to be associated with a history of medication which might modulate the variables of interest. This will be discussed later.

LITERATURE ON INFECTION AND BIPOLAR DISORDER

The cycling course of bipolar disorder has prompted psychiatrists to consider an infectious etiology of this disease.[8] Table 14.1 provides an overview of infections screened for in bipolar patients or reported concurrent with bipolar symptomatology. As can be seen, several viral, bacterial, and parasitic infections have been investigated. However, there are no consistent and convincing results supporting a role for infections causing bipolar disorder. Latent infections with a relapsing-remitting course have also been implicated.

Reactivation of latent herpes simplex virus (HSV) infection was hypothesized in the etiology of bipolar disorder without further substantiation to date.[9] Cytomegalovirus (CMV), another herpes virus, was also investigated. Whereas older studies demonstrated increased prevalence of this infection in bipolar patients or patients with depressive episodes of bipolar disorder,[10–12] a more recent investigation in postmortem brains could not detect CMV viral sequences in these patients.[13] Retroviral and endogenous retroviral infection has been hypothesized in bipolar disorder as well as in schizophrenia.[14–18] However, so far there are no substantial data supporting such an infection in bipolar disorder, whereas there are some positive data for schizophrenia.[8,19] Results on Borna virus in patients with bipolar disorder are inconsistent.[20–24]

Parasitic infections have also been implicated in psychiatric disorders. Increased prevalence of *Toxoplasma gondii* infection has been reported in schizophrenic patients.[17,25] However, very preliminary data (including our own unpublished observations) do not support an increase in the prevalence of toxoplasmosis in bipolar patients,[27] although symptomatic toxoplasma encephalitis might also yield bipolar symptomatology.[28,29] One investigation of a particular mutation of a prion protein that has been associated with bipolar symptomatology did not find it in a population with a high prevalence of bipolar disorder.[30]

Using different approaches, affective, cognitive, and behavioral symptoms have been detected in patients or animals infected with certain infectious agents. With respect to HIV, AIDS mania has become a key term.[31–33] *Borrelia burgdorferi* may cause affective symptoms similar to bipolar symptoms,[34] but there

Table 14.1 Bipolar disorder and infections

Infection	Material	Finding (compared to non-psychiatric controls)
HSV-1/2	Serology, blood	Increased specific antibodies[10,35]
HSV-1/2	Serology, blood	Negative[36]
HSV-1/2	Serology, blood	Case reports in herpes encephalitis mimicking bipolar symptomatology[37]
CMV	Serology, blood	Increased specific antibodies[10]
CMV	CSF	Increased percentage of patients with detection of specific antibodies[12]
CMV stealth virus	Brain, CSF	Detection[11]
CMV	Brain	No detection of CMV sequences[13]
Retrovirus	Blood, brain, CSF	Negative[13–16,18,38]
Borna	Blood	Increased specific antibodies, increased detection of Borna sequences[20–22,24]
Borna	Blood	Negative[23]
Toxoplasma gondii	Blood	Preliminary data without hints on increased percentage of infected individuals[39]
Prion protein	Blood	Particular mutation absent[30]
HIV	Serology, blood	Case reports in HIV patients with bipolar symptomatology, AIDS mania[31,32]
Borrelia burgdorferi	Serology, blood	Case reports in Lyme disease patients with bipolar symptomatology[34]

are no systematic data on this infection in patients with bipolar disorder.

Thus, so far there are no consistent and convincing data that there is any particular infection specifically associated with bipolar disorder. Results on unipolar depression and schizophrenia are more detailed, although lack specific associations.

From these data and some general thoughts on the epidemiology of the infections investigated, it appears unlikely that the presence of any of these infections is sufficient to account for the pathophysiology of bipolar disorder or any of the other major psychiatric disorders. However, infections might play a more complex role in their pathophysiology. This will be discussed in more detail later.

LITERATURE ON IMMUNITY AND BIPOLAR DISORDER

A further hypothesis on the cycling course of bipolar disorder deals with disturbances in immunity and autoimmunity.[40] However, there are very limited data connecting bipolar disorder with immunity. Increased *in vitro* stimulated proliferation of peripheral blood mononuclear cells (PBMC) and increased plasma levels of soluble interleukin-2 receptor (sIL-2R) have been demonstrated in bipolar patients during acute mania.[41] Another study reported increased plasma levels of sIL-2R and sIL-6R in patients with mania.[42] More recently, researches did not find any effects on IL-12 plasma levels in bipolar patients, whereas there were increases in patients with unipolar depression, with medication decreasing IL-12 levels after eight weeks in all patient groups.[43] Acute phase proteins were increased in the plasma of bipolar patients, and their levels were more pronounced during the manic than the depressive episode.[44] Histone synthesis by PBMC (indicative of cell cycle state) was found to be different in patients with either depressive or manic episodes compared to the normothymic state or control subjects.[45] The expression of the neuronal adhesion molecule N-CAM was different in various brain regions in postmortem brain samples of patients with bipolar disorder versus brains of patients with schizophrenia or healthy controls.[46] Some studies on autoimmune variables and antibody levels in general could not demonstrate significant effects in bipolar patients compared to healthy controls or patients with the other major disorders (see Table 14.2).

Unfortunately, immune variables mentioned previously may be modulated by many factors. We demonstrated that certain psychotropic medications, cigarette smoking, and experimental *in vitro* conditions affect these variables and might thereby confound data with respect to the etiology of the disorder.[50–52]

Thus, so far there are no specific and significant associations between bipolar disorder and immune variables. However, as with the issue of infection, immunity may still play a role in the pathophysiology of bipolar disorder.

EFFECT OF MEDICATIONS

Certain antidepressants and antipsychotics modulate cytokine systems such as TNF, leptin, and IL-2.[51,53–55] There are also some data on mood stabilizers such as lithium, valproate, and carbamazepine affecting the cytokine system. Oral lithium treatment might be effective in treating recurrent HSV infections.[56] Lithium[57] added to various *in vitro* settings was shown to affect tumor growth,[58] modulate IL-2 secretion,[59] increase superoxide dismutase activity in various brain regions,[60] modulate LPS response *in vitro*,[61] and modulate megakaryocytogenesis by GM-CSF.[62] Valproate may affect HIV infection;[63] long-term treatment with valproate in mice modulated immune parameters *in vitro*.[64] Carbamazepine also modulates various immune functions *in vitro*.[65,66] In a recent study, valproic acid was as efficient as the gold standard trimethoprim in inhibiting the parasite *Toxoplasma gondii* in an *in vitro* paradigm.[67]

Thus, medications typically used in patients with bipolar disorder have immunomodulatory and anti-infectious properties. While it may be concluded that these properties are relevant for the treatment response, it cannot be concluded that immunity and infection are etiologically involved in the genesis of bipolar disorder.

PATHOPHYSIOLOGY

Infection and immunity might play a role in bipolar disorder, but this may not be due to a specific infection or a particular immune modulation causing bipolar disorder. So, how could infection and immunity be involved?

Neurotransmitters and infection/immunity

Lipkin and coworkers were the first to describe that somatostatin positive neurons in mice infected with lymphocytic choriomeningitis virus (LCV) contain this virus without any morphological abnormalities; the LCV infected mice, however, show significantly reduced mRNA levels of somatostatin and display significant behavioral changes.[68] Thus, this persistent neurotropic infection causes severe behavioral symptomatology and modulates a particular neurotransmitter system without any obvious morphological changes. This very much reflects what we are confronted with in psychiatric disorders – severe symptomatology and modulation of neurotransmitter systems, but without attendant significant cellular pathomorphology. More recent publications support this line of evidence. Rats infected with Borna virus display long-lasting modulations of their serotonin, norepinephrin, and enkephalinergic neurotransmitter systems. After infection, they also show stable abnormal behaviour.[69,70] Moreover, psychotropic medications seem to interact differentially in these models

Table 14.2 Bipolar disorder and immunity

Immune parameter	Material	Finding
PBMC proliferation	Cross-sectional PBMC of bipolar patients	Increased during mania[41]
SIL-2R	Blood concentration	Increased during mania[41,42]
SIL-6R	Blood concentration	Increased during mania[42]
IL-12	Blood	No effect in bipolar patients, increased in monopolar depression compared to controls
		Decrease in all patient groups (bipolar, monopolar depression, schizophrenia) after eight weeks of medication[43]
Acute phase proteins	Blood concentrations	Increase more pronounced during mania than during depression only in non-medicated individuals[44]
Histone proteins	Production of histone proteins by PBMC	Different between manic and depressive and normothymic states or healthy controls[45]
N-CAM	Postmortem brain	Different expression in different regions and with different diagnosis (bipolar disorder, schizophrenia, healthy controls)[46]
Panel of autoantibodies	Blood, cross-sectional	No significant effects in bipolar or monopolar patients compared with controls but age and gender effects found across all groups[47]
Cold agglutinin autoantibodies	Blood, cross-sectional	No difference compared to controls[48]
IgM	Blood, cross-sectional	Increased in all patients (monopolar depression, bipolar disorder, schizophrenia) compared with controls[49]
CRP, ANA	Blood, cross-sectional	No effect in bipolar patients compared to increases in monopolar depression patients[49]

depending on the presence or absence of infection and depending on the rat strain. Whereas fluoxetine inhibited hyperactivity in infected Lewis rats, it did not have this effect in infected Fisher344 rats. Noninfected rats of either strain were not hyperactive in response to fluoxetine. Toxoplasmosis is a parasitic infection which interacts with the serotonin neurotransmitter system;[71–74] the parasite consumes tryptophane, decreasing brain serotonin levels as shown in a mouse model.[75] This observation confirms the serotonin hypothesis of depression in a potential mouse model of the disorder.[76] So, one might speculate that relapsing depressive symptomatology depends on the activity of the persistent intracellular parasite *Toxoplasma gondii*.

While these issues appear to elucidate further the pathophysiology of bipolar disorder, they are difficult to investigate because:

1) The main site of action is in the brain which cannot be analyzed sufficiently *in vivo* with respect to intracellular neurotransmitter levels.
2) Different animal models yield different results, which point to further individual predispositions.

Neurodevelopment and infection/immunity

Another putative link between infection/immunity and psychiatric disorders is the neurodevelopmental history. The neurodevelopmental hypothesis of schizophrenia states that modified neurodevelopment is causally linked with schizophrenia later in life.[77] There is a vast body of literature on morphological abnormalities in the brains of adult patients pointing to disrupting events during neurodevelopment. How then might infections and immunity be linked with neurodevelopment?

It has been shown that viruses may interact with the neurodevelopmental timetable and adversely affect adult neurodifferentiation. A well investigated animal model is the murine infection with Semliki forest virus (SLV). In differentiated neurons this virus leads to a particular immune reaction, whereas in nondifferentiated neurons this virus seems to switch the intracellular pathway of differentiation and cell death towards cell death by apoptosis.[78] Thus, this viral infection interferes on an individual cellular basis with neuronal differentiation, neuronal death, and immune response.[78,79] In this particular animal model, it is the immune response which may lead to the devastating course of the disease;[79] in athymic mice the virus persists intracellularly but there are no signs of demyelination and further symptoms. In contrast, in immunocompetent mice, there is a full-blown cellular and humoral immune response. Thus, this animal model demonstrates that a viral infection may lead to various effects on neurodevelopment and neurodifferentiation and that the severity of symptoms depends on the time point of infection during brain development and ongoing neurodifferentiation, and the predisposition for a specific immune response.

Similar observations have been made with respect to perinatal toxoplasmosis which leads to a severe debilitating disease, compared to postnatal, adult toxoplasmosis which does not yield any relevant infectious symptomatology in immunocompetent individuals.[80] Mice prenatally infected with influenza virus displayed significantly reduced intracellular levels of Reelin, an extracellular glycoprotein that plays a major role in neurodevelopment/neurodifferentiation.[81] This effect on Reelin was reflected in a mild maldevelopment of the neocortex,[82] whereas postnatal influenza infection does not have these effects. Reelin was shown to be altered in patients with psychiatric disorders including bipolar disorder.[83] Thus, these latent infections may differentially interfere with the predisposition of the infected individual concerning time point of infection, cells infected, and the immunologic condition of the individual. One might speculate that this particular network is responsible for some type of symptomatology.

Signal transduction and infection/immunity

Intracellular signal transduction has demonstrated to be dependent on associations between extracellular events that were believed to be independent of one another. The neuroplasticity hypothesis of major depression is an example of integration between abnormalities in the hypothalamic-pituitary-adrenal (HPA) axis and the regulation of neurotrophic factors, and metabolism of calcium intracellularly by the signal transduction pathway of cyclic AMP responsive element binding (CREB) protein/calmodulin.[84–86] Thus, these essential intracellular mediating pathways may also provide an integrating view on the infectious and immunologic phenomena discussed previously with respect to the pathophysiology and etiology of bipolar and other psychiatric disorders.

A group of intraneuronal proteins and peptides, called synaptophysins, SNAREs, and SNAPs, is essentially involved in modulating the formation of synapses and the exocytosis of neurotransmitters.[87] SNAP-25 was altered in patients with mood disorders or schizophrenia.[88] Certain infections, such as retroviral, viral, and prion infections, as well as cytokines and growth factors such as tumor necrosis factor (TNF)-α and brain-derived neurotrophic factor

(BDNF), modify these systems and lead to disturbed synaptic signaling.[89–93]

Intracellular pathways such as the CREB and calcium dependent mechanisms[86] or Wnt[94–96] are relevant with respect to the regulation of brain development and neurodifferentiation. Various latent infections have been shown to interfere with these systems. HIV infection modulated certain CREB-dependent reactions,[97,98] leading to particular responses in neuronal and glial cells via immune modulators. CMV infection was shown to modulate signal transduction significantly if infected neurons were depolarized.[99] It was suggested that the CMV promotor region acts as a molecular switch in neurons affecting the consequent reaction of the neurons towards activation/depolarization by a CREB-dependent pathway. Oncogenesis and pathology caused by the neurotropic JC virus or the hepatitis C virus are most likely due to deregulation of the Wnt pathway.[100,101]

Thus, various infections interfere with intracellular signal transduction pathways that play pivotal roles in cell development and differentiation. The immunologic reaction in response to the infection interferes with these intracellular pathways on one hand, and on the other, induction of these pathways by the infectious agents may lead to activation of cytokines and growth factors modulating cellular development and differentiation.

DISCUSSION

Conventional data on the prevalence of various infections and immune variations in patients with bipolar disorder yield results that do not support a pathogenetic and pathophysiological role of infections and immunity in bipolar disorder. We now have recent molecular data that encourage a revisitation of the infectious and immune hypothesis of bipolar disorder. Additional hypotheses are the traditional and generalized neurotransmitter hypothesis of psychiatric syndromes, and the neurodevelopmental, neuroplasticity, genetic, and environmental hypotheses. These hypotheses were believed to be mutually exclusive. However, the data presented demonstrate that the impact of infection, immunity, neurodevelopment, neuroplasticity, genetics, environment, and the regulation of neurotransmitters can all be integrated intracellularly. Furthermore, the issue of latency can also be explained. A particular genetic background, a specific timetable for infection, and individual cellular activation and activity provide the scenario whereby a particular infection could cause neurodevelopmental changes, impair neuroplasticity, dysregulate neurotransmitter systems, and lead to psychiatric symptomatology at particular time points. Thus, the presence of specific latent infections is not sufficient to understand psychiatric pathology, but the complex interplay of various factors might provide a key to unravel the etiopathogenesis of disorders such as bipolar disorder.

Another field of recent research supports the tenet that the modulation of various intracellular signaling pathways might play a pivotal role in the pathophysiology of psychiatric disorders and particularly bipolar disorder. Mood stabilizing and relapse preventing agents, such as lithium and valproate, modulate and stabilize signal transducing pathways such as calcium/CREB-dependent and Wnt pathways.[26,102–105] These substances were also shown to modulate infections and immune variables. Whereas other psychotropic medications, such as clozapine, olanzapine, and amitriptylline, have variable effects on cytokines and infections, only lithium and valproate have shown consistent and strong effects. This might underline the pathophysiological relevance of the modulated systems in the cycling course of bipolar disorder. The stabilization of intracellular signaling may be more essential in bipolar disorder than in the non-cycling disorders of major depression and schizophrenia.

The research results may provide explanations or rationales for the clinical observation of affective instability in bipolar disorder. Moreover, the intracellular stabilizing effects of lithium and valproate may be essential for correct treatment of bipolar disorder. Thus, the research results further support the position that misdiagnosis of bipolar disorder may have a significant effect on clinical outcome.

In summary, etiopathogenetic hypotheses for psychiatric and bipolar disorders, encompassing the infectious and immune hypotheses, were formerly mutually exclusive and antagonistic but now 'merge intracellularly'.

CONCLUSION

The traditional descriptive prevalence data on individual infections and immune variables, for the most part gathered from sera of patients, do not support a role for infection and immunity in bipolar disorder, schizophrenia, or major depression. However, recent data on intracellular networking by signal transducing systems, modulated in a complex interdependent network by infections, immunity, genes, and individual cellular activity, provide a new and exciting perspective. Infection and immunity might play a pivotal role in etiopathogenesis and pathophysiology of bipolar disorder by modulating intracellular signal

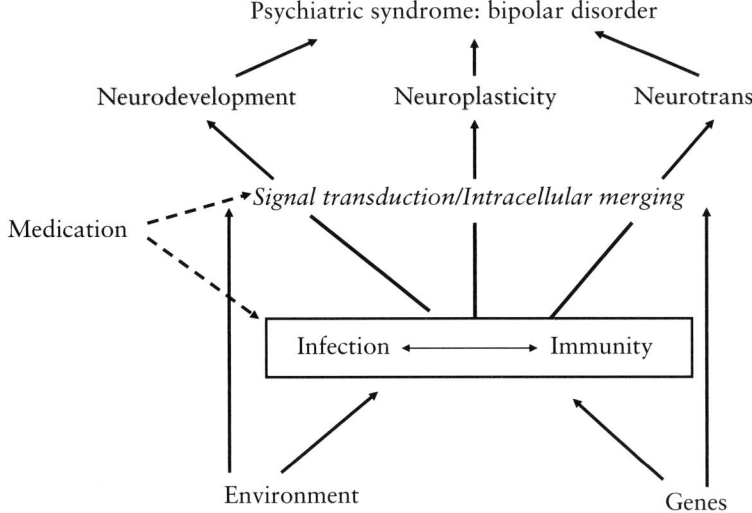

Figure 14.1 Simplified diagram of intracellular convergence of multiple factors leading to the development of bipolar symptoms.

transducing systems with respect to neurodevelopment, neuroplasticity, and neurotransmitter regulation. Additional factors such as environment and genetic predisposition could also be involved in this network. Clinically effective medications typically used in bipolar disorder, such as lithium and valproate, may be integrated in this complex system and may interplay with the same signal transducing systems relevant to the etiopathogenesis of bipolar disorder. The antimicrobial effects of these substances may also be mediated by this intracellular network, or might have additional causes. Figure 14.1 will attempt to summarize and simplify this complex network.

Further research is needed and encouraged. From our point of view, the following issues warrant further research:

1) The brains of affected patients need to be studied since several relevant infections are latent and neuro-/glio-tropic; the cellular modulations might not be present peripherally, and consequently peripheral cells may not serve as relevant cellular models.
2) If a panel of infections causes the same modulations of intracellular signal transducing systems, these infections should be examined as a group rather than individually. One might compare individuals positive for the 'panel infections' with individuals negative for these infections, and one might compare psychiatric patients with various specific diagnoses for the panel of infections. Thus, the design of clinical studies might change significantly.
3) Treatment trials in infected versus non infected patients might be feasible.
4) New agents should be designed and tested with respect to their modulation of particular intracellular signal transducing systems.

REFERENCES

1. American Psychiatric Association. *Diagnostic and Statistical Manual of Mental Disorders*. Washington DC: American Psychiatric Association, 1994.
2. World Health Organization. *International Classification of Diseases* (10th revision). 1993.
3. Rihmer Z, Rutz W, Pihlgren H. Depression and suicide on Gotland. An intensive study of all suicides before and after a depression-training programme for general practitioners. *J Affective Disorders* 1995; **35**: 147–52.
4. Angst J, Gamma A. A new bipolar spectrum concept: a brief review. *Bipolar Disorder* 2002; **4(S1)**: 11–4.
5. Bowden CL. Strategies to reduce misdiagnosis of bipolar depression. *Psychiatr Serv* 2001; **52**: 51–5.
6. Rihmer Z, Kiss Z. Bipolar disorder and suicidal behaviour. *Bipolar Disorder* 2002; **4(S1)**: 21–5.
7. Rihmer Z, Barsi J, Arato M, Demeter E. Suicide in subtypes of primary major depression. *J Affective Disorders* 1990; **18**: 221–5.
8. Yolken RH, Torrey EF. Viruses, schizophrenia, and bipolar disorder. *Clin Microbiol Rev* 1995; **8**: 131–45.
9. Rimon R, Halonen P. Herpes simplex virus infection and depressive illness. *Dis Nervous Sys* 1969; **30**: 338–40.
10. Lycke E, Norrby R, Roos BE. A serological study on mentally ill patients with particular reference to the prevalence of herpes virus infections. *Br J Psychiatry* 1974; **124**: 273–9.
11. Martin WJ. Simian cytomegalovirus-related stealth virus isolated from the cerebrospinal fluid of a patient with bipolar psychosis and acute encephalopathy. *Pathobiol* 1996; **64**: 64–6.
12. Torrey EF, Yolken RH, Winfrey CJ. Cytomegalovirus antibody in cerebrospinal fluid of schizophrenic patients detected by enzyme immunoassay. *Science* 1982; **216**: 892–4.

13. Sierra-Honigmann AM, Carbone KM, Yolken RH. Polymerase-chain reaction (PCR) search for viral nucleic acid sequences in schizophrenia. *Br J Psychiatry* 1995; **166**: 55–60.
14. Crow TJ. A re-evaluation of the viral hypothesis: is psychosis the result of retroviral integration at a site close to the cerebral dominance gene? *Br J Psychiatry* 1984; **145**: 243–53.
15. Torrey EF, Peterson MR. Slow and latent viruses in schizophrenia. *Lancet* 1973; **2**: 22–4.
16. Torrey EF, Yolken RH. At issue: is household crowding a risk factor for schizophrenia and bipolar disorder? *Schizophr Bull* 1998; **24**: 321–4.
17. Torrey EF, Yolken RH. The schizophrenia-rheumatoid arthritis connection: infectious, immune, or both? *Brain Behav Immunity* 2001; **15**: 401–10.
18. Yolken RH, Karlsson H, Yee F et al. Endogenous retroviruses and schizophrenia. *Brain Res Rev* 2000; **31**: 193–9.
19. Hinze-Selch D. Infection, treatment and immune response in patients with bipolar disorder versus patients with major depression, schizophrenia or healthy controls. *Bipolar Disorder* 2002; **4**(S1): 81–3.
20. Amsterdam JD, Winokur W, Dyson A et al. Borna disease virus: a possible etiologic factor in human affective disorders? *Arch Gen Psychiatry* 1985; **42**: 1093–6.
21. Bode L, Reckwald P, Severus WE et al. Borna disease virus-specific circulating immune complexes, antigenemia and free antibodies – the key marker triplet determining infection and prevailing in severe mood disorders. *Mol Psychiatry* 2001; **6**: 481–91.
22. Fu ZF, Amsterdam JD, Kao M et al. Detection of Borna disease virus-reactive antibodies from patients with affective disorder by western immunoblot technique. *J Affective Disorders* 1993; **27**: 61–8.
23. Kim YK, Kim SH, Choi SH et al. Failure to demonstrate Borna disease virus genome in peripheral blood mononuclear cells from psychiatric patients in Korea. *J Neurovirol* 1999; **5**: 196–9.
24. Taieb O, Baleyte JM, Mazet P, Fillet AM. Borna disease virus and psychiatry. *Eur Psychiatry* 2001; **16**: 3–10.
25. Yolken RH, Bachmann S, Ruslanova I et al. Antibodies to *Toxoplasma gondii* in individuals with first-episode schizophrenia. *Clin Infec Dis* 2001; **32**: 842–44.
26. Willmoth F, Spleiβ O, Wiesmann K et al. Expression of G-proteins and regulators of G-protein signalling in neutrophils of patients with bipolar disorder: effects of mood stabilizers. *Bipolar Disorder* 2002; **4**(S1): 75–6.
27. Wilms S, Bozkurt B, Vogel T et al. Toxoplasmosis in schizophrenia, bipolar and depressive disorders versus healthy controls: immunologic and epidemiologic findings. *Pharmacopsychiatry* 2003; **36**: 272–3.
28. Alla P, de Jaureguiberry JP, Galzin M et al. Hemiballism with manic access caused by toxoplasmic abscess in AIDS. *Ann Med Interne* 1997; **148**: 507–9.
29. Delgado Garcia G. Garcia Landa J. Reactivity of the intradermal test with toxoplasmosis in schizophrenic patients. *Revista Cubana Medicin Tropical* 1979; **31**: 225–33.
30. Korczyn AD, Chapman J, Belmaker RH et al. Absence of the prion protein mutation in bipolar manic-depressive patients. *Br J Psychiatry* 1992; **161**: 132.
31. Ellen SR, Judd FK, Mijch AM, Cockram A. Secondary mania in patients with HIV infection. *Aust NZ J Psychiatry* 1999; **33**: 353–60.
32. Mijch AM, Judd FK, Lyketsos CG et al. Secondary mania in patients with HIV infection: are antiretrovirals protective? *J Neuropsychiatry Clin Neurosci* 1999; **11**: 475–80.
33. Rundell JR, Wise MG. Causes of organic mood disorder. *J Neuropsychiatry Clin Neurosci* 1989; **1**: 398–400.
34. Fallon BA, Nields JA. Lyme disease: a neuropsychiatric illness. *Am J Psychiatry* 1994; **151**: 1571–83.
35. Halonen PE, Rimon R, Arohonka K, Jäntti V. Antibody levels to herpes simplex type 1, measles and rubella viruses in psychiatric patients. *Br J Psychiatry* 1974; **125**: 461–5.
36. Torrey EF, Peterson MR, Brannon WL et al. Immunoglobulins and viral antibodies in psychiatric patients. *Br J Psychiatry* 1978; **132**: 342–8.
37. Koehler K, Guth W. The mimicking of mania in 'benign' herpes simplex encephalitis. *Biol Psychiatry* 1979; **14**: 405–11.
38. Hart DJ, Heath RG, Sautter FJ Jr et al. Antiretroviral antibodies: implications for schizophrenia, schizophrenia spectrum disorders, and bipolar disorder. *Biol Psychiatry* 1999; **45**: 704–14.
39. Wilms S, Stoltenberg R, Kell S et al. Toxoplasmosis in individuals with schizophrenia versus bipolar and depressive disorders versus healthy controls: preliminary immunologic and epidemiologic results. *Bipolar Disorder* 2002; **4**(S1): 139.
40. Hurlock EC. Interferons: potential roles in affect. *Med Hypotheses* 2001; **56**: 558–66.
41. Tsai SY, Chen KP, Yang YY et al. Activation of indices of cell-mediated immunity in bipolar mania. *Biol Psychiatry* 1999; **45**: 989–94.
42. Maes M, Bosmans E, Calabrese J et al. Interleukin-2 and interleukin-6 in schizophrenia and mania: effects of neuroleptics and mood stabilizers. *J Psychiatric Res* 1995; **29**: 141–52.
43. Kim YK, Suh IB, Kim H et al. The plasma levels of interleukin-12 in schizophrenia, major depresion and bipolar mania: effects of psychotropic medication. *Mol Psychiatry* 2002; **7**: 1108–14.
44. Maes M, Delange J, Ranjan R et al. Acute phase proteins in schizophrenia, mania and major depression: modulation by psychotropic drugs. *Psychiatry Res* 1997; **66**: 1–11.
45. Sourlingas TG, Issidorides MR, Havaki S et al. Peripheral blood lymphocytes of bipolar affective patients have a histone synthetic profile indicative of an active cell state. *Prog Neuropsychopharmacol Biol Psychiatry* 1998; **22**: 81–96.
46. Vawter MP, Howard AL, Hyde TM et al. Alterations of hippocampal secreted N-CAM in bipolar disorder and synaptophysin in schizophrenia. *Mol Psychiatry* 1999; **4**: 467–75.
47. Hornig M, Amsterdam JD, Kamoun M, Goodman DB. Autoantibody disturbances in affective disorders: a function of age and gender? *J Affective Disorders* 1999; **55**: 29–37.
48. Spivak B, Radwan M, Brandon J et al. Clod agglutinin autoantibodies in psychiatric patients: their relation to diagnosis and pharmacological treatment. *Am J Psychiatry* 1991; **148**: 244–7.
49. Legros S, Mendlewicz J, Wybran J. Immunoglobulins, autoantibodies and other serum protein fractions in psychiatric disorders. *Eur Arch Psychiatry Neurol Sci* 1985; **235**: 9–11.
50. Haack M, Hinze-Selch D, Fenzel T et al. Plasma levels of cytokines and soluble cytokine receptors in psychiatric patients upon hospital admission: effects of confounding factors and diagnosis. *J Psychiatric Res* 1999; **33**: 407–11.
51. Hinze-Selch D, Pollmächer T. In vitro cytokine secretion in individuals with schizophrenia: results, confounding factors and implications for further research. *Brain Behav Immunity* 2001; **15**: 282–318.
52. Pollmächer T, Hinze-Selch D. Factors confounding studies of circulating soluble interleukin-2 receptor levels in schizophrenia. *Schizophr Res* 1998; **33**: 123–4.
53. Hinze-Selch D, Schuld A, Kraus T et al. Effects of antidepressants on weight and on the plasma levels of leptin, TNF-α and soluble TNF receptors: a longitudinal study in patients treated with amitriptyline or paroxetine. *Neuropsychopharmacol* 2000; **23**: 13–9.

54. Pollmächer T, Hinze-Selch D, Mullington J. Effects of clozapine on plasma cytokine and soluble cytokine receptor levels. *J Clin Psychopharmacol* 1996; **16**: 403–9.
55. Schuld A, Kraus T, Haack M et al. Plasma levels of cytokines and soluble cytokine receptors during treatment with olanzapine. *Schizophr Res* 2000; **43**: 154–66.
56. Amsterdam JD, Maislin G, Hooper MB. Suppression of herpes simplex virus infection with oral lithium carbonate – a possible antiviral activity. *Pharmacotherapy* 1996; **16**: 1070–5.
57. Rybakowski JK. Antiviral and immunomodulatory effect of lithium. *Pharmacopsychiatry* 2000; **33**: 159–64.
58. Wu Y, Cai D. Study of the effect of lithium on lymphokine-activated killer cell activity and its antitumor growth. *Proc Soc Exp Biol Med* 1992; **201**: 284–8.
59. Wilson R, Fraser WD, McKillop JH et al. The in vitro effects of lithium on the immune system. *Autoimmunity* 1989; **4**: 109–14.
60. Shukla GS. Mechanism of lithium action: in vivo and in vitro effects of alkali metals on brain superoxide dismutase. *Pharmacol Biochem Behav* 1987; **26**: 235–40.
61. Ishizaka S, Moller G. Lithium chloride induces partial responsiveness to LPS in nonresponder B cells. *Nature* 1982; **299**: 363–5.
62. Gallicchio VS, Chen MG, Watts TD. Specificity of lithium (Li+) to enhance the production of colony stimulating factor (GM-CSF) from mitogen-stimulated lymphocytes in vitro. *Cellular Immunol* 1984; **85**: 58–66.
63. Witvrouw M, Schmit JC, Van Remoortel B et al. Cell type-dependent effect of sodium valproate on human immunodeficiency virus type 1 replication in vitro. *AIDS Res Human Retroviruses* 1997; **13**: 187–92.
64. Queiroz ML, Mullen PW. Effects of sodium valproate on the immune response. *Int J Immunopharmacol* 1992; **14**: 1133–7.
65. Furst SM, Uetrecht JP. The effect of carbamazepine and its reactive metabolite, 9-acridine carboxaldehyde, on immune cell function in vitro. *Int J Immunopharmacol* 1995; **17**: 445–52.
66. Gilhus NE. The in vitro effect of phenytoin and carbamazepine on subpopulations of human blood mononuclear cells. *Int J Immunopharmacol* 1983; **5**: 283–8.
67. Jones-Brando LV, Torrey EF, Yolken RH. Drugs used in the treatment of schizophrenia and bipolar disorder inhibit the replication of *Toxoplasma gondii*. *Schizophr Res* 2003; **62**: 237–44.
68. Lipkin WI, Battenberg EL, Bloom FE, Oldstone MB. Viral infection of neurons can depress neurotransmitter mRNA levels without histologic injury. *Brain Res* 1988; **451**: 333–9.
69. Pletnikov MV, Rubin SA, Vogel MW et al. Effects of genetic background on neonatal Borna disease virus infection-induced neurodevelopmental damage. II. Neurochemical alterations and responses to pharmacological treatments. *Brain Res* 2002; **944**: 108–23.
70. Solbrig MV, Koob GF, Lipkin WI. Key role for enkephalinergic tone in cortico-striatal-thalamic function. *Eur J Neurosci* 2002; **16**: 1819–22.
71. Däubener W, Hadding U. Cellular immune reactions directed against *Toxoplasma gondii* with special emphasis on the central nervous system. *Med Microbiol Immunol* 1997; **185**: 195–206.
72. Däubener W, MacKenzie CR. IFN-gamma activated indoleamine 2,3-dioxygenase activity in human cells is an antiparasitic and an antibacterial effector mechanism. *Adv Exp Med Biol* 1999; **467**: 517–24.
73. Däubener W, Posdziech V, Hadding U, MacKenzie CR. Inducible anti-parasitic effector mechanisms in human uroepithelial cells: tryptophan degradation vs. NO production. *Med Microbiol Immunol* 1999; **187**: 143–7.
74. Däubener W, Spors B, Hucke C et al. Restriction of *Toxoplasma gondii* growth in human brain microvascular endothelial cells by activation of indoleamine 2,3-dioxygenase. *Infect Immunity* 2001; **69**: 6527–31.
75. Stibbs HH. Changes in brain concentrations of catecholamines and indoleamines in *Toxoplasma gondii* infected mice. *Ann Tropical Med Parasitol* 1985; **79**: 153–7.
76. Nemeroff CB. Recent advances in the neurobiology of depression. *Psychopharmacol Bull* 2000; **36**(S2): 6–23.
77. Marenco S, Weinberger DR. The neurodevelopmental hypothesis of schizophrenia: following a trail of evidence from cradle to grave. *Dev Psychopathol* 2000; **12**: 501–27.
78. Allsopp TE, Fazakerley JK. Altruistic cell suicide and the specialized case of the virus-infected nervous system. *Trends Neurosci* 2000; **23**: 284–90.
79. Fazakerley JK. Pathogenesis of Semliki Forest virus encephalitis. *Neurovirol* 2002; **8**: 66–74.
80. Zygmunt DJ. *Toxoplasma gondii*. *Inf Control Hospital Epidemiol* 1990; **11**: 207–11.
81. Fairen A, Morante-Oria J, Frassoni C. The surface of the developing cerebral cortex: still special cells one century later. *Prog Brain Res* 2002; **136**: 281–91.
82. Fatemi SH, Emamian ES, Kist D et al. Defective corticogenesis and reduction in Reelin immunoreactivity in cortex and hippocampus of prenatally infected neonatal mice. *Mol Psychiatry* 1999; **4**: 145–54.
83. Fatemi SH, Kroll JL, Stary JM. Altered levels of Reelin and its isoforms in schizophrenia and mood disorders. *Neuroreport* 2001; **12**: 3209–15.
84. Aldenhoff JB. Imbalance of neuronal excitability as a cause of psychic disorder. *Pharmacopsychiatry* 1989; **22**: 227–40.
85. Aldenhoff JB, Gruol DL, Rivier J et al. Corticotropin releasing factor decreases postburst hyperpolarizations and excites hippocampal neurons. *Science* 1983; **221**: 875–7.
86. Duman RS, Heninger GR, Nestler EJ. A molecular and cellular hypothesis of depression. *Arch Gen Psychiatry* 1997; **54**: 597–606.
87. Sudhof TC. The synaptic vesicle cycle revisited. *Neuron* 2000; **28**: 317–20.
88. Fatemi SH, Earle JA, Stary JM et al. Altered levels of the synaptosomal associated protein SNAP-25 in hippocampus of subjects with mood disorders and schizophrenia. *Neuroreport* 2001; **12**: 3257–62.
89. Fatemi SH, Sidwell R, Kist D et al. Differential expression of synaptosome-associated protein 25 kDa (SNAP-25) in hippocampi of neonatal mice following exposure to human influenza virus in utero. *Brain Res* 1998; **800**: 1–9.
90. Poli A, Pistello M, Carli MA et al. Tumor necrosis factor-alpha and virus expression in the central nervous system of cats infected with feline immunodeficiency virus. *J Neurovirol* 1999; **5**: 465–73.
91. Siso S, Puig B, Varea R et al. Abnormal synaptic protein expression and cell death in murine scrapie. *Acta Neuropathologica* 2002; **103**: 615–26.
92. Takei N, Sasaoka K, Inoue K et al. Brain-derived neurotrophic factor increases the stimulation-evoked release of glutamate and the levels of exocytosis-associated proteins in cultured cortical neurons from embryonic rats. *J Neurochem* 1997; **68**: 370–5.
93. Tartaglia N, Du J, Tyler WJ et al. Protein synthesis-dependent and -independent regulation of hippocampal synapses by brain-derived neurotrophic factor. *J Biol Chemistry* 2001; **276**: 37585–93.
94. Huelsken J, Birchmeier W. New aspects of Wnt signaling pathways in higher vertebrates. *Curr Opin Genet Dev* 2001; **11**: 547–53.

95. Pandur P, Maurus D, Kühl M. Increasingly complex: new players enter the Wnt signaling network. *Bioessays* 2002; **24**: 881–4.
96. Reya T, Duncan AW, Ailles L et al. A role for Wnt signaling in self-renewal of haematopoietic stem cells. *Nature* 2003; **423**: 409–14.
97. Flora G, Lee YW, Nath A et al. Methamphetamine potentiates HIV-1 Tat protein-mediated activation of redox-sensitive pathways in discrete regions of the brain. *Exp Neurol* 2003; **179**: 60–70.
98. Wortman MJ, Krachmatov CP, Kim JH et al. Interaction of HIV-1 Tat with puralpha in nuclei of human glia cells: characterization of RNA-mediated protein-protein binding. *J Cellular Biochem* 2000; **77**: 65–74.
99. Wheeler DG, Cooper E. Depolarization strongly induces human cytomegalovirus major immediate-early promoter/enhancer activity in neurons. *J Biol Chemistry* 2001; **276**: 31978–85.
100. Khalili K. Human neurotropic JC virus and its association with brain tumors. *Dis Markers* 2001; **17**: 143–7.
101. Shackel NA, McGuiness PH, Abbott CA et al. Insights into the pathobiology of hepatitis C virus-associated cirrhosis: analysis of intrahepatic differential gene expression. *Am J Pathol* 2002; **160**: 641–54.
102. Chen G, Huang LD, Jiang YM, Manji HK. The mood-stabilizing agent valproate inhibits the activity of glycogen synthase kinase-2. *J Neurochem* 1999; **72**: 1327–30.
103. Blaheta RA, Cinatl J Jr. Anti-tumor mechanisms of valproate: a novel role for an old drug. *Med Res Rev* 2002; **22**: 492–511.
104. Gould TD, Manji HK. The Wnt signaling pathway in bipolar disorder. *Neuroscientist* 2002; **8**: 497–511.
105. Jope RS, Bijur GN. Mood stabilizers, glycogen synthase kinase-3beta and cell survival. *Mol Psychiatry* 2002; **7(S1)**: 35–45.

15

Role of Borna disease virus in neuropsychiatric disorders

Oliver Planz and Lothar Stitz

SUMMARY

The discovery of Borna disease virus (BDV) specific antibodies in sera of psychiatric patients encouraged many scientists all over the world to investigate a possible correlation of psychiatric disorders with BDV infection. However, after almost 20 years of research in this field, many reports with controversial views have resulted in uncertainty as to whether BDV is indeed a causative agent for some psychiatric diseases. In the following chapter, we critically summarize the current knowledge on BDV infection in man, including methods used for diagnosis of BDV infection.

INTRODUCTION

Borna disease was first described in the veterinary literature at the end of the 18th century as a disease characterized by central nervous symptoms in horses. More precise reports on a 'disease of the head' (hitzige Kopfkrankheit), brain fever, subacute meningitis, or 'hypersomnia of horses' can be found at the beginning of the 19th century. The name of the disease refers to an epidemic in the town of Borna in Saxony near Leipzig in 1895, when almost all horses in a cavalry regiment died with severe central nervous system symptoms.[1] The experimental transmission of the disease to animals using homogenized brain material from diseased horses led to the detection of a filterable entity, Borna disease virus (BDV), as the etiological agent of the disease.[2] Although these studies were undertaken in the 1920s, the nature of this virus remained obscure for a long time. Work on the type of nucleic acid, the organization of the genome, the characterization of virus-coded proteins, and the classification of the virus, has increased our understanding of the agent causing a defined neurological disease in animals. Today, BDV has been detected in many warm-blooded animal species including horses, sheep, cattle, cats, and dogs.[1,3,4]

In addition to its relevance for veterinary science, BD is an important experimental model for virus-induced degenerative CNS disease in rats and mice and it has been shown to be useful for the investigation of immunopathological mechanisms in the central nervous system.[5–9] The issue of whether BDV could be involved in psychiatric disorders was first addressed when Rudolf Rott, Hilary Koprowski, and others reported that serum antibodies to BDV were found in patients with bipolar disorders.[10] Since then numerous reports from research groups worldwide have been published presenting data in favour of an involvement of BDV or a BDV-like agent in psychiatric disorders. However, several papers have also been published that report a failure to detect BDV in patients with psychiatric disorders, leading to a discussion on whether indeed BDV or a BDV-related agent can cause psychiatric diseases. This led to discussions about whether this virus should be regarded as a zoonotic agent. In this chapter we will provide a critical overview of current knowledge on the association of diagnostic markers of BDV infection with psychiatric disorders.

BORNA DISEASE VIRUS

BDV is a non-cytolytic single-stranded RNA virus, representing the only member of *Bornaviridae* in the order of *Mononegavirales*. It is highly associated with neuronal cells. The approximately 8.9 kb size BDV

This work is dedicated to Professor Dr Rudolf Rott, one of the pioneers in Borna disease virus research, who died at the age of 77.

genome with negative polarity is replicated in the nucleus of the infected cell and represents six different open reading frames (ORFs).

ORF I encodes the nucleoprotein (NP) which exists as 40 kDa and 38 kDa proteins, the latter resulting from translation of a second AUG codon of the same mRNA 13 amino acids downstream of the first AUG codon. Due to an N-terminal nuclear localization signal (NLS) located between the first 13 amino acids of NP, p40 is detectable in the nucleus, while p38 is only found in the cytoplasm.[11,12]

ORF II codes for the phosphoprotein p24 (P). Although the function of this protein has not been fully investigated, it is proposed that the phosphoprotein functions as a cofactor of viral RNA transcription for virus replication. This protein is phosphorylated in its serine residues, suggesting that its function could be controlled by cellular kinases.[13,14] It apparently plays a major role in the nucleoplasmic transport of BDV ribonucleoprotein complex (RNP). The nucleoprotein and the phosphoprotein are the first viral proteins that can be detected after *in vivo* or *in vitro* infection, and are also the major targets to be recognized by the antibodies of infected individuals. Consequently, these two viral proteins are used intensively for serological diagnostics. The phosphoprotein interacts with itself, with the nucleoprotein, and with a third protein, the nonglycosylated X protein or p10. ORF X overlaps with ORF II. The X protein is also localized in the nucleus of infected cells, even though it does not have an NLS.[15–17]

The ORF III encodes the p16 protein and represents the putative matrix protein (M). It has been proposed that the matrix protein is located on the viral surface and is involved in virus attachment to the cell.[18,19] It contains hydrophobic sequences characteristic for membrane spanning proteins and can form stable tetramers.[19] The glycosylation of the matrix protein is still under discussion.[20,21]

The ORF IV encodes for the glycoprotein (G, described as gp94) that is found in its N-glycosylated form at approximately 94 kDa. A C-terminal cleavage product of G has been identified with a molecular mass of approximately 43 kD (described as gp43). Both the full length G protein and the gp43 are detectable in the virion, while only the cleavage product is translocated to the membrane of the host cell.[22,23] There is some evidence that G mediates penetration by membrane fusion after the fusion peptide becomes exposed by proteolytic cleavage of the glycoprotein.

Finally the L protein, the gene product of ORF V, which is localized at the 5'-end of the viral antigenome, has been identified as a 180–190 kD protein and represents a RNA-dependent RNA polymerase.[24,25] The L-polymerase is located in the nucleus of infected cells. In addition to the phosphoprotein, the L-polymerase is also phosphorylated at serine residues, making this protein a further candidate for BDV-host cell interactions.[24]

The unique feature of BDV, namely that replication occurs in the nucleus of infected cells, demands a nuclear localization and export function of the viral proteins. However, the consecutive steps involved in virus replication and, consequently, the role of the viral proteins, are not fully understood. The nuclear localization signals (NLSs) of the NP and P make these proteins suitable for nuclear localization activity.[12,15,16,26,27] In contrast, the nuclear export function of the X protein is not fully investigated and controversially discussed.[15,17,28] More recently, it was suggested that the NP protein has export activity due to a leucine rich motif in its NES.[27] Cellular splicing machinery is required to process some of the primary RNA transcripts. A variety of mechanisms are used to regulate gene expression, including the use of overlapping reading frames, overlapping transcription units, alternative RNA splicing, and leaky ribosome scanning during protein translation.[29] The replication cycle seems to be completed within 24 hours. It is proposed that only one to three infectious virus particles are produced and released by budding on the cell surface of the infected cells. The BDV particles are 70–130 nm in diameter and have spikes approximately 7 nm long.[30,31]

BORNA DISEASE VIRUS INFECTION IN ANIMALS

The classic hosts for BDV are horses and sheep. Nevertheless, in the last three decades, natural BDV infection was investigated in a wide variety of wild and domestic animals.[1] Several recent publications report the presence of BDV or anti-BDV antibodies in pets like cats and dogs.[32–39] In addition to the natural infection, BDV was transferred after experimental infection to various animal species including primates. In the following section the clinical outcome of BDV infection and the role of immunopathogenesis after BDV infection in natural and experimentally infected animals is summarized.

Natural infection

In natural hosts, the disease occurs sporadically after incubation times varying from weeks to months and possibly even longer. If the infection becomes manifest, the disease is characterized during the early phase by disturbances of the sensory functions, impaired posture of the limbs, temporary immobility and excitations, ataxia, hyperesthesia, vision disorders and nystagmus, together with anorexia, fever, and colics. The early neurological symptoms are mainly disorders of functions governed by the limbic system, whereas during the later stages of the disease dysfunctions of the motor system, such as paralysis and paresis, predominate. Most naturally infected animals die one to two weeks after onset of the disease, but recoveries or recurrence have also been observed.

Experimental infection

Essentially, the same sequence and comparable disease symptoms as described above for natural hosts can be observed after infection of experimental animals like rats, rabbits, chicken, and monkeys, with a virus obtained from naturally infected horses and sheep. The disease starts with alertness and loss of fear, followed by lack of coordination, hyperactivity, aggressiveness, and later passiveness and hypersomnia.

It was not until the 1980s that research by Rudolf Rott, Opendra Narayan, and Hanns Ludwig revealed that Borna disease is an immune-mediated disease. Experiments on the immunopathological mechanisms were performed in the Lewis rat, which is presently the most intensively and best investigated animal model.[5,7,9,40–44] After infection of adult rats by various routes, including intracerebral, intraocular, intranasal, and intramuscular injection, infectious virus and virus-specific antigens can be detected in high concentrations in the cerebrospinal fluid, brain, retina, peripheral nerves, and adrenal gland.[5,43,45–48]

Histological studies on the brains of diseased rats reveal perivascular and parenchymal infiltrates. Immunohistological observations revealed the phenotype of cells present in the encephalitic lesions. CD4-positive T cells and, to a lower extent, CD8 positive T cells make up about 50% of the cells found in the brain infiltrates, whereas macrophages represent the majority of a single inflammatory cell type in the perivascular and parenchymal infiltrates. The CD8 positive T cells are the main effector cells, recognizing predominately the nucleoprotein, and are responsible for MHC class I restricted lysis of BDV infected cells, while CD4 positive T cells provide help for BDV-specific B cells and cytotoxic T cells.

Immunohistological examinations of brains from naturally infected horses and donkeys showed perivascular and parenchymal infiltrates very similar to those found after experimental infection of rats, making this system an excellent model to study BDV induced immunopathology. In the chronic stage of the disease, signs of dementia, chronic debility, and behavioral abnormalities, including severe learning deficiencies, prevail. However, infection without overt clinical signs but with behavioral alterations has also been reported in experimentally infected animals. In some studies, learning deficiencies and slight behavioral changes (such as alterations in social behavior) have been reported in tree shrews and rhesus monkeys.[49,50]

DIAGNOSIS OF BORNA DISEASE VIRUS

Currently, there is no validated diagnostic tool available for BDV. The screening systems are divided into tests allowing the detection of either BDV-specific antibodies, viral antigens, or virus-specific nucleic acids. In the following section these different systems and their strengths or weaknesses for BDV diagnosis are summarized.

Detection of BDV-specific antibodies

For the detection of BDV-specific antibodies, indirect immunofluorescence assay (IFA), western blot analysis (WB), enzyme linked immunoabsorbant assay (ELISA), and electrochemiluminescence immunoassay (ELICA) are the most commonly used tests.[51]

For IFA, BDV infected cells are incubated with different dilutions of sera. Since NP and P proteins are the major targets for the humoral immune response, and these proteins are present in the nuclei of infected cells due to nuclear localization,[52–54] BDV-reactive antibodies are diagnosed by a typical punctate immunostaining of most likely RNPs in the nucleoplasm.[55] The titers of human BDV-specific antibodies are frequently below 1:40. These low titers are also found in naturally infected horses or sheep.[56,57] IFA with BDV-infected Madin Darby kidney cells was used for the first documentation of BDV-reactive antibodies in sera of psychiatric patients.[10] Different cell lines with variation in expression of BDV antigen are used for IFA, which may account for some of the differences in the prevalence rates. Nevertheless, the reproducibility of IFA was confirmed in various multi-center studies.[58] Using IFA, it is not possible to distinguish whether the corresponding human sera do indeed contain BDV-specific or cross-reactive antibodies, since autoantibodies have been detected in many cases of psychiatric disorder.[59–61]

For western blotting, various sources of antigen are used – for example, BDV cell lysate, recombinant protein or BDV brain homogenates.[62–65] WB allows us to investigate the specificity of BDV reactive sera. Some studies revealed that human antibodies directed against only one of these proteins showed positive reactivity,[66,67] whereas in other studies human sera were found to contain antibodies that recognized more than one viral protein.[63,68–71] These latter studies argue against cross-reactive antibodies and support specific BDV seropositivity. Therefore, a restrictive criterion was proposed where seropositivity was only assessed if more than one BDV protein is specifically recognized by human sera, as is successfully used for the detection of other viral infections.[63] Whether similar restrictive criteria should apply for BDV is questionable. After experimental BDV infection in some strains of mice, BDV-specific antibodies directed against NP and P can be found while sera from other strains only react with one BDV protein (authors' unpublished data).

During the few last years, ELISAs or modified ELISAs such as ELICA or EIA have been favorably used to detect BDV reactive human sera.[51,66,71–73] Recombinant, purified viral proteins were used in most of these assays; therefore, the risk of false positive results due to cross-reactive or autoantibodies was reduced.[51,62,66–70,74–76] The advantage of these assay systems is the defined source of reagents like monoclonal antibodies or recombinant viral proteins, making these assays good candidates for an evaluated test system. Furthermore, since the assays are performed in microtiter plates, high throughput can be achieved, allowing one to test high numbers of human sera.

Nevertheless, the diagnostic value of serological tests in general was questioned when the observation was published that human BDV antibodies bind their antigens with low avidity whereas antibodies from various animals bind BDV with high avidity, arguing for nonspecific binding of all serological test methods using human sera.[77] However, a recent report using peptide arrays suggested that these antibodies with low affinity found in psychiatric patients are indeed specific for BDV or a BDV-like agent and indicate infection.[78]

Detection of BDV or viral proteins

Two methods were used for the detection of BDV-specific antigens in psychiatric patients: antigen capture ELISA and fluorocytometry (FACS). Using monoclonal antibodies against NP and P, BDV antigen was first detected in the peripheral blood mononuclear cells (PBMC) of psychiatric patients by FACS;[79] the study revealed that 15–17% of analyzed monocytes expressed BDV antigens. Unfortunately, PBMCs of normal control cases were not included in this pilot study. Furthermore, a discrepancy exists between these findings and the amount of viral RNA detected by RT-nested PCR.[80] RT-nested PCR is required for the detection of BDV RNA in some of the FACS-positive PBMC samples. Thus, the RNA detection data in humans are in concert with findings in neonatally BDV-infected rats where the number of infected PBMCs is very low and thus generally requires RT-nested PCR.[81–84] Although caution is needed when comparing the results of human and animal studies, these data imply that the viral load in human PBMC is lower than suggested from the FACS analysis, questioning the reliability of this test. Without further data on the specificity and sensitivity of BDV antigen detection by FACS (for example, testing the PBMCs of BDV-infected rats), the diagnostic value of this tool remains uncertain.

To measure BDV antigens in the CSF and blood, an antigen-captured ELISA has been developed which uses monoclonal antibodies and polyclonal antiserum to capture and detect the antigen, respectively.[72] With the help of this assay researchers were able to detect BDV-specific circulating immune complexes and their interaction with BDV-specific antibodies and viral antigens.[72] After evaluation, this assay could be a good candidate for a diagnostic tool to detect BDV-specific antigens and, as described above, BDV reactive sera.

So far, only a few groups have succeeded in isolating BDV from blood or brain tissue using either complicated *in vitro* or *in vivo* procedures.[85,86] Since accidental contamination of human samples with laboratory strain viruses cannot be formally excluded, the significance of these findings is questionable.[87,88] Unfortunately, the human isolates in question have not been available for examination by the general scientific community.

Detection of BDV-specific nucleic acid

Two methods are most suitable for detecting BDV-specific nucleic acid: reverse transcriptase polymerase chain reaction (RT-PCR) and *in situ* hybridization. While RT-PCR is mostly used to detect BDV-specific nucleic acid from blood and also to a lesser extent from postmortem brain material, *in situ* hybridization is most suitable for histology. The use of RT-PCR in BDV diagnosis has lead to controversial results and consequently to various discussions on the reliability of this method for BDV diagnosis. Two reasons are behind this. First, RT-PCR is an amplification method. Therefore, contamination of the samples with laboratory BDV nucleic acid is possible. Second, sensitivities in different laboratories resulting from different methods are likely. In a multicenter study in Germany, different RT-PCR methods were compared, resulting in the finding that the method by Vahlenkamp and coworkers[83] was the most reliable and the most sensitive (Borna study group unpublished results). Nevertheless, until recently this method has not been used as the standard method of BDV diagnosis.

In conclusion, for diagnostic purposes, reliable, reproducible, and easy-to-use screening systems are required. Serological tests on the basis of ELISA, EIA, or ECLIA allow high throughput and with the use of monoclonal antibodies or recombinant viral protein a general standard should be possible, which would allow us to compare samples in different laboratories. The same is true for the detection of viral antigens by EIA. After evaluation and standardization, these tests do not require extra skill or techniques and can be easily performed in any diagnostic laboratory. In contrast, although the RT-PCR described by Vahlenkamp and colleagues is a first step to standardize this method for BDV diagnosis, the source and the preparation of RNA is still controversial. Furthermore, RNA preparation and the complete RT-PCR requires certain skills to avoid cross-contamination or production of false negative results.[83,89] This problem could be solved in the near future, when fully automated purification of nucleic acid will be routinely available.

BDV INFECTION IN HUMANS

The first reports of detection of BDV specific antibodies in the sera of human psychiatric patients led to an intense discussion about whether this virus causes disease in man.[10,90–92] Nevertheless, our knowledge about the epidemiology of BDV infection in humans is still preliminary. The mode of transmission, the distribution, and the natural reservoir remain unknown. Furthermore, the causative role of BDV in disease is unclear.

Infections have been reported in Europe, North America, and in a few parts of Asia. Most recently the presence of BDV in Australia has been debated. Nevertheless, it is plausible that BDV infection is even more distributed as indicated by subclinical infections of various animals. This is mostly due to the lack of a standardized method for detection and a lack of experience in linking disease symptoms to BDV infection. Since Rott and colleagues first published the detection of BDV-specific antibodies in human psychiatric patients,[10] detection of BDV infection in humans has mostly focused on patients with neuropsychiatric disorders including affective disorders and schizophrenia. In addition, investigations were also carried out to detect BDV in patients with AIDS, chronic fatigue syndrome, multiple sclerosis, motor neuron diseases, and brain tumors.[55,69,70,93–99]

Here, we would like to focus on the current status of BDV infection in psychiatric patients and summarize the current knowledge of BDV infection in schizophrenia, affective disorders, and other various disorders separately.

BDV in schizophrenia

Most investigations on the detection of BDV footprints were performed with patients with schizophrenia. Several reports exist showing a correlation of BDV with this disease. An early study screened 71 sera from various psychiatric patients, including some patients with schizophrenia, using IFA. Overall, in a follow up study, 20% of patients were found to have positive sera.[100] IFA and WB showed a higher rate of positive samples from schizophrenic patients as compared to healthy controls.[63] Moreover, using a restrictive criterion of specific recognition of more than one BDV protein, serum positivity was found in 14.4% of patients, whereas none of the sera from controls was considered positive.[63] In one study IFA, WB, ECLIA, and RT-PCR were combined with a PBMC proliferation assay for screening of BDV-reactive human antibodies. None of the 45 psychiatric patients with schizophrenia were positive in all five assays. BDV-reactive antibodies of four patients were directed against the P protein only in western blot.[66] Recently, a study was performed in Poland testing sera of 617 schizophrenic patients and 412 healthy individuals with the ECLIA method.[73] Here, 13 out of 617 (2.1%) and four out of 412 control samples (1%) gave positive reactions.

Various publications have concluded that BDV-RNA was present in the PBMCs of schizophrenic patients.[64,66,67,75,83,101–104] In one report, RT-PCR was performed independently in Europe and in the USA. While seven out of 11 samples were positive in one lab, three samples gave positive reactions in both labs. Nevertheless, after sequence analysis a high similarity to the laboratory strain was found.[64] In contrast, inter- and intrapatient BDV sequence variability was found when analyzing PBMC from schizophrenic patients.[102] In another study, 45% of schizophrenic patients had either BDV antibodies and/or BDV RNA, while no positive reaction was found in control samples.[67]

In this and other studies, no association of BDV infection and age, hospitalization, and family history could be found.[63,64,67,73]

In contrast, several groups have failed to detect BDV-RNA in the PBMCs of schizophrenic patients or

Table 15.1 Detection of BDV markers in patients with schizophrenia

Reference	Number of samples	Source	Prevalence Disease	Prevalence Control	Assay
99	4	Serum	25% (1/4)	–	IFA
62	110	Serum	24.4% (22/90)	20% (4/20)	IFA
	110	Serum	32.2% (29/90)	20% (4/20)	WB
105	6	Brain	0 (0/3)	0% (0/3)	RT-PCR
	48	CSF	0 (0/48)	–	RT-PCR
64	337	Serum	14% (16/114)	1.5% (3/203)	WB
	34	PBMC	64% (7/11)	0% (0/23)	RT-PCR
101	85	PBMC	10% (5/49)	0% (0/36)	RT-PCR
102	3	PBMC	100% (3/3)	–	RT-PCR
65	10	Serum	20% (2/10)	0% (0/10)	WB
	48	PBMC	0% (4/34)	0% (0/14)	RT-PCR
106	249	Serum	2% (2/179)	0% (0/70)	IFA
	249	PBMC	0% (0/179)	0% (0/70)	RT-PCR
	14	PBMC	0% (0/7)	0% (0/7)	RT-PCR
110	27	Brain	53% (9/17)	0% (0/10)	RT-PCR
67	93	PBMC	45% (30/67)	0% (0/26)	RT/PCR WB
104	161	PBMC	4% (3/77)	2% (2/84)	RT-PCR
75	143	PBMC	14% (10/74)	1% (1/69)	RT-PCR
108	39	PBMC	0% (0/39)	–	RT-PCR
34	4	Brain	25% (1/4)	0% (0/2)	RT-PCR
76	217	PBMC	1.8% (1/44)	0.6% (1/173)	RT-PCR
	264	Serum	0% (0/54)	0% (0/210)	WB
109	55	Serum	(3/29)	(6/26)	IFA
	55	PBMC	(4/29)	(7/26)	RT-PCR
66	90	Serum	9% (4/45)	0% (0/45)	WB, IFA ECLIA
73	1029	Serum	2.1% (13/617)	1% (4/412)	ECLIA

in the PBMCs of patients suffering from other psychiatric diseases.[65,105–108] In one report the prevalence of BDV-RNA in psychiatric patients was not significantly different from that in healthy volunteers.[76] Another report revealed that the frequencies of BDV-RNA positivity in a group of healthy controls exceeded that in a group of patients.[109]

In conclusion, in the various test systems and studies (summarized in Table 15.1) used, the evidence remains that either BDV-reactive antibodies or BDV-specific nucleic acid are found more frequently in schizophrenic patients than in normal controls.

BDV virus in affective disorders

The affective-anxiety disorder spectrum includes patients suffering from bipolar affective disorders, recurrent depression, or anxiety disorders. In 1985 the two classical papers by Rott et al and Amsterdam et al were published.[10,90] They examined serum samples from 285 and 265 psychiatric patients with affective disorders and 200 and 105 normal volunteers respectively, using the indirect immunofluorescence focus assay for the presence of Borna virus-specific antibodies. They found 4–4.5% reactive sera in the psychiatric patients, whereas sera from the control group did not show any reaction. In principle, these early findings were confirmed by one study using the same technique and another using western blot analysis.[62,100] By western blotting, serum antibodies were reactive against either the nucleoprotein (38% patient/16% control), the phosphoprotein (12% patient/4% control), or against both viral proteins (7% patient/1% control). Most surprisingly, in the confirmatory immunofluorescence study, 37% of the patient sera showed reaction with BDV.[100]

In a WB analysis study of patients with affective disorders, researchers found six out of 52 patients (12%) to have reactive sera, whereas three out of 203 (1.5%) control sera were reactive against BDV.[64] In addition, they tested five patients by RT-PCR in two different laboratories. Surprisingly, in three out of five samples BDV-specific nucleic acid could be recovered. Nevertheless, the nucleic acid sequence was almost identical to the standard laboratory viral sequence. In contrast, all RT-PCR positive patients were also reactive by WB analysis, arguing against nucleic acid contamination.[64] In a recent work using ECLIA, seven seropositive samples were found out of 158 (4.4%) from patients in Poland, consistent with the percentage found in the early investigations by Rott and Amsterdam.[73] Nevertheless, four out of 412 (1%) sera from healthy volunteers gave a positive reaction in the ECLIA. Using serological techniques, only one report clearly demonstrated a failure to detect BDV-specific antibodies in patients with affective disorders.[106] In this work, in sera from 122 patients and 70 controls only one patient's serum was weakly reactive by IFA, but failed to give a positive signal in WB analysis.

Following the study with schizophrenic patients, Fukuda and colleagues also investigated 45 patients with affective disorders and 45 healthy volunteers using the combination of WB, ELICA, IFA, RT-PCR, and proliferation assay. Here, they were able to identify one patient who showed a PBMC proliferative response against NP and P proteins. In addition, serum of this patient was reactive by IFA, WB analysis, and ECLIA, but only against the NP protein. Unfortunately, the P-specific RT-PCR failed to give a positive result.[66] Since serum reactivity was directed only against the NP protein, one might argue that an NP-specific RT-PCR would be more appropriate in this case. Two reports supported the finding that by using RT-PCR the BDV-specific nucleic acid can be detected in PBMCs of patients with affective disorders.[101,104] Furthermore, the detection of BDV-specific nucleic acid in brains and the detection of BDV antigen in CSF has been reported.[97,110]

As summarized in Table 15.2, except for a few reports, BDV-specific antibodies or viral nucleic acid were found more frequently in patients with affective disorders than in controls.

BDV in psychiatric disorders

The early studies were all performed by IFA, including two reports by Rott and coworkers whose first study tested 894 samples, and their second tested more than 6000 samples. In the first study the rate of seropositivity in the patient group was 0.6%, while none of the sera from the control group showed reactivity.[10] In the second study, 4–7% seropositive samples were detected in patients while less than 1% of the control donors were positive. Interestingly, most positive sera of this control group came from BDV endemic areas. Therefore, it was speculated that the infection might take an unapparent course similar to that occasionally occurring after the natural infection of horses.[56,111] This observation was supported by further reports and could explain negative results in follow up studies.[85,112] Since the seropositive findings had to be interpreted with caution, the findings were supplemented with the detection of what appeared to be BDV or a related agent after co-culture of BDV susceptible cells with CSF from the patients. A small number of discrete foci of immunofluorescent-positive cells could be detected 10–12 days

Table 15.2 Detection of BDV markers in patients with affective disorders

Reference	Number of samples	Source	Prevalence Disease	Control	Assay
90	370	Serum	4.5% (12/265)	0% (0/105)	IFA
10	485	Serum	4% (12/285)	0% (0/200)	IFA
62	255	Serum	7% (9/138)	1% (1/117)	WB
100	27	Serum	37% (10/27)	–	IFA
64	255	Serum	12% (6/52)	1.5% (3/203)	WB
	26	PBMC	60% (3/5)	0% (0/23)	RT-PCR
101	42	PBMC	17% (1/6)	0% (0/36)	RT-PCR
106	179	Serum	1% (1/122)	0% (0/70)	IFA, WB
110	15	Brain	40% (2/5)	0% (0/10)	RT-PCR
104	133	PBMC	4% (2/49)	2% (2/84)	RT-PCR
97	134	CSF	5% (3/65)	0% (0/69)	ELISA
66	90	Serum	2% (1/45)	0% (0/45)	WB
	90	PBMC	2% (1/45)	0% (0/45)	RT-PCR
73	570	Serum	4.4% (7/158)	1% (4/412)	ECLIA

after co-culture. Unfortunately after several passages the positive cells disappeared.[111] Since PCR was not established at this time, they were not able to rescue BDV-specific nucleic acid. Further investigations using IFA showed either no[93,106] or only slight differences in seropositive samples from patients compared with controls (24%/11%).[101]

Using RT-PCR and WB analysis, one study found BDV-specific RNA in PBMCs from psychiatric patients (45%) but not in controls. Seropositivity was 14% in the patient group and 1.5% in controls. One sample showed a positive RT-PCR in two different laboratories and a positive reaction by WB analysis.[64] While other studies supported the finding of BDV-specific nucleic acid by RT-PCR from PBMCs of various psychiatric patients,[83,102] others failed to show this correlation.[65,106] In addition to these reports, a further study was not able to correlate BDV infection with various psychiatric diseases (1.8% patients/1% controls) using the ECLIA method.[73]

As summarized in Table 15.3, BDV antigens or BDV-specific antibodies can be found in patients with various psychiatric diseases. Nevertheless, these reports are outnumbered by papers that report no correlation of BDV with disease. The positive findings can be explained by the fact that disease diagnosis was only partial and that these patients would belong to other groups.[111]

CONCLUSION

Numerous studies report the detection of BDV in psychiatric patients, while various reports fail to replicate this correlation. The interpretation of some of these results is difficult, but in some cases the discrepancies can be explained. The inconsistent detection of BDV-

Table 15.3 Detection of BDV markers in patients with various psychiatric disorders					
Reference	Number of samples	Source	Prevalence Disease	Control	Assay
10	894	Serum	0.6% (4/694)	0% (0/200)	IFA
93	1182	Serum	2% (13/642)	2% (11/540)	IFA
111	>6000	Serum	4–7% (>5000)	≤1% (≤10/1000)	IFA
100	49	Serum	12% (6/49)	–	IFA
68	60	Serum	30% (18/60)	–	WB
	60	PBMC	37% (22/60)	–	RT-PCR
64	335	Serum	14% (18/132)	1.5% (3/203)	WB
	35	PBMC	42% (5/12)	0% (0/23)	RT-PCR
101	91	Serum	24% (13/55)	11% (4/36)	IFA
106	114	Serum	0% (0/44)	0% (0/70)	IFA/WB
	118	PBMC	2% (2/106)	0% (0/12)	RT-PCR
65	28	PBMC	0% (0/24)	0% (0/4)	RT-PCR
83	40	PBMC	37% (10/27)	15% (2/13)	RT-PCR
73	583	Serum	1.8% (3/171)	1% (4/412)	ECLIA

RNA in human blood samples could be due to differences in the initial amount of blood or the sensitivity of the RT-PCR technique used. Clearly, the negative findings do not exclude the possibility that BDV can infect humans. Furthermore, these results may also indicate that both the percentage of BDV-positive patients and the amount of RNA in the blood is very low or that patient selection methods are not identifying the correct population for testing. In serological studies, conflicting results could be due to the use of different methods or reagents. This can be solved in the future since standardized, evaluated test systems should be designed.

Based on review papers summarized in this chapter it would be tempting to speculate that a correlation exists between the presence of BDV or a BDV-like agent and the presence of affective disorders and, to a lesser extent, schizophrenia, while no obvious correlation exists in patients with other psychiatric disorders. Nevertheless, it is absolutely necessary that more studies or multicenter studies are performed using standardized diagnostic assays, which need to be designed, before a definitive correlation can be made.

REFERENCES

1. Ludwig H, Bode L. Borna disease virus: new aspects on infection, disease, diagnosis and epidemiology. *Rev Sci Tech* 2000; **19**: 259–88.
2. Zwick W, Seifried O. Übertragbarkeit der seuchenhaften Gehirn- und Rückenmarksentzündung des Pferdes (Borna'schen Krankheit) auf kleine Versuchstiere (Kaninchen). *Berl Münch Tierärztl Wochenschr* 1924; **41**: 129–32.
3. Rott R, Becht H. Natural and experimental Borna disease in animals. *Curr Top Microbiol Immunol* 1995; **190**: 17–30.
4. Stitz L, Rott R. Borna disease virus (*Bornaviridae*). In: *Encyclopedia of Virology* (Granoff A, Webster RG, eds). Academic Press, 1999: 167–73.
5. Narayan O, Herzog S, Frese K et al. Behavioral disease in rats caused by immunopathological responses to persistent borna virus in the brain. *Science* 1983; **220**: 1401–3.

6. Planz O, Bilzer T, Sobbe M, Stitz L. Lysis of major histocompatibility complex class I-bearing cells in Borna disease virus-induced degenerative encephalopathy. *J Exp Med* 1993; **178**: 163–74.
7. Stitz L, Dietzschold B, Carbone KM. Immunopathogenesis of Borna disease. *Curr Top Microbiol Immunol* 1995; **190**: 75–92.
8. Briese T, Hornig M, Lipkin WI. Borna virus immunopathogenesis in rodents: models for human neurological diseases. *J Neurovirol* 1999; **5**: 604–12.
9. Stitz L, Bilzer T, Planz O. The immunopathogenesis of Borna disease virus infection. *Front Biosci* 2002; **7**: d541–55.
10. Rott R, Herzog S, Fleischer B et al. Detection of serum antibodies to Borna disease virus in patients with psychiatric disorders. *Science* 1985; **228**: 755–6.
11. Pyper JM, Gartner AE. Molecular basis for the differential subcellular localization of the 38- and 39-kilodalton structural proteins of Borna disease virus. *J Virol* 1997; **71**: 5133–9.
12. Kobayashi T, Shoya Y, Koda T et al. Nuclear targeting activity associated with the amino terminal region of the Borna disease virus nucleoprotein. *Virology* 1998; **243**: 188–97.
13. Thiedemann N, Presek P, Rott R, Stitz L. Antigenic relationship and further characterization of two major Borna disease virus-specific proteins. *J Gen Virol* 1992; **73**: 1057–64.
14. Schwemmle M, De B, Shi L et al. Borna disease virus P-protein is phosphorylated by protein kinase Cepsilon and casein kinase II. *J Biol Chem* 1997; **272**: 21818–23.
15. Schwemmle M, Salvatore M, Shi L et al. Interactions of the borna disease virus P, N, and X proteins and their functional implications. *J Biol Chem* 1998; **273**: 9007–12.
16. Malik TH, Kobayashi T, Ghosh M et al. Nuclear localization of the protein from the open reading frame x1 of the Borna disease virus was through interactions with the viral nucleoprotein. *Virology* 1999; **258**: 65–72.
17. Wolff T, Pfleger R, Wehner T et al. A short leucine-rich sequence in the Borna disease virus p10 protein mediates association with the viral phospho- and nucleoproteins. *J Gen Virol* 2000; **81**: 939–47.
18. Kliche S, Briese T, Henschen AH et al. Characterization of a Borna disease virus glycoprotein, gp18. *J Virol* 1994; **68**: 6918–23.
19. Stoyloff R, Strecker A, Bode L et al. The glycosylated matrix protein of Borna disease virus is a tetrameric membrane-bound viral component essential for infection. *Eur J Biochem* 1997; **246**: 252–7.
20. Stoyloff R, Bode L, Borchers K, Ludwig H. Neutralization of Borna disease virus depends upon terminal carbohydrate residues (alpha-D-man, beta-D-GlcNAc) of glycoproteins gp17 and gp94. *Intervirology* 1998; **41**: 135–40.
21. Kraus I, Eickmann M, Kiermayer S et al. Open reading frame III of borna disease virus encodes a nonglycosylated matrix protein. *J Virol* 2001; **75**: 12098–104.
22. Richt JA, Furbringer T, Koch A et al. Processing of the Borna disease virus glycoprotein gp94 by the subtilisin-like endoprotease furin. *J Virol* 1998; **72**: 4528–33.
23. Gonzalez-Dunia D, Cubitt B, de la Torre JC. Mechanism of Borna disease virus entry into cells. *J Virol* 1998; **72**: 783–8.
24. Walker MP, Jordan I, Briese T et al. Expression and characterization of the Borna disease virus polymerase. *J Virol* 2000; **74**: 4425–8.
25. Walker MP, Lipkin WI. Characterization of the nuclear localization signal of the Borna disease virus polymerase. *J Virol* 2002; **76**: 8460–7.
26. Shoya Y, Kobayashi T, Koda T et al. Two proline-rich nuclear localization signals in the amino- and carboxyl-terminal regions of the Borna disease virus phosphoprotein. *J Virol* 1998; **72**: 9755–62.
27. Kobayashi T, Kamitani W, Zhang G et al. Borna disease virus nucleoprotein requires both nuclear localization and export activities for viral nucleocytoplasmic shuttling. *J Virol* 2001; **75**: 3404–12.
28. Malik TH, Kishi M, Lai PK. Characterization of the P protein-binding domain on the 10-kilodalton protein of Borna disease virus. *J Virol* 2000; **74**: 3413–7.
29. Hornig M, Briese T, Lipkin WI. Borna disease virus. *J Neurovirol* 2003; **9**: 259–73.
30. Briese T, Lipkin WI, de la Torre JC. Molecular biology of Borna disease virus. *Curr Top Microbiol Immunol* 1995; **190**: 1–16.
31. Kohno T, Goto T, Takasaki T et al. Fine structure and morphogenesis of borna disease virus. *J Virol* 1999; **73**: 760–6.
32. Weissenbock H, Nowotny N, Caplazi P et al. Borna disease in a dog with lethal meningoencephalitis. *J Clin Microbiol* 1998; **36**: 2127–30.
33. Berg AL. Borna disease in cats. *Vet Rec* 1999; **145**: 87.
34. Nakamura Y, Watanabe M, Kamitani W et al. High prevalence of Borna disease virus in domestic cats with neurological disorders in Japan. *Vet Microbiol* 1999; **70**: 153–69.
35. Helps CR, Turan N, Bilal T et al. Detection of antibodies to Borna disease virus in Turkish cats by using recombinant p40. *Vet Rec* 2001; **149**: 647–50.
36. Ouchi A, Kishi M, Kobayashi T et al. Prevalence of circulating antibodies to p10, a non-structural protein of the Borna disease virus in cats with ataxia. *J Vet Med Sci* 2001; **63**: 1279–85.
37. Dauphin G, Legay V, Sailleau C et al. Evidence of Borna disease virus genome detection in French domestic animals and in foxes (*Vulpes vulpes*). *J Gen Virol* 2001; **82**: 2199–204.
38. Okamoto M, Kagawa Y, Kamitani W et al. Borna disease in a dog in Japan. *J Comp Pathol* 2002; **126**: 312–7.
39. Johansson M, Berg M, Berg AL. Humoral immune response against Borna disease virus (BDV) in experimentally and naturally infected cats. *Vet Immunol Immunopathol* 2002; **90**: 23–33.
40. Hirano N, Kao M, Ludwig H. Persistent, tolerant or subacute infection in Borna disease virus-infected rats. *J Gen Virol* 1983; **64**: 1521–30.
41. Herzog S, Kompter C, Frese K, Rott R. Replication of Borna disease virus in rats: age-dependent differences in tissue distribution. *Med Microbiol Immunol (Berl)* 1984; **173**: 171–7.
42. Herzog S, Wonigeit K, Frese K et al. Effect of Borna disease virus infection on athymic rats. *J Gen Virol* 1985; **66**: 503–8.
43. Carbone KM, Duchala CS, Griffin JW et al. Pathogenesis of Borna disease in rats: evidence that intra-axonal spread is the major route for virus dissemination and the determinant for disease incubation. *J Virol* 1987; **61**: 3431–40.
44. Carbone KM, Duchala CS, Narayan O. Borna disease. An immunopathologic response to viral infection in the CNS. *Ann NY Acad Sci* 1988; **540**: 661–2.
45. Narayan O, Herzog S, Frese K et al. Pathogenesis of Borna disease in rats: immune-mediated viral ophthalmoencephalopathy causing blindness and behavioral abnormalities. *J Infect Dis* 1983; **148**: 305–15.
46. Carbone KM, Trapp BD, Griffin JW et al. Astrocytes and Schwann cells are virus-host cells in the nervous system of rats with Borna disease. *J Neuropathol Exp Neurol* 1989; **48**: 631–44.
47. Morales JA, Herzog S, Kompter C et al. Axonal transport of Borna disease virus along olfactory pathways in spontaneously and experimentally infected rats. *Med Microbiol Immunol (Berl)* 1988; **177**: 51–64.
48. Deschl U, Stitz L, Herzog S et al. Determination of immune cells and expression of major histocompatibility complex class II antigen in encephalitic lesions of experimental Borna disease. *Acta Neuropathol* 1990; **81**: 41–50.

49. Sprankel H, Richarz K, Ludwig H, Rott R. Behavior alterations in tree shrews (*Tupaia glis*, Diard 1820) induced by Borna disease virus. *Med Microbiol Immunol (Berl)* 1978; **165**: 1–18.
50. Stitz L, Krey H, Ludwig H. Borna disease in rhesus monkeys as a models for uveo-cerebral symptoms. *J Med Virol* 1981; **6**: 333–40.
51. Yamaguchi K, Sawada T, Naraki T et al. Detection of Borna disease virus-reactive antibodies from patients with psychiatric disorders and from horses by electrochemiluminescence immunoassay. *Clin Diag Lab Immunol* 1999; **6**: 696–700.
52. Carbone KM, Moench TR, Lipkin WI. Borna disease virus replicates in astrocytes, Schwann cells and ependymal cells in persistently infected rats: location of viral genomic and messenger RNAs by in situ hybridization. *J Neuropathol Exp Neurol* 1991; **50**: 205–14.
53. Briese T, de la Torre JC, Lewis A et al. Borna disease virus, a negative-strand RNA virus, transcribes in the nucleus of infected cells. *Proc Natl Acad Sci USA* 1992; **89**: 11486–9.
54. Cubitt B, Oldstone C, de la Torre JC. Sequence and genome organization of Borna disease virus. *J Virol* 1994; **68**: 1382–96.
55. Bode L, Komaroff AL, Ludwig H. No serologic evidence of Borna disease virus in patients with chronic fatigue syndrome. *Clin Infect Dis* 1992; **15**: 1049.
56. Lange W, Jaeschke G. Influenza epidemic in horses in West Berlin 1983–1985. 2. Virological and serological findings. *Dtsch Tierarztl Wochenschr* 1987; **94**: 157–60.
57. Bechter K, Bauer M, Estler HC et al. Expanded nuclear magnetic resonance studies in Borna disease virus seropositive psychiatric patients and control probands. *Nervenarzt* 1994; **65**: 169–74.
58. Planz O, Bechter KA, Schwemmle M. Human Borna disease virus infection. In: *Borna Disease Virus and its Role in Neuropsychiatric Disease* (Carbone KM, ed). 2002: 179–225.
59. Ganguli R, Brar JS, Solomon W et al. Altered interleukin-2 production in schizophrenia: association between clinical state and autoantibody production. *Psychiatry Res* 1992; **44**: 113–23.
60. Legros S, Mendlewicz J, Wybran J. Immunoglobulins, autoantibodies and other serum protein fractions in psychiatric disorders. *Eur Arch Psychiatry Neurol Sci* 1985; **235**: 9–11.
61. Shinitzky M, Deckmann M, Kessler A et al. Platelet autoantibodies in dementia and schizophrenia. Possible implication for mental disorders. *Ann NY Acad Sci* 1991; **621**: 205–17.
62. Fu ZF, Amsterdam JD, Kao M et al. Detection of Borna disease virus-reactive antibodies from patients with affective disorders by western immunoblot technique. *J Affect Disord* 1993; **27**: 61–8.
63. Waltrip RW, Buchanan RW, Summerfelt A et al. Borna disease virus and schizophrenia. *Psychiatry Res* 1995; **56**: 33–44.
64. Sauder C, Muller A, Cubitt B et al. Detection of Borna disease virus (BDV) antibodies and BDV RNA in psychiatric patients: evidence for high sequence conservation of human blood-derived BDV RNA. *J Virol* 1996; **70**: 7713–24.
65. Richt JA, Alexander RC, Herzog S et al. Failure to detect Borna disease virus infection in peripheral blood leukocytes from humans with psychiatric disorders. *J Neurovirol* 1997; **3**: 174–8.
66. Fukuda K, Takahashi K, Iwata Y et al. Immunological and PCR analyses for Borna disease virus in psychiatric patients and blood donors in Japan. *J Clin Microbiol* 2001; **39**: 419–29.
67. Iwahashi K, Watanabe M, Nakamura K et al. Clinical investigation of the relationship between Borna disease virus (BDV) infection and schizophrenia in 67 patients in Japan. *Acta Psychiatr Scand* 1997; **96**: 412–5.
68. Kishi M, Nakaya T, Nakamura Y et al. Prevalence of Borna disease virus RNA in peripheral blood mononuclear cells from blood donors. *Med Microbiol Immunol* 1995; **184**: 135–8.
69. Auwanit W, Ayutthaya PI, Nakaya T et al. Unusually high seroprevalence of Borna disease virus in clade E human immunodeficiency virus type 1-infected patients with sexually transmitted diseases in Thailand. *Clin Diag Lab Immunol* 1996; **3**: 590–3.
70. Kitani T, Kuratsune H, Fuke I et al. Possible correlation between Borna disease virus infection and Japanese patients with chronic fatigue syndrome. *Microbiol Immunol* 1996; **40**: 459–62.
71. Horimoto T, Takahashi H, Sakaguchi M et al. A reverse-type sandwich enzyme-linked immunosorbent assay for detecting antibodies to Borna disease virus. *J Clin Microbiol* 1997; **35**: 1661–6.
72. Bode L, Reckwald P, Severus WE et al. Borna disease virus-specific circulating immune complexes, antigenemia, and free antibodies – the key marker triplet determining infection and prevailing in severe mood disorders. *Mol Psychiatry* 2001; **6**: 481–91.
73. Rybakowski F, Sawada T, Yamaguchi K et al. Borna disease virus – reactive antibodies in Polish psychiatric patients. *Med Sci Monit* 2002; **8**: 642–6.
74. Takahashi H, Nakaya T, Nakamura Y et al. Higher prevalence of Borna disease virus infection in blood donors living near thoroughbred horse farms. *J Med Virol* 1997; **52**: 330–5.
75. Chen CH, Chiu YL, Shaw CK et al. Detection of Borna disease virus RNA from peripheral blood cells in schizophrenic patients and mental health workers. *Mol Psychiatry* 1999; **4**: 566–71.
76. Tsuji K, Toyomasu K, Imamura Y et al. No association of Borna disease virus with psychiatric disorders among patients in northern Kyushu, Japan. *J Med Virol* 2000; **61**: 336–40.
77. Allmang U, Hofer M, Herzog S et al. Low avidity of human serum antibodies for Borna disease virus antigens questions their diagnostic value. *Mol Psychiatry* 2001; **6**: 329–33.
78. Billich C, Sauder C, Frank R et al. High-avidity human serum antibodies recognizing linear epitopes of Borna disease virus proteins. *Biol Psychiatry* 2002; **51**: 979–87.
79. Bode L, Steinbach F, Ludwig H. A novel marker for Borna disease virus infection. *Lancet* 1994; **343**: 297–8.
80. Gonzalez-Dunia D, Sauder C, de la Torre JC. Borna disease virus and the brain. *Brain Res Bull* 1997; **44**: 647–64.
81. Sierra-Honigmann AM, Rubin SA, Estafanous MG et al. Borna disease virus in peripheral blood mononuclear and bone marrow cells of neonatally and chronically infected rats. *J Neuroimmunol* 1993; **45**: 31–6.
82. Sauder C, de la Torre JC. Sensitivity and reproducibility of RT-PCR to detect Borna disease virus (BDV) RNA in blood: implications for BDV epidemiology. *J Virol Methods* 1998; **71**: 229–45.
83. Vahlenkamp TW, Enbergs HK, Muller H. Experimental and natural Borna disease virus infections: presence of viral RNA in cells of the peripheral blood. *Vet Microbiol* 2000; **76**: 229–44.
84. Furrer E, Bilzer T, Stitz L, Planz O. Neutralizing antibodies in persistent Borna disease virus infection: prophylactic effect of gp94-specific monoclonal antibodies in preventing encephalitis. *J Virol* 2001; **75**: 943–51.
85. Bode L, Durrwald R, Rantam FA et al. First isolates of infectious human Borna disease virus from patients with mood disorders. *Mol Psychiatry* 1996; **1**: 200–12.
86. Nakamura Y. Isolation of Borna disease virus from the autopsy brain of a schizophrenia patient. *Hokkaido Igaku Zasshi* 1998; **73**: 287–97.

87. Schwemmle M, Jehle C, Formella S, Staeheli P. Sequence similarities between human Borna virus isolates and laboratory strains question human origin. *Lancet* 1999; **354**: 1973–4.
88. Planz O, Rziha HJ, Stitz L. Genetic relationship of Borna disease virus isolates. *Virus Genes* 2003; **26**: 25–30.
89. Planz O, Rentzsch C, Batra A et al. Pathogenesis of Borna disease virus: granulocyte fractions of psychiatric patients harbor infectious virus in the absence of antiviral antibodies. *J Virol* 1999; **73**: 6251–6.
90. Amsterdam JD, Winokur A, Dyson W et al. Borna disease virus. A possible etiologic factor in human affective disorders? *Arch Gen Psychiatry* 1985; **42**: 1093–6.
91. Bechter K, Herzog S, Schuttler R, Rott R. MRI in psychiatric patients with serum antibodies against Borna disease virus. *Psychiatry Res* 1989; **29**: 281–2.
92. Bode L, Riegel S, Lange W, Ludwig H. Human infections with Borna disease virus: seroprevalence in patients with chronic diseases and healthy individuals. *J Med Virol* 1992; **36**: 309–15.
93. Bode L, Riegel S, Ludwig H et al. Borna disease virus-specific antibodies in patients with HIV infection and with mental disorders. *Lancet* 1988; **2**: 689.
94. Kitze B, Herzog S, Rieckmann P et al. No evidence of Borna disease virus-specific antibodies in multiple sclerosis patients in Germany. *J Neurol* 1996; **243**: 660–2.
95. Nakaya T, Takahashi H, Nakamura Y et al. Demonstration of Borna disease virus RNA in peripheral blood mononuclear cells derived from Japanese patients with chronic fatigue syndrome. *FEBS Lett* 1996; **378**: 145–9.
96. de la Torre JC, Gonzalez-Dunia D, Cubitt B et al. Detection of Borna disease virus antigen and RNA in human autopsy brain samples from neuropsychiatric patients. *Virology* 1996; **223**: 272–82.
97. Deuschle M, Bode L, Heuser I et al. Borna disease virus proteins in cerebrospinal fluid of patients with recurrent depression and multiple sclerosis. *Lancet* 1998; **352**: 1828–9.
98. Evengard B, Briese T, Lindh G et al. Absence of evidence of Borna disease virus infection in Swedish patients with chronic fatigue syndrome. *J Neurovirol* 1999; **5**: 495–9.
99. Bachmann S, Caplazi P, Fischer M et al. Lack of association between Borna disease virus infection and neurological disorders among HIV-infected individuals. *J Neurovirol* 1999; **5**: 190–5.
100. Bode L, Ferszt R, Czech G. Borna disease virus infection and affective disorders in man. *Arch Virol Suppl* 1993; **7**: 159–67.
101. Igata-Yi R, Yamaguchi K, Yoshiki K et al. Borna disease virus and the consumption of raw horse meat. *Nat Med* 1996; **2**: 948–9.
102. Kishi M, Arimura Y, Ikuta K et al. Sequence variability of Borna disease virus open reading frame II found in human peripheral blood mononuclear cells. *J Virol* 1996; **70**: 635–40.
103. Iwahashi K, Watanabe M, Nakamura K et al. Borna disease virus infection and schizophrenia: seroprevalence in schizophrenia patients. *Can J Psychiatry* 1998; **43**: 197.
104. Iwata Y, Takahashi K, Peng X et al. Detection and sequence analysis of borna disease virus p24 RNA from peripheral blood mononuclear cells of patients with mood disorders or schizophrenia and of blood donors. *J Virol* 1998; **72**: 10044–9.
105. Sierra-Honigmann AM, Carbone KM, Yolken RH. Polymerase chain reaction (PCR) search for viral nucleic acid sequences in schizophrenia. *Br J Psychiatry* 1995; **166**: 55–60.
106. Kubo K, Fujiyoshi T, Yokoyama MM et al. Lack of association of Borna disease virus and human T-cell leukemia virus type 1 infections with psychiatric disorders among Japanese patients. *Clin Diag Lab Immunol* 1997; **4**: 189–94.
107. Lieb K, Hallensleben W, Czygan M et al. No Borna disease virus-specific RNA detected in blood from psychiatric patients in different regions of Germany. The Bornavirus Study Group [letter]. *Lancet* 1997; **350**: 1002.
108. Kim YK, Kim SH, Choi SH et al. Failure to demonstrate Borna disease virus genome in peripheral blood mononuclear cells from psychiatric patients in Korea. *J Neurovirol* 1999; **5**: 196–9.
109. Selten JP, van Vliet K, Pleyte W et al. Borna disease virus and schizophrenia in Surinamese immigrants to the Netherlands. *Med Microbiol Immunol* 2000; **189**: 55–7.
110. Salvatore M, Morzunov S, Schwemmle M, Lipkin WI. Borna disease virus in brains of North American and European people with schizophrenia and bipolar disorder. Bornavirus Study Group. *Lancet* 1997; **349**: 1813–4.
111. Rott R, Herzog S, Bechter K, Frese K. Borna disease, a possible hazard for man? *Arch Virol* 1991; **118**: 143–9.
112. Bode L, Ludwig H. Clinical similarities and close genetic relationship of human and animal Borna disease virus. *Arch Virol Suppl* 1997; **13**: 167–82.

16

Infectious trigger in obsessive compulsive and tic disorders

Tanya K Murphy, Deborah M Herbstman, and Paula J Edge

INTRODUCTION

Two neuropsychiatric illnesses that have prompted research over the last decade into possible infectious triggers are obsessive compulsive disorder (OCD) and Tourette syndrome (TS). With a lifetime prevalence of 2–3%, OCD is an anxiety disorder characterized by recurrent, unwanted, and distressing thoughts, images, or impulses (obsessions) and/or complex, repetitive, rule-governed behaviors that the patient feels driven to perform (compulsions). Childhood-onset OCD accounts for approximately half of all OCD patients,[1] and is associated with a high rate of comorbid tic disorders, along with disruptive and developmental disorders. Higher familial risk and poorer treatment response are also frequently associated with childhood-onset OCD. Tourette syndrome is a chronic neuropsychiatric disorder characterized by multiple motor and phonic tics that wax and wane in both type and severity, and by an array of behavioral problems including symptoms of attention deficit hyperactivity disorder (ADHD) and OCD. The clinical manifestations of TS include movements such as shoulder shrugging, head turning, eye-blinking, and uncontrolled vocalizations of both a simple and complex nature.[2] The prevalence of tics can be as high as 18.5% in school age children and 23.4% in classrooms for children with learning disabilities.[3]

The age of onset for OCD is typically 10 years old, although a younger OCD onset age was found in children with both OCD and tics.[4] In a study that documented the course of tic severity over two decades, onset was followed by an initial progressive pattern of tic worsening with many remitting by their late teens. The most severe period of tic worsening occurred at 10 years of age.[2] The course of OCD/tic symptoms in children varies considerably. A child with only OCD or only tics may develop additional symptoms months or years later. Although OCD is often chronic and disabling, in some cases OCD has an episodic course.[5] Unlike OCD, DSM-IV includes a specific diagnosis of transient tic disorder, recognizing that many tic patients are likely to meet the criteria for this diagnostic classification early in the course of the illness and subsequently remit entirely or develop a more chronic, waxing and waning course.

OCD and TS are currently viewed as types of developmental brain dysfunction, resulting in an imbalance between voluntary and involuntary activation and inhibition with specific influences in cortico-striato-thalamocortical (CSTC) loops.[6] Neurochemical studies suggest an abnormal metabolism of the neurotransmitters dopamine and serotonin may be involved in both disorders.[7–9]

PEDIATRIC AUTOIMMUNE NEUROPSYCHIATRIC DISORDERS ASSOCIATED WITH STREPTOCOCCUS (PANDAS)

The modern story of PANDAS began in 1987 with the unexpected resurgence of rheumatic fever (RF) in geographically diverse parts of the United States.[10] Prior to these cases, the disease seemed virtually eradicated when the rate of RF fell dramatically in the 40 years following World War II. In several respects, these recent outbreaks were unlike previous ones.[11] In contrast to earlier reports, these RF cases were generally associated with a greater proportion of individuals who developed Sydenham chorea (SC), a major manifestation of RF that is thought to occur when antibodies directed against group A streptococcus (GAS) cross-react with epitopes on neurons of the basal ganglia (and other brain areas) causing motoric and behavioral disturbances.[12-15]

Around the time of the RF resurgence, Susan Swedo, a National Institutes of Mental Health (NIMH) researcher, and colleagues Leonard, Garvey, and Kiessling, among others, became interested in the relationship between SC and OCD, noting a high prevalence of OC symptoms in patients with SC.[16] This interest was prompted by several considerations, among them:[17]

1) Evidence that basal ganglia dysfunction was involved in both conditions
2) Historical accounts of patients with SC having increased obsessionality and emotional lability.[18]

Swedo and colleagues then conducted several systematic investigations into the neuropsychiatric aspects of SC.[16,19] In one study, OC symptoms were assessed and compared in two age- and sex-matched groups of patients with RF: one with SC and another without SC.[16] The group with SC had significantly more OC symptoms. Subsequent studies have shown that over 70% of patients with SC exhibit OC symptoms that resemble classic cases of OCD.[17,20] Although patients that have SC appear to have the greatest risk for developing OCD, those with RF without chorea also have increased risk for developing OCD over expected prevalence.[21] Other psychiatric symptoms frequently reported in patients with SC were separation anxiety, hyperactivity, inattention, and emotional lability.[19] This work then led Swedo and colleagues to coin the term PANDAS (pediatric autoimmune neuropsychiatric disorders associated with streptococcus) to describe cases of childhood-onset OCD whose onset/exacerbations appear to be linked to GAS. While PANDAS was named in 1997, 68 years earlier a phenotype similar to PANDAS was reported by Selling.[22] He described three cases where he attributed tic symptoms to a concurrent sinusitis.

Confusion has long existed on distinguishing Tourette syndrome from Sydenham chorea. While classification by symptom became the prevailing maxim by the late 19th century, a continuing debate has persisted among neurologists and psychiatrists who believed that classification boundaries should be set by common underlying causes.[23] The noted French physician, Jean Itard, insisted that pathological evidence pointed to 'the white part of the striate cortices' (the basal ganglia) and rheumatic fever as being underlying causes of movement disorders. Many distinguished English and French physicians such as Richard Bright and CMS Sandras held to the view that movement disorders with the same underlying pathology were probably variations of the same disorder. Taranta and Stollerman first established the role of GAS in 1956 when they demonstrated the connection between prior throat infection and later sequelae of a movement disorder. The debate continues today, but recent clinical findings increasingly lend support to the role of infections in tic and OCD symptom development.[23]

PHENOTYPE CHARACTERISTICS

The current diagnostic criteria for PANDAS are:

1) The presence of obsessive compulsive disorder and/or a tic disorder
2) Pediatric onset of symptoms (age three years to puberty)
3) Episodic or sawtooth course of symptom severity
4) An association with group A streptococcal infection (a positive throat culture for strep or history of scarlet fever)
5) An association with neurological abnormalities (motoric hyperactivity or adventitious movements, such as choreiform movements).

Swedo and colleagues reported on 50 PANDAS cases;[24] many had an acute and dramatic onset that was frequently associated with preceding streptococcal pharyngitis (44%). When followed prospectively, 31% of the 144 observed neuropsychiatric exacerbations were associated with documented GAS infection, and only 33 episodes (22.9%) had no evidence of infectious trigger including viral illness, suspected GAS infection, or exposure to GAS. In addition to a diagnosis of OCD and/or TS, these children were frequently observed to have symptoms of separation anxiety, nightmares, personality change, oppositional behaviors, and deterioration in math skills and handwriting.

Another PANDAS characteristic is average age of onset at age seven,[24] which parallels that of TS, but is earlier than that of childhood OCD (at 10 years). Gender may also influence symptom presentation, with boys more likely to present with tics and girls more likely to present with chorea-like movements. Whether the course of PANDAS remits or progresses to a more chronic illness is not yet known; however, the symptom course characteristic of PANDAS may be typical of OCD and tics early in the illness. Table 16.1 illustrates the similarities and differences among OCD, tics, SC, and PANDAS.

Table 16.1 Comparison of OCD, tics, PANDAS, and SC				
Variable	OCD	TS/Tic disorders	SC	PANDAS
Typical age of onset	10 years	7 years	5–15 years	7 years
Gender relatedness	Under age 15, males slightly higher, female:male ratio increases post-puberty	2:1 male to female ratio	1.7:1 female to male	Nearly 5:1 male:female ratio under age 8; thereafter, males slightly outnumber females
Course	Typically unremitting, though some episodic cases reported	Peak severity age 10, 50% of cases remit by late teens	Typically remits in 2 years	Episodic or sawtooth course, long-term prognosis unknown
Involvement of basal ganglia	Strong support	Strong support	Strong support	Good support
GAS trigger	Reported, causation uncertain	Reported in some cases, causation uncertain	Clear evidence	Proposed association
Neurological findings	Increased findings of NSS, including 'choreiform' movements	Increased findings of NSS, including 'choreiform' movements	Frank chorea	'Choreiform' movements

OCD, obsessive compulsive disorder; TS, Tourette syndrome; SC, Sydenham chorea; PANDAS, pediatric autoimmune neuropsychiatric disorders associated with streptococcus; GAS, group A streptococcus; NSS, neurological soft signs.

GAS PATHOGENESIS

Strong support exists for GAS as the inciting agent in the development of rheumatic fever (RF) and its neuropsychiatric expression, Sydenham chorea (SC).[12] PANDAS could be considered as a broadening of SC, or this subtype of OCD/TS may yet have a unique pathophysiology distinct from SC.[25] A possible prototype for examining PANDAS is based on post-streptococcal reactive arthritis (PSRA).[26,27] PSRA has similarities to the arthritis seen in RF but the criteria for RF are not met; notably, there are few reports of carditis and no CNS involvement. Pathophysiologically, PSRA may differ from RF in that PSRA has been associated with non-group A streptococcus and may have serotypes of GAS different from those associated with RF.

The CNS manifestations characteristic of SC are thought to be related to production of antibodies to streptococcal antigens associated with the M protein of streptococcus that cross-react with epitopes on neuronal tissue.[13,14] Remarkable homology among various epitopes of the streptococcal M protein and tissue molecules (such as tropomyosin) suggests a humoral-mediated mechanism of autoimmunity in the pathogenesis of RF. Studies have found increased antineuronal antibody binding to basal ganglia tissue in SC patients that correlate with symptom severity.[14,28] New research supports antibody-mediated neuronal cell signaling in the pathogenesis of SC.[29] The exact mechanism whereby autoantibodies gain access across the blood brain barrier is not known. Cross-reactive B cells, possibly to a CNS epitope, could lead to intrathecal productivity of antibody.[30]

The role of bacterial superantigens in the pathogenesis of autoimmune disorders has received increased attention. Recently, Kotb and colleagues have begun to study streptococcal superantigens and their role in rheumatic fever.[31,32] Superantigens (SAgs) are molecules that exert a dramatic immunostimulatory response by interacting with the class II MHC and the variable region of the beta chain (V_β) of the T cell receptor (TCR). This interaction bypasses the typical immune response and causes an oligoclonal expansion of one or more V_β components. This activation leads to a prodigious production of cytokines,[33] which is thought to be at least partly responsible for the associated toxicity of SAgs. Some elements thought to have superantigenic activity include the streptococcal pyrotoxins (SPE A, B, and C) as well as components of the cell, particularly the M protein.[34–36] In the last few years, many discoveries have been made regarding GAS genetics and virulence factors. Some of these suspected virulence factors were not present in earlier strains of GAS.[37] Some of these proteins, such as streptococcal phospholipase (Sla), share homology with the C subunit of textilotoxin, a neurotoxin from the Australian common brown snake.[38,39] Although many superantigens (aka exotoxins) have been recently discovered, their exact role in GAS virulence is not well understood. Clinical evidence that GAS may be changing is reflected in changes in the clinical manifestations of illnesses caused by GAS. Scarlet fever and necrotizing fasciitis have increased dramatically in incidence.[40,41] In the outbreaks of RF in the mid-1980s, a higher representation of certain serotypes and mucoid strains of GAS was noted,[42] and a large proportion (75% in one study) of individuals had only mild or no history of prior pharyngitis.[43]

STREPTOCOCCAL ANTIBODIES

Many associations of GAS with OCD and/or tic disorders have been described.[24,44–51] See Table 16.2 for details. Observations have been made that attributed tics and/or OCD onset/exacerbation to recent strep or respiratory infection or to categorically elevated GAS titers. For example, in a retrospective survey of 80 children (5–17 years of age) diagnosed with a tic disorder, 53% of patients described acute and severe onset or worsening of their tic symptoms. Of those, 21% reported their abrupt changes occurred within six weeks of a preceding streptococcal infection.[45] A study examining children for first evaluation of tic disorders found a significant increase in antistreptolysin O (ASO) titer elevations with 38% of 150 children with tics having ASO>500 IU/ml compared with 2% of healthy controls ($n = 150$).[52] A pediatric group examined all children who presented with a sudden onset of a neuropsychiatric problem (such as OCD, a tic disorder, or late age-onset ADHD), for group A streptococcus and found 12 over a three-year period, all with OC symptoms. They reported that these children also had high prevalence of urinary frequency, and two children had high anti-deoxyribonuclease B (DNAB) titers. They found that the neuropsychiatric symptoms rapidly remitted with antibiotic therapy.[48]

After streptococcal infections, titers may remain elevated for six months to a year. Those with a dramatically fluctuating neuropsychiatric symptom course had more evidence of persistent elevations in one or more strep titers compared to those that had a course inconsistent with PANDAS.[53] This finding may be due to the relative proximity of the streptococcal infection and repeated streptococcal exposures leading to more severe and turbulent symptoms.

Persistent immune activation to GAS is a possibility and may be a consequence of multiple factors including developmental and/or environmental influences. Young age at time of streptococcal infection may alter future immune responses to group A streptococcus. An innate response to GAS antigens leading to higher than typical antibody levels may also be possible. Additionally, exclusive association to GAS is provisional because other types of infection are believed to trigger neuropsychiatric symptoms (see Table 16.3) consistent with OCD/TS.[54,55]

SEASONALITY

Observations that tic symptoms are increased in fall and winter months correlate with peak streptococcal pharyngitis rates.[53,84] RF incidence peaks from January to March, with lower rates reported in the summer months.[85] Seasonal variation in GAS and tic symptoms reflects increased exposure rates during school winter months. Seasonal variation of infections

Table 16.2 Evidence of immune basis in OCD and tic disorders

Reference	Sample characteristics	Findings/conclusions
22	Case report of two 14-year-old males and one 11-year-old male	Tic disorders with evidence of sinus infection. Radical removal of the foci resulted in remitted tics. Suggested tics are due to infectious origin, particularly of sinuses.
56	Case study of 11-year-old male	Developed severe tics after illness with high fever. Treated with corticosteroid therapy and tics resolved.
46	Case study of 14-year-old female	Following pharyngitis, pre-existing motor tics were exacerbated by the onset of chorea. All movements improved after 8 months' antibiotic prophylaxis.
57	IF staining of antibody to caudate in 38 pediatric cases without tics, 19 with OCS and ADHD, 19 with ADHD without OCS	The sera from OCS cases showed antibodies directed against caudate at a rate significantly higher than that of clinical controls.
44	IF staining of antibody to caudate in one group of 50 children referred for evaluation of ADHD, behavior disorders, and learning disabilities (24 with an associated movement disorder) Replicated in 33 children (21 with an associated movement disorder)	In both samples, those with movement disorders were significantly more likely to have evidence of ANeA and to have at least one antistreptococcal titer elevated than were those without movement disorders. 44% were strongly positive for ANeA.
54	Case study of four males aged 10–14 years	Infection-triggered OCD and tics treated with plasmapheresis ($n = 2$), IVIG ($n = 1$), and immunosuppressive doses of prednisone ($n = 1$). All subjects had a clinically significant response immediately after treatment.
58	Case study of 12-year-old male with severe OCD	BG volumes correlated with severity of OCD symptoms and decreased following plasmapheresis with corresponding improvement in OCD.
47	Case study of 12-year-old female	Treatment resistant OCD and chronic tics associated with strep infection treated multimodally. Significant improvement after plasmapheresis and prophylactic antibiotics.
59	Two males with TS/OCD aged two and nine	IgA deficiency found in 10% of authors' patients with OCD/tics, recommend better understanding of immune status before initiating immune therapies.

Table 16.2 Continued

Reference	Sample characteristics	Findings/conclusions
60	CSF cytokine in 24 OCD children, 22 schizophrenic children, and 42 ADHD children	OCD preponderance of type 1 cytokines, schizophrenia preponderance of type 2 cytokines.
61	31 patients with childhood-onset OCD and/or tics and 21 HC; GAS, ANeA, and D8/17 levels measured	Study done in summer: no difference in GAS titer levels, trend towards increased ANeA binding.
62	Case study of 10-year-old male with infection-triggered severe OCD and chronic tics	Improvement of OCD/tics after antibiotic treatment. Argued for need of treatment guidelines in PANDAS cases.
51	Five-year-old female with sudden and dramatic onset of tics and OCD following a GAS throat infection	Subject improved after treatment with IVIG followed by antibiotic prophylaxis.
24	50 children who met PANDAS criteria; systematic clinical evaluation	111 of 144 symptom exacerbations suggested GAS infection as trigger.
63	Double-blind, cross-over penicillin prophylaxis in 37 PANDAS children	Equal number of infections seen in both active and placebo phases. No significant change seen in OC or tic symptom severity between the two phases.
64	29 children with severe infection-triggered exacerbations of OCD or tic; 10 received plasma exchange, nine received IVIG, and 10 got placebo	Plasma exchange and IVIG were both effective in lessening symptom severity for children with infection-triggered OCD and tic disorders.
65	ANeA study in 41 TS children and 39 control subjects	Children with TS have a higher median but not mean levels of ANeA. Assay failed to identify a relationship between antibodies and clinical phenotype or one-time markers for streptococcal infection
66	19 streptococcal-triggered OCD and/or tic children and 19 age/gender matched HC; assessment of neuromotor functioning	Motor performance was significantly slower during exacerbations of streptococcal triggered OCD and/or tics and these motor skills improved when the neuropsychiatric symptoms were in remission.
67	Volumetric MRIs in 34 children with PANDAS and 82 HC children	BG volumes were higher in PANDAS than in healthy children.

Table 16.2 Continued

Reference	Sample characteristics	Findings/conclusions
68	Animal study of five subject rats and five control rats; subject rats infused with sera from TS children; control rats received sera from HC children	Immunohistochemical analysis confirmed presence of IgG selectively bound to striatal neurons.
69	Proband = 54 children with PANDAS and 157 first degree relatives interviewed	Rates of tic disorders and OCD in first-degree relatives of pediatric probands with PANDAS are higher than those reported in the general population.
50	Streptococcal titers studied in 13 TS and 13 HC children, 23 TS and 23 HC adults, and 17 schizophrenics	TS patients exhibited higher antistreptococcal titers than age-matched comparison groups of both children and adults.
70	105 subjects aged seven to 55 years old with diagnosis of CTD, OCD, or ADHD, and 37 HC; antistreptococcal antibody titers and BG volumes measured	ADHD was associated significantly with streptococcal titers. No significant association found between antibody titers and CTD or OCD. BG volumes were significantly different in OCD and ADHD subjects compared to other groups.
45	Assessment of onset characteristics in 80 TS children aged five to 17 years	42 subjects had sudden, explosive onset or worsening of tic symptoms; nine subjects had sudden, explosive onset or worsening of tic symptoms specifically associated with a streptococcal infection.
71	25-year-old adult male with onset of OCD after severe antibiotic responsive pharyngitis	In all aspects except age, patient fulfilled established criteria for PANDAS. Poststreptococcal disease may result in adult onset OCD.
52	300 children (150 with tics and 150 without tics) with ASO titers compared	ASO titers were significantly higher compared to control subjects. Relationship exists between severity of tic disorder and magnitude of serologic response to GAS antigen.
72	Autoantibody assessment of 103 female, 124 male children and adults aged 8–85 years; TS = 81, SC = 27, autoimmune illness = 52, and HC = 67	TS patients had significantly higher mean rank of total ANeA, ANA; strep titers were higher in adults than HC.

Table 16.2 Continued

Reference	Sample characteristics	Findings/conclusions
73	Antibodies against M proteins studied in 25 TS adults and 25 HC	Increased titers of antibodies against the streptococcal M12 and M19 proteins (RF associated serotypes) in TS patients compared with HC.
74	Onset and exacerbations strep-triggered OCD in 12-year-old female and tics in eight-year-old male sibling	Tonsillectomy performed with significant symptom improvement.
75	Serum antibodies assayed in 20 TS children and 21 control subjects	Data demonstrate significant differences between the autoantibody patterns in normal serum and serum from TS patients against striatal antigens.
49	Onset assessment in 83 children aged six to 17 years with primary diagnosis of OCD and primary caregivers	In URI present versus URI absent group, more patients experienced a sudden rather than insidious onset of symptoms; those associated with sudden onset exhibited a comorbid tic disorder. Specific inquiry about OCD onset around time of URI should clue clinician to look prospectively for PANDAS.
76	20-year-old female with adult onset of tics and OC; case study following sore throat	Tics had abdominal muscle involvement. Except for age of onset, subject met all criteria for PANDAS.
77	36 rats infused with sera from 12 TS patients with high levels of autoantibodies, 12 TS patients with low levels of autoantibodies, and 12 healthy controls	Oral stereotypies significantly increased in rats infused with sera from patients with high levels of autoantibodies. The results are consistent with an autoimmune etiology in a subset of cases of TS.
78	41 TS children and 38 controls; ANeA, ANA antistreptococcal antibodies measured	Inconclusive: suggest that longitudinal measurements should be evaluated before definitive conclusions are drawn on associations between TS, ADHD, or OCD and ANeA, ANA streptococcal titers.

OBSESSIVE COMPULSIVE AND TIC DISORDERS 143

Table 16.2 Continued

Reference	Sample characteristics	Findings/conclusions
79	100 patients with TS; 50 children with neurological disease, 40 recent uncomplicated streptococcal infection, 50 adults with neurological disease, and 50 HC adults; ASO ANeA were detected using WB and indirect IF	ASO was raised in 64% of children with TS, 15% of pediatric neurological disease controls, 68% of adults with TS, 12% of adult neurological controls, and 8% of adult HC. WB showed positive binding in 20% of children and 27% of adults with TS, compared with 2–4% of control groups. The most common BG binding was to a 60 kDa antigen.
53	25 OCD and/or tic disorder children (12 female, 13 male) evaluated for symptom severity and GAS antibody titers at six-week intervals for up to two years	In subjects with large symptom changes, positive correlations were found between ACHO and OCD severity rating changes. Patients with marked OCD/tic symptom changes may be characterized by prolonged GAS

OCS, obsessive compulsive symptoms; ADHD, attention deficit hyperactivity disorder; AneA, antineuronal antibody; OCD, obsessive compulsive disorder; TS, Tourette syndrome; CTD, chronic tic disorder; IVIG, intravenous immunoglobulin; BG, basal ganglia; IgA, immunoglobulin A; CSF, cerebral spinal fluid; GAS, group A streptococcus; HC, healthy controls; PANDAS, pediatric autoimmune neuropsychiatric disorders associated with streptococcus; IgG, immunoglobulin G; ASO, anti-streptolysin O; ANA, antinuclear antibody; RF, rheumatic fever; URI, upper respiratory infection; IF, immunofluorescence; WB, western blot; ACHO, anti-carbohydrate A.

Table 16.3 Thinking outside the boundaries of PANDAS		
Possible immune/infectious triggers	Other possible neuropsychiatric manifestations	Onset/course/age
Mycoplasma pneumonia[50]	Trichotillomania	Insidious onset
Coxsackie	Mania[80]	Adult onset[71]
Influenza[54]	Psychosis[81]	Chronic course
Non-GAS	Depression[82]	
Immunizations	Learning disabilities	
Allergies	ADHD[24,70]	
	Separation anxiety disorder[24]	
	Autistic symptoms	
	Anorexia nervosa[83]	

GAS, group A streptococcus; ADHD, attention deficit hyperactivity disorder.

and neuropsychiatric exacerbations may also be due to cycles of host susceptibility due to alterations in melatonin levels or immune function.[86]

VULNERABILITY

Many factors come into play that may make a child more likely to develop immune sequelae to GAS including maternal immunity, age of infection, recurrent infections, genetic susceptibility, and pathogen-specific attributes. Maternal immunity may have unknown influence on disease development. One possibility is that maternal antibodies to GAS are cross-reactive to fetal CNS tissue, leading to subtle alterations in brain development.[87,88] Another mechanism could be that presence or absence of maternal antibodies may influence future immune defense against microbes.[89] Age at first streptococcal infection may play an important role in susceptibility to developing neuropsychiatric sequelae due to atypical clinical presentation leading to misdiagnosis, or an immature immune system.

Streptococcal pharyngitis may be more likely to be missed in clinical assessment of very young patients. In a study of children age 24–36 months presenting to an emergency department, one third of children with pharyngeal erythema had positive throat cultures for GAS.[90] Strep pharyngitis in preschool children presents with less evidence of tonsillar exudates and cervical adenopathy and more evidence of gastroenteritis than that seen in school age children.[91] Although development of RF is rare in children under five,[92] the impact of early GAS infections on future immune response to GAS and neuropsychiatric vulnerability is unknown.

Frequent GAS infections may also predispose to sequelae. Reasons for GAS recurrence are likely to be complex and numerous. Most of the recurrences are relapses, in other words infection by the same streptococcal type as opposed to new infections of a different type. Possible causes could include poor compliance or inadequate duration of antibiotic therapy, poor antibiotic penetration into tonsillar tissue, inactivation of antibiotic due to beta-lactamase-producing bacteria, lack of protective oral flora, or immunological defects.[93] The consequences of recurrent tonsillopharyngitis are largely unknown. Several of our OCD/tic patients report onset of their neuropsychiatric symptoms after repeated streptococcal infections over the course of a few months (unpublished data). One study of 12 patients found that the number of prior GAS infections correlated with a more severe course and a greater incidence of relapse.[48]

Many children with OCD/TS have a history of tonsillectomy at an early age.[53] Many children undergo tonsillectomy and adenoidectomy secondary to sleep apnea from adenoid hypertrophy or recurrent pharyngeal GAS infections. Although symptomatic GAS infections have been shown to decrease after tonsillectomy,[94] the role of non-carrier state subclinical infections has not been documented. Recent research has shown that children with hypertrophy of adenoids and tonsils exhibit both local and general changes in immunological parameters.[95,96] Both humoral and cellular parameters significantly decreased postoperatively, but at six months postoperative examination these parameters had normalized.[96] The impact of tonsillectomy and adenoidectomy on the development of autoimmune sequelae has not been studied.

Genetics probably play an important role in understanding an individual's vulnerability to infection-triggered neuropsychiatric disorders. Since Sydenham chorea is a model for understanding PANDAS, looking at the genetics of SC may give insights into hereditary susceptibility to PANDAS. For more than 100 years, it has been suspected that individuals who contract RF are so predisposed.[97] The observation that rheumatic fever is more prevalent among relatives than unrelated controls supports the hypothesis that susceptibility to RF is, in part, genetically determined.[98,99] Specifically, an individual's human leukocyte antigen class II haplotypes (HLA) are hypothesized to impact the type and severity of illness developed when exposed to streptococcal infections.[100] However, studies using modern molecular techniques to locate the specific genes involved in RF have not yet been done.

The genetics of OCD and TS have been studied more extensively than RF, and while there is clear evidence to support a hereditary predisposition,[101–105] more needs to be done to understand further the genetic vulnerability involved in these illnesses. Positive findings about the genetic risk factors for OCD and tics lend support to a genetic component in PANDAS; more studies are needed to examine the specific genes that may contribute to PANDAS. To date, there has been only one report looking specifically at the family histories of PANDAS patients.[69] The first-degree relatives of 54 PANDAS probands were evaluated for tics, OCD, subclinical OCD, and other DMS-IV Axis I disorders. It was shown that the rates of OCD and tic disorders in first-degree relatives of PANDAS patients mirrored those previously reported in probands with childhood onset OCD and TS. Other psychiatric disorders that are commonly comorbid with all cases of OCD and TS, including ADHD, major depressive disorder, and phobias, were observed in a number of the family members of PANDAS patients. A child's risk of developing PANDAS is probably due to his/her genetic predisposition and pathogen/environmental factors. Figure 16.1 illustrates these risk factors.

AUTOANTIBODIES AND IMMUNE PARAMETERS

When it was hypothesized that children with OCD or tics may share pathophysiology with SC, researchers began searching for antineuronal antibodies in these patients. The finding of increased antineuronal antibodies to caudate in patients with Tourette syndrome[44] parallels findings of increased antineuronal antibodies in patients with Sydenham chorea.[14,28]

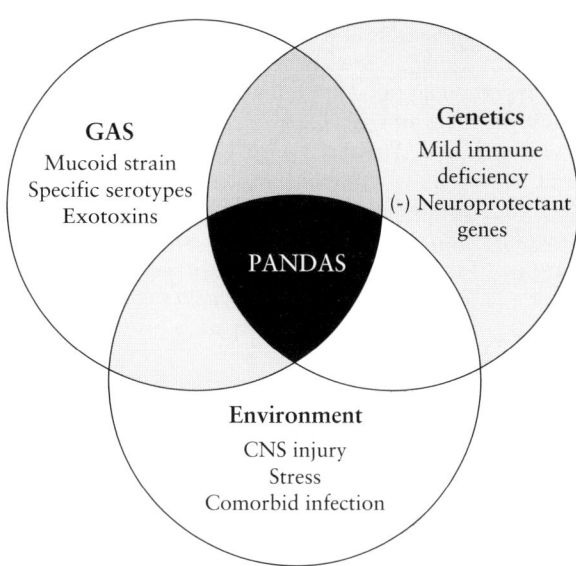

Figure 16.1 PANDAS vulnerability.

Evidence of antineuronal antibodies in patients with tic disorders implies a humorally-mediated mechanism of CNS pathology,[44,106] but the specificity to the disease process has yet to be determined. Some studies in OCD or TS (see Table 16.2) show antibody binding in the control groups that suggests lack of test sensitivity, or possibly controls with benign autoimmunity.[57,61,106]

Measurement of peripheral cytokine profiles, lymphocyte subsets, and antibodies to viruses and self-proteins have been the primary focus of efforts made to study alterations in immune indices in adults with OCD,[107–110] following in the steps of studies that support the role of cell-mediated mechanisms in the pathogenesis of RF.[34,111] Some studies found evidence of an altered or imbalanced immune function in adult OCD patients,[60,108] while others failed to find humoral evidence of autoimmunity[107,110] or cytokine alterations.[107,112,113] However, a chart review study concluded that adult OCD patients appeared to have an increased rate of immune-related diseases beyond that seen in other psychiatric disorders.[114] These studies highlight the need for further exploration of the role immune processes play in the development and maintenance of OCD and/or tic symptoms, as previous study sample sizes have often been small and the degree to which hypothalamo-pituitary-axis alterations (due to stress vs. autoimmunity) have affected results has yet to be resolved.

The search for markers of central nervous system (CNS) injury in neurological illnesses has led to findings of increased levels of CNS proteins, S100, and enolase in cerebral spinal fluid and/or serum.[115,116] Identification of an immune marker in OCD/TS could aid in subtyping phenotypes into those best suited for immune therapies. A study examining peripheral levels of S100B in patients with TS found that S100B was elevated in comparison to an age-matched reference group.[117] More studies will be needed to elucidate further the significance of this finding. Peripheral markers of disease could result from CNS injury or inflammation via a breached blood brain barrier, or from overproduction of a protein in the CNS or peripherally.

The hope of finding a marker for immune-mediated OCD/tics began as an extension of studies of a putative peripheral marker of susceptibility to RF. Monoclonal antibody (mAb) D8/17, which was originally isolated from a patient with rheumatic carditis, reacts with epitopes expressed on expanded populations of B lymphocytes from the majority of patients with documented RF.[118,119] Based on cross-reactivity experiments using the D8/17 antibody, studies attempting to identify this B cell antigen suggest homology to helical coiled-coil molecules such as myosin, tropomyosin, and M6 protein of GAS. Strong binding has been reported to smooth muscle, whereas weak fluorescence in the cytoplasm of cortical and caudate neuronal cells was detected.[120] Otherwise, no other work has been reported on D8/17 expression within various areas of the central nervous system or on the characterization of the putative antigen.

As the diagnosis of SC is often a diagnosis of exclusion, increased expression of D8/17 has been proposed to help differentiate SC from other forms of chorea.[121] Subsequently, the possibility of an immune-mediated pathogenesis of OCD/TS has generated interest (Table 16.4) in the potential of mAb D8/17 for identifying patients at risk for streptococcal-precipitated neuropsychiatric disorders. In two recent flow cytometric studies, increased binding was observed in neuropsychiatric patients compared to controls but a subpopulation of D8/17-positive B cells was not found.[122,123] The diagnostic potential of this antibody and its relationship to the pathophysiology of psychiatric disorders has yet to be established. However, we are aware of a number of studies where group differences were not obtained.

NEUROLOGICAL FACTORS

There is a high comorbidity among childhood onset OCD, tics, ADHD, and the presence of neurological soft signs (NSS), such as choreiform movements and pronator sign/drift. In a recent study 21 of 25 subjects had both OCD and a tic disorder, and 15 had comorbid ADHD.[53] Twelve of these 25 subjects showed choreiform movements that represented an overall worsening of neurological performance that was concurrent with or followed neuropsychiatric symptom exacerbations. In addition, a positive correlation was noted between increase in tic severity as measured by the Yale Global Tic Severity Scale (YGTSS) and worsening in choreiform assessment two visits later ($p = .029$). This pattern is consistent with the finding in a study of RF that OCD symptoms precede the appearance of any motoric manifestation by days or weeks.[21]

More recently, neurological sequelae including myoclonus,[132] poststreptococcal basal ganglia encephalopathy,[133] obsessive compulsive disorder,[19] and tic disorders[44] have been associated with GAS. The clinical neurological picture of a PANDAS child can be both subtle and complicated: subtle in that neurological soft signs may only present intermittently in a particular child, and complicated because the clinical significance of these findings is unknown and no causal relationship has been identified to account for these neurological performance fluctuations, although associations with OCD/tic symptom exacerbation and GAS infections have been postulated.[24] In a comparison of fine motor functioning of 19 children with PANDAS and 19 age- and gender-matched controls, motor performance was significantly slower during exacerbations of streptococcal-triggered OCD and/or tics and these motor skills improved when neuropsychiatric symptoms were in remission.[66]

Signs of worsening neurological performance may not be noticed by parents, although some parents may comment on deterioration in handwriting (bigger, sloppier letters) or a decrease in motor skills (a good baseball player becomes a mediocre player). However, parents are more likely to focus on increased OCD and/or tic symptoms and increased moodiness or on increased attention deficit behaviors such as inability to focus, increased hyperactivity, or more distractibility. Neurological soft signs are usually elicited only upon stressed neurological examination. Choreiform movements, pronator sign/drift, difficulties in balance, or changes in fine motor skills may be present. It may be that neurological fluctuations are characteristic of all children with OCD/tics, but this theory has been neither verified nor disproved at this time. More research is needed in this area to clarify the neurological issues. Assessments need to be developed that will best differentiate choreiform movements from those consistent with chorea and choreiform from tic movements. This distinction has troubled physicians for years, as suggested by Selling, '... of evidence already

OBSESSIVE COMPULSIVE AND TIC DISORDERS 147

Table 16.4 D8/17 studies (n = 11)

Reference	Sample characteristics	Method/site	Findings/conclusions
124	43 children and adults with OCD and/or TS and 31 healthy children and adults as controls	IFM and FC/RU	FACS assay had sensitivity of 77% and specificity of 87%.
123	33 Dutch tic disorder patients and 20 healthy volunteers	FC/Groningen	D8/17 overexpression in patient group (20/33) was significantly higher than in comparison group. FC analysis did not indicate a separate subpopulation of D8/17-positive B cells.
125	18 patients with childhood autism and 14 comparable medically ill subjects	IFM/RU	78% of patients were positive for D8/17 compared to 21% of comparison group. Severity of repetitive behaviors significantly correlated with D8/17 positivity.
61	31 patients with childhood-onset OCD and/or tics and 21 healthy subjects	IFM/UF	Assays performed without complete blinding. All patients were considered positive compared with one control.
126	32 patients with OCD and/or tics and 12 healthy controls	FC/UF	Mean B cell binding for 26% tics/OCD, 9% HC; 66% of patients were positive compared with 8% of controls. 'Many methodological issues will need to be addressed before generalized use of assay for diagnostic purposes.'
127	12 OCD subjects, 17 trichotillomania subjects, and 22 healthy controls	IFM/S Africa	Subjects with OCD showed increased cell binding; however, controls showed higher binding than trichotillomania subjects.
83	16 subjects 7–21 years old with possible PANDAS anorexia nervosa (AN); comparison subjects were 17 psychiatric patients with no eating disorder and no PANDAS characteristics	IFM/RU	D8/17+ in 81% of AN and 12% of comparison subjects: mean B cell binding was 27.1% in AN compared to 5.3% in comparison group.

148 NEUROPSYCHIATRIC DISORDERS AND INFECTION

Table 16.4 Continued

Reference	Sample characteristics	Method/site	Findings/conclusions
128	27 PANDAS children, nine SC children, and 24 HC children.	IFM/RU	D8/17+ in 89% of SC, 85% of PANDAS, and 17% of HC
129	2631 children from Mexico City for D8/17; 108 positive children were compared to 132 negative children for psychiatric symptoms	IFM/Mexico— 0.15 ml blood	For one child with tics and two with OCD there was no association to D8/17, but in 10 children with depression there was a significant association.
130	42 with PANDAS, 26 with SC, and 19 HC (216 samples evaluated)	IFM and FC/RU	Sensitivity of assay dropped over time; test-retest agreement was 61%.
131	29 adults with OCD, 26 healthy controls	IFM/RU	58.6% of OCD and 42.3% of controls were positive (ns). When both groups were combined, males were significantly more likely to be positive. No relationship to presence of tics or age of onset

RU, Rockefeller University; UF, University of Florida; IFM, immunofluorescence microscopy; FC, flow cytometry; SC, Sydenham chorea; HC, healthy controls; OCD, obsessive compulsive disorder; TS, Tourette syndrome; PANDAS, pediatric autoimmune neuropsychiatric disorders associated with streptococcus; AN, anorexia nervosa; ns, not statistically significant.

at hand, there is the relationship of tic and chorea. While the movements in the two diseases differ, one can always pick out isolated movements in chorea identical with those of tic, and conversely in cases of tic some movements identical with chorea.'[22]

DIAGNOSIS AND TREATMENT ISSUES

As a definitive association between GAS and OCD/tics has yet to be established, protocols for diagnosis and treatment are provisional. During the history gathering process, careful attention should be given to reports of repeated, frequent infections, evidence of GAS in a young child (e.g. unexplained abdominal pain accompanied by fever), scarlet fever, brief episodes of tics, OCD, or compulsive urination that remitted, and especially sudden onset of OCD or tics accompanying an infectious illness. In patients with abnormal neurological examination evidenced by muscle weakness, abnormal reflexes ('hung up' patellar reflex) or chorea, further workup is indicated. In patients with new onset OCD or tics, or recent symptom exacerbation, a throat culture is a relatively benign procedure that will help rule out the possibility of symptoms being triggered by a subclinical GAS infection. Streptococcal titers obtained at symptom onset should be repeated to examine for a rise in titers four to six weeks later. In patients with onset exceeding four weeks prior, streptococcal titers add support but do not provide definitive proof of a streptococcal trigger. Examples of typical PANDAS cases are provided below.

Case 1

At five years of age, John presented with a two-day complaint of urinary frequency to his pediatrician. While being evaluated, the pediatrician noticed the boy had signs of scarlet fever and subsequently obtained a throat culture that was positive for GAS. Two weeks later, John developed obsessional thoughts about neatness and his appearance and had difficulty concentrating. These symptoms remitted fully. A careful review of John's medical history revealed two other strep infections at ages two and six and a history of transient tic symptoms between the ages of three and five. At age seven, he had a tic exacerbation and when evaluated by neurology two months later for diagnosis, his strep titers were ASO = 240 and DNAB = 960, and three months later ASO = 120 and DNAB = 960.

At age nine, John developed concerns about germs, cleanliness, and fear of harm to himself or others.

Shortly after his OCD flare-up, John's tic symptoms markedly increased to include complex motor and vocal tics. This tic exacerbation coincided with nosebleeds. At the suggestion of his psychiatrist, a throat culture was obtained which was positive for GAS although he had no symptoms of pharyngitis. Standard therapy was given and his tics significantly remitted by day eight of the antibiotic. His OC symptoms gradually remitted over the next two months. A later ear and sinus infection triggered another tic exacerbation; this time a throat culture was negative for GAS.

Case 2

Jane presented at age nine to her pediatrician with acute onset of incapacitating OCD one week after complaining of a sore throat that was treated with homeopathic remedies. She had a past history of separation anxiety disorder at age eight that resolved completely without treatment and no other past psychiatric illnesses. Her obsessive thoughts were of symmetry and neatness, religion, and fears of social inappropriateness. Jane would compulsively repeat prayers and ask forgiveness and order/arrange objects. OC symptoms were so severe that they prevented Jane from attending school and functioning normally in social and family situations.

One week after onset of OC symptoms, Jane had a positive throat culture and no increase in ASO, but had an elevated DNAB titer. Three days later, Jane developed an eye-blinking tic. Her OCD symptoms stabilized after treatment with penicillin for GAS and addition of an atypical antipsychotic.

While the PANDAS hypothesis remains unsettled, the current treatment for patients meeting the PANDAS criteria continues to be the standard of care practices for patients with OCD and/or TS. Although there is increasing evidence to support a link between GAS and neuropsychiatric disorders, it must be considered that there is an extremely high incidence of pediatric streptococcal infections, not all streptococcal infections are detected, and only a minority of children develops a neuropsychiatric illness. Proof that antimicrobial prophylaxis significantly reduces recurrence and/or exacerbation of OC/tic symptoms would suggest a supportive role for infectious agents in the onset or worsening of these conditions. The use of prophylactic antibiotics in the prevention of neuropsychiatric exacerbations in patients with SC suggests that about a third will continue to have a recurrence.[134] One study where SC patients received monthly prophylactic injections of benzathine penicillin G showed that not all SC recurrences appear to be strep-triggered, and that recurrences may occur after infections too mild or too brief to be easily detected.[135] At NIMH, a placebo-controlled trial of penicillin prophylaxis for children with episodic OCD and/or tic disorders did not prove that penicillin was superior to placebo as prophylaxis against GAS.[63] However, this study was marked by several design confounds including concerns about subject compliance, length of the protocol, and streptococcal infections occurring frequently in both the active and placebo phases. Given these potential confounds, the NIMH study was changed to a 12-month parallel design comparing penicillin and azithromycin with initial promising results that antibiotics may decrease the frequency of neuropsychiatric exacerbation.[136] More work is needed to support the initial data from the ongoing NIMH study before widespread use of prophylactic antibiotics can be endorsed.

The results of a plasmapheresis or intravenous immunoglobulin (IVIG) trial in the treatment of children with PANDAS add additional support for an immune-mediated pathology of OCD and tics.[64] Study participants showed marked improvements in OCD severity, anxiety, and overall functioning, and tic symptoms significantly improved in those receiving plasma exchange. These improvements were noted in the first week with plasma exchange and in three weeks with IVIG therapy, and maintained at one-year follow-up in 82% of the children (subjects received prophylactic antibiotics after immune therapy was completed). Approximately half of the children were able to decrease or discontinue their neuropsychotropic medications. These treatment gains, however, appear to be specific to children who clearly meet the criteria for PANDAS, as plasma exchange in four children with severe chronic OCD did not result in significant improvements.[137] For these patients, it is possible that an immune-mediated process resulted in irreversible neurologic insults that are less responsive to immune therapies. However, this group could represent children with non-immune-mediated etiologies of their illness. Also, neuropsychiatric symptom response to immune therapies is not specific to streptococcal-triggered symptoms. One study reported on two children with evidence of viral-triggered symptoms that improved after immune therapies.[54]

CONCLUSIONS

In conclusion, the exact role that streptococcal infections play in OCD/TS and possibly other childhood-onset neuropsychiatric disorders is unknown. The nosology of PANDAS offers a framework on which to compare the spectrum of 'standard' OCD/TS. At least in a subgroup of patients, evidence is accumulating to support an association of GAS to neuropsychiatric symptom onset and/or exacerbations. However, it is likely that the validity of PANDAS will continue to be questioned since determining a clear causation is difficult against a background of a common childhood illness and the frequent occurrence of both related and unrelated neuropsychiatric exacerbations. However, continuing to search for immune markers and following these children closely for changes in clinical symptoms and immune measures is likely to provide a more applicable understanding of this association.

REFERENCES

1. Karno M, Golding JM, Sorenson SB, Burnam MA. The epidemiology of obsessive-compulsive disorder in five US communities. *Arch Gen Psychiatry* 1988; **45**: 1094–9.
2. Leckman JF, Peterson BS. The pathogenesis of Tourette's syndrome: epigenetic factors active in early CNS development. *Biol Psychiatry* 1993; **34**: 425–7.
3. Kurlan R, McDermott MP, Deeley C et al. Prevalence of tics in schoolchildren and association with placement in special education. *Neurology* 2001; **57**: 1383–8.
4. Leonard HL, Lenane MC, Swedo SE et al. Tics and Tourette's disorder: a 2- to 7-year follow-up of 54 obsessive-compulsive children. *Am J Psychiatry* 1992; **149**: 1244–51.
5. Perugi G, Akiskal HS, Gemignani A et al. Episodic course in obsessive-compulsive disorder. *Eur Arch Psychiatry Clin Neurosci* 1998; **248**: 240–4.
6. Leckman JF, Riddle MA. Tourette's syndrome: when habit-forming systems form habits of their own? *Neuron* 2000; **28**: 349–54.
7. Ernst M, Zametkin AJ, Jons PH et al. High presynaptic dopaminergic activity in children with Tourette's disorder. *J Am Acad Child Adolesc Psychiatry* 1999; **38**: 86–94.
8. McDougle CJ, Goodman WK, Leckman JF et al. The efficacy of fluvoxamine in obsessive-compulsive disorder: effects of comorbid chronic tic disorder. *J Clin Psychopharmacol* 1993; **13**: 354–8.
9. Anderson GM, Leckman JF, Cohen DJ. Neurochemical and neuropeptide systems. In: *Tourette's Syndrome Tics, Obsessions, Compulsions – Developmental Psychopathology and Clinical Care* (Leckman JF, Cohen DJ, eds). New York: John Wiley and Sons, 1998: 261–81.
10. Hosier DM, Craenen JM, Teske DW, Wheller JJ. Resurgence of acute rheumatic fever. *Am J Dis Child* 1987; **141**: 730–3.
11. Ayoub EM. Resurgence of rheumatic fever in the United States. The changing picture of a preventable illness. *Postgrad Med* 1992; **92**: 133–6, 139–42.
12. Taranta A, Stollerman GH. The relationship of Sydenham's chorea to infection with group A streptococci. *Am J Med* 1956; **20**: 170.
13. Bronze MS, Dale JB. Epitopes of streptococcal M proteins that evoke antibodies that cross-react with human brain. *J Immunol* 1993; **151**: 2820–8.
14. Husby G, van de Rijn I, Zabriskie JB et al. Antibodies reacting with cytoplasm of subthalamic and caudate nuclei neurons in

15. Stollerman GH. Rheumatic fever. *Lancet* 1997; **349**: 935–42.
16. Swedo SE, Rapoport JL, Cheslow DL et al. High prevalence of obsessive-compulsive symptoms in patients with Sydenham's chorea. *Am J Psychiatry* 1989; **146**: 246–9.
17. Swedo SE. Sydenham's chorea. A model for childhood autoimmune neuropsychiatric disorders. *JAMA* 1994; **272**: 1788–91.
18. Osler W. *On Chorea and Choreiform Affections*. Philadelphia: HK Lewis, 1894.
19. Swedo SE, Leonard HL, Schapiro MB et al. Sydenham's chorea: physical and psychological symptoms of St Vitus dance. *Pediatrics* 1993; **91**: 706–13.
20. Asbahr FR, Negrao AB, Gentil V et al. Obsessive-compulsive and related symptoms in children and adolescents with rheumatic fever with and without chorea: a prospective 6-month study. *Am J Psychiatry* 1998; **155**: 1122–4.
21. Mercadante MT, Busatto GF, Lombroso PJ et al. The psychiatric symptoms of rheumatic fever. *Am J Psychiatry* 2000; **157**: 2036–8.
22. Selling L. The role of infection in the etiology of tics. *Arch Neurol Psychiatry* 1929; **22**: 1163–71.
23. Kushner HI, Kiessling LS. The controversy over the classification of Gilles de la Tourette's syndrome, 1800–1995. *Perspect Biol Med* 1996; **39**: 409–35.
24. Swedo SE, Leonard HL, Garvey M et al. Pediatric autoimmune neuropsychiatric disorders associated with streptococcal infections: clinical description of the first 50 cases. *Am J Psychiatry* 1998; **155**: 264–71.
25. Murphy TK, Goodman WK, Ayoub EM, Voeller KK. On defining Sydenham's chorea: where do we draw the line? *Biol Psychiatry* 2000; **47**: 851–7.
26. Ahmed S, Ayoub EM, Scornik JC et al. Poststreptococcal reactive arthritis: clinical characteristics and association with HLA-DR alleles. *Arthritis Rheum* 1998; **41**: 1096–102.
27. Jansen TL, Janssen M, van Riel PL. Grand rounds in rheumatology: acute rheumatic fever or post-streptococcal reactive arthritis: a clinical problem revisited. *Br J Rheumatol* 1998; **37**: 335–40.
28. Kotby AA, El Badawy N, El Sokkary S et al. Antineuronal antibodies in rheumatic chorea. *Clin Diagn Lab Immunol* 1998; **5**: 836–9.
29. Kirvan CA, Swedo SE, Heuser JS, Cunningham MW. Mimicry and autoantibody-mediated neuronal cell signaling in Sydenham chorea. *Nat Med* 2003; **9**: 914–20.
30. Knopf PM, Harling-Berg CJ, Cserr HF et al. Antigen-dependent intrathecal antibody synthesis in the normal rat brain: tissue entry and local retention of antigen-specific B cells. *J Immunol* 1998; **161**: 692–701.
31. Kotb M. Bacterial pyrogenic exotoxins as superantigens. *Clin Microbiol Rev* 1995; **8**: 411–26.
32. Abbott WG, Skinner MA, Voss L et al. Repertoire of transcribed peripheral blood T-cell receptor beta chain variable-region genes in acute rheumatic fever. *Infect Immun* 1996; **64**: 2842–5.
33. Torres BA, Johnson HM. Modulation of disease by superantigens. *Curr Opin Immunol* 1998; **10**: 465–70.
34. Tomai M, Kotb M, Majumdar G, Beachey EH. Superantigenicity of streptococcal M protein. *J Exp Med* 1990; **172**: 359–62.
35. Tomai MA, Aelion JA, Dockter ME et al. T cell receptor V gene usage by human T cells stimulated with the superantigen streptococcal M protein. *J Exp Med* 1991; **174**: 285–8.
36. Tomai MA, Beachey EH, Majumdar G, Kotb M. Metabolically active antigen presenting cells are required for human T cell proliferation in response to the superantigen streptococcal M protein. *FEMS Microbiol Immunol* 1992; **4**: 155–64.
37. Proft T, Webb PD, Handley V, Fraser JD. Two novel superantigens found in both group A and group C streptococcus. *Infect Immun* 2003; **71**: 1361–9.
38. Pearson JA, Tyler MI, Retson KV, Howden ME. Studies on the subunit structure of textilotoxin, a potent presynaptic neurotoxin from the venom of the Australian common brown snake (*Pseudonaja textilis*). 3. The complete amino-acid sequences of all the subunits. *Biochim Biophys Acta* 1993; **1161**: 223–9.
39. Beres SB, Sylva GL, Barbian KD et al. Genome sequence of a serotype M3 strain of group A streptococcus: phage-encoded toxins, the high-virulence phenotype, and clone emergence. *Proc Natl Acad Sci USA* 2002; **99**: 10078–83.
40. Krause RM. Evolving microbes and re-emerging streptococcal disease. *Clin Lab Med* 2002; **22**: 835–48.
41. Efstratiou A. Group A streptococci in the 1990s. *J Antimicrob Chemother* 2000; **45**: 3–12.
42. Schwartz B, Facklam RR, Breiman RF. Changing epidemiology of group A streptococcal infection in the USA. *Lancet* 1990; **336**: 1167–71.
43. Congeni BL. The resurgence of acute rheumatic fever in the United States. *Pediatr Ann* 1992; **21**: 816–20.
44. Kiessling LS, Marcotte AC, Culpepper L. Antineuronal antibodies: tics and obsessive-compulsive symptoms. *J Dev Behav Pediatr* 1994; **15**: 421–5.
45. Singer HS, Giuliano JD, Zimmerman AM, Walkup JT. Infection: a stimulus for tic disorders. *Pediatr Neurol* 2000; **22**: 380–3.
46. Kerbeshian J, Burd L, Pettit R. A possible post-streptococcal movement disorder with chorea and tics. *Dev Med Child Neurol* 1990; **32**: 642–4.
47. Tucker DM, Leckman JF, Scahill L et al. A putative poststreptococcal case of OCD with chronic tic disorder, not otherwise specified. *J Am Acad Child Adolesc Psychiatry* 1996; **35**: 1684–91.
48. Murphy ML, Pichichero ME. Prospective identification and treatment of children with pediatric autoimmune neuropsychiatric disorder associated with group A streptococcal infection (PANDAS). *Arch Pediatr Adolesc Med* 2002; **156**: 356–61.
49. Giulino L, Gammon P, Sullivan K et al. Is parental report of upper respiratory infection at the onset of obsessive-compulsive disorder suggestive of pediatric autoimmune neuropsychiatric disorder associated with streptococcal infection? *J Child Adolesc Psychopharmacol* 2002; **12**: 157–64.
50. Muller N, Riedel M, Forderreuther S et al. Tourette's syndrome and mycoplasma pneumoniae infection. *Am J Psychiatry* 2000; **157**: 481–2.
51. Perlmutter SJ, Garvey MA, Castellanos X et al. A case of pediatric autoimmune neuropsychiatric disorders associated with streptococcal infections. *Am J Psychiatry* 1998; **155**: 1592–8.
52. Cardona F, Orefici G. Group A streptococcal infections and tic disorders in an Italian pediatric population. *J Pediatr* 2001; **138**: 71–5.
53. Murphy TK, Sajid M, Soto O et al. Detecting pediatric autoimmune neuropsychiatric disorders associated with streptococcus in children with obsessive-compulsive disorder and tics. *Biol Psychiatry* 2004; **55**: 61–8.
54. Allen AJ, Leonard HL, Swedo SE. Case study: a new infection-triggered, autoimmune subtype of pediatric OCD and Tourette's syndrome. *J Am Acad Child Adolesc Psychiatry* 1995; **34**: 307–11.
55. Fallon BA, Nields JA. Lyme disease: a neuropsychiatric illness. *Am J Psychiatry* 1994; **151**: 1571–83.
56. Kondo K, Kabasawa T. Improvement in Gilles de la Tourette syndrome after corticosteroid therapy. *Ann Neurol* 1978; **4**: 387.

57. Kiessling LS, Marcotte AC, Culpepper L. Antineuronal antibodies in movement disorders. *Pediatrics* 1993; **92**: 39–43.
58. Giedd JN, Rapoport JL, Leonard HL et al. Case study: acute basal ganglia enlargement and obsessive-compulsive symptoms in an adolescent boy. *J Am Acad Child Adolesc Psychiatry* 1996; **35**: 913–5.
59. Hansen CR, Bershow SA. Immunology of TS/OCD. *J Am Acad Child Adolesc Psychiatry* 1997; **36**: 1648–9.
60. Mittleman BB, Castellanos FX, Jacobsen LK et al. Cerebrospinal fluid cytokines in pediatric neuropsychiatric disease. *J Immunol* 1997; **159**: 2994–9.
61. Murphy TK, Goodman WK, Fudge MW et al. B lymphocyte antigen D8/17: a peripheral marker for childhood-onset obsessive-compulsive disorder and Tourette's syndrome? *Am J Psychiatry* 1997; **154**: 402–7.
62. Weiss M, Garland J. More on PANDAS [letter]. *J Am Acad Child Adolesc Psychiatry* 1997; **36**: 1163–5.
63. Garvey MA, Perlmutter SJ, Allen AJ et al. A pilot study of penicillin prophylaxis for neuropsychiatric exacerbations triggered by streptococcal infections. *Biol Psychiatry* 1999; **45**: 1564–71.
64. Perlmutter SJ, Leitman SF, Garvey MA et al. Therapeutic plasma exchange and intravenous immunoglobulin for obsessive-compulsive disorder and tic disorders in childhood. *Lancet* 1999; **354**: 1153–8.
65. Singer HS, Giuliano JD, Hansen BH et al. Antibodies against a neuron-like (HTB-10 neuroblastoma) cell in children with Tourette syndrome. *Biol Psychiatry* 1999; **46**: 775–80.
66. Becker D. Personal communication. Spring 2000: Meeting of the American Academy of Neurology.
67. Giedd JN, Rapoport JL, Garvey MA et al. MRI assessment of children with obsessive-compulsive disorder or tics associated with streptococcal infection. *Am J Psychiatry* 2000; **157**: 281–3.
68. Hallett JJ, Harling-Berg CJ, Knopf PM et al. Anti-striatal antibodies in Tourette syndrome cause neuronal dysfunction. *J Neuroimmunol* 2000; **111**: 195–202.
69. Lougee L, Perlmutter SJ, Nicolson R et al. Psychiatric disorders in first-degree relatives of children with pediatric autoimmune neuropsychiatric disorders associated with streptococcal infections (PANDAS). *J Am Acad Child Adolesc Psychiatry* 2000; **39**: 1120–6.
70. Peterson BS, Leckman JF, Tucker D et al. Preliminary findings of antistreptococcal antibody titers and basal ganglia volumes in tic, obsessive-compulsive, and attention deficit/hyperactivity disorders. *Arch Gen Psychiatry* 2000; **57**: 364–72.
71. Bodner SM, Morshed SA, Peterson BS. The question of PANDAS in adults. *Biol Psychiatry* 2001; **49**: 807–10.
72. Morshed SA, Parveen S, Leckman JF et al. Antibodies against neural, nuclear, cytoskeletal, and streptococcal epitopes in children and adults with Tourette's syndrome, Sydenham's chorea, and autoimmune disorders. *Biol Psychiatry* 2001; **50**: 566–77.
73. Muller N, Kroll B, Schwarz MJ et al. Increased titers of antibodies against streptococcal M12 and M19 proteins in patients with Tourette's syndrome. *Psychiatry Res* 2001; **101**: 187–93.
74. Orvidas LJ, Slattery MJ. Pediatric autoimmune neuropsychiatric disorders and streptococcal infections: role of otolaryngologist. *Laryngoscope* 2001; **111**: 1515–9.
75. Wendlandt JT, Grus FH, Hansen BH, Singer HS. Striatal antibodies in children with Tourette's syndrome: multivariate discriminant analysis of IgG repertoires. *J Neuroimmunol* 2001; **119**: 106–13.
76. Martinelli P, Ambrosetto G, Minguzzi E et al. Late-onset PANDAS syndrome with abdominal muscle involvement. *Eur Neurol* 2002; **48**: 49–51.
77. Taylor JR, Morshed SA, Parveen S et al. An animal model of Tourette's syndrome. *Am J Psychiatry* 2002; **159**: 657–60.
78. Loiselle CR, Wendlandt JT, Rohde CA, Singer HS. Antistreptococcal, neuronal, and nuclear antibodies in Tourette syndrome. *Pediatr Neurol* 2003; **28**: 119–25.
79. Church AJ, Dale RC, Lees AJ et al. Tourette's syndrome: a cross sectional study to examine the PANDAS hypothesis. *J Neurol Neurosurg Psychiatry* 2003; **74**: 602–7.
80. Soto O, Murphy TK. Bipolar affective disorder and the immune system. In: *Child and Early Adolescent Bipolar Disorder: Theory, Assessment, and Treatment* (Geller B, DelBello M, eds). New York: Guilford Press, 2002.
81. Casanova MF et al. Sydenham's chorea and schizophrenia: a case report. *Schizophr Res* 1995; **16**: 73–6.
82. Fernandez-Rivas A et al. Recurrent depression: infections-autoimmune etiology? *J Am Acad Child Adolesc Psychiatry* 2000; **39**: 810–2.
83. Sokol MS, Ward PE, Tamiya H et al. D8/17 expression on B lymphocytes in anorexia nervosa. *Am J Psychiatry* 2002; **159**: 1430–2.
84. Snider LA, Seligman LD, Ketchen BR et al. Tics and problem behaviors in schoolchildren: prevalence, characterization, and associations. *Pediatrics* 2002; **110**: 331–6.
85. Tolaymat A, Goudarzi T, Soler GP et al. Acute rheumatic fever in north Florida. *South Med J* 1984; **77**: 819–23.
86. Dowell SF. Seasonal variation in host susceptibility and cycles of certain infectious diseases. *Emerg Infect Dis* 2001; **7**: 369–74.
87. Vincent A, Deacon R, Dalton P et al. Maternal antibody-mediated dyslexia? Evidence for a pathogenic serum factor in a mother of two dyslexic children shown by transfer to mice using behavioural studies and magnetic resonance spectroscopy. *J Neuroimmunol* 2002; **130**: 243–7.
88. Patterson PH. Maternal infection: window on neuroimmune interactions in fetal brain development and mental illness. *Curr Opin Neurobiol* 2002; **12**: 115–8.
89. Zinkernagel RM. Maternal antibodies, childhood infections, and autoimmune diseases. *N Engl J Med* 2001; **345**: 1331–5.
90. Woods WA, Carter CT, Schlager TA. Detection of group A streptococci in children under 3 years of age with pharyngitis. *Pediatr Emerg Care* 1999; **15**: 338–40.
91. Schwartz RH, Hayden GF, Wientzen R. Children less than three-years-old with pharyngitis. Are group A streptococci really that uncommon? *Clin Pediatr (Phila)* 1986; **25**: 185–8.
92. Denny FW Jr. A 45-year perspective on the streptococcus and rheumatic fever: the Edward H. Kass Lecture in infectious disease history. *Clin Infect Dis* 1994; **19**: 1110–22.
93. Holm SE. Treatment of recurrent tonsillopharyngitis. *J Antimicrob Chemother* 2000; **45** (Suppl): 31–5.
94. Paradise JL, Bluestone CD, Colborn DK et al. Tonsillectomy and adenotonsillectomy for recurrent throat infection in moderately affected children. *Pediatrics* 2002; **110**: 7–15.
95. Ikinciogullari A, Dogu F, Egin Y, Babacan E. Is immune system influenced by adenotonsillectomy in children? *Int J Pediatr Otorhinolaryngol* 2002; **66**: 251–7.
96. Zielnik-Jurkiewicz B, Jurkiewicz D. Implication of immunological abnormalities after adenotonsillotomy. *Int J Pediatr Otorhinolaryngol* 2002; **64**: 127–32.
97. Cheadle WB. Various manifestations of the rheumatic state as exemplified in childhood and early life. *Lancet* 1889; **1**: 821–7, 871–7.
98. Taranta A, Toorsdag S, Metrakos JD et al. Rheumatic fever in monozygotic and dizygotic twins. *Circulation* 1959; **20**: 778–92.
99. Pickles W, Lond M. A rheumatic family. *Lancet* 1943; **245**: 241–2.

100. Kotb M, Norrby-Teglund A, McGeer A et al. An immunogenetic and molecular basis for differences in outcomes of invasive group A streptococcal infections. *Nat Med* 2002; **8**: 1398–404.
101. Rasmussen SA, Tsuang MT. The epidemiology of obsessive compulsive disorder. *J Clin Psychiatry* 1984; **45**: 450–7.
102. Reddy PS, Reddy YC, Srinath S et al. A family study of juvenile obsessive-compulsive disorder. *Can J Psychiatry* 2001; **46**: 346–51.
103. Hanna GL. Clinical and family-genetic studies of childhood obsessive-compulsive disorder. In: *Obsessive-Compulsive Disorder: Contemporary Issues in Treatment* (Goodman WK, Rudorfer MV, Maser JD, eds). Mahwah, NJ: Lawrence Erlbaum Associates, 2000: 87–103.
104. Devor EJ. Complex segregation analysis of Gilles de la Tourette syndrome: further evidence for a major locus mode of transmission. *Am J Hum Genet* 1984; **36**: 704–9.
105. Pauls DL, Leckman JF. The inheritance of Gilles de la Tourette's syndrome and associated behaviors. Evidence for autosomal dominant transmission. *N Engl J Med* 1986; **315**: 993–7.
106. Singer HS, Giuliano JD, Hansen BH et al. Antibodies against human putamen in children with Tourette syndrome. *Neurology* 1998; **50**: 1618–24.
107. Carpenter LL, Heninger GR, McDougle CJ et al. Cerebrospinal fluid interleukin-6 in obsessive-compulsive disorder and trichotillomania. *Psychiatry Res* 2002; **112**: 257–62.
108. Marazziti D, Presta S, Pfanner C et al. Immunological alterations in adult obsessive-compulsive disorder. *Biol Psychiatry* 1999; **46**: 810–4.
109. Ravindran AV, Griffiths J, Merali Z, Anisman H. Circulating lymphocyte subsets in obsessive compulsive disorder, major depression and normal controls. *J Affect Disord* 1999; **52**: 1–10.
110. Black JL, Lamke GT, Walikonis JE. Serologic survey of adult patients with obsessive-compulsive disorder for neuron-specific and other autoantibodies. *Psychiatry Res* 1998; **81**: 371–80.
111. Hutto JH, Ayoub EM. Cytotoxicity of lymphocytes from patients with rheumatic carditis in vitro. In: *Streptococcal Diseases and the Immune Response* (Read SE, Zabriskie JB, eds). New York: Academic Press, 1987: 733–8.
112. Maes M, Meltzer HY, Bosmans E. Psychoimmune investigation in obsessive-compulsive disorder: assays of plasma transferrin, IL-2 and IL-6 receptor, and IL-1 beta and IL-6 concentrations. *Neuropsychobiology* 1994; **30**: 57–60.
113. Monteleone P, Catapano F, Fabrazzo M et al. Decreased blood levels of tumor necrosis factor-alpha in patients with obsessive-compulsive disorder. *Neuropsychobiology* 1998; **37**: 182–5.
114. Dinn WM, Harris CL, McGonigal KM, Raynard RC. Obsessive-compulsive disorder and immunocompetence. *Int J Psychiatry Med* 2001; **31**: 311–20.
115. Persson L, Hardemark HG, Gustafsson J et al. S-100 protein and neuron-specific enolase in cerebrospinal fluid and serum: markers of cell damage in human central nervous system. *Stroke* 1987; **18**: 911–8.
116. Lamers KJ, van Engelen BG, Gabreels FJ et al. Cerebrospinal neuron-specific enolase, S-100 and myelin basic protein in neurological disorders. *Acta Neurol Scand* 1995; **92**: 247–51.
117. van Passel R, Schlooz WA, Lamers KJ et al. S100B protein, glia and Gilles de la Tourette syndrome. *Euro J Paediatr Neurol* 2001; **5**: 15–9.
118. Zabriskie JB. Rheumatic fever: a model for the pathological consequences of microbial-host mimicry. *Clin Exp Rheumatol* 1986; **4**: 65–73.
119. Patarroyo ME, Winchester RJ, Vejerano A et al. Association of a B-cell alloantigen with susceptibility to rheumatic fever. *Nature* 1979; **278**: 173–4.
120. Kemeny E, Husby G, Williams RC, Zabriskie JB. Tissue distribution of antigen(s) defined by monoclonal antibody D8/17 reacting with B lymphocytes of patients with rheumatic heart disease. *Clin Immunol Immunopathol* 1994; **72**: 35–43.
121. Feldman BM, Zabriskie JB, Silverman ED, Laxer RM. Diagnostic use of B-cell alloantigen D8/17 in rheumatic chorea. *J Pediatr* 1993; **123**: 84–6.
122. Murphy T, Goodman W. Genetics of childhood disorders: XXXIV. Autoimmune disorders, part 7: D8/17 reactivity as an immunological marker of susceptibility to neuropsychiatric disorders. *J Am Acad Child Adolesc Psychiatry* 2002; **41**: 98–100.
123. Hoekstra PJ, Bijzet J, Limburg PC et al. Elevated D8/17 expression on B lymphocytes, a marker of rheumatic fever, measured with flow cytometry in tic disorder patients. *Am J Psychiatry* 2001; **158**: 605–10.
124. Chapman F, Visvanathan K, Carreno-Manjarrez R, Zabriskie JB. A flow cytometric assay for D8/17 B cell marker in patients with Tourette's syndrome and obsessive compulsive disorder. *J Immunol Methods* 1998; **219**: 181–6.
125. Hollander E, DelGiudice-Asch G, Simon L et al. B lymphocyte antigen D8/17 and repetitive behaviors in autism. *Am J Psychiatry* 1999; **156**: 317–20.
126. Murphy TK, Benson N, Zaytoun A et al. Progress toward analysis of D8/17 binding to B cells in children with obsessive compulsive disorder and/or chronic tic disorder. *J Neuroimmunol* 2001; **120**: 146–51.
127. Niehaus DJ, Knowles JA, van Kradenberg J et al. D8/17 in obsessive-compulsive disorder and trichotillomania. *S Afr Med J* 1999; **89**: 755–6.
128. Swedo SE, Leonard HL, Mittleman BB et al. Identification of children with pediatric autoimmune neuropsychiatric disorders associated with streptococcal infections by a marker associated with rheumatic fever. *Am J Psychiatry* 1997; **154**: 110–2.
129. Inoff-Germain G, Rodriguez RS, Torres-Alcantara S et al. An immunological marker (D8/17) associated with rheumatic fever as a predictor of childhood psychiatric disorders in a community sample. *J Child Psychol Psychiatry* 2003; **44**: 782–90.
130. Hamilton CS, Garvey MA, Swedo SE. Sensitivity of the D8/17 assay. *Am J Psychiatry* 2003; **160**: 1193–4; author reply 1194.
131. Eisen JL, Leonard HL, Swedo SE et al. The use of antibody D8/17 to identify B cells in adults with obsessive-compulsive disorder. *Psychiatry Res* 2001; **104**: 221–5.
132. DiFazio MP, Morales J, Davis R. Acute myoclonus secondary to group A beta-hemolytic streptococcus infection: a PANDAS variant. *J Child Neurol* 1998; **13**: 516–8.
133. Dale RC, Church AJ, Surtees RA et al. Post-streptococcal autoimmune neuropsychiatric disease presenting as paroxysmal dystonic choreoathetosis. *Mov Disord* 2002; **17**: 817–20.
134. Terreri MT, Roja SC, Len CA et al. Sydenham's chorea – clinical and evolutive characteristics. *Sao Paulo Med J* 2002; **120**: 16–9.
135. Berrios X, Quesney F, Morales A et al. Are all recurrences of 'pure' Sydenham chorea true recurrences of acute rheumatic fever? *J Pediatr* 1985; **107**: 867–72.
136. Swedo SE. Personal communication, 2001.
137. Nicolson R, Swedo SE, Lenane M et al. An open trial of plasma exchange in childhood-onset obsessive-compulsive disorder without poststreptococcal exacerbations. *J Am Acad Child Adolesc Psychiatry* 2000; **39**: 1313–5.

17

Post-streptococcal neuropsychiatric disease: Sydenham's chorea and beyond

Russell C Dale and Andrew J Church

INTRODUCTION

The classic description of Sydenham's chorea (SC) by Thomas Sydenham in 1686 described a 'change in personality' in addition to a dancing movement disorder. However, two centuries passed before SC was associated with rheumatism and rheumatic carditis.[1] Subsequently, during the 20th century, group A streptococcus was identified as the main disease precipitant. SC is now accepted as a major criterion of rheumatic fever (Jones criteria). It is proposed that immune reactivity against the streptococcal organism induces an aberrant autoimmune attack directed against the brain rather than infection of the brain, although the exact pathogenesis remains unknown. Recently, interest in Sydenham's chorea has been re-ignited due to the proposed recognition of a broader spectrum of neuropsychiatric outcomes after streptococcal infection which include tics, obsessive-compulsive disorder and attention deficit hyperactivity disorder.[2] This has led to speculations that post-streptococcal neuropsychiatric diseases may be autoimmune models of common childhood diseases, and that even 'idiopathic' Tourette syndrome and obsessive-compulsive disorder could also be secondary to post-streptococcal autoimmunity.[3]

We will critically appraise the current understanding of this spectrum of disorders, but start first with historical descriptions over the last four centuries.

HISTORICAL DESCRIPTIONS

Thomas Sydenham (1624–1689) published his landmark book *Schedula Monitoria de Novae Febris Ingressa* in 1686.[4] He described a childhood movement disorder that became known as Sydenham's chorea. He attempted to distinguish this disorder from a dancing mania which was common in medieval Europe that was presumed to be secondary to hysteria provoked by religious superstition.[5] The term chorea is derived from the Greek word for dancing and has come to describe fast, involuntary, purposeless, extrapyramidal movements. In addition to the abnormal movements, Sydenham also described emotional lability and a change in temperament, but did not note the association with rheumatic fever.[4]

It was not until 1810 that Bouteille recognized the association between arthritic rheumatism and chorea.[6] In 1899, diplococcus was grown from the body fluids of a child who died of rheumatic carditis and chorea.[7] Then in the first decade of the 20th century, a series of experiments in rabbits showed that intravenous injection of the diplococcus resulted in carditis and chorea, supporting a direct link between the micro-organism and disease.[8] By 1968, it was generally believed that rheumatic fever and SC were 'immune-allergic' complications of the streptococcal organisms.[9] In the last half of the 20th century, the incidence of SC significantly reduced in the developed world, although it remains endemic in the developing world. However, interest in post-streptococcal neuropsychiatric conditions was re-ignited after an epidemic of group A streptococcal infections in Rhode Island, USA, during the 1980s, that was associated with a dramatic increase in movement disorders and psychiatric disease amongst children.[10] However, rather than chorea, the patients manifested a different movement disorder – motor tics. Subsequent detailed psychometric analysis demonstrated psychiatric disorders (particularly obsessive-compulsive disorder or OCD) were commonly associated with the movement disorders, and sometimes occurred in isolation.[2] In view of this apparently new clinical phenotype, a new term was used to describe post-streptococcal tics and OCD –

PANDAS (pediatric autoimmune neuropsychiatric disorders associated with streptococcal infections).[2]

CLINICAL FEATURES

Movement disorders and other neurological signs

Chorea remains the classic movement disorder occurring after streptococcal infections. SC is most common in children aged between five and 15, and is more common in girls.[11,12] Due to the controversy surrounding the concept of PANDAS, some would argue that chorea is the only proven post-streptococcal movement disorder.[13] However, it is not unusual for multiple movement disorder phenotypes to be observed in neurological disease. The best example is Huntington's disease: although chorea is the classical phenotype, tics, dystonia, and Parkinsonism are also recognized in Huntington's disease.[14,15] Indeed, different movement disorders have been described in patients with 'Sydenham's chorea' throughout the 20th century including tics, myoclonus, and tremor.[16,17] Furthermore, a recent report described motor tics in 73% of patients with SC.[18]

However, the description of motor tics secondary to streptococcal infection has been met with skepticism and controversy.[13] In order to improve the diagnostic specificity, patients with PANDAS are required to have at least two exacerbations of motor tics and/or OCD with microbiologically defined streptococcal infections.[2] Some patients have been reported to have multiple relapses precipitated by infections.[2] Appropriate skepticism over the concept of PANDAS has arisen primarily due to the difficulty making a temporal association between two common childhood problems; motor tics can occur in up to 5% of children, and typically wax and wane in severity.[13] Likewise, streptococcal infections are endemic in school age populations and are the most common single cause of tonsillitis. Therefore, an association between tics and streptococcal infection could, it is argued, occur by chance. It is for this reason that robust biological markers are required to improve diagnostic sensitivity and specificity in post-streptococcal brain disorders (discussed later). However, a number of groups from around the world have now published data supporting a proposed link between streptococcal infections and motor tics,[2,19–21] and the concept of PANDAS remains an active and important area of research.

Apart from chorea, other extrapyramidal movement disorders have also been described after streptococcal infection including case reports of myoclonus, dystonia, and paroxysmal dystonic choreoathetosis.[22–24] Whilst other neurological signs are less common, muscular weakness and hypotonia may occur,[25] and may in extremes present as an apparent tetraparesis (without spasticity), termed chorea paralytic or chorea mollis.[26] Dysarthria is also not unusual in SC, and is thought to be extrapyramidal in origin. Other neurological signs would be considered atypical, such as seizures, pyramidal signs,[27] and dementia. Although school difficulties are quite common in PANDAS, it is unclear whether these are secondary to cognitive problems or are a consequence of comorbid psychiatric disturbance such as attention deficit hyperactivity disorder.[2] Only detailed neuropsychological examination could define the nature of these school difficulties.

An interesting recent phenomenon is the presence of enuresis.[2,28] Again, whether this is secondary to associated emotional problems, or has an alternative biological origin, requires further examination.

In conclusion, it would appear that a broad spectrum of movement disorders are precipitated by streptococcal infection, although neurological signs are relatively restricted to extrapyramidal movements. This has added to the hypothesis that the basal ganglia is particularly vulnerable to the immunological insult after group A streptococcal infection. Finally, with regard to outcome, approximately 50% of SC patients make a complete recovery from the movement disorder, although residual psychiatric disorders may remain.[29,30]

Psychiatric disorders

Thomas Sydenham noted during his original clinical descriptions an 'emotional lability' during SC. Further observation confirmed the behavioral abnormalities that became known as the 'choreic temperament'. A follow-up study of patients up to 20 years after SC presentation demonstrated a high incidence of residual psychiatric symptoms, suggesting that psychiatric disorders may remain long after resolution of the movement disorder.[30] Although psychiatric manifestations associated with SC were initially attributed to hysteria or psychological trauma, it is now accepted that the psychiatric symptoms are secondary to the brain insult. Recent detailed psychometric examination of patient cohorts with SC and PANDAS have defined the psychiatric complications using international diagnostic criteria.[18,31–34] Table 17.1 reviews the studies that have examined the incidence of obsessive-compulsive disorder in SC. All the studies reported an incidence of OCD higher than the expected incidence of OCD in childhood (approximately 1%).[35] An interesting observation is that the

Table 17.1 Incidence of obsessive-compulsive disorder (OCD) in Sydenham's chorea (SC) and rheumatic fever (RhF)

Study reference	Cohort (number)	Percentage with OCD
31	SC (n = 20)	20%
32	SC (n = 23)	13%
33	SC (n = 30)	17%
18	SC (n = 22)	14%
34	SC (n = 20)	10%
32	RhF (n = 14)	0%
33	RhF (n = 20)	0%
18	RhF (n = 20)	10%

risk of OCD appears to increase with relapses or chronicity of disease.[36] The incidence of OCD in PANDAS is more difficult to define as OCD is a criterion for a diagnosis of PANDAS.[2] However, we have reported a high incidence of OCD (50%) in patients with post-streptococcal tics (n = 16).[34] These patients had a relapsing and persistent course as described by Swedo. The relapsing nature of disease in these patients may have directly contributed to the high rate of OCD seen. The higher incidence of OCD in SC and post-streptococcal tics suggests that these movement and emotional disorders could be biologically linked. This association is well described in Tourette syndrome, but is also described in other movement disorders such as Parkinson's disease and Huntington's disease.[37,38]

The emotional correlates in post-streptococcal neuropsychiatric disease are not restricted to OCD. Indeed other emotional disorders such as generalized anxiety, separation anxiety, and major depressive disorder are more common in SC and PANDAS than normal controls.[2,18]

Although emotional disorders appear to be the most common psychiatric outcome of post-streptococcal brain disorders, other psychiatric disorders are significantly over-represented in populations with SC and PANDAS. Attention deficit hyperactivity disorder (ADHD) and oppositional defiant disorder are significantly higher in both SC and PANDAS than normal populations.[2,18] By contrast, psychotic disorders such as mania and schizophrenia would be considered atypical and are rarely described.[39] Attempting to correlate the psychiatric diseases with a specific neuroanatomical site is more difficult. Although obsessive-compulsive disorder is thought to be associated with basal ganglia dysfunction and related cortico-striatal circuits,[40] neither ADHD nor conduct disorders are thought to derive from basal ganglia dysfunction. This may suggest that the CNS dysfunction may be more widespread than the basal ganglia alone.

Multi-organ involvement

Sydenham's chorea is one of the major Jones criteria of rheumatic fever, and often exists as part of a multi-organ disease involving the heart, joints, and skin, in addition to the brain.[26] SC does however occur in isolation. The incidence of chorea in rheumatic fever appears to demonstrate annual fluctuation (ranging from 7–60%) that may be related to variations in specific rheumatogenic streptococcal strains.[41] It appears that in PANDAS and other post-streptococcal brain syndromes, pathology is isolated to the brain. The cause of this important difference is not known.

PATHOGENESIS

The exact pathogenesis of post-streptococcal neuropsychiatric disease is not known. However, we will now review the current understanding of disease pathogenesis with particular reference to the neuroanatomical localization, and the proposed immune mediators of disease.

Neuroanatomy and neuropathology

The basal ganglia include the following nuclei: caudate and putamen (collectively known as the striatum), globus pallidus, and the substantia nigra. The basal ganglia are part of the neuronal circuits communicating with the cerebral cortex and the thalamus. There are relatively few pathological reports of SC, partly due to the non-fatal nature of the acute disease. Two historical reports described inflammatory infiltrate of the perivascular parenchyma, an appearance commonly seen in encephalitis.[42,43] In these reports, the inflammatory changes were most striking in the basal ganglia, although the cerebral cortex and thalamus were also significantly involved. One further report found neuronal degeneration only (rather than inflammation),[44] suggesting heterogeneity may exist in the pathogenesis of post-streptococcal brain disease. Alternatively, these reports may be atypical given their fatal nature.

Speculations on neurochemistry

The exact neurochemical alterations have not been defined in post-streptococcal disorders. However, hypotheses have focused on an imbalance of neurochemicals, particularly dopamine or GABA (gamma aminobutyric acid). The dopamine hypothesis states that dopamine exists in excess in SC, or there is increased dopamine sensitivity. This dopamine hypothesis derives from the recognition that L-dopa and dopamine derivatives can induce dyskinesias such as chorea and tics in Parkinson's disease. Furthermore, dopamine antagonists such as haloperidol are effective agents in the treatment of Sydenham's chorea and tics, although this agent is not currently considered a first line agent due to significant side effects. Further support for the dopamine hypothesis derives from the recognition that estrogen can exacerbate Sydenham's chorea (both oral contraceptives and pregnancy can precipitate relapses).[45,46] It is proposed that female sex hormones may modify or sensitize post-synaptic dopaminergic receptors in the striatum.

An alternative hypothesis is that the inhibitory effects of GABA are diminished, resulting in overstimulation of thalamo-cortical neurones. GABAergic projection neurons are precociously damaged in the course of acute metabolic insults (e.g. hypoxia, hypoglycaemia) and chronic neurodegenerative disorders (e.g. Huntington's disease),[47] and appear to be particularly vulnerable to these insults. A similar process may be occurring in post-streptococcal neuropsychiatric disorders. Sodium valproate enhances the activity of GABA and has been reported to be effective in SC.[48] Other than dopamine or GABA, alternative hypotheses would include alterations in serotonin metabolism, a neurochemical incriminated in the pathogenesis of obsessive-compulsive disorder (OCD).[40]

Neuroimaging

Magnetic resonance neuroimaging is usually normal in SC and PANDAS.[49,50] Occasionally, enhancing lesions may be observed that are usually localized to the basal ganglia.[51–53] We have previously described 10 patients with acute disseminated encephalomyelitis (ADEM) after streptococcal infection with basal ganglia involvement.[27] These patients had dystonia and behavioral alteration as the predominant clinical features. Although there were disseminated inflammatory lesions, the basal ganglia were most markedly affected.[27] Volumetric measurement of brain regions in SC and PANDAS has shown that the basal ganglia are selectively enlarged in acute disease,[49,54] and return to normal during remission.[55] One MR spectrometry case report showed changes in basal ganglia n-acetyl aspartate, a finding consistent with neuronal dysfunction or loss.[52] Furthermore, SPECT imaging has demonstrated alterations in blood flow and metabolism predominantly restricted to the basal ganglia.[56–58] A further SPECT study that labeled dopamine-2 receptors showed reduced basal ganglia uptake during further relapses suggestive of progressive damage.[59] These abnormal imaging findings (when present) are commonly reversible, although there are descriptions of irreversible changes with secondary permanent damage or necrosis.[34,60] In conclusion, conventional MR imaging is usually normal in post-streptococcal neuropsychiatric disease although more sophisticated measurements have identified that the basal ganglia is the predominant brain region affected by disease.

Immunopathogenesis

It is proposed that group A streptococcus infection induces an immune response in the host that cross-reacts with brain epitopes due to structural or amino acid similarities. This hypothesis is termed molecular mimicry and is a favored theory in other neurological disorders such as Guillain Barre syndrome (which is often precipitated by campylobacter infection).

Group A streptococcus is also capable of producing a number of complications in humans, including invasive disease and importantly other autoimmune diseases (such as glomerulonephritis and arthritis). However, group A streptococcus most commonly causes self-limiting episodes of tonsillitis or skin infections.

The precipitating streptococcal infection in SC and PANDAS usually presents as a pharyngeal infection. The latency between infection and neurological onset is variable but is often between two and three weeks.[2,27] A number of different immune mediators could be theoretically capable of producing brain disease, including T-lymphocytes, B-lymphocytes and antibodies, complement, cytokines, or bacterial toxins. To date, most attention has focused on antineuronal antibodies as possible mediators of disease. Husby initially described antineuronal antibodies in 46% of acute SC patients compared to only 1–4% of controls.[61] Using an immunofluorescent method, he showed that these antibodies bound mainly to caudate and subthalamus neurons, and to a lesser extent cortical neurons. Further recent work has confirmed the high incidence of antineuronal antibodies (95–100%) in acute SC with a reduction of antibodies in persistent or chronic SC.[62,63] Using human basal ganglia in a western immunoblotting method, we have proposed that a restricted group of neuronal antigens that have molecular weights of 40, 45, and 60 kDa are involved in antibody binding.[62] Singer has also found antineuronal antibodies in SC although the candidate autoantigens are of higher molecular weights using his methods.[64] It must be noted that differing methodologies including antigen preparation and antibody detection make direct comparisons difficult.[62,64] Immunofluorescent staining has localized the antibody binding primarily to the cytoplasm.[61,62] It has been argued previously that autoantibodies are more likely to be pathogenic if they bind to antigens on the (membrane) surface of cells. Identifying these autoantigens would be of great interest and may help interpret their potential pathogenicity. Recent studies have shown that the antibodies are predominantly of the IgG1 subclass and also exist in the cerebrospinal fluid.[65] Similar antibody findings have been demonstrated in PANDAS using immunofluorescent studies,[10] although more detailed examination in PANDAS is lacking. Whether PANDAS and SC have a similar immunopathogenesis remains to be determined.

The presence of antibodies in patient serum does not necessarily infer pathogenicity, as antineuronal antibodies could be produced as a consequence of neural damage (although imaging studies do not suggest this). For antibodies to be deemed pathogenic, they need to have 'effector' function.[66] To demonstrate effector function, one criterion is the induction of disease after transfer of antibodies to an animal model. Antibodies from PANDAS patients have been shown to induce stereotypical tic-like movements in rats after direct infusion into rat striatum.[67,68] In addition, in a placebo-controlled trial, PANDAS patients showed clinical improvements after treatment with intravenous immunoglobulin or plasma exchange but not with a placebo treatment.[69] Although these findings support the pathogenicity of antineuronal antibodies, further criteria are required before these syndromes can be confidently defined as antibody-mediated diseases.

Alternative immune mechanisms could include T-lymphocyte cell-mediated cytotoxicity or cytokine-mediated neuronal damage. We have previously investigated the cytokine environment in the CSF and serum of SC patients. No SC patients had detectable interferon-gamma (a cytokine associated with cell-mediated cytotoxicity) in the CSF.[65] In contrast, the cytokines IL-4 and IL-10 were modestly elevated in both CSF and serum. IL-4 and IL-10 are anti-inflammatory cytokines and also have a role in autoimmunity and B-lymphocyte production of antibodies. This provisional cytokine study supports an autoantibody hypothesis, although more extensive cytokine examination is needed to establish further the possible role of cytokines.[65]

One unanswered question is: How do the immune mediators cross the blood brain barrier? Possible explanations include damage to the blood brain barrier with consequent passive transfer of autoreactive lymphocytes or antibodies into the brain. Alternatively, if the blood brain barrier remains intact, how could immune mediators gain access to the brain? Recent findings have shown that activated lymphocytes are capable of passing through the intact blood brain barrier and surveying the brain parenchyma.[70] This 'immune surveillance' occurs at a very low level in the brain compared to other organs, and will be unremarkable as long as the lymphocytes do not recognise an autoantigen. If an autoantigen is recognized by the activated lymphocytes, a cascade of cell recruitment and cytokine induction may occur.

A further question is: Why are streptococcal organisms immunogenic to the brain? This important question is not fully answered. M-proteins, complex helical proteins on the surface of group A streptococci, are considered possible mediators of post-streptococcal brain syndromes, predominantly due to their recognized immunogenicity.[71] Particular M-serotypes (M5, M6, and M19) have been associated with outbreaks of rheumatic fever and SC, supporting the concept of rheumatogenic strains. Further support for this hypothesis is the demonstration that some antibrain antibodies cross-react with epitopes from M-proteins.[71] However, definitive evidence that M-proteins are the mediators of disease is lacking and other cell surface streptococcal proteins could be capable of disease induction. Indeed, a number of streptococcal surface proteins share homology with human brain proteins.

Alternative immunogenic factors could include toxin-mediated inflammation, a process recently proposed as important in post-streptococcal glomerulonephritis.[72]

GENETICS

Despite group A streptococcal infections being remarkably common, relatively few people appear vulnerable to post-streptococcal autoimmune disease. Studies have shown that there is an increased incidence of rheumatic fever and SC in family members of SC patients.[11] Likewise, the incidence of obsessive-compulsive disorder and tic disorders is higher in family members of patients with PANDAS than in the general population.[73] It would therefore appear that a genetic predisposition is important in disease induction. The possible mechanisms of this genetic predisposition could be diverse, such as a neurochemical or immunological vulnerability. A genetic predisposition to autoimmunity is the most favored hypothesis. Limited studies of HLA loci have not revealed any association in SC.[74] Instead, attention has focused on a B-lymphocyte marker, D8/17, that is highly expressed in patients with SC, PANDAS, and rheumatic fever.[75,76] As the function of this lymphocyte marker is unknown, it is unclear whether this marker represents a pathogenic autoimmune predisposition, or is an epiphenomenon.

TREATMENT

Two separate approaches exist in the treatment of post-streptococcal brain syndromes: treatment to correct the immune abnormalities or correct the secondary neurochemical alterations. Penicillin is accepted as a prophylactic agent in SC, to reduce further streptococcus-mediated relapses. Immunotherapies such as steroids have been shown to be efficacious in SC.[77] Intravenous immunoglobulin and plasma exchange have also been effective in a controlled trial in PANDAS.[69] There have been no large trials comparing all three immune treatments. It should be kept in mind that at least half of SC patients will have a self-limiting disorder and arguably do not warrant immune therapies that may cause significant side effects.[29] Alternative therapies that alter neurochemistry have been shown to be effective in SC. Haloperidol and other dopamine antagonists are effective in treating acute chorea in SC, although they do have potential side effects.[78] In addition, haloperidol can induce apoptosis in striatal neurons.[79] Other agents such as sodium valproate and carbamazepine are efficacious in SC and have potentially useful mood stabilizing effects.[48,80,81]

IMPLICATIONS FOR COMMON NEUROPSYCHIATRIC DISORDERS

The recognition of the PANDAS phenotype has lead to speculation that post-streptococcal autoimmunity may be important in common neuropsychiatric disorders such as Tourette syndrome, tic disorders, obsessive-compulsive disorder, and attention deficit hyperactivity disorder (ADHD). A number of studies have attempted to address this possible association.

Cross-sectional studies have revealed higher mean antistreptolysin O (ASO) titers in patients with tics and Tourette syndrome,[19–21] although other studies have found no association.[3,82,83] Two studies that found no association in the whole TS cohort did show that the subgroup with comorbid ADHD had statistically elevated ASO titers.[82,84] As antineuronal antibodies are the proposed mediators of SC and PANDAS, there have been cross-sectional studies of antineuronal antibodies in Tourette syndrome. The results have been mixed and conflicting. Although some studies have demonstrated more prevalent antineuronal antibodies in TS,[3,21,85] other studies have failed to find an association.[82,83,86] It is of interest that the three positive studies have proposed a basal ganglia protein of 60 kDa to be the most discriminating antigen in TS compared to controls.[3,21,85] We have reported that this 60 kDa antigen appears to be common to both SC and TS, supporting the hypothesis that post-streptococcal autoimmunity may also be important in TS.[21] It is acknowledged that longitudinal studies comparing clinical, microbiological, and immunological markers are essential to define whether a true association exists.[82]

CONCLUSION

The spectrum of post-streptococcal brain disorders has broadened beyond Sydenham's chorea to include other movement and psychiatric disorders. This group of disorders offers the opportunity to examine the complex immune relationship between microorganisms and the host. Tic disorders, TS, OCD, and ADHD are very common in childhood (up to 5% of children in total). If definitive evidence can be provided for a role of streptococcus in these disorders, it will transform our treatment approach to these common neuropsychiatric disorders in the future.

REFERENCES

1. Jummani R, Okun M. Sydenham chorea. *Arch Neurol* 2001; 58: 311–3.
2. Swedo SE, Leonard HL, Garvey M et al. Pediatric autoimmune neuropsychiatric disorders associated with streptococcal infections: clinical description of the first 50 cases. *Am J Psychiatry* 1998; 155: 264–71.
3. Singer HS, Giuliano JD, Hansen BH et al. Antibodies against human putamen in children with Tourette syndrome. *Neurology* 1998; 50: 1618–24.
4. Sydenham T. *The Entire Works of Thomas Sydenham. Vols 1 and 2*. London: Sydenham Society, 1848. Reprinted Birmingham, AL: Classics in Medicine Society, 1979.

5. Straton CR. The prechoreic stages of chorea. *BMJ* 1885; **2**: 437–8.
6. Bouteille EM. *Traite de la Choree, ou Danse de St. Guy*. Paris: Vincard, 1810.
7. Wesphal P, Wasserman, Malkoff. Ueber den infectiosen Charakter und den Zusammenhang von acutem Gelenkrheumatismus und Chorea. *Berl Klin Wochenschr* 1899; **29**: 638–40.
8. Poynton F, Paine A. *Researches on Rheumatism*. London: Churchill Livingstone Inc, 1913.
9. Thiebaut F. Sydenham's chorea. In: *Handbook of Clinical Neurology: Diseases of the Basal Ganglia*. Vol 6 (Vinken PJ, Bruyn GW, eds). Amsterdam: North Holland Publishing Co, 1968: 409–34.
10. Kiessling LS, Marcotte AC, Culpepper L. Antineuronal antibodies in movement disorders. *Pediatrics* 1993; **92**: 39–43.
11. Nausieda PA, Grossman BJ, Koller WC et al. Sydenham chorea: an update. *Neurology* 1980; **30**: 331–4.
12. Schwartzman J. Chorea minor: review of 175 cases with reference to etiology, treatment and sequelae. *Rheumatology* 1950; **6**: 89.
13. Kurlan R. Tourette's syndrome and 'PANDAS': will the relation bear out? Pediatric autoimmune neuropsychiatric disorders associated with streptococcal infection. *Neurology* 1998; **50**: 1530–4.
14. Jankovic J, Ashizawa T. Tourettism associated with Huntington's disease. *Mov Disord* 1995; **10**: 103–5.
15. van Dijk JG, van der Velde EA, Roos RA, Bruyn GW. Juvenile Huntington disease. *Hum Genet* 1986; **73**: 235–9.
16. Creak M, Guttman E. Chorea, tics, compulsive utterances. *J Med Sci* 1935; **81**: 834.
17. Kerbeshian J, Burd L, Pettit R. A possible post-streptococcal movement disorder with chorea and tics. *Dev Med Child Neurol* 1990; **32**: 642–4.
18. Mercadante MT, Busatto GF, Lombroso PJ et al. The psychiatric symptoms of rheumatic fever. *Am J Psychiatry* 2000; **157**: 2036–8.
19. Muller N, Riedel M, Straube A et al. Increased anti-streptococcal antibodies in patients with Tourette's syndrome. *Psychiatry Res* 2000; **94**: 43–9.
20. Cardona F, Orefici G. Group A streptococcal infections and tic disorders in an Italian pediatric population. *J Pediatr* 2001; **138**: 71–5.
21. Church AJ, Dale RC, Lees AJ et al. Tourette's syndrome: a cross sectional study to examine the PANDAS hypothesis. *J Neurol Neurosurg Psychiatry* 2003; **74**: 602–7.
22. DiFazio MP, Morales J, Davis R. Acute myoclonus secondary to group A beta-hemolytic streptococcus infection: a PANDAS variant. *J Child Neurol* 1998; **13**: 516–8.
23. Dale RC, Church AJ, Benton S et al. Post-streptococcal autoimmune dystonia with isolated bilateral striatal necrosis. *Dev Med Child Neurol* 2002; **44**: 485–9.
24. Dale RC, Church AJ, Surtees RA et al. Post-streptococcal autoimmune neuropsychiatric disease presenting as paroxysmal dystonic choreoathetosis. *Mov Disord* 2002; **17**: 817–20.
25. Cardoso F, Eduardo C, Silva AP, Mota CC. Chorea in fifty consecutive patients with rheumatic fever. *Mov Disord* 1997; **12**: 701–3.
26. Marques-Dias MJ, Mercadante MT, Tucker D, Lombroso P. Sydenham's chorea. *Psychiatr Clin North Am* 1997; **20**: 809–20.
27. Dale RC, Church AJ, Cardoso F et al. Poststreptococcal acute disseminated encephalomyelitis with basal ganglia involvement and auto-reactive antibasal ganglia antibodies. *Ann Neurol* 2001; **50**: 588–95.
28. Murphy ML, Pichichero ME. Prospective identification and treatment of children with pediatric autoimmune neuropsychiatric disorder associated with group A streptococcal infection (PANDAS). *Arch Pediatr Adolesc Med* 2002; **156**: 356–61.
29. Cardoso F, Vargas AP, Oliveira LD et al. Persistent Sydenham's chorea. *Mov Disord* 1999; **14**: 805–7.
30. Freeman JM, Aron AM, Collard JE, MacKay MC. The emotional correlates of Sydenham's chorea. *Pediatrics* 1965; **35**: 42–9.
31. Abbas S, Khanna S, Taly AB. Obsessive-compulsive disorder and rheumatic chorea: is there a connection? *Psychopathology* 1996; **29**: 193–7.
32. Swedo SE, Rapoport JL, Cheslow DL et al. High prevalence of obsessive-compulsive symptoms in patients with Sydenham's chorea. *Am J Psychiatry* 1989; **146**: 246–9.
33. Asbahr FR, Negrao AB, Gentil V et al. Obsessive-compulsive and related symptoms in children and adolescents with rheumatic fever with and without chorea: a prospective 6-month study. *Am J Psychiatry* 1998; **155**: 1122–4.
34. Dale RC, Church AJ, Heyman I et al. Poststreptococcal autoimmune hyperkinetic movement disorders. *Dev Med Child Neurol* 2002; **43**(Suppl. 90): 42.
35. Meltzer H, Gatward R, Goodman R et al. *The Mental Health of Children and Adolescents in Great Britain*. London: HMSO, 2000.
36. Asbahr FR, Ramos RT, Negrao AB, Gentil V. Case series: increased vulnerability to obsessive-compulsive symptoms with repeated episodes of Sydenham chorea. *J Am Acad Child Adolesc Psychiatry* 1999; **38**: 1522–5.
37. Alegret M, Junque C, Valldeoriola F et al. Obsessive-compulsive symptoms in Parkinson's disease. *J Neurol Neurosurg Psychiatry* 2001; **70**: 394–6.
38. De Marchi N, Mennella R. Huntington's disease and its association with psychopathology. *Harv Rev Psychiatry* 2000; **7**: 278–89.
39. Lewis A, Minski L. Chorea and psychosis. *Lancet* 1935; **1**: 536.
40. Stein DJ. Obsessive-compulsive disorder. *Lancet* 2002; **360**: 397–405.
41. Goldenberg J, Ferraz MB, Fonseca ASM et al. Sydenham's chorea: clinical and laboratory findings: analysis of 187 cases. *Rev Paul Med* 1992; **110**: 152–7.
42. Greenfield JG, Wolfsohn JM. The pathology of Sydenham's chorea. *Lancet* 1922; **2**: 603–6.
43. Marie P, Tretiakoff C. Examen histologique des centres nerveux dans un cas de choree aigue de Sydenham. *Rev Neurol* 1920; **36**: 428–38.
44. Colony HS, Malamud N. Sydenham's chorea. a clinicopathologic study. *Neurology* 1956; **6**: 672–6.
45. Nausieda PA, Koller WC, Weiner WJ, Klawans HL. Chorea induced by oral contraceptives. *Neurology* 1979; **29**: 1605–9.
46. Nausieda PA, Koller WC, Weiner WJ, Klawans HL. Modification of postsynaptic dopaminergic sensitivity by female sex hormones. *Life Sci* 1979; **25**: 521–6.
47. Calabresi P, Centonze D, Bernardi G. Cellular factors controlling neuronal vulnerability in the brain: a lesson from the striatum. *Neurology* 2000; **55**: 1249–55.
48. Daoud AS, Zaki M, Shakir R, al-Saleh Q. Effectiveness of sodium valproate in the treatment of Sydenham's chorea. *Neurology* 1990; **40**: 1140–1.
49. Giedd JN, Rapoport JL, Kruesi MJ et al. Sydenham's chorea: magnetic resonance imaging of the basal ganglia. *Neurology* 1995; **45**: 2199–202.
50. Swedo SE, Leonard HL, Schapiro MB et al. Sydenham's chorea: physical and psychological symptoms of St Vitus dance. *Pediatrics* 1993; **91**: 706–13.
51. Kienzle GD, Breger RK, Chun RW et al. Sydenham chorea: MR manifestations in two cases. *AJNR Am J Neuroradiol* 1991; **12**: 73–6.

52. Castillo M, Kwock L, Arbelaez A. Sydenham's chorea: MRI and proton spectroscopy. *Neuroradiology* 1999; **41**: 943–5.
53. Traill Z, Pike M, Byrne J. Sydenham's chorea: a case showing reversible striatal abnormalities on CT and MRI. *Dev Med Child Neurol* 1995; **37**: 270–3.
54. Giedd JN, Rapoport JL, Garvey MA et al. MRI assessment of children with obsessive-compulsive disorder or tics associated with streptococcal infection. *Am J Psychiatry* 2000; **157**: 281–3.
55. Giedd JN, Rapoport JL, Leonard HL et al. Case study: acute basal ganglia enlargement and obsessive-compulsive symptoms in an adolescent boy. *J Am Acad Child Adolesc Psychiatry* 1996; **35**: 913–5.
56. Weindl A, Kuwert T, Leenders KL et al. Increased striatal glucose consumption in Sydenham's chorea. *Mov Disord* 1993; **8**: 437–44.
57. Goldman S, Amrom D, Szliwowski HB et al. Reversible striatal hypermetabolism in a case of Sydenham's chorea. *Mov Disord* 1993; **8**: 355–8.
58. Lee PH, Nam HS, Lee KY et al. Serial brain SPECT images in a case of Sydenham chorea. *Arch Neurol* 1999; **56**: 237–40.
59. Kornek B, Asenbaum S, Dale R et al. Affection of striatal neurons in Sydenham's chorea as demonstrated by IBZM-SPECT and anti-basal ganglia antibodies. *Neuropediatrics* 2002; **33**: A86.
60. Emery ES, Vieco PT. Sydenham chorea: magnetic resonance imaging reveals permanent basal ganglia injury. *Neurology* 1997; **48**: 531–3.
61. Husby G, van de Rijn I, Zabriskie JB et al. Antibodies reacting with cytoplasm of subthalamic and caudate nuclei neurons in chorea and acute rheumatic fever. *J Exp Med* 1976; **144**: 1094–110.
62. Church AJ, Cardoso F, Dale RC et al. Anti-basal ganglia antibodies in acute and persistent Sydenham's chorea. *Neurology* 2002; **59**: 227–31.
63. Kotby AA, El Badawy N, El Sokkary S et al. Antineuronal antibodies in rheumatic chorea. *Clin Diagn Lab Immunol* 1998; **5**: 836–9.
64. Singer HS, Loiselle CR, Lee O et al. Anti-basal ganglia antibody abnormalities in Sydenham chorea. *J Neuroimmunol* 2003; **136**: 154–61.
65. Church AJ, Dale RC, Cardoso F et al. CSF and serum immune parameters in Sydenham's chorea: evidence of an autoimmune syndrome? *J Neuroimmunol* 2003; **136**: 149–53.
66. Archelos JJ, Hartung HP. Pathogenetic role of autoantibodies in neurological diseases. *Trends Neurosci* 2000; **23**: 317–27.
67. Taylor JR, Morshed SA, Parveen S et al. An animal model of Tourette's syndrome. *Am J Psychiatry* 2002; **159**: 657–60.
68. Hallett JJ, Harling-Berg CJ, Knopf PM et al. Anti-striatal antibodies in Tourette syndrome cause neuronal dysfunction. *J Neuroimmunol* 2000; **111**: 195–202.
69. Perlmutter SJ, Leitman SF, Garvey MA et al. Therapeutic plasma exchange and intravenous immunoglobulin for obsessive-compulsive disorder and tic disorders in childhood. *Lancet* 1999; **354**: 1153–8.
70. Knopf PM, Harling-Berg CJ, Cserr HF et al. Antigen-dependent intrathecal antibody synthesis in the normal rat brain: tissue entry and local retention of antigen-specific B cells. *J Immunol* 1998; **161**: 692–701.
71. Bronze MS, Dale JB. Epitopes of streptococcal M proteins that evoke antibodies that cross-react with human brain. *J Immunol* 1993; **151**: 2820–8.
72. Romero M, Mosquera J, Novo E et al. Erythrogenic toxin type B and its precursor isolated from nephritogenic streptococci induce leukocyte infiltration in normal rat kidneys. *Nephrol Dial Transplant* 1999; **14**: 1867–74.
73. Lougee L, Perlmutter SJ, Nicolson R et al. Psychiatric disorders in first-degree relatives of children with pediatric autoimmune neuropsychiatric disorders associated with streptococcal infections (PANDAS). *J Am Acad Child Adolesc Psychiatry* 2000; **39**: 1120–6.
74. Donadi EA, Smith AG, Louzada-Junior P et al. HLA class I and class II profiles of patients presenting with Sydenham's chorea. *J Neurol* 2000; **247**: 122–8.
75. Khanna AK, Buskirk DR, Williams RC Jr et al. Presence of a non-HLA B cell antigen in rheumatic fever patients and their families as defined by a monoclonal antibody. *J Clin Invest* 1989; **83**: 1710–6.
76. Swedo SE, Leonard HL, Mittleman BB et al. Identification of children with pediatric autoimmune neuropsychiatric disorders associated with streptococcal infections by a marker associated with rheumatic fever. *Am J Psychiatry* 1997; **154**: 110–2.
77. Green LN. Corticosteroids in the treatment of Sydenham's chorea. *Arch Neurol* 1978; **35**: 53–4.
78. Shannon KM, Fenichel GM. Pimozide treatment of Sydenham's chorea. *Neurology* 1990; **40**: 186.
79. Mitchell IJ, Cooper AJ, Griffiths MR. The selective vulnerability of striatopallidal neurons. *Prog Neurobiol* 1999; **59**: 691–719.
80. Marques-Dias MJ, Paz J. Aspectos clinicos e tratamento da coreia reumatica. *Revista da Sociedade Cardiologia Estado de Sao Paulo* 1993; **3**: 7.
81. Pena J, Mora E, Cardozo J et al. Comparison of the efficacy of carbamazepine, haloperidol and valproic acid in the treatment of children with Sydenham's chorea: clinical follow-up of 18 patients. *Arq Neuropsiquiatr* 2002; **60**: 374–7.
82. Loiselle CR, Wendlandt JT, Rohde CA, Singer HS. Antistreptococcal, neuronal, and nuclear antibodies in Tourette syndrome. *Pediatr Neurol* 2003; **28**: 119–25.
83. Morshed SA, Parveen S, Leckman JF et al. Antibodies against neural, nuclear, cytoskeletal, and streptococcal epitopes in children and adults with Tourette's syndrome, Sydenham's chorea, and autoimmune disorders. *Biol Psychiatry* 2001; **50**: 566–77.
84. Peterson BS, Leckman JF, Tucker D et al. Preliminary findings of antistreptococcal antibody titers and basal ganglia volumes in tic, obsessive-compulsive, and attention deficit/hyperactivity disorders. *Arch Gen Psychiatry* 2000; **57**: 364–72.
85. Wendlandt JT, Grus FH, Hansen BH, Singer HS. Striatal antibodies in children with Tourette's syndrome: multivariate discriminant analysis of IgG repertoires. *J Neuroimmunol* 2001; **119**: 106–13.
86. Singer HS, Giuliano JD, Hansen BH et al. Antibodies against a neuron-like (HTB-10 neuroblastoma) cell in children with Tourette syndrome. *Biol Psychiatry* 1999; **46**: 775–80.

18

Exploring the pathophysiology of PANDAS: Streptococcus, Sydenham's, and superantigens

Kyle A Williams, Jon E Grant, Patrick Schlievert, and Suck-Won Kim

INTRODUCTION

The past five years have seen an increased interest in the association between *Streptococcus pyogenes* infections and a constellation of neuropsychiatric diseases including Sydenham's chorea (SC), obsessive compulsive disorder (OCD), Tourette syndrome (TS), and pediatric autoimmune neuropsychiatric disorder associated with streptococcal infection (PANDAS). With the landmark publication of the first 50 PANDAS cases in 1998, Swedo and colleagues expanded the landscape of pediatric psychiatry from genetic and environmental factors to bacterial pathogens in the origin of neuropsychiatric disease.[1] This inclusion continues to incite considerable controversy. While numerous studies have supported the association between group A β-hemolytic streptococcus (GABHS) infection and neuropsychiatric sequelae, few investigators have identified reliable streptococcal virulence factors or accepted disease markers; moreover no studies have identified a genetic locus candidate, and the PANDAS phenotype remains debatable.[2–5]

The difficulties in elucidating the pathogenesis of PANDAS are reflective of the complexity of the organism in question and the ubiquity of childhood exposure to GABHS. *Streptococcus pyogenes* is a diverse organism capable of initiating an array of clinical diseases, from uncomplicated pharyngitis to toxic shock syndrome with or without necrotizing fasciitis, and delayed sequelae, including acute rheumatic fever (ARF), Sydenham's chorea, and acute glomerulonephritis. A comprehensive review of streptococcal disease, however, is beyond the scope of this chapter.[6]

Recent advances in our understanding of the GABHS organism, most notably the sequencing of three highly virulent serotypes of GABHS,[7–9] require a re-analysis of the proposed role of GABHS in the etiology of PANDAS. The purpose of this chapter is to clarify our current understanding of the PANDAS phenotype and its related syndromes with emphasis on Sydenham's chorea (SC), review current evidence suggesting an autoimmune etiology in PANDAS and SC, and provide a rationale for the investigation of superantigens (SAGs) in the pathophysiology of PANDAS.

PANDAS

The criteria for PANDAS (see Box 18.1) put forward by Swedo and colleagues share a significant degree of symptomatology with OCD, TS, and SC. Evidence suggests that PANDAS incorporates the psychiatric symptoms of OCD, the motoric hyperactivity of TS and SC, and the temporal association with GABHS infection characteristic of SC.[10,11]

The proposed role of a GABHS-induced autoimmune etiology in PANDAS remains highly contro-

---

Box 18.1 Criteria for PANDAS

1) Presence of obsessive compulsive disorder (OCD) and/or tic disorder
2) Pediatric onset (age three years to puberty)
3) Episodic course of symptom severity
4) Association with group A beta-hemolytic streptococcal infections (GABHS)
5) Association with neurological abnormalities (motor hyperactivity, adventitious movements, or choreiform movements).

Table 18.1 Antineuronal antibody assays for OCD and/or Tourette syndrome, Sydenham's chorea, anorexia nervosa, and healthy controls

Reference	Groups studied	Number positive/ number studied
15	SC	10/11 (91%)
	Controls	9/18 (50%)
16	Movement disorders*	36/45 (80%)
	Non-movement disorders	16/38 (42%)
3	OCD, TS, tics	12/31 (39%)
	Healthy controls	5/21 (24%)
17	RF with chorea	10/21 (47%)
18	TS	25/41 (61%)
	Controls	13/39 (33%)
19	SC (Acute)	10/10 (100%)
	SC (Chronic)	13/14 (92%)
	Controls	0/40
20	SC (Acute)	19/20 (95%)
	SC (Persistent)	9/16 (56%)
	Controls	0/12

* Tics, Tourette, chorea, choreiform movements

versial. Numerous investigators have isolated antibodies that react to neuronal components of the basal ganglia in an array of tic and/or obsessive compulsive disorders. A brief summary of this work is highlighted in Table 18.1, and readers are pointed towards a recent review by Hoekstra and colleagues.[12] No studies to date have characterized antineuronal antibody profiles in a cohort of PANDAS patients. As such, the proposed role for autoimmune involvement in PANDAS borrows heavily from the symptom homology with SC and temporal involvement with GABHS. The predominant theory of streptococcal induction of autoimmune phenomena in SC and PANDAS centers on a process termed molecular mimicry. It is hypothesized that antibodies directed against immunogenic streptococcal proteins bind to endogenous antigens on neurons, cardiac myocytes, and so on, due to a high degree of sequence or structural homology between the streptococcal protein and endogenous proteins.[13] In particular, the M protein, a cell surface streptococcal protein, has been implicated as the streptococcal target and promoter of molecular mimicry due to its sequence homology with basal ganglia epitopes and cross-reactivity with antineuronal antibodies.[14]

Multiple studies have identified antineuronal (ANAs) and anti-basal ganglia antibodies (ABGAs) in SC and tic disorders using indirect immunofluoresence. Husby and colleagues discovered ANAs directed against the caudate and subthalamic nuclei using indirect immunofluoresence and provided preliminary evidence for cross-reactivity between these ANAs and streptococcal M proteins.[21] Using similar methods, Kiessling and colleagues characterized ANAs in children with recent onset of movement disorders; 44% of the movement disorders group were positive for antibodies directed against human caudate, as were 21% of controls.[16] Similarly high false positive rates have been found in studies of ANAs using immunofluoresence in SC and TS.[3,22] Kotby and colleagues reported ABGAs in 100% of SC patients without any false positives in a study using sera from SC patients applied to basal ganglia tissue from a 34-week-old stillborn fetus.[19]

Recent ANAs/ABGAs studies employing western blotting and enzyme-linked immunosorbent assay (ELISA) to improve both specificity and objectivity have met with conflicting results. The first of these studies identified ABGAs in 20 acute and 16 persistent SC patients; ABGAs were detected in 95% of acute SC patients, 56% of chronic SC patients, and 0% of controls using ELISA with whole basal ganglia tissue (caudate, putamen, globus pallidus, and subthalamic nucleus). The investigators reported antibodies directed at antigens of 40, 45, and 60 kilodaltons (kDa) using western blotting.[20] A more recent study failed to identify any difference in antibodies to caudate, putamen, and globus pallidus using ELISA and multiple different tissue preparations in SC.[23] However, when these same tissue preparation methods were used in assessing ABGAs in TS, an increase in ELISA ABGAs reactivity was found in the putamen, but not the caudate or globus pallidus, and western blots revealed binding to antigens of 83, 67, and 60 kDa.[18]

Improvement in tic and OC symptoms in all PANDAS patients treated with either plasma exchange or intravenous immunoglobulin (IVIG) lends further support to an autoimmune etiology for PANDAS.[24] In this study, 10 patients treated with plasma exchange demonstrated significant improvements in OC symptoms and tics compared to 10 receiving saline infusions. The IVIG group showed a 45% decrease in OC symptoms (measured using the Children's Yale-Brown obsessive compulsive scale), but tic levels failed to show significant responses based upon a Tourette syndrome unified rating scale. Furthermore, the decrease in OC symptoms was maintained one year post-treatment in 82% of the treatment groups.[24]

These treatments may represent a removal (plasma exchange), or blockade/dilution (IVIG) of ANAs. It is hypothesized that plasma exchange may induce a return to normal immune function with the removal of the offending autoimmune antibodies. The long-term improvement in the IVIG group, however, is difficult to interpret, and the authors caution against overanalysis of this study due to the broad possible mechanisms of action involved in both treatments.[24] These findings are supported by a study of therapeutic plasma exchange in a group of five non-PANDAS pediatric OCD patients that failed to demonstrate efficacy in reducing OC or tic symptoms based upon the Yale-Brown obsessive compulsive scale.[25]

A recent prospective PANDAS study conducted by Murphy and Pichechero has lent credence to the temporal association between GABHS infection and PANDAS emergence, as well as the ability to identify PANDAS patients in a non-retrograde fashion.[11] The 12 patients in this study demonstrated an abrupt (≈1 week) onset of OCD behavior, 10 were GABHS culture-positive at symptom onset, and six demonstrated a significant relapse in obsessive compulsive symptoms during a six month follow-up period. Interestingly, 75% of the patients in this study did not exhibit motoric involvement, and all patients showed a marked decrease in obsessive compulsive symptoms after antibiotic therapy.

Despite a suggested autoimmune etiology, the T cell response remains largely unclassified in PANDAS and SC. One study examining cytokines (soluble substances associated with T cell activation) in the CSF of 24 pediatric OCD patients found elevations in IL-2 in comparison to attention deficit hyperactivity disorder ($n = 42$) and schizophrenic patients ($n = 22$).[26] Another study reported CSF elevations of both IL-4 and IL-10 in 31% of acute SC patients ($n = 14$) and serum elevations of IL-4, IL-10, and IL-12.[20]

THE IMMUNE RESPONSE IN PANDAS AND SYDENHAM'S CHOREA

While no studies have detected an overwhelming T cell response in either PANDAS or SC, early evidence suggests that T cells may play a central role in the etiology of both. T cells, through activation and specific roles as T helper 1 cells (Th1) and T helper 2 cells (Th2), act as regulators of immune function and, through activation of B cells, regulate antibody production. ABGAs appear to belong to the IgG class of immunoglobulins, the primary anamnestic (memory) immunoglobulin of the immune system.[20] B cells are unable to undergo class switching from IgM to IgG immunoglobulin production without co-stimulatory support from activated Th2 helper cells,[27] which suggests that T cells are involved in the production of IgG class ABGAs.

T cells, which migrate as lymphocytic stem cells from production in the bone marrow, undergo maturation and antigen selectivity in the thymus. Self-antigens are displayed to developing T cells by the antigen presenting cells of the thymus (primarily thymic cortical epithelial cells) by displaying peptides bound to MHC I and MHC II complexes to the T cells. An intricate 'thymic education' system of positive (T cells which do not respond too vigorously) and negative (T cells which respond strongly to self-antigens) selection is employed to ensure mature T cells recognize, but do not respond to, self-antigens before they migrate from the thymus.[28]

B cells, however, undergo maturation and selection in the bone marrow and secondary lymphoid tissues, and autoreactive B cells are deleted through display of low levels of self-antigens in these tissues.[27] As B cells respond to native, non-MHC bound antigens, they are not selected due to reactivity based upon MHC processing and display. B cell activation, characterized by immunoglobulin class switching and antibody production, is dependent upon the display of a recognized antigen bound to MHC II on its surface and subsequent activation of a Th2 cell that recognizes the MHC-antigen complex.[29] Thus T cells, particularly of the Th2 class, are the ultimate guardians against autoimmunity in the immune system.

With respect to GABHS infection and molecular mimicry, any process that potentially interferes with T cell activation may provide the basis for a failure of self-tolerance. *Streptococcus pyogenes* is known to encode multiple virulence factors that interfere with the ability of the immune system to process streptococcal proteins to promote survival *in vivo*.[6] These virulence factors range from mucoid-phenotypes and C5a peptidase, which prevent opsonization and phagocytosis by macrophages, to hyaluronidase, which degrades hyaluronic acid and promotes tissue invasion.[6] One class of GABHS virulence factors currently under intense investigation is a class of T cell stimulatory exotoxins termed superantigens. The following section describes the origin and mechanisms of streptococcal superantigens, the pathogenesis of acute rheumatic fever and SC with respect to GABHS, and is followed by a hypothesized role for superantigens in the etiology of PANDAS and SC.

SUPERANTIGENS

Superantigens are a family of immunostimulatory protein exotoxins produced primarily by GABHS and *Staphylococcus aureus*. Originally isolated from strains of *S. aureus* in patients with menstrual-associated toxic shock syndrome,[30,31] SAGs have since been identified as major virulence factors in invasive serotypes of *S. pyogenes* and *S. aureus*.[32] SAGs are highly implicated in a growing list of autoimmune diseases of varying severity, such as atopic dermatitis,[32,33] guttate psoriasis,[34,35] and multiple sclerosis.[36]

Unlike nominal peptide antigens, SAGs are capable of nonspecifically stimulating vast numbers of CD4+ T cells, resulting in excessive cytokine release and host-tissue destruction. Conventional antigens, when presented to T cells by antigen-presenting cells (APCs), such as macrophages and B-cells, require recognition by all five variable regions (Vβ, Dβ, Jβ, Vα, Jα) of the T cell receptor (TCR).[37] These five elements of the TCR interact with the major histocompatibility complex (MHC) and the antigen bound to the MHC on the APC. Bacterial SAGs bind both the class II major histocompatibility complex (MHC II) molecule on APCs and specific Vβ regions on the TCR, disrupting the normal APC-antigen-TCR interactions that regulate T cell activation.[38] Furthermore, SAGs bind to the TCR outside the antigen-binding groove, thus activating T cells irrespective of the composition of the bound MHC.[39,40]

This SAG-induced cross linking of TCR and the APC activates T cells at orders of magnitude higher than conventional antigens. A normal T cell response to an antigen may activate 1 in 10,000 T cells, while certain SAGs can nonspecifically induce activation of 20% of T cells in a lymphocyte population.[41,42] Additionally, SAGs exhibit extraordinary potency; significant T cell proliferation can be detected with administration of picogram (10^{-12} g/ml) concentrations.[43,44] Binding of the SAG to the TCR-MHC II complex induces a powerful mitogenic response, resulting in massive T cell proliferation and cytokine release, namely interferon-γ, IL-2, and TNF-β from T cells, and IL-1 and TNF-α from macrophages. This SAG-induced cytokine response is far greater than in antigen-driven stimulation of T cells, presumably as a result of the polyclonal activation and proliferation of T cells. In the most severe situations, such as toxic shock syndrome, this cytokine release may result in hypotensive shock, organ failure, and death.

Of the numerous SAGs identified to date, each demonstrates activation of a unique repertoire of the approximately 25 identified human Vβ T cell subsets; while different SAGs may expand the same Vβ subset, each SAG shows a unique profile of Vβ T cell expansion. When analyzed according to amino acid sequence homology and three-dimensional structure, the large family of staphylococcal and streptococcal SAGs segregate into five subgroups. The majority of the streptococcal SAGs fall into a subgroup of bacterial SAGs based upon structural homogeneity. The streptococcal SAGs, classified as streptococcal pyrogenic exotoxins (Spes), contain SpeA, SpeC, SpeJ, SpeK, and the recently discovered SpeL and SpeM.[45] This streptococcal subgroup of SAGs recognize a small number of Vβ T cell subsets (around three Vβ subsets on average), while some staphylococcal SAGs may bind as many as nine Vβ subsets. These SAG divisions are not simply academic; the subgroups reveal a functional homogeneity and evolutionary lineage which, as will be discussed, have important implications in clinical disease.

Distribution of SAGs varies among streptococcal M serotypes because certain SAGs, such as SpeJ, are chromosomally encoded and found in all GABHS serotypes, while the majority of streptococcal SAGs are present on mobile, bacteriophage-encoded elements, and are thus found at varying degrees among GABHS serotypes. Bacteriophage-encoded elements are generated by viral (i.e. bacteriophage) infection of a bacterial host; small sections of bacterial DNA are 'accidentally' packaged, along with viral genetic material, into the replicating virions. The resulting mature virions, termed prophages, carry a piece of the host bacterial genome, which can be transferred and incorporated into the next bacterial host infected by the bacteriophage.

Recent genomic sequencing of three highly invasive serotypes of GABHS (M1, M3, and M18) has revealed that significant portions of these streptococcal genomes comprise prophage-encoded elements.[9,45,46] These prophages encode for streptococcal SAGs and virulence factors almost exclusively, and prophage elements account for as much as 50% of the genomic diversity between these invasive streptococcal serotypes.[46] The mobile nature of prophage-encoded SAG genes results in transfer of these genes between and within M serotypes, resulting in M strain serotypes with unique SAG production profiles.[47] Analysis of invasive M3 serotypes collected over the past century also indicates these prophages mutate, giving rise to variant SAGs with distinct properties.[46] For example, M3 serotypes isolated in the 1920s encode the SAG SpeA1; a single nucleotide substitution, resulting in a single amino acid substitution, has given rise to SpeA3, an SAG currently produced by M3 isolates which demonstrates 50% more mitogenic activity *in vitro* than its predecessor.[46]

The result of this evolution and gene transfer among GABHS serotypes appears to be the emergence of a small number of high-virulence streptococcal phenotypes.[8,46] Epidemiological support for this theory is derived from records of streptococcal disease outbreaks throughout the last century; while over 100 unique M types have been identified, certain M serotypes have repeatedly shown non-random pairing with specific streptococcal diseases.[48] With respect to acute rheumatic fever, the M18 strain has been repeatedly associated with ARF outbreaks in the United States.[46,49,50]

LESSONS FROM SALT LAKE CITY

There have been nine outbreaks of ARF in the United States in the last 18 years, two of them in the intermountain region surrounding Salt Lake City, Utah.[50] Serological data collected from ARF patients in Utah strongly implicate an M18 strain, serotype MGAS8232, as the causative organism in both outbreaks occurring in 1985–86 and 1997–98.[7,51,52] Each recorded peak in the incidence of MGAS8232 among GABHS serotypes was reflected by a 100% increase in the incidence of ARF in the region.[51] Interestingly, analysis of MGAS8232 isolates obtained during both outbreaks indicates the organism remained nearly genetically identical in the 13 years between outbreaks.[7,51]

The outbreaks of ARF in Salt Lake City, Utah, represent a departure from previous US ARF outbreaks in a number of ways. First, the outbreaks occurred in a unique patient demographic; whereas previous outbreaks of ARF have been largely confined to military bases and patients with limited medical and economic resources,[52] the two Utah outbreaks occurred in largely white (97%), middle-class patients with adequate access to medical care. Also, the outbreak was twice due to an M18 organism that has since been highly characterized, as both outbreaks have been ascribed to a genetically identical MGAS8232 strain.[51] This organism also displayed a streptococcal mucoid phenotype, conferring protection against conventional penicillin antibiotics. Finally, an increased incidence of SC over previous ARF outbreaks was observed during both outbreaks, with estimates ranging from a 5–27% increase in SC incidence during both outbreaks.[52]

DNA microarray analysis of 36 M18 serotypes collected over the past 78 years indicates MGAS8232 carries two widely distributed phage-encoded SAG genes, *speA* and *speC* (which code for SAGs speA and speC, respectively), as well as two novel phage-encoded SAG genes, *speL* and *speM* (coding for the novel SAGs speL and speM), which are specific to the M18 strain. Recent characterization of speL and speM indicates they preferentially expand T cells expressing Vβ1, Vβ5.1, Vβ23 (speL), Vβ1, Vβ23 (speM), and, like speC (which is also made by M18 serotypes), are superantigenic at picogram amounts.[45] SpeL and speM share a highly conserved structural architecture with speC, as well as a significant amount of sequence identity (47% and 48%, respectively).[45] SpeC is known to activate T cells that express the Vβ8.2 receptor through a novel mechanism among SAGs, and exhibits a much higher degree of Vβ specificity than other SAGs.[53] Protein crystallography shows speC binds to a high-affinity, zinc-dependent site on MHC II molecules, a unique mechanism among SAGs.[54,55] SpeL and speM also express zinc-binding regions, and their high degree of structural homology with speC suggests they interact with the MHC II-peptide-T cell receptor in the same way as speC.[45]

The increased incidence of SC in the Utah outbreaks may be a consequence of the virulence factors of the M18 MGAS8232 strain, in particular host effects elicited by the superantigens encoded by MGAS8232. In the following section, we describe a hypothesis for the pathogenesis of SC and PANDAS using the MGAS8232 as a model for infection. Finally, we suggest additional directions for research for refining our understanding of PANDAS and SC.

SUPERANTIGENS AND PSYCHIATRIC DISEASE

In a general model for the etiology of PANDAS, Swedo has argued that four conditions must be met; GABHS infection, a susceptible host, an abnormal immune response, and CNS and clinical manifestations.[56] A SAG-mediated etiology in PANDAS and SC fulfills these criteria.

While the streptococcal M protein is an attractive candidate for the establishment of molecular mimicry and production of ABGAs, it is unlikely that the M protein is the sole factor required for establishing an autoimmune disease. Even in ARF outbreaks with highly rheumatogenic M serotypes, such as in Utah, the prevalence of ARF rarely exceeds 1% of the population, and there are probably numerous cases of M18 MGAS8232 per year which do not progress to post-streptococcal sequelae. If M protein was the major determinant of molecular mimicry we would expect to see higher rates of GABHS-induced autoimmune disease. However, the M protein may play a significant role, as specific M serotypes are repeatedly and reliably associated with ARF.[57]

If the clinical manifestations of PANDAS and SC are indeed due to anti-basal ganglia antibodies (ABGAs), analysis of the antibodies themselves may yield insight into their origins. The isolated ABGAs have uniformly been of the IgG class of immunoglobulins (discussed earlier), which indicates an anamnestic, Th2-mediated response over an acute IgM response to streptococcal M protein. Furthermore, investigators have isolated ABGAs which respond to multiple, albeit unknown, neuronal epitopes. This suggests one of three possibilities: these antibodies do not display a high degree of specificity and are capable of binding multiple epitopes, antibodies are binding the same epitope expressed on multiple different neuronal proteins, or these antibodies represent multiple antibodies from distinct B cell lines. The last scenario represents polyclonal B cell activation directed against multiple antigens, a frequent finding in autoimmune diseases known as epitope spreading.

When an antigenic protein, like M protein, is presented to the immune system, one or multiple immunodominant regions are selected by the immune system for recognition and attack. For example, when mice are injected with 167 amino acid length myelin basic protein (MBP) in an animal model of multiple sclerosis called experimental autoimmune encephalomyelitis (EAE), the immune system mounts the greatest T cell response against MBP amino acids 1–11.[58] Inoculation of the mice with MBP causes demyelination and limited hypotonia and paralysis; this paralysis resolves over weeks and the mice regain function. However, injection with the superantigen SEA (staphylococcal enterotoxin A) or SEB (staphylococcal enterotoxin B) causes an immediate relapse in EAE symptoms. Analysis of the immune response following administration of SEA or SEB shows that the immunodominant region of MBP has shifted; the T cell response after SAG injection shows three other distinct regions of the MBP molecule now elicit the greatest T cell response.[58] Furthermore, the T cell response to the original immunodominant region has been downregulated, and the immunodominant region selected after SAG administration stimulates T cells at far higher magnitudes than the original immunodominant peptide.[58]

This SAG-mediated upregulation and shift in the T cell response may have important implications for the B cell response and antibody generation. Indeed, recent evidence indicated SEB can stimulate antibody production three to four-fold against proteins injected one week prior to SAG administration.[59] This upregulation in antibody production is CD4+ T cell dependent, as co-administration of the CD4+ T cell inhibitory interleukin IL-10 with the SAGs completely abrogates the increased antibody production.[59]

With respect to PANDAS and SC, the combination of potentially cross-reactive M protein epitopes and streptococcal SAG production may provide the necessary factors for the induction of an autoimmune disorder. We hypothesize that a synergistic effect between M protein epitopes, SAGs, and the immune system is responsible for antineuronal antibody production and the CNS involvement seen in both diseases.

In this hypothesized model, the GABHS organism must meet two criteria. First, it must contain M protein epitopes that evoke antibodies which cross-react with human neuronal tissue. Second, it must produce SAGs capable of expanding Vβ T cell subsets which bind these cross-reactive epitopes when displayed on MHC II molecules, leading to B cell activation and antineuronal antibody production. We hypothesize that, due to evolution and phage encoded gene transfer, certain high virulence streptococcal serotypes are more likely to express both of these traits, thus increasing the likelihood that infection with these organisms will result in post-streptococcal autoimmune disease.

In this model, the host must also meet certain criteria. It is widely hypothesized that autoreactive T cells may survive selection in the thymus and lay dormant in the periphery, only resulting in expansion upon antigen encounter and by, once again, escaping anergic selection in the periphery.[60] If these 'forbidden clones' encounter a cross-reactive GABHS epitope displayed on an MHC molecule, they may proliferate and drive an antibody response. It is unlikely that these forbidden clones would be involved in the immunodominant response to the streptococcal M protein or, alternatively, that the immunodominant region of the M protein is cross-reactive. However, if SAG production downregulates the immunodominant T cell response, the forbidden clone is bound to the MHC II-displayed epitope of the M protein which it recognizes, and the clone displays a Vβ subset which can be expanded by the SAG, this may result in a massive proliferation of the cross-reactive T cells.

This may result in widespread B cell activation and high levels of autoantibody production. Host susceptibility in this model would thus be a result of faulty T cell selection in the thymus, or due to differences in host susceptibility to the effects of SAGs; evidence exists for both scenarios.[60,61]

This scenario fits with many aspects of PANDAS and SC, and there is indirect evidence to suggest SAG involvement in both disorders. While not yet investigated, it is possible that SAGs have a deleterious effect on the human thymus such that exposure to SAGs in childhood may predispose one to errors in thymic selection and autoimmune disorders. This may explain why multiple GABHS infections seem to be required in patients before they develop PANDAS, or the time lapse between development of ARF and clinical signs of SC. A rush of antineuronal antibodies, driven by SAG T cell expansion, may also explain the explosive onset of symptoms seen in PANDAS, although this may also represent attainment of a threshold of damage before symptoms appear.

Finally, this model may also explain the explosive recurrence in symptoms seen in subsequent GABHS infections in PANDAS patients. It may be possible that once the GABHS infection and SAGs are eliminated from the host, the autoreactive clones are once again downregulated to dormant status by the immune system. Yet, if one is exposed to streptococcal SAGs that overlap in Vβ expansion with SAGs that previously resulted in T cell proliferation and neuropsychiatric disease, the second SAG exposure may result in another round of autoantibody production and clinical disease.

FUTURE DIRECTIONS

While much focus has been placed on antineuronal antibodies and molecular mimicry, very little attention has been focused on streptococcal virulence factors that may account for these processes. Numerous questions remain to be answered in PANDAS and SC. If these are autoimmune disorders, why are they, at times, self-limited and not progressive? Why are children mainly at risk? Against what cell type and specific region are the antineuronal antibodies directed, and why are these structures/proteins immunogenic? Are streptococcal antigens the only microbial pathogens which contribute to PANDAS pathology?

Genomic sequencing and technological advancements in analyzing streptococcal gene products have vastly increased the feasibility of analyzing the effects of streptococcal virulence factors on the human immune system. Future studies directed at these interactions may clarify factors that predispose susceptible hosts to post-streptococcal autoimmune disorders, identify areas for therapeutic intervention, and delineate the pathology of PANDAS and SC.

REFERENCES

1. Swedo SE, Leonard HL, Garvey M et al. Pediatric autoimmune neuropsychiatric disorders associated with streptococcal infections: clinical description of the first 50 cases. *Am J Psychiatry* 1998; **155**: 264–71.
2. Kaplan EL. PANDAS? or PAND? Or both? Or neither? *Contemp Pediatrics* 2000; **17**: 81–96.
3. Murphy TK, Goodman WK, Fudge MW et al. B lymphocyte antigen D8/17: a peripheral marker for childhood-onset obsessive-compulsive disorder and Tourette's syndrome? *Am J Psychiatry* 1997; **154**: 402–7.
4. Shulman ST. Pediatric autoimmune neuropsychiatric disorders associated with streptococci (PANDAS). *Pediatr Infect Dis J* 1999; **18**: 281–2.
5. Kurlan R. Tourette's syndrome and 'PANDAS': will the relation bear out? Pediatric autoimmune neuropsychiatric disorders associated with streptococcal infection. *Neurology* 1998; **50**: 1530–4.
6. Cunningham MW. Pathogenesis of group A streptococcal infections. *Clin Microbiol Rev* 2000; **13**: 470–511.
7. Smoot JC, Barbian KD, Van Gompel JJ et al. Genome sequence and comparative microarray analysis of serotype M18 group A streptococcus strains associated with acute rheumatic fever outbreaks. *Proc Natl Acad Sci* 2002; **99**: 4668–73.
8. Beres SB, Sylva GL, Barbian KD et al. Genome sequence of a serotype M3 strain of group A streptococcus: phage-encoded toxins, the high-virulence phenotype, and clone emergence. *Proc Natl Acad Sci* 2002; **99**: 10078–83.
9. Ferretti JF, McShan WM, Ajdic D et al. Complete sequence of an M1 strain of *Streptococcus pyogenes*. *Proc Natl Acad Sci* 2001; **98**: 4658–63.
10. Snider LA, Swedo SE. Post-streptococcal autoimmune disorders of the central nervous system. *Curr Opin Neurol* 2003; **16**: 359–65.
11. Murphy ML, Pichichero ME. Prospective identification and treatment of children with pediatric autoimmune neuropsychiatric disorder associated with group A streptococcal infection (PANDAS). *Arch Pediatr Adolesc Med* 2002; **156**: 356–61.
12. Hoekstra PJ, Kallenberg CGM, Korf J, Minderaa RB. Is Tourette's syndrome an autoimmune disease? *Mol Psychiatry* 2002; **7**: 437–45.
13. Dale RC, Heyman I. Post-streptococcal autoimmune psychiatric and movement disorders in children. *Br J Psychiatry* 2002; **181**: 188–90.
14. Bronze MS, Dale JB. Epitopes of streptococcal M proteins that evoke antibodies that cross-react with human brain. *J Immunol* 1993; **151**: 2820–8.
15. Swedo SE, Rapoport JL, Cheslow DL et al. High prevalence of obsessive-compulsive symptoms in patients with Sydenham's chorea. *Am J Psychiatry* 1989; **146**: 246–9.
16. Kiessling LS, Marcotte AC, Culpepper L. Antineuronal antibodies in movement disorders. *Pediatrics* 1993; **92**: 39–43.
17. Asbahr FR, Negrao AB, Gentil V et al. Obsessive-compulsive and related symptoms in children and adolescents with rheumatic fever with and without chorea: A prospective 6-month study. *Am J Psychiatry* 1998; **155**: 1122–4.

18. Singer HS, Giuliano JD, Hansen BH et al. Antibodies against human putamen in children with Tourette syndrome. *Neurology* 1998; **50**: 1618–24.
19. Kotby AA, El Badawy N, El Sokkary S et al. Antineuronal antibodies in rheumatic chorea. *Clin Diagn Lab Immunol* 1998; **5**: 836–9.
20. Church AJ, Dale RC, Cardoso F et al. CSF and serum immune parameters in Sydenham's chorea: evidence of an autoimmune syndrome? *J Neuroimmunol* 2003; **136**: 149–53.
21. Husby G, van de Rijn I, Zabriskie JB et al. Antibodies reacting with cytoplasm of subthalamic and caudate nuclei neurons in chorea and acute rheumatic fever. *J Exp Med* 1976; **144**: 1094–110.
22. Swedo SE, Leonard HL, Schapiro MB et al. Sydenham chorea: physical and psychological symptoms of St. Vitus dance. *Pediatrics* 1993; **91**: 706–13.
23. Singer HS, Loiselle CR, Lee O et al. Anti-basal ganglia antibody abnormalities in Sydenham chorea. *J Neuroimmunol* 2003; **136**: 154–61.
24. Perlmutter SJ, Leitman SF, Garvey MA et al. Therapeutic plasma exchange and intravenous immunoglobulin for obsessive-compulsive disorder and tic disorders in childhood. *Lancet* 1999; **354**: 1153–58.
25. Nicolson R, Swedo SE, Lenane M et al. An open trial of plasma exchange in childhood-onset obsessive-compulsive disorder without poststreptococcal exacerbations. *J Am Acad Child Adolesc Psychiatry* 2000; **39**: 1313–5.
26. Mittleman BB, Castellanos FX, Jacobsen LK et al. Cerebrospinal fluid cytokines in pediatric neuropsychiatric disease. *J Immunol* 1997; **159**: 2994–9.
27. Delves PJ, Roitt IM. The immune system. First of two parts. *N Engl J Med* 2000; **343**: 37–49.
28. Fink PJ, Bevan MJ. Positive selection of thymocytes. *Adv Immunol* 1995; **59**: 99–133.
29. Delves PJ, Roitt IM. The immune system. Second of two parts. *N Engl J Med* 2000; **343**: 108–17.
30. Barsumian EL, Schlievert PM, Watson DW. A new staphylococcal enterotoxin, enterotoxin F, associated with toxic-shock-syndrome *Staphylococcus aureus* isolates. *Lancet* 1978; **1**: 1017–21.
31. Schlievert PM, Shands KN, Dan BB et al. Identification and characterization of an exotoxin from *Staphylococcus aureus* associated with toxic-shock syndrome. *J Infec Dis* 1981; **143**: 509–16.
32. Yarwood JM, Leung DY, Schlievert PM. Evidence for the involvement of bacterial superantigens in psoriasis, atopic dermatitis, and Kawasaki syndrome. *FEMS Microbiol Lett* 2000; **192**: 1–7.
33. Travers JB, Hamid QA, Norris DA et al. Epidermal HLA-DR and the enhancement of cutaneous reactivity to superantigenic toxins in psoriasis. *J Clin Invest* 1999; **104**: 1181–9.
34. Leung DY, Meissner HC, Fulton DR et al. Toxic shock syndrome toxin-secreting *Staphylococcus aureus* in Kawasaki syndrome. *Lancet* 1993; **342**: 1385–8.
35. Leung DY, Sullivan KE, Brown-Whitehorn TF et al. Association of toxic shock syndrome toxin- and exfoliative toxin-secreting *Staphylococcus aureus* with Kawasaki syndrome complicated by coronary artery disease. *Pediatr Res* 1997; **42**: 268–72.
36. Soos JM, Schiffenbauer J, Johnson HM. Treatment of PL/J mice with the superantigen, staphycoccal enterotoxin B, prevents development of experimental allergic encephalomyelitis. *J Neuroimmunol* 1993; **43**: 39–43.
37. Davis MM, Bjorkman PJ. T-cell antigen receptor genes and T-cell recognition. *Nature* 1988; **334**: 395–402.
38. McCormick JK, Yarwood JM, Schlievert PM. Toxic shock syndrome and bacterial superantigens: an update. *Ann Rev Microbiol* 2001; **55**: 77–104.
39. Russell JK, Pontzer CH, Johnson HM. The I-Aβb region (65–85) is a binding site for the superantigen staphylococcal enterotoxin A. *Biochem Biophys Res Commun* 1990; **168**: 696–701.
40. Russell JK, Pontzer CH, Johnson HM. Both α-helices along the major histocompatibility complex binding cleft are required for staphylococcal enterotoxin A function. *Proc Natl Acad Sci* 1991; **88**: 7228–32.
41. Schlievert PM. Staphylococcal and streptococcal superantigens. In: *Bacterial Protein Toxins* (Burns DL, Barbieri JT, Iglewski BH, Rappuoli R, eds). Washington DC: ASM Press, 2003: 293–308.
42. Llewelyn M, Cohen J. Superantigens: microbial agents that corrupt immunity. *Lancet Infec Dis* 2002; **2**: 156–62.
43. Dinges MM, Orwin PM, Fast DJ et al. Toxic shock syndrome-associated staphylococcal and streptococcal pyrogenic toxins are potent inducers of tumor necrosis factor production. *Infec Immunol* 1989; **57**: 291–4.
44. Hackett SP, Stevens DL. Superantigens associated with staphylococcal and streptococcal toxic shock syndrome are potent inducers of tumor necrosis factor-beta synthesis. *J Infec Dis* 1993; **168**: 232–5.
45. Smoot LM, McCormick JK, Smoot JC et al. Characterization of two novel superantigens made by an acute rheumatic fever strain of *Streptococcus pyogenes*. *Infec Immunol* 2002; **70**: 7095–104.
46. Banks DJ, Beres SB, Musser JM. The fundamental contribution of phages to GAS evolution, genome diversification and strain emergence. *Trends Microbiol* 2002; **10**: 515–21.
47. Norrby-Teglund A, Thulin P, Gan BS et al. Evidence for superantigen involvement in severe group A streptococcal tissue infections. *J Infec Dis* 2001; **184**: 853–60.
48. Efstratiou A. Group A streptococci in the 1990s. *J Antimicrobial Chemother* 2000; **45**(Suppl): 3–12.
49. Johnson DR, Stevens DL, Kaplan EL. Epidemiologic analysis of group A streptococcal serotypes associated with severe systemic infections, rheumatic fever, or uncomplicated pharyngitis. *J Infec Dis* 1992; **166**: 374–82.
50. Musser JM, Krause R. The revival of group A streptococcal diseases, with a commentary on staphylococcal toxic shock syndrome. In: *Emerging Infections* (Krause RM, ed). San Diego, CA: Academic Press, 1998: 185–218.
51. Smoot JC, Korgenski EK, Daly JA et al. Molecular analysis of group A streptococcus type emm 18 isolates temporally associated with acute rheumatic fever outbreaks in Salt Lake City, Utah. *J Clin Microbiol* 2002; **40**: 1805–10.
52. Veasy LG, Wiedmeier SE, Orsmond GS et al. Resurgence of acute rheumatic fever in the intermountain area of the United States. *N Engl J Med* 1987; **316**: 421–7.
53. Li P-L, Tiedemann RE, Moffat SL, Fraser JD. The superantigen streptococcal pyrogenic exotoxin C (SPE-C) exhibits a novel mode of action. *J Exp Med* 1997; **186**: 375–83.
54. Sundberg EJ, Hongmin L, Llera AS et al. Structures of two streptococcal superantigens bound to TCR β chains reveal diversity in the architecture of T cell signaling complexes. *Structure* 2002; **10**: 687–99.
55. Li Y, Li H, Dimasi N et al. Crystal structure of a superantigen bound to the high-affinity, zinc-dependent site on MHC class II. *Immunity* 2001; **14**: 93–104.
56. Swedo SE. Pediatric autoimmune neuropsychiatric disorders associated with streptococcal infections (PANDAS). *Mol Psychiatry* 2002; 7 Suppl 2: S24–5.
57. Bessen DE, Veasy LG, Hill HR et al. Serologic evidence for a class I group A streptococcal infection among rheumatic fever patients. *J Infec Dis* 1995; **172**: 608–11.
58. Soos JM, Mujtaba MG, Schiffenbauer J et al. Intramolecular epitope spreading induced by staphylococcal entertoxin super-

antigen reactivation of experimental allergic encephalomyelitis. *J Neuroimmunol* 2002; **123**: 30–4.
59. Torres BA, Perrin GQ, Mujtaba MG et al. Superantigen enhancement of specific immunity: antibody production and signaling pathways. *J Immunol* 2002; **169**: 2907–14.
60. Karlsen AE, Dyrberg T. Molecular mimicry between non-self, modified self and self in autoimmunity. *Semin Immunol* 1998; **10**: 25–34.
61. Kotb M. Bacterial pyrogenic exotoxins as superantigens. *Clin Microbiol Rev* 1995; **8**: 411–26.

19

Antibodies against CNS antigens in autism: Possible cross-reaction with dietary proteins and infectious agent antigens

Aristo Vojdani and Edwin L Cooper

INTRODUCTION

One of the advantages of working for 25 years in a research and clinical laboratory is having the opportunity to observe the evolution of a test assay from a crude and nonspecific to a pure and specific level. Between 1975 and 1980, we started our testing in relation to antibodies to CNS antigens with antibrain antibodies using a section of the mammalian brain and immunofluorescent examinations. Due to many false positive results, we began looking for a more specific assay for detecting antibodies against different components of nervous system antigens. Due to advancements in biochemistry, affinity purification, and the development of enzyme-linked immunoassay (ELISA) in the early 1980s, detection of antibodies against pure antigens such as myelin basic protein (MBP), myelin associated glycoprotein (MAG), myelin oligodendrocyte glycoprotein (MOG), ganglioside, sulfatide, glutamate receptor, tubulin, and neurofilaments (NFT) became possible in our laboratory. During the past 10 years, thanks to genetic engineering and recombinant antigens, different encephalitogenic peptides became available and are used in our assays. These recombinant antigens and peptides did not only render the antibody assays specific but helped us to investigate the source of antibodies and to understand the mechanisms behind the root causes underlying autoimmune reactions to antigens of the nervous system.

AUTOIMMUNE NEUROLOGICAL DISORDERS

Autoimmune neurological disorders occur when immunologic tolerance to myelin and other neurologic antigens of Schwann cells, axons, and the motor or ganglioside neurons are lost. The resulting demyelinating disease shares the pathologic features of myelin destruction, accompanied by an inflammatory infiltration into the brain, spinal cord, or the optic nerve.[1,2]

The most common demyelinating disease is multiple sclerosis. Multiple sclerosis (MS) is a disease of the myelin CNS that is clinically characterized by episodes of neurologic dysfunction separated by time and space. Pathologically, multiple sclerosis may be diagnosed by measuring the infiltration of monocytes, helper T-cells, and demyelination, as well as the appearance of measurable antibody levels against MBP, MOG, and α-B-crystallin. The striking appearance of inflammatory cells in the brain, spinal cord, and cerebrospinal fluid in MS patients further indicates that an attack against the immune system, directed at certain components of CNS myelin, is central to the pathogenesis of MS.[3–5]

Activated T-cells, activated monocytes/macrophages and their cytokines play a special role in the pathogenesis of disease. Activated T-helper cells release interleukin-2, interferon-γ, and lymphotoxins, while monocytes release tumor necrosis factor-α (TNF-α). The monocytes are primed by T-cell-derived interferon-γ to release TNF-α. TNF-α and lymphotoxins have been reported to be injurious to myelin and oligodendrocytes.

Using immunogold-labeled peptides of myelin antigens and high-resolution microscopy, techniques that can detect antigen-specific antibodies *in situ*, immunologists have identified autoantibodies specific for myelin antigen myelin/oligodendrocyte glycoprotein of the CNS. These autoantibodies are specifically bound to disintegrating myelin around axons in lesions of acute MS and in the marmoset model of allergic encephalomyelitis. These findings represent direct evidence that autoantibodies against a specific myelin protein mediate target membrane damage in CNS demyelinating disease.[6-8]

In the complete collection of proteins extracted from MS-affected myelin, the dominant human antigen for CD4+ T-cells appears to be α-B-crystallin, a small heat shock protein. Enhanced levels of α-B-crystallin are present in the cytosol of oligodendrocytes and astrocytes in MS lesions, where it is upregulated at the earliest stages of lesional formation. After myelin phagocytosis in MS lesions, α-B-crystallin becomes available to T-cells, suggesting the important role of this autoantigen in the pathogenesis of MS. The presentation of these antigens by T-cells to B-cells results in autoantibody production. It can therefore be postulated that IgG, IgM, and IgA antibodies against MBP, MOG, and α-B-crystallin will aid in the diagnosis of MS and other demyelinating diseases.[9-11]

Based on these immunological mechanisms that contribute to injury of neurons, it is possible to culture lymphocytes from patients with questionable neurological disorders and antigens, and to replicate a majority of these steps *in vitro*. Only lymphocytes of patients with neurological disorders that possess prior memory of exposure to these antigens *in vivo* will be stimulated when they are exposed to them in the test tube. Such experiments should result in the production of a significant amount of pro-inflammatory cytokines – interferon-γ, TNF-α, TNF-β, or all three cytokines.

Due to repeated injury to neurons by cytokines, activated helper cells, macrophages, complement, and proteases, neuron-specific antigens are released into the circulation. The release of these brain antigens and initiation of immune response against them results in IgG, IgM, and IgA antibodies in the blood of patients with neurological disorders against one or all of the following CNS antigens:

1) Myelin basic protein
2) Myelin associated glycoprotein
3) Myelin oligodendrocyte glycoprotein
4) Proteolipid protein
5) α-B-crystallin
6) Phosphodiesterase
7) Transaldolase
8) Glutamate receptor
9) S-100 protein
10) Ganglioside
11) Sulfatide
12) Tubulin
13) Cerebellar peptide
14) Neurofilaments
15) Muscarinic acetylcholine receptor
16) Acetylcholine receptor.

Antibodies to these and other nervous system antigens have been found in a variety of neuroimmune conditions. These antibodies and their occurrences in different conditions are shown in Table 19.1.

ANTIBODIES IN CHILDREN WITH AUTISM

The etiology and pathogenesis of autism is not well understood. The disorder may have a variety of causes including environmental, neural, genetic, immune, and biochemical. Structural abnormalities have been identified in areas of the autistic brain, with a pattern suggesting that a neurodevelopmental abnormality may have occurred.[12,13] Immunological research has suggested autoimmunity as a pathogenic factor in autism.[14-16] Circulating autoantibodies are produced against brain tissue antigens and hence aid in the diagnosis of different autoimmune neurological disorders.

Recently, we measured autoantibodies against nine different neuron-specific antigens and three cross-reactive peptides in the sera of autistic subjects and healthy controls by means of enzyme-linked immunosorbent assay (ELISA) testing. The antigens were MBP, MAG, ganglioside (GM_1), sulfatide (SULF), chondroitin sulfate ($CONSO_4$), MOG, α-B-crystallin (α-B-CRYS), neurofilament proteins (NAFP), tubulin and three cross-reactive peptides, *Chlamydia pneumoniae* (CPP), streptococcal M protein (STM6P), and milk butyrophilin (BTN). Autistic children showed the highest levels of IgG, IgM, and IgA antibodies against all neurologic antigens as well as the three cross-reactive peptides. These antibodies were shown to be specific, since immune absorption demonstrated that only neuron-specific antigens or their cross-reactive epitopes could significantly reduce antibody levels. These antibodies may have been synthesized as a result of an alteration in the blood brain barrier. The barrier promotes access of preexisting T-cells and central nervous system antigens to immunocompetent cells, which may initiate inflammatory/immune responses.[17]

Detecting antibodies against CNS antigens in autism

Forty subjects (23 males and 17 females), from three to 12 years of age (mean 6.4 years), with a diagnosis of autism, were sent by different clinicians to our laboratory for immunological examination. The clinical diagnosis of autism was made according to the DSM-III-R criteria, established by the American

Table 19.1 Antibodies to nervous system antigens in different conditions	
Antigens	**Disease occurrences**
Myelin basic protein Myelin oligodendrocyte α-B-crystallin Transaldolase	Multiple sclerosis
Myelin associated glycoprotein (MAG – GM1, LM1, GD1b, GQ1b) and sulfatide	Demyelinating sensorimotor neuropathies or polyneuropathy with paraproteinemias
Campylobactor jejuni	Guillain Barre syndrome
Sulfatide and chondroitin sulfate	Chronic sensory neuropathy
Glutamate receptors	Amyotrophic lateral sclerosis or Lou Gehrig's disease
Ion channel	Rassmussen's encephalitis
Cerebellar tissue and Purkinje cells	Paraneoplastic cerebellar degeneration and autism
Myelin basic protein, neuron-axon filament protein (NFP), glial fibrillary acidic protein (GFAP), and tubulin	Neurotoxicity and autism
S-100 protein	Alzheimer's, brain aging, and vascular dementia
Muscarinic acetylcholine receptor	Schizophrenia
Acetylcholine receptor	Myasthenia Gravis

Psychiatric Association (Washington DC), as well as by a developmental pediatrician, a pediatric neurologist, and/or a licensed psychologist. Blood samples were excluded if their medical histories included head injury, evidence of gliomas, failure to thrive, and other known factors that may contribute to abnormal development. For comparison, blood samples from 40 healthy, age- and sex-matched controls were included in this analysis. ELISA assay antibodies (IgG, IgM, and IgA) against nine different neuron-specific antigens and cross-reactive peptides were measured in both groups according to the method described by Vojdani and colleagues.[17]

Levels of IgG

Using ELISA assays, sera from 40 healthy subjects and 40 autistic children were analyzed for the presence of IgG, IgM, and IgA antibodies against nine neuron-specific antigens and three encephalitogenic and cross-reactive proteins. The OD for IgG antibody values obtained with 1:100 dilution of healthy control sera ranged from .01 to .84, varying among subjects and antigens. The mean ± standard deviation (SD) of these OD values ranged from .13 ± .09 to .23 ± .18. The corresponding IgG OD values from autistic children's sera ranged from .05 to 2.47 with the mean ± SD of IgG values ranging from .41 ± .33 to .72 ± .65. The differences between mean ± SD of control sera and mean ± SD of autistic children's sera were highly significant ($p < .001$). At a cut-off value of .3 OD, levels of IgG antibody against these antigens were calculated in control and patient sera and it was found that while 5–22.5% of control sera had IgG values higher than .3 OD, the autistic children's group showed elevated IgG values in 47.5–57.5% ($p < .001$) (see Table 19.2).

Table 19.2 Percent elevation of IgG, IgM, and IgA antibody levels against nine different neural antigens in controls (C) and children with autism at a cut-off of two SDs above the mean of controls

Antigen	IgG		IgM		IgA	
	Controls	Patients	Controls	Patients	Controls	Patients
MBP	14	57	16	61	12	48
MAG	9	49	12	56	5	29
GM_1	6	52	9	59	3	37
SULF	4	51	13	64	6	41
$CONSO_4$	7	46	12	60	5	42
MOG	11	43	11	58	7	39
α-B-CRYS	4	53	9	56	3	21
NFT	6	49	8	53	6	27
Tubulin	12	50	10	56	8	36

Levels of IgM and IgA

In comparison, levels of IgM and IgA antineuron-specific antigens in sera of autistic children were significantly higher against all tested antigens ($p < .001$) when the .3 OD cut-off point was used; 10–20% of controls versus 57.5–72.55% of autistic children's sera showed elevated IgM antibody levels ($p < .001$) (see Table 19.2). Likewise, percent elevated serum IgA antineuronal autoantibodies at the OD value of greater than .3 were significantly higher in autistic children than in controls. The percent positive for IgA antibodies in controls ranged from 5–15%, and in patients, from 20–52.5% ($p < .001$) (see Table 19.2).

Origin of antibodies to neuron-specific antigens

In demyelinating sensorimotor neuropathies, such as Guillain-Barre syndrome (GBS) and chronic inflammatory demyelinating polyneuropathy, IgG, IgM, and IgA antibodies have been detected against myelin and acidic glycolipids (GM_1, LM_1, GQ_1, and GD_1b) and sulfatide.[18–20] These antibodies cross-react with Campylobacter jejuni and GM_1 has been observed in acute GBS.[21,22] In patients with polyneuropathy associated with paraproteinemias, IgM against MAG and IgM or IgA monoclonal gammopathy have been observed.[23] Antibodies against sulfatide and chondroitin sulfate are found in the blood of subjects suffering from chronic sensory neuropathy. These antibodies are polyreactive and react with neurons on the surface of dorsal root ganglia where the blood nerve barrier is relatively permeable.[24,25]

NEUROIMMUNE ABNORMALITIES INDUCED BY XENOBIOTICS AND METALS

It is of considerable interest that antibodies to neuron-specific antigens are prevalent in populations exposed to environmental and occupational chemicals and in patients with neurodegenerative diseases in which viruses or other infectious agents are the suspected etiological agents. For example, IgG antibodies to MBP, neuronal cytoskeletal proteins, and neurofilaments are detected in workers exposed to lead or mercury.[26] The titer of these antibodies is significantly correlated with blood lead or urinary mercury, which are the typical indices of exposure. Moreover, the level of these antibodies is correlated with the degree of sensorimotor deficits, because these antibodies interfere with neuromuscular function.[27]

Toxic chemicals (such as polychlorinated biphenyl or PCBs, mercury, lead, and others) can induce alteration or overexpression of genes involved in regional brain GFAP and astroglial GRP. Overexpression of these genes results in a change in the structural differentiation of astrocytes and hence autoimmune responses to neurofilament proteins.[28–30]

Edelson and Cantor demonstrated a body burden of neurotoxins in more than 90% of autistic children.[31,32] These authors presented evidence for genetic and environmental aspects of a hypothetical process believed to cause immune system injury secondary to exposure to the immunotoxins. Activation of the immune system is caused by toxins leading to the production of autoantibodies against haptens (the toxic chemicals attached to brain proteins). The subsequent damage may be considered a component in the etiologic process of neurotoxicity in the autistic spectrum disorders.

INFECTIONS AND NEUROIMMUNOLOGICAL DISORDERS

Numerous recent studies have attempted to associate infectious agents with neurological disorders, including paramyxoviruses, cytomegalovirus, T-lymphotropic viruses, and herpes virus type 6. For example, the cerebrospinal fluid (CSF) of 17 patients with relapsing remitting MS, 20 patients with progressive MS, and 27 patients suffering from other neurological diseases has been examined by polymerase chain reaction (PCR). Results revealed *Chlamydia pneumoniae* DNA in 97% of MS patients, versus only 18% controls or patients with other neurological disorders. Moreover, *C. pneumoniae* was isolated from the CFS of 64% of MS patients, versus 11% of controls. The mere presence of *C. pneumoniae* or other infectious agents in the CNS does not necessarily prove that the organism triggers the disease. Rather, the presence of the organism may exacerbate a pathogenic process initiated by other mechanisms.[33–37]

One explanation for disease development postulates that specific antigenic epitopes from an unspecified infectious agent or agents induce(s) a host immune response in which cross-reactivity with myelin triggers disease, a concept referred to as molecular mimicry. In this scenario, certain T cells and/or antibodies elicited in response to antigens of the infectious agent also recognize relevant self-antigens in the CNS, thereby initiating the destructive autoimmune process.[38–43]

Until recently, there has been little direct evidence readily available in support of the molecular mimicry hypothesis to clearly delineate the role of infectious agents as a cause for neurological disorders. For example, studies in mice have shown that infection with Theiler's virus elicits an inflammatory response in the CNS that progresses to chronic experimental autoimmune encephalomyelitis.[44] Epitopes of streptococcal M proteins have also been shown to evoke antibodies that cross-react with human brain neuronal cell basal ganglia, which are potentially involved in the pathogenesis of Sydenham's chorea (associated with acute rheumatic fever). Very recently, a rather elaborate experiment of a well-characterized rat model of MS has been used to investigate the causal relationship between infections and MS. Investigators identified a 20-mer peptide from a protein specific to *C. pneumoniae* which shares a seven-amino acid motif with a critical epitope of myelin basic protein, a major CNS antigen targeted by the autoimmune response in MS. This bacterial peptide induces a Th1 response, accompanied by severe clinical and histological experimental autoimmune encephalomyelitis in Lewis rats, a condition closely reflective of many aspects of MS. Studies with peptide analogues suggest that different populations of encephalitogenic T cells are activated by the *C. pneumoniae* and myelin basic protein antigens.[45,46]

Many infectious agents including measles,[47] rubella virus,[48] and cytomegalovirus[49] have long been suspected as etiologic factors in autism. However, whether these viruses induce brain autoantibodies has not yet been explored.[16] For this reason, we reviewed the literature and found that over 60 different microbial peptides have been reported to cross-react with human brain tissue and MBP. Furthermore, these peptides not only cross-react with MBP and induce T-cell responses but they can also induce experimental autoimmune encephalomyelitis.[45,46,50]

Based upon the observation that maternal infection increases the risk for schizophrenia and autism in offspring, it has been shown that respiratory infection of pregnant mice (both BALB/c and C57BL/6 strains) with the human influenza virus resulted in offspring that displayed highly abnormal behavioral responses as adults. As in schizophrenia and autism, these offspring displayed deficits in pre-pulse inhibition (PPI) in the acoustic startle response. Compared with control mice, the infected mice also showed striking responses to the acute administration of antipsychotic and psychomimetic drugs. Moreover, these mice were deficient in exploratory behavior in both open-field and novel-object tests, and they were deficient in social interaction. At least some of these behavioral changes were probably attributable to the maternal immune response itself. Researchers concluded that abnormal levels of cytokine production, which interfere with neuroimmune communications, are responsible for abnormal development of the brain.[51,52]

DIETARY PROTEINS AND NEUROIMMUNOLOGICAL DISORDERS

Among families with autistic children, it is well known that elimination of milk and wheat from a diet significantly improves the child's condition. This clinical finding correlates with laboratory results reported by Stefferl and colleagues, who found that an encephalitogenic T-cell response to MOG can be either induced or alternatively suppressed as a consequence of immunological cross-reactivity or molecular mimicry with the extracellular IV-like domain of milk protein butyrophilin.[53] All of these clinical laboratory findings shed light on our detection of higher levels of antibodies against milk antigens in autistic sera. Based on previous research,[45,46,50,53] we chose streptococcus synthetic peptide containing the conserved M protein or brain cross-reactive epitope, a *C. pneumoniae* specific peptide, and the butyrophilin milk peptide, which modulates the encephalitogenic T-cell response to MOG in experimental autoimmune encephalomyelitis, for our cross-reactivity study.

Indeed, when we tested IgG, IgM, and IgA antibodies against milk peptides, we found that every single serum with ELISA values higher than .3 OD against neurological antigens also exhibited high levels of antibodies against neurological antigens and antibodies against milk peptides in a higher percentage of experimental sera (see Table 19.3). These antibodies appear to be specific since in our absorption studies, milk butyrophilin had a similar effect to MBP or MOG in reducing antibody levels from highly positive sera.[17] Similar to milk peptides, antibodies against different gliadin peptides have also been described in celiac disease, gluten ataxia, and recently in children with autism.

POSSIBLE MECHANISM FOR NEUROIMMUNE ABNORMALITIES IN AUTISM

One of the most frequent presentations of gluten sensitivity is neurologic dysfunction called gluten ataxia. Up to 33% of patients presenting with neurologic dysfunction and 90% of patients presenting with pruritic vesicular rash of dermatitis herpetiformis associated with gluten sensitivity also have celiac disease.[54] While the remaining patients have serologic markers or anti-gliadin antibodies and genetic susceptibility (HLADQ2), they do not have histologic evidence of small bowel involvement. Based on a major epidemiologic study involving more than 200 patients, gluten ataxia was found to account for 40% of cases with idiopathic sporadic cerebellar degeneration. When patients with gluten ataxia were autopsied, perivascular cuffing with inflammatory cells, predominantly affecting the cerebellum, and loss of Purkinje cells were detected. These inflammatory reactions resulting in Purkinje cell loss imply that the neurologic insult may be immune-mediated.[55–58] It is not clear whether such immune-mediated damage is primarily cellular or antibody-driven.

In a recent study, investigators assessed the reactivity of sera from patients with gluten ataxia, patients newly diagnosed with celiac disease without neurologic dysfunction, and healthy control subjects.[58] Using indirect immunocytochemisty on human cerebellar and rat CNS tissue, cross-reactivity of a commercial IgA antigliadin antibody with cerebellar tissue was analyzed. Sera from 12 of 13 patients with gluten ataxia strongly presented stained Purkinje cells. Less intense staining was observed in some but not all sera from patients with newly diagnosed celiac disease without neurologic dysfunction. At high dilutions (1:800) staining was observed only using sera from patients with gluten ataxia but not from control subjects. Sera from patients with gluten ataxia also stained some brainstem and cortical neurons in rat CNS tissue. Commercial anti-gliadin antibody stained human Purkinje cells in a similar manner. Absorption of the antigliadin antibodies using crude gliadin abolished the staining in patients with celiac disease without neurologic dysfunction, but not in those with gluten ataxia. The study's conclusion suggested that patients with gluten ataxia have antibodies against Purkinje cells that cross-react with epitopes on Purkinje cells, and humoral immune responses are involved in the pathogenesis of gluten ataxia.[58]

STRUCTURAL SIMILARITY BETWEEN GLIADIN PEPTIDES AND CEREBELLAR ANTIGENS

Several distinctive neurologic disorders occur in patients with paraneoplastic cerebellar degeneration (PCD). The syndrome of PCD generally occurs in

Table 19.3 Serum levels of gliadin and cerebellar peptide antibodies (IgG, IgM, and IgA) in controls (C) and in patients with autism, expressed as OD in ELISA

Specimen	Gliadin		Cerebellar	
	C	Autism	C	Autism
1	.01	.10	.11	.21
2	.13	.02	.08	.03
3	.02	.65	.09	.88
4	.18	.15	.27	.05
5	.12	.23	.14	.11
6	.09	.37	.03	.29
7	.01	.07	.07	.04
8	.13	.54	.09	.12
9	.46	.85	.06	.54
10	.02	.71	.04	.62
11	.58	.23	.46	.16
12	.05	.12	.04	.07
13	.13	.06	.08	.14
14	.11	.13	.16	.12
15	.21	.20	.07	.11
16	.16	.57	.13	.16
17	.14	.16	.18	.13
18	.35	.11	.39	.18
19	.15	.17	.12	.16
20	.21	.13	.19	.12
21	.07	.79	.05	.38
22	.08	1.25	.06	.67
23	.12	.41	.05	.35
24	.14	1.34	.13	.61
25	.18	.21	.12	.14
26	.38	.16	.17	.21
27	.11	.08	.23	.03
28	.15	.21	.09	.15
29	.08	.85	.02	.98
30	.05	.57	.04	.89
31	.22	.21	.17	.09
32	.01	.98	.04	.12
33	.05	.06	.06	.15
34	.03	.21	.02	.56
35	.09	.17	.07	.22
36	.14	1.36	.28	.58
37	.17	.09	.12	.06
38	.10	.81	.09	.63
39	.02	.09	.11	.06
40	.07	.21	.05	.12

Table 19.3 Continued

Specimen	Gliadin		Cerebellar	
	C	Autism	C	Autism
41	.26	.17	.14	.15
42	.49	.12	.58	.16
43	.02	.99	.08	.48
44	.08	1.24	.17	.67
45	.74	.62	.14	.45
46	.09	.08	.21	.07
47	.14	1.45	.08	.18
48	.18	.75	.05	.69
49	.53	.13	.67	.12
50	.21	1.18	.14	.94
Mean	.17	.45	.14	.32
±	±	±	±	±
SD	.16	.42	.13	.33
p value		.000000		.000247

patients with neoplasms of the lung, breast, ovary, or with Hodgkin's disease. Neuropathologic features of PCD include extensive loss of Purkinje cells, degenerative changes in the remaining Purkinje cells, and variable losses of granule and basket neurons.

The presence of anti-Purkinje cell antibodies in some PCD patients suggests an autoimmune etiology. To identify the molecular targets for these autoantibodies, an Agt11 cDNA expression library from human cerebellum was constructed and screened with IgG from a patient with paraneoplastic cerebellar degeneration. A single clone, pCDR2, produced a fusion protein that reacted strongly with the patient's IgG. Sequencing the pCDR clones revealed six amino acids repeated in tandem along the entire cDNA sequence (VAL, PRO, LEU, LEU, GLU, ASP). This gene was expressed predominantly in neuroectodermal tissues.[59]

Similarly, by studying amino acid sequences of α-gliadin, several peptides, in particular A 33 MER, were discovered to be responsible for cellular and humoral immune reactions in celiac disease. These identified peptides LQLQPFPQPQLPYPQPQLPYPQ PQLPYPQPQPF (33 MER), PLVQQQQFLGQQQPF PPQ (18 MER), GSVQPQQQLPQFEIR (15 MER) and Q, Q, G, Y, Y, PT (gluteomorphins) had several characteristics suggesting that they are primary initiators of the inflammatory response to gluten in Celiac Sprue patients.[60]

In vitro and *in vivo* studies in rats and humans demonstrated that gliadin is resistant to breakdown by all gastric, pancreatic, and intestinal brush-border membrane proteases. Gliadin reacted with tissue transglutaminase, the major autoantigen in Celiac Sprue, with substantially greater selectivity than known natural substrates of this extracellular enzyme. It was a potent inducer of gut-derived human T-cell lines from 14 of 14 Celiac Sprue patients. Homologs of this peptide were found in all food grains that are toxic to Celiac Sprue patients but are absent from all nontoxic food grains.[60]

Therefore, we developed peptide-based ELISA assays for measuring antibodies against gliadin and cerebellar peptides simultaneously in children with autism. For this, the peptides gliadin 33 MER, 18 MER, 15 MER, and gluteormorphin (7 MER) were dissolved in methanol in equal amounts at concentrations of 1 mg/ml for measurement of gliadin peptide antibodies. For measurement of anticerebellar antibodies, two peptides – Phe Leu Glu Asp Val Pro Leu Leu Glu Asp Ile Pro Leu Glu Asp Val Pro and Leu Leu Glu Asp Thr Asp Phe Leu Glu Asp Pro Asp

Phe Leu Glu Ala Ile Asp – were dissolved in methanol concentration of 1 mg/ml. After dilution of these peptides (1:100 in .01 M PBS) 100 μl was added to each microtiter well and other ELISA steps were followed. Sera from 50 patients with autism were measured for simultaneous presence of IgG, IgM, and IgA antibodies against gliadin and cerebellar peptides and compared to healthy controls. Results summarized in Table 19.3 showed that at two SDs above the mean of controls, 21 or 42% of patients with autism had elevated antibody levels against gliadin peptides, and only six or 12% of control subjects had elevated antibodies against these peptides. In comparison, 18 or 36% of patients and four or 8% of controls demonstrated significantly elevated antibodies against cerebellar peptides. And 17 of 21 subjects (80%) with autism had simultaneous elevation in antigliadin and anticerebellar peptides, indicating cross-reaction between gliadin and cerebellar antigens, which results in these antibodies in a majority of gliadin-reactive patients with autism. The remaining four patients (20%) had significant elevation in IgG, IgM, and IgA antibodies against gliadin but not against cerebellar peptides. Finally, one patient demonstrated elevation in antibodies against cerebellar but not gliadin peptides (see Table 19.3 and Figure 19.1).

In celiac disease, these antibodies are produced according to a sequence of different amino acids such as GLn-Xaa-Pro or GLn-Xaa-Pro-iLEU, LEU, VAL, Phe, TYR, TRP, THR, SER preferred by transglutaminase,[61] resulting in antibody production against gliadin peptides and the target tissue antigen. In children with autism, we found that these and other gliadin peptides were specific not only for transglutaminase but also for different aminopeptidases (DPP I, DPP IV, CD13) and lymphocyte receptors (DPP IV = CD26, CD69).[62] In addition to molecular mimicry, antibody production against dietary proteins and tissue antigens may be possible due to different mechanisms of action, as described below.

POSSIBLE BINDING OF GLIADIN, CASEIN, AND STREPTOKINASE TO DPP IV

It has been shown that streptokinase (SK), a protein secreted by streptococcus, binds to DPP IV and results in antibody production against DPP IV and SK in patients with autoimmune diseases.[63,64] Since interaction of CD26 with SK has been associated with SK and antiCD26 autoantibodies, we sought to determine whether possible binding of other peptides to DPP IV (CD26) occurred in children with autism. A series of ELISA experiments was performed to establish the binding specificity of gliadin, casein peptides, and SK to CD26. The plates was coated with CD26 and then with 1% BSA or HSA, for inhibition of nonspecific binding to microplate wells. Gliadin, casein peptides, and SK were then added. Plates were incubated for one hour at 37°C and washed five times for removal of unbound competing antigens. Then, for demonstration of casein, gliadin, and SK binding to CD26, purified enzyme labeled rabbit anti-CD26 was added to different wells.

After proper incubation and washing, binding of these peptides and proteins to CD26 was measured by adding peroxidase substrate and measuring color

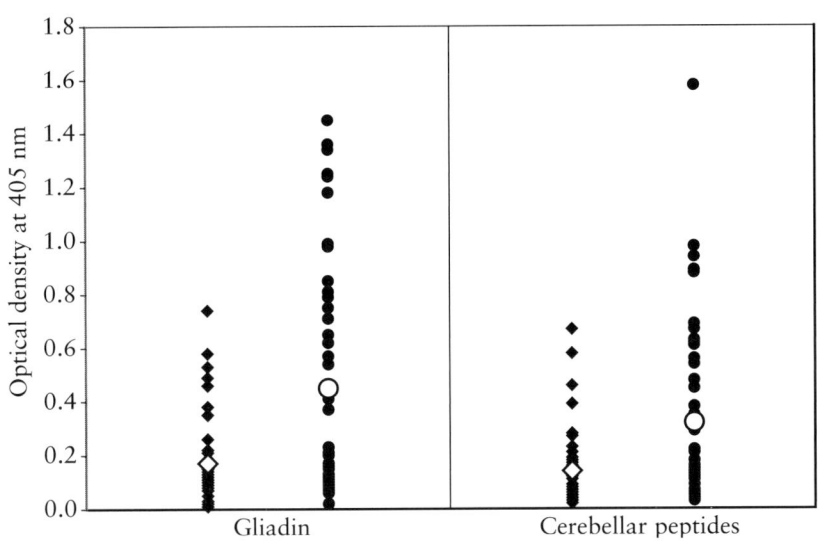

Figure 19.1 Scattergram of serum titer of IgG, IgM, and IgA antibodies against gliadin and cerebellar peptides in healthy control subjects ◆ and autistic patients ● expressed as optical density in ELISA.

Table 19.4 Inhibition of anti-CD26 binding to CD26 by gliadin, casein, and streptokinase, which reflects the binding of these molecules to CD26 coated plates

Microwell coated with:	Peroxidase labeled rabbit anti-	ELISA OD at 492 nm	% Binding of gliadin, casein, and streptokinase to CD26
BSA + HSA	CD26	.28	BG
BSA + HSA	Gliadin	.31	BG
BSA + HSA	Casein	.29	BG
BSA + HSA	SK	.33	BG
CD26 + BSA + HSA	CD26	2.16	–
CD26 + Gliadin	CD26	1.19	52
CD26 + Casein	CD26	1.34	44
CD26 + SK	CD26	.72	77

BG, background.

development at 492 nm. Binding of dietary peptides and SK to CD26 was demonstrated by % inhibition in binding of CD26 to anti-CD26. This % inhibition of CD26 binding to its specific antibody by different peptides and SK was calculated and is summarized in Table 19.4. Results showed that binding of casein, gliadin peptides, and SK was 44%, 52%, and 77%, respectively. This binding of bacterial toxins, gliadin, and casein peptides results in anti-gliadin, casein, SK, and anti-DPP IV autoantibodies.

ANTI-DPP IV (CD26), AUTOANTIBODY LEVELS IN CONTROLS AND SUBJECTS WITH AUTISM

We investigated whether autoantibodies to CD26 exist in the sera of patients with autism by ELISA using highly purified CD26. As shown in Figure 19.2, at a cutoff of .3 OD and sera dilution of 1:100, IgG, IgM, and IgA isotype anti-CD26 autoantibodies were detected in 24 of 50 (48%) patient serum samples for

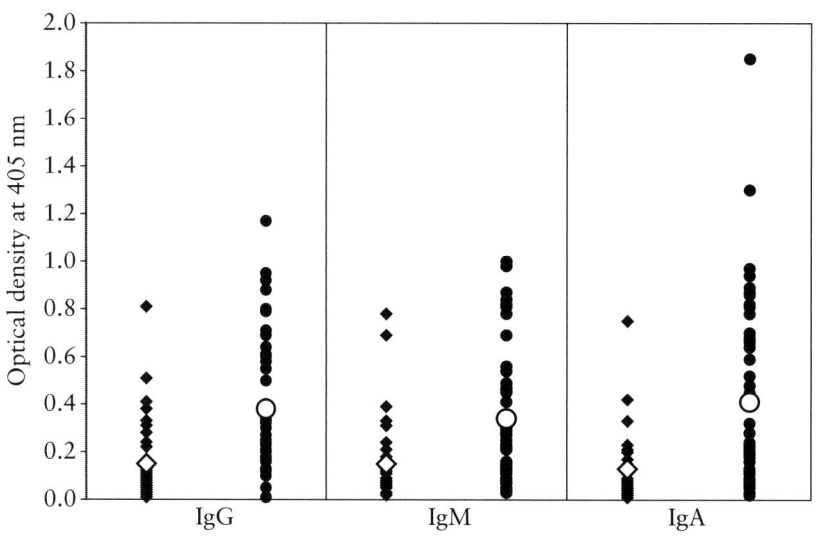

Figure 19.2 Scattergram of serum titer of IgG, IgM, and IgA antibodies against dipeptidyl peptidase IV (CD26) in healthy control subjects ◆ and autistic patients ● expressed as optical density in ELISA test.

IgG, 20 of 50 (40%) for IgM, and 22 of 50 (44%) for IgA. In contrast, autoantibodies to CD26 were detected in 14%, 10%, and 8% of healthy donors, respectively. The mean ± SD for these antibodies in controls ranged from .13 ± .13 to .15 ± .14 and in patients, significantly elevated and ranged from .34 ± .27 to .41 ± .39 with p value being highly significant ($p < .0001$).

ANTIBODIES AGAINST GLUTEN, CASEIN PEPTIDES, AND SK

Having shown that a subpopulation of children with autism exhibited antibodies against CD26, we then set out to show that these antibodies are generated due to dietary peptides and infectious agent antigens (SK). Using similar ELISA methods, the results of IgG, IgM, and IgA antibodies against gluten peptides are shown in Figure 19.3. The OD for IgG antibody values with 1:100 dilutions of healthy control sera ranged from .01–.84, varying among subjects. The mean ± SD values were .17 ± .17. The corresponding IgG OD values from autistic children's sera ranged from .03–1.18 with a mean ± SD of .34 ± .29. At a cutoff value of .3 OD, levels of IgG antibody against gliadin peptides were calculated. While six of 50 controls (12%) had high IgG values, 22 or 44% of patients showed IgG elevation ($p < .0001$). Levels of IgM and IgA anti-gliadin peptides in controls and children with autism are also shown in Figure 19.3. Similar to IgG, these antibodies were significantly higher in patients, 36% for IgM and 46% for IgA, while in controls 10% were elevated for IgM and 12% for IgA ($p < .0001$).

Concomitant with the increase of IgG, IgM, and IgA antibodies against gliadin peptides, we also observed a statistically significant increase of anti-casein peptide and anti-SK antibodies in patients' sera. The mean ± SD of antibodies against casein peptide for controls was .16 ± .17 for IgG, .16 ± .13 for IgM, and .14 ± .09 for IgA antibodies. The corresponding values in patients with autism were .39 ± .38 for IgG, .40 ± .41 for IgM, and the highest value, .52 ± .52 for IgA antibodies (Figure 19.4). Percent elevations of IgG, IgM, and IgA antibodies in controls were 10%, 8%, and 8%, while 42%, 34%, and 42% of patients' sera at the cutoff of .3 OD showed IgG, IgM, or IgA antibodies against casein peptides.

Analysis of anti-SK IgG, IgM, and IgA levels (Figure 19.5) shows that while only 1–2 of 50 control specimens (2–4%) had elevated antibodies, a significant percent of patients (18%, 48%, and 24%) demonstrated IgG, IgM, or IgA elevation. The mean ± SD of anti-SK antibodies was significantly elevated in patients compared to controls, for IgA and IgM ($p < .0001$) and for IgG ($p < .008$) (Figure 19.5).

SIMULTANEOUS DETECTION OF ANTIBODIES

For examination of possible involvement of gliadin, casein peptides, and SK in the production of auto-antibodies against CD26, calculation of simultaneous elevation in these antibodies in patients' sera were performed. Analysis of the data showed that while some patients had elevation in IgG, IgM, or IgA against one or two of four tested antigens,

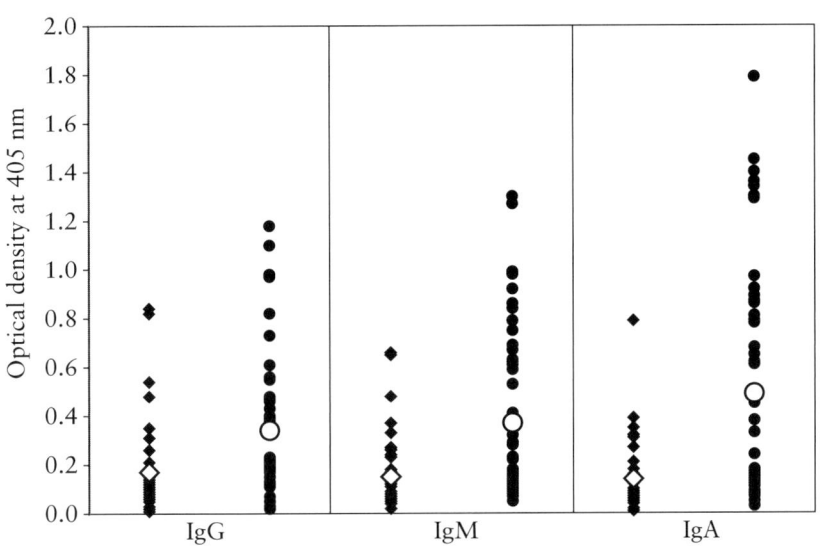

Figure 19.3 Scattergram of serum titer of IgG, IgM, and IgA antibodies against gliadin peptides in healthy control subjects ◆ and autistic patients ● expressed as optical density in ELISA test.

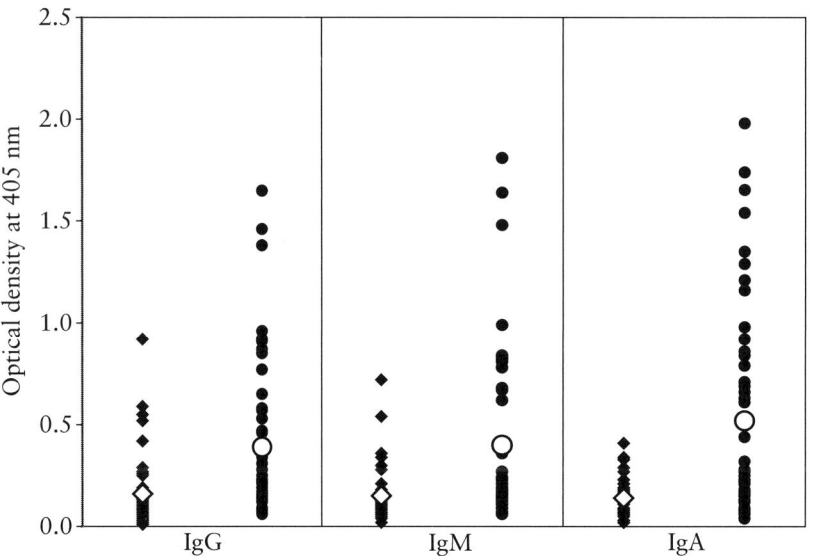

Figure 19.4 Scattergram of serum titer of IgG, IgM, and IgA antibodies against casein peptides in healthy control subjects ◆ and autistic patients ● expressed as optical density in ELISA test.

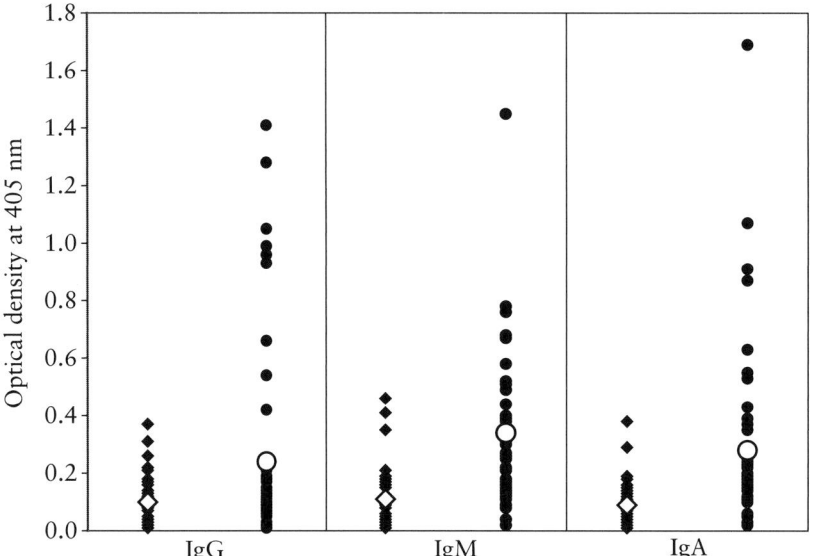

Figure 19.5 Scattergram of serum titer of IgG, IgM, and IgA antibodies against streptokinase in healthy control subjects ◆ and autistic patients ● expressed as optical density in ELISA test.

different subgroups showed simultaneous elevation in IgG, IgM, or IgA antibodies not only against CD26 but also against gliadin, casein peptides, or SK. This simultaneous elevation of anti-CD26, casein, gliadin, and SK in children with autism further supports the argument for the binding of these dietary and bacterial peptides or antigens to tissue enzymes (dipeptidylpeptidase) or lymphocyte receptors (CD26). The possible mechanism of action for DPP IV binding of dietary peptides, infections, and xenobiotics resulting in antibody production against DPP IV, gliadin, casein, and SK is shown in Figure 19.6.

TRIGGERS FOR AUTOANTIBODIES AND AUTISM

From these results, we learn that autoantibodies to different tissue antigens in autism are produced by two different mechanisms of action:

1) By direct binding of infectious agent antigens or peptides, or dietary proteins or peptides, or by binding of xenobiotics or their metabolites to tissue enzymes or cell receptors and inducing antibody production against the tissue antigens as well as bacterial, dietary, or xenobiotics.

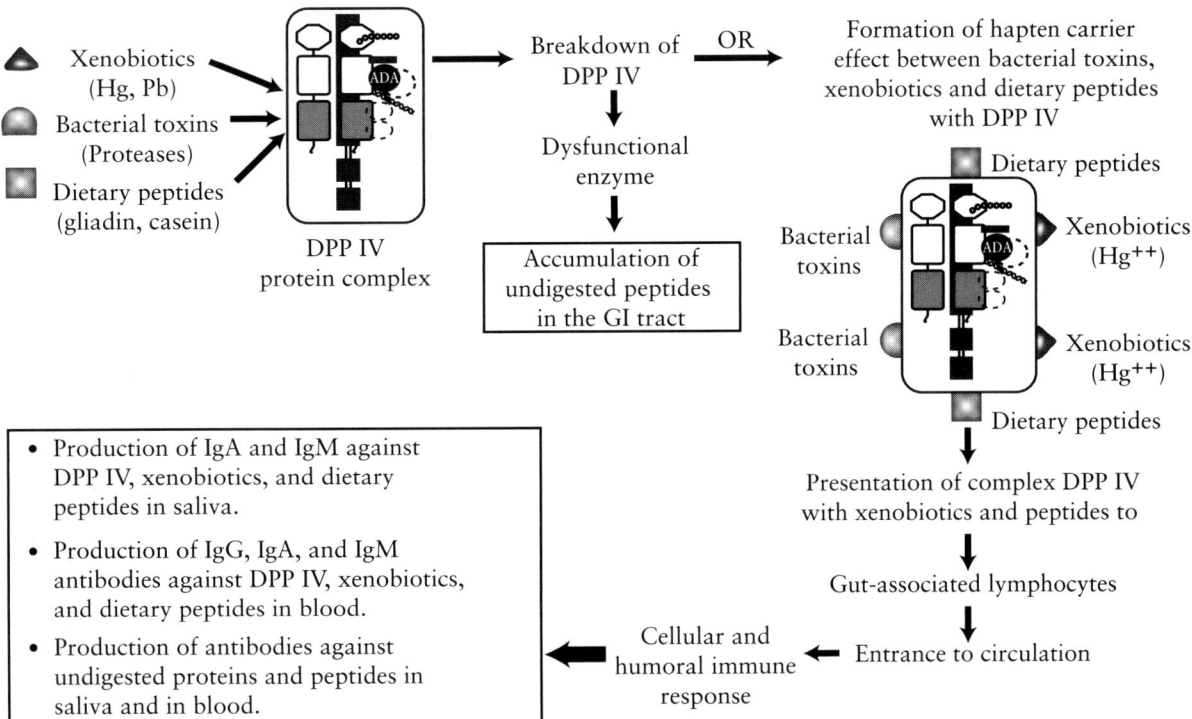

Figure 19.6 Xenobiotics, bacterial toxins, and dietary peptides binding to DPP IV, formation of hapten carrier effect, and production of antibodies against DPP IV, xenobiotics, peptides, and bacterial toxins. This may result in dysfunction of the DPP IV molecule and accumulation of peptides in the GI tract and in circulation.

2) Many infectious agents and dietary proteins and peptides share similar epitopes with different tissue antigens. Therefore, immune responses against the infectious agents or dietary proteins result in autoimmune reactions with different tissue antigens including brain cells.

Based on these findings, we postulate that dietary and infectious antigens and xenobiotics play a role in the pathophysiology of autism. It is likely that environmental factors, including infection-induced injury, cause release of neuronal antigens, which through activation of inflammatory cells could lead to autoimmune reactions in genetically susceptible individuals.

PATHOGENESIS AND MECHANISM OF AUTOIMMUNITY AND AUTISM

For cross-reactive circulating antibodies to become pathogenic, they must cross the blood brain barrier. It is now known that permeability of the blood brain barrier increases after major histocompatibility complex class I expression,[65] activated lymphocyte interaction,[16] and change in neuronal cell adhesion molecules.[13] Based on a review of literature and results reported here, we propose the following 10 events, as shown in Figure 19.7, that may explain possible mechanisms of injury in autism:

1) In the course of a lifetime, the body is exposed to infectious agents, which mimic neuron-specific antigens, such as EBV, CMV, HHV-6, HTLV-1, HTLV-2, streptococcus, *Chlamydia pneumoniae* or even milk and gluten peptides.
2) Pre-existing autoreactive T cells are generated by molecular mimicry as a result of contact with dietary proteins and viral, bacterial, and parasitic antigens, which have sequence homologies or matched motifs with autoantigens.
3) Bacterial enterotoxins, viral antigens, and metals such as mercury and lead, may increase adhesion molecules on brain endothelial cells. Toxic chemicals may also increase leukocyte function-associated antigens on activated T cells.
4) Pre-existing autoreactive T cells may transmigrate across the blood brain barrier and induce

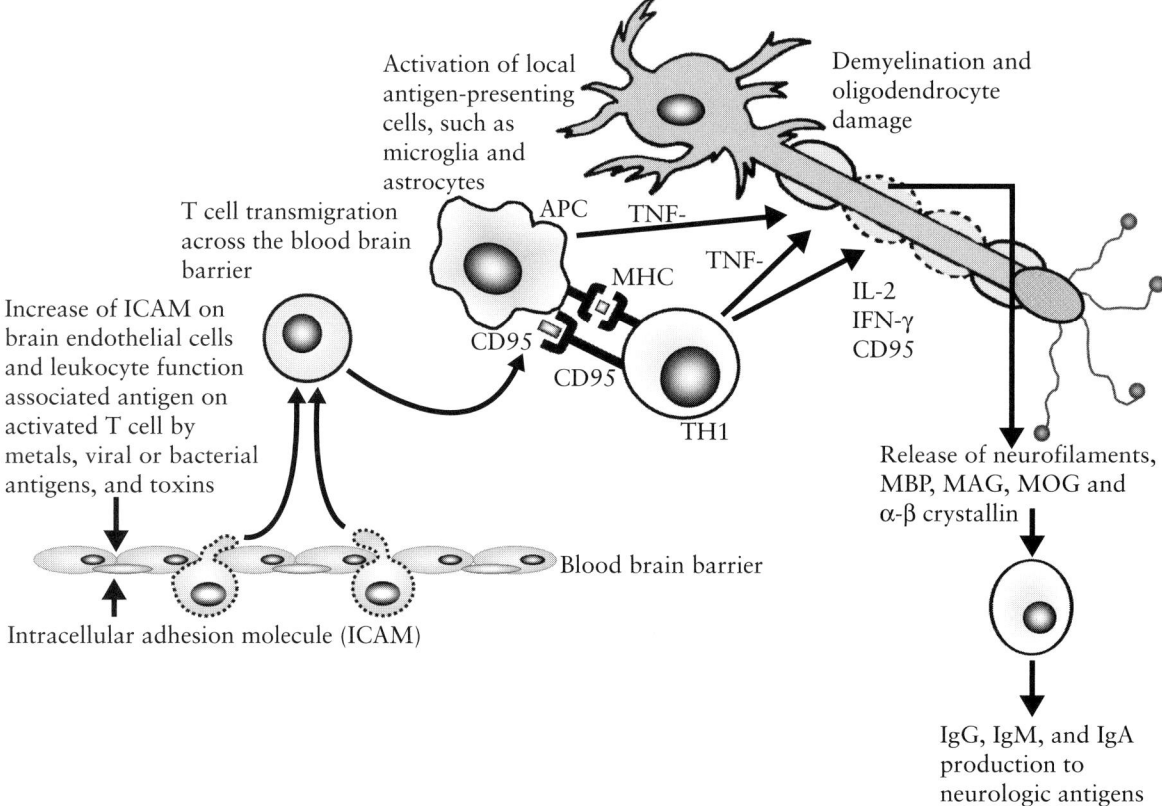

Figure 19.7 Cellular and humoral immune mechanisms in infection- and xenobiotics-induced neurotoxicity, which includes neuronal degeneration, secondary demyelination, and possibly reactive astrogliosis. Under pathological conditions, pre-existing autoreactive T cells are generated by molecular mimicry as a result of sequence homologies or matched motifs between autoantigen and viral, bacterial, or parasitic proteins. Increased ICAM on endothelial cells by xenobiotics and bacterial toxins may allow transmigration of these auto-reactive T cells across the blood brain barrier, resulting in cellular and humoral immune responses against nerve cells.

the activation of local antigen-presenting cells, such as microglia and astrocytes.

5) By reacting to μ, δ, and κ opioid receptors on both lymphocytes and nerve cells, dietary peptides such as casomorphins, gluteomorphins, and others may change the level of cytokine production and interfere with neuroimmune communication.[51,52,66,67]

6) Production of IL-2, INF-γ, and TNF-α by T-helper-1 autoreactive cells and TNF-α by the antigen-presenting cells (astrocytes and microglia) may result in oligodendrocyte damage and demyelination.

7) As a result of this sequence of events, MBP, MAG, MOG, α-B-crystallin, and other antigens are released from neurofilaments and enter the circulatory system. This results in immune reactions, such as the formation of plasma cells with the capacity to produce IgG, IgM, and IgA antibodies against neuron-specific antigens.

8) These antibodies may cross the blood brain barrier and combine with brain tissue antigens to form immune complexes, thus causing further damage to the neurological tissue. These antibodies, along with toxic biological weaponry such as arachidonic acid and free radicals, can erode neuron myelin and impair electrical transmission between a muscle and the central nervous system.

9) This hypothesis may explain significant differences in levels of pathogenic anti-neurological

autoantibodies between control subjects and patients exposed to toxic chemicals and metals.

10) Finally, a broad analysis across the living spectrum would reveal rather universal similarities.[68,69]

REFERENCES

1. Noronha A, Arnason B. Demyelinating diseases. In: *Clinical Immunology* (Rich R, Fleisher TA, Schwartz B et al, eds). St Louis, MO: Mosby, 1995: 1364–76.
2. Steinman L. Multiple sclerosis: a coordinated immunological attack against myelin in the central nervous system. *Cell* 1996; **85**: 299–302.
3. Amor S, Baker D, Layward L et al. Multiple sclerosis: variations on a theme. *Immunol Today* 1997; **18**: 368–71.
4. Raine CS, Cannella SL, Hauser CP. Genain demyelination in primate autoimmune encephalomyelitis and acute multiple sclerosis lesions: a case for antigen-specific antibody mediation. *Ann Neurol* 1999; **46**: 144–60.
5. Noseworthy JH, Lucchinetti C, Rodriguez M, Weinshenker BJ. Multiple sclerosis, a review. *N Engl J Med* 2000; **343**: 938–52.
6. Genain CP, Cannella B, Hauser SL, Raine CS. Identification of autoantibodies associated with myelin damage in multiple sclerosis. *Nature Med* 1999; **5**: 170–5.
7. Holz A, Bielekova B, Martin R, Oldstone MBA. Myelin-associated oligodendrocytic basic protein: identification of an encephalitogenic epitope and association with multiple sclerosis. *J Immunol* 2000; **164**: 1103–9.
8. Bajramovic JJ, Plomp AC, Van Der Goes A et al. Presentation of α-β-crystallin to T-cells in active multiple sclerosis lesions: an early event following inflammatory demyelination. *J Immunol* 2000; **164**: 4359–66.
9. Chou YK, Bourdette DN, Offner H et al. Frequency of T-cells specific for myelin basic protein and myelin proteolipid protein in blood and cerebrospinal fluid in multiple sclerosis. *J Neuroimmunol* 1992; **38**: 105.
10. Brock HPM, Uccelli A, Kerlero de Rosbo N et al. Myelin/oligodendrocyte glycoprotein-induced autoimmune encephalomyelitis in common marmosets: the encephalitogenic T-cell epitope P-MOG 24-36 is present by a monomorphic MHC class II molecule. *J Immunol* 2000; **165**: 1093–101.
11. Von Büdingen H, Tanuman N, Villaslada P et al. Immune response against the myelin/oligodendrocyte glycoprotein in experimental autoimmune demyelination. *J Clin Immunol* 2001; **21**: 155–60.
12. Rodier PM, Ingram JL, Tisdale B et al. Embryological origin for autism: development abnormalities of the cranial nerve motor nuclei. *J Comp Neurol* 1996; **370**: 247–61.
13. Purcell AE, Rocco MM, Lenhart JA et al. Assessment of neuronal cell adhesion molecule (NCAM) in autistic serum and postmortem brain. *J Autism Dev Discord* 2001; **31**: 183–93.
14. Weizman A, Weizman R, Szekely GA et al. Abnormal immune response to brain tissue antigen in the syndrome of autism. *Am J Psychiatry* 1982; **139**: 1462–5.
15. Singh VK, Warren RP, Odell JD et al. Antibodies to myelin basic protein in children with autistic behavior. *Brain Behav Immun* 1993; **7**: 97–103.
16. Singh VK, Warren RP, Averett R, Ghaziuddin M. Circulating autoantibodies to neuronal and glial filament protein in autism. *Pediatr Neurol* 1997; **17**: 88–90.
17. Vojdani A, Campbell AW, Anyanwu E et al. Antibodies to neuron-specific antigens in children with autism: possible cross-reaction with encephalitogenic proteins from milk, *Chlamydia pneumoniae* and streptococcus group A. *J Neuroimmunol* 2002; **129**: 168–77.
18. Baba H, Daune GC, Ilyas A et al. Anti-GM$_1$ ganglioside antibodies with differing fine specificities in patients with multifocal motor neuropathy. *J Neuroimmunol* 1989; **25**: 143–50.
19. Chabraoui F, Derrington EA, Mallie-Didier F et al. Dot-blot immunodetection of antibodies against GM$_1$ and other gangliosides on PVDF-P membrane. *J Immunol Methods* 1993; **165**: 225–30.
20. Isoardo G, Ferrero B, Barbero P et al. Anti-GM$_1$ and anti-sulfatide antibodies in polyneuropathies. *Acta Neurol Scand* 2001; **103**: 180–7.
21. Kaldor J, Speed BR. Guillain-Barre syndrome and *Campylobacter jejuni*: a serological study. *BMJ* 1984; **288**: 1867–70.
22. Greunewald R, Ropper AH, Lior H. Serologic evidence of *Campylobacter jejuni* coli enteritis in patients with Guillain-Barre syndrome. *Arch Neurol* 1991; **48**: 1080–2.
23. Ropper AH, Gorson KC. Neuropathies associated with paraproteinemia. *N Engl J Med* 1998; **338**: 1601–7.
24. Nemni R, Fazio R, Quattrini A et al. Antibodies to sulfatide and chondroitin sulfate in patients with chronic sensory neuropathy. *J Neuroimmunol* 1993; **43**: 79–86.
25. Fredman P, Lycke J, Anderson O et al. Peripheral neuropathy associated with monoclonal IgM antibody to glycolipids with a terminal glucoronyl-3-sulfate epitope. *J Neurol* 1993; **240**: 381–7.
26. El-Fawal HAN, Gong Z, Little AR, Evans HL. Exposure to mercury results in serum autoantibodies to neurotype and gliotypic proteins. *Neurotoxicology* 1996; **17**: 267–76.
27. El-Fawal HAN, Waterman SJ, DeFeo A, Shamy MY. Neuroimmunology: humoral assessment of neurotoxicity and autoimmune mechanism. *Environ Health Perspect* 1999; **5**: 767–75.
28. Morse DC, Plug A, Wesseling W et al. Persistent alterations in regional brain glial fibrillary acidic protein and synpatophsin levels following pre- and postnatal polychlorinated biphenyl exposure. *Toxic Appl Pharmacol* 1996; **139**: 252–61.
29. Partl S, Herbst H, Schaeper F et al. GFAP gene expression is altered in young rats following developmental low level lead exposure. *Neurotoxicity* 1998; **19**: 547–52.
30. Qian Y, Harris ED, Zheng Y, Tiffany-Castiglioni E. Lead targets GRP78, a molecular chaperone, in C6 rat glioma cells. *Toxicol Pharmacol* 2000; **163**: 260–6.
31. Edelson SB, Cantor DS. Autism: xenobiotic influences. *Toxicol Ind Health* 1998; **14**: 799–811.
32. Edelson SB, Cantor DS. The neurotoxic etiology of the autistic spectrum disorder: a replicative study. *Toxicol Ind Health* 2000; **16**: 239–47.
33. Sibley WA, Bamford CR, Clark K. Clinical viral infections and multiple sclerosis. *Lancet* 1985; **1**: 1313–5.
34. Johnson RT, Griffin DE. Virus-induced autoimmune demyelinating disease of the central nervous system. In: *Concepts in Viral Pathogenesis II* (Notkins AL, Oldstone MBA, eds). New York: Springer, 1986: 203–9.
35. Rösener M, Harms F, Dichgans J, Martin R. Chickenpox and multiple sclerosis: a case report. *J Neurol Neurosurgery Psychiatry* 1995; **58**: 637–8.
36. Zimmer C. Do chronic diseases have an infectious root? *Science* 2001; **293**: 1974–7.
37. Wucherpfenning KW. Infectious trigger for inflammatory neurological disease. *Nature Med* 2002; **8**: 455–7.
38. Fujunami RS, Oldstone MBA. Amino acid homology between the encephalitogenic site of myelin basic protein and virus: mechanism for autoimmunity. *Science* 1985; **203**: 1043–5.
39. Wucherpfenning KW, Strominger JL. Molecular mimicry in T cell-mediated autoimmunity: viral peptides activate human T

cell clones specific for myelin basic protein. *Cell* 1995; **80**: 695–705.
40. Rajeswari MH, Ravindranath H, Graves MC. Monoclonal IgM antibodies from CMV-infected mice recognize the GlCNAC-containing receptor determinant of murine CMV as well as neutralizing anti-CMV IgG antibodies. *Virology* 1992; **188**: 143–51.
41. Moktarian F, Zhang Z, Shi Y et al. Molecular mimicry between a viral peptide and a myelin oligodendrocyte glycoprotein induces autoimmune demyelinating disease in mice. *J Neuroimmunol* 1999; **95**: 43–8.
42. Esposito M, Venkatesh V, Otvos L et al. Human transaldolase and cross-reactive viral epitopes identified by autoantibodies of multiple sclerosis patients. *J Immunol* 1999; **163**: 4027–32.
43. Caselli E, Boni M, Bracci A et al. Detection of antibodies directed against human herpesvirus-6 U 94/REP in sera of patients affected by multiple sclerosis. *J Clin Microbiol* 2002; **40**: 4131–7.
44. Olson JK, Eagar TN, Miller SD. Functional activation of myelin-specific T-cells by virus-induced mimicry. *J Immunol* 2002; **169**: 2719–26.
45. Bronze MS, Dale JB. Epitope of streptococcal M proteins that evoke antibodies that cross-react with the human brain. *J Immunol* 1993; **151**: 2820–8.
46. Lenz DC, Lu L, Conant SB et al. A *Chlamydia pneumoniae*-specific peptide induces experimental autoimmune encephalomyelitis in rats. *J Immunol* 2001; **167**: 1803–8.
47. Wakefield AJ, Murch SH, Anthony A et al. Ileal-lymphoid-nodular hyperplasia, non-specific colitis, and pervasive developmental disorder in children. *Lancet* 1998; **351**: 637–41.
48. Chess S, Fernandez P, Korn S. Behavioral consequences of congenital rubella. *J Pediatr* 1978; **93**: 669–703.
49. Ivarsson SA, Bjerre L, Vegfors P, Ahlfors K. Autism as one of several abnormalities in two children with congenital cytomegalovirus infection. *Neuropediatrics* 1990; **21**: 102–3.
50. Grogan JL, Kramer A, Nogai A et al. Cross-reactivity of myelin basic protein-specific T-cells with multiple microbial peptides: experimental autoimmune encephalomyelitis induction in TCR transgenic mice. *J Immunol* 1999; **163**: 3764–70.
51. Fatemi SH, Earle J, Kanodia R et al. Prenatal viral infection leads to pyramidal cell atrophy and macrocephaly in adulthood: implications for genesis of autism and schizophrenia. *Cell Mol Neurobiol* 2002; **22**: 25–33.
52. Shi L, Fatemi SH, Sidwell RW, Patterson PH. Maternal influenza infection causes marked behavorial and pharmacological changes in the offspring. *J Neurosciences* 2003; **23**: 297.
53. Stefferl A, Schubart A, Storch M et al. Butyrophilin, a milk protein, modulates the encephalitogenic T-cell response to myelin oligodendrocyte glycoprotein in experimental autoimmune encephalomyelitis. *J Immunol* 2000; **165**: 2859–65.
54. Hadjivassiliou M, Grünewald RA, Lawden M et al. Headache and CNS white matter abnormalities related with gluten sensitivity. *Neurology* 2001; **56**: 385–8.
55. Bürk L, Bösch, S, Müller CA. Sporadic cerebellar ataxia associated with gluten sensitivity. *Brain* 2001; **124**: 1013–9.
56. Bushara KO, Goebel SU, Shill H et al. Gluten sensitivity in sporadic and hereditary cerebellar ataxia. *Ann Neurol* 2001; **49**: 540–3.
57. Sblattero D, Berti I, Trevisiol C. Human recombinant tissue transglutaminase ELISA: an innovative diagnostic assay for coeliac disease. *Am J Gastroenterol* 2000; **95**: 1253–7.
58. Hadjivassiliou M, Boscolos S, Davies-Jones GAB et al. The humoral response in the pathogenesis of gluten ataxia. *Neurology* 2002; **58**: 1221–6.
59. Dropcho EJ, Chen Y, Posner JB, Old LJ. Cloning of a brain protein identified by autoantibodies from a patient with paraneoplastic cerebellar degeneration. *Proc Natl Acad* 1987; **84**: 4552–6.
60. Shan L, Molberg Ø, Parrot I et al. Structural basis for gluten intolerance in Celiac Sprue. *Science* 2002; **297**: 2275–9.
61. Sollid LM. Coeliac disease: dissecting a complex inflammatory disorder. *Nature Rev Immunol* 2002; **2**: 647–55.
62. Vojdani A, Pangborn JB, Vojdani E, Cooper EL. Infections, toxic chemicals and dietary peptides binding to lymphocyte receptors and tissue enzymes are responsible for autoimmunity in autism. *Int J Immunopath Pharmacol* 2003; **16**: 189–99.
63. Gonzalez-Gronow M, Weber MR, Gawdi G, Pizzo SV. Dipeptidylpeptidase IV (CD26) is a receptor for streptokinase on rheumatoid synovial fibroblasts. *Fibrinol Proteol* 1998; **12**: 129–35.
64. Chuchacovich M, Gatica H, Pizzo HSV, Gonzalez-Gronow M. Characterization of human serum dipeptidylpeptidase IV (CD26) and analysis of its autoantibodies in patients with rheumatoid arthritis and other autoimmune diseases. *Clin Exp Rheumatol* 2001; **19**: 673–80.
65. Fabry Z, Raine CS, Hart MN. Nervous tissues as an immune compartment: the dialect of the immune response in the CNS. *Immunol Today* 1994; **15**: 218–24.
66. Wang J, Charboneau R, Barke RA et al. μ-opoid receptor mediates chronic restraint stress-induced lymphocyte apoptosis. *J Immunol* 2002; **168**: 3630–6.
67. Rogers TJ, Peterson PK. Opioid G protein-coupled receptors: signals at the crossroads of inflammation. *Trends Immunol* 2003; **24**: 116–21.
68. Cooper EL, Parrinello N. Invertebrates, ectotherms, immunonotoxicology: extrapolation to human health. In: *Modulators of Immune Responses: The Evolutionary Trail* (Stolen JS, Fletcher TC, Bayne CJ et al, eds). Fair Haven NJ: SOS Publications, 1996: 331–42.
69. Cooper EL, Parrinello N. Comparative immunological models can enhance analyses of environmental immunotoxicity. *Ann Rev Fish Dis* 1996; **6**: 179–91.

20

Immunological issues in patients with autism spectrum disorders

Harumi Jyonouchi

INTRODUCTION

Autism spectrum disorders (ASD) are umbrella terms for a group of developmental disorders diagnosed on the basis of behavioral phenomena without presence of objective biomarkers.[1] Behavioral symptoms of ASD are most likely the results of expression of various etiological and pathological factors and they probably vary at different stages of development, leading to markedly variable behavioral manifestations and degrees of cognitive impairment. This makes it difficult to analyze a role for each etiological factor in ASD.

Apart from behavioral symptoms, ASD children often exhibit medical problems that are probably associated with immune abnormalities. For example, a number of ASD children suffer from recurrent otitis media (OM), rhinosinusitis (RS), and pharyngitis. ASD children tend to have a prolonged and more severe course of illness with benign microbial infection when compared to their siblings. Young ASD children also frequently exhibit apparent intolerance to certain foods with accompanying gastrointestinal (GI) symptoms.[2] These problems may coincide with or precede the onset of autistic symptoms in some ASD children. However, as opposed to primary immune or autoimmune disorders, these medical problems are not necessarily progressive or expanding. In fact, a fair number of ASD children appear to experience partial resolution or amelioration of these symptoms with age, indicating that adaptive or counterregulatory immune mechanisms may be developed with age. Nevertheless, immune abnormalities manifested in early life can be detrimental, affecting the immature central nervous system (CNS) and leading to persistent or irreversible impairment of CNS functions.

Immune abnormalities reported in ASD children are variable and lack a consistent pattern specific for ASD children. This could be attributed to two facts. First, most studies were cross-sectional and included ASD children of a wide age range. Second, some ASD children have been treated with neuropsychiatric medications that could modulate immune functions. Even so, reported immune abnormalities indicate immunodysregulatory conditions.[3] Other relatively consistent findings in ASD children are abnormalities of neurotransmitters that could modulate the immune functions directly or indirectly. To date, we do not know whether the immune abnormalities reported in ASD children are primary defects or secondary to defects of neuroendocrine or other organ systems, or how such immune abnormalities are associated with clinical features of ASD. Obvious heterogeneity of the etiology and pathogenesis of ASD makes it unlikely that one mechanism of immune abnormalities is applicable to the whole ASD population. Instead, it is more realistic to think that multiple underlying mechanisms lead to various immune abnormalities and these vary considerably in each patient and at each time point.

In infants and young children, innate immunity exerts a significant role prior to the development of adaptive immunity. Aberrant innate (nonspecific) immunity could lead to the symptoms often described in ASD children prior to the development of effective antigen (Ag)-specific adaptive immunity. In this chapter, we will first discuss innate and adaptive immunity and interactions of the immune system with the neuroendocrine system. Then we will discuss potential immune mechanisms in the development of ASD with special emphasis on the role of innate immune abnormalities.

INNATE AND ADAPTIVE IMMUNITY AND NEUROIMMUNE INTERACTIONS

Innate immunity and the CNS

Immune responses against foreign Ags consist of initial, nonspecific, immune responses (innate immunity) and subsequent Ag-specific immune responses (adaptive immunity). Innate immunity provides initial immune responses by activating first-line immune cells (macrophage/monocytes, dendritic cells, natural killer or NK cells, and so on).[4] These cells mount nonspecific immune responses by recognizing pathogen-associated molecular patterns (PAMPs) and perhaps tissue-derived danger signals through pattern recognition receptors (PRRs) and other receptors.[4–6] Innate immune responses produce proinflammatory cytokines, including tumor necrosis factor-α (TNF-α), interleukin-6 (IL-6), IL-1β, and IL-8, that help suppress the systemic dissemination of microbes. These proinflammatory cytokines also affect the hypothalamo-pituitary-adrenocortical (HPA) axis and modulate stress responses.[7,8] Effects of proinflammatory cytokines are counterregulated by suppressive cytokines and soluble receptors including IL-10, transforming growth factor-β (TGF-β), soluble TNF-receptor I (sTNFRI), sTNFRII, and IL-1 receptor antagonists (IL-1ra). Thus, these mediators present in the periphery and the CNS comprise a link between peripheral immune stimulation and CNS-mediated behaviors. Dysregulated production of these mediators could lead to changes in the CNS-mediated behaviors. For example, patients with excessive production of proinflammatory cytokines may experience unrefreshing sleep and fatigue.[9]

Innate immunity and adaptive immunity

To generate effective Ag-specific (adaptive) immune responses, Ag-presenting cells (APC; dendritic cells, macrophage/monocytes, and so on) must be activated in order to present Ags properly to T cells. Innate immunity plays a crucial role for activation of APC and subsequent Ag-specific adaptive immune responses.[4] PAMPs and other stimulants of innate immunity facilitate activation and maturation of APC that leads to augmentation of Ag processing and upregulation of costimulatory and adhesion molecules. Activated APC will migrate to the regional draining lymph nodes (LN) where Ag will be presented to naïve T cells. The degree of innate immune responses thus partly determines subsequent adaptive immune responses.

Upon Ag presentation, resting T-helper (Th) cells are activated into effector-stage Th cells with distinguished patterns of cytokine production with complex processes of intracellular signaling.[10–12] Th1 responses induce phagocytic cell-mediated immune responses by producing Th1 cytokines (IFN-γ, IL-2, and TNF-β) and facilitating production of IgG1/IgG3 antibodies (Abs) that enhance opsonization. Type 2 T cell (T2) responses induce eosinophil-mediated inflammatory responses by production of Th2 cytokines (IL-4, IL-5, and IL-13) and augmenting production of IgG4/IgE Abs.[10–12] Th1 and Th2 cytokines counterregulate each other and innate immune responses also partly determine processes of Th cell differentiation.[4,11] For example, production of IL-12 by innate immune cells preferentially promotes differentiation of Th1 cells.[10,11]

Imbalance of Th1/Th2 responses has been implicated in the pathogenesis of various disorders. Skewed T1 responses may be associated with organ-specific autoimmune diseases including CNS autoimmune disorders (such as multiple sclerosis).[13] On the other hand, excessive T2 responses may predispose individuals to allergic disorders.[14,15] Types of cytokine produced by innate immune cells are partly determined by stimulants of innate immunity (such as PAMPs). That is, the kinds of microbial infection exposure in early life (exposure to certain types of stimulants of innate immunity) profoundly affect initial Th1 and Th2 differentiation[13,16] and determine subsequent Th cell responses (Th cell memory). Therefore, aberrant innate immune responses to common microbes and other environmental factors in early life could lead to skewed Th1 or Th2 responses and predispose individuals to certain diseases. Skewed Th1 or Th2 responses have also been postulated in ASD children[17,18] but the results of various studies are inconclusive.

Innate immunity and immune tolerance

The immune system does not react to benign environmental factors such as food Ags under normal circumstances, since these environmental factors lack stimulants of innate immunity and hence they are poorly capable of activating APC. When activation of APC is insufficient, T cells presented with Ag will become unresponsive or go through apoptosis, instead of being activated (peripheral tolerance). The immune system is also capable of developing regulatory T cells to suppress undesired immune responses actively.[19–21] The gut immune system is generally well equipped for inducing immune tolerance, partly due to the presence of intestinal flora and hence more frequent presence of stimuli of innate immunity (mainly PAMPs such as endotoxin) in other organs. However, when innate immune responses are excessive or dysregulated, T and B cells may become aberrantly reactive to benign environmental factors and even to autoantigens. As a result, undesired immune responses against DPs, medications, and food additives could occur. Such immune reactions could lead to various GI symptoms, skin rash, respiratory symptoms, and even behavioral changes; it is reported that patients with celiac disease, a disease caused by immune reactivity to wheat protein (gliadin), often present with neurological manifestations including memory impairment, cerebellar ataxia, and neuropathy.[22] Aberrant innate immune responses could also lead to autoimmunity.[13,16,23]

INTERACTION BETWEEN THE GUT, RESPIRATORY MUCOSAL IMMUNE SYSTEM, AND CNS

It has been postulated that primary and/or secondary GI inflammatory conditions may trigger and/or aggravate clinical features of ASD.[24] This may be partly attributed to neuroendocrine mediators produced in the GI tract with or without involvement of the gut immune system. This may also be true for respiratory inflammatory pathology. Autoimmunity triggered by molecular mimicry (as seen in celiac disease) and bystander effects have also been frequently postulated as the potential immune mechanisms of enterocolonic encephalopathy and also infection-triggered neuroimmune disorders (CNS Lyme diseases, Sydenham's chorea, and so on). However, there are no known autoantigens or microbial Ags cross-reactive to human tissues associated with ASD.

We have previously reported frequent innate immune abnormalities in ASD children.[25] On the basis of our findings, we speculate that such innate immune abnormalities may make their gut and possibly respiratory mucosal immune systems more easily activated by relatively benign microbes. This may lead to the production of various inflammatory mediators by the mucosal immune system, leading to a prolonged course of illness. These mediators may subsequently affect the neuroendocrine system. In this section, we summarize the potential effects of the gut and respiratory mucosa-derived mediators on the CNS response, focusing on the immune activation.

Peptide hormones and neurotransmitters

A number of neuroendocrine peptide hormones and neurotransmitters are found in the immune system. Recent evidence supports that these peptides and transmitters are also produced by the immune system. These mediators are used for both intra-immune system regulation and bidirectional communication between the immune and neuroendocrine systems, and include peptide hormones such as corticotropin (ACTH), endorphins, TSH (thyrotropin), growth hormone (GH), prolactin, corticotropin releasing factor (CRF), and neuropeptides (vasoactive intestinal peptides or VIP, substance P, calcitonin gene related peptides or CGRP, and somatostatin).

The immune system appears to produce these mediators upon stimulation by microbial products including endotoxins (LPS).[26] These mediators produced by the immune system affect the CNS directly or indirectly. For instance, CRF stimulates macrophages to produce IL-1 that will affect the HPA axis by stimulating CRF release from the hypothalamus and sensitize the pituitary gland to direct ACTH-releasing activity of IL-1.[27] Microbial products are potent stimulants of innate immunity.[4–6] The apparent innate immune abnormalities in a subset of ASD children[25] may affect the production of peptide hormones and neurotransmitters by the mucosal immune system, leading to changes in the CNS response.

Reciprocally, immune cells also express receptors for these peptide hormones and neurotransmitters. The immune system and CNS derived by these mediators could alter the mucosal immune responses positively and/or negatively. Innate immune abnormalities triggered by PAMPs and tissue-released products could disrupt homeostasis of neuroendocrine-immune interactions that could lead to aberrant behaviors.

Cytokines: influences on microglial cells

Microglial cells are regarded as quiescent tissue macrophage-like cells which can be activated by migrated activated T cells, dendritic cells, and macrophages infiltrated from the periphery through direct interaction and by soluble factors. Activation of microglial cells is implicated in the pathogenesis of various neurodegenerative disorders.[28] Mediators produced by microglial cells can be proinflammatory (IFN-γ, TNF-α, IL-1, and IL-12), and also counter-regulatory (IL-10, TGF-β, and IFN-α/β).[29] Cytokines associated with innate immunity (IL-1, IL-6, and TNF-α) can cross the blood brain barrier (BBB) and could influence microglial cells and astrocytes in the CNS in addition to affecting the HPA axis. Taken together, chronic inflammatory conditions in the gut and respiratory mucosa could potentially affect the CNS response through activating CNS immune cells in addition to affecting the HPA axis. There is a controversy regarding the presence of inflammatory mediators in the brain of autism patients.[2,30] However, in a limited number of ASD children with evidence of innate immune abnormalities and concurrent

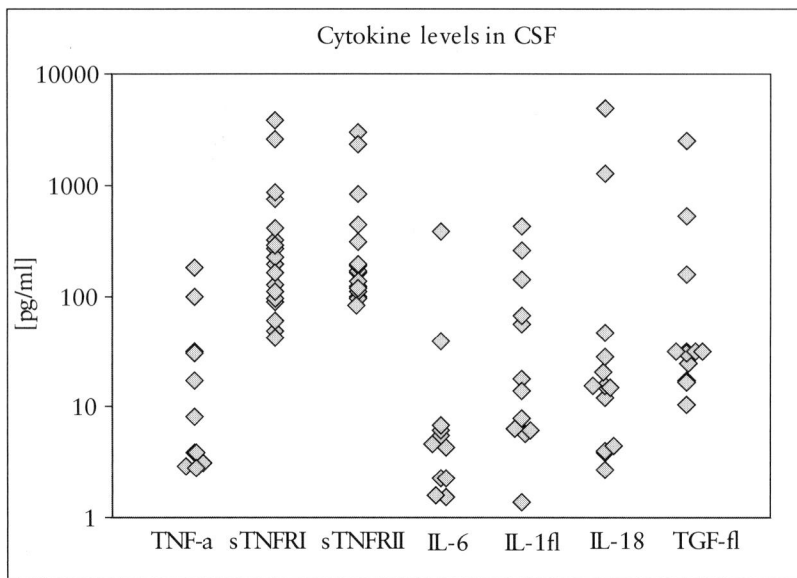

Figure 20.1 Proinflammatory and counterregulatory cytokines levels in CSF of ASD children. In a limited number of control samples obtained for workup of seizure disorders, we did not detect TNF-α, IL-6, IL-1β, IL-18, or TGF-β. sTNFRI and sTNFRII levels are elevated similar to the levels observed in multiple sclerosis patients. sTNFRI/II were used as indicators for TNF-α overproduction, since a half-life of TNF-α *in vivo* is relatively short (<1 h).

GI and/or respiratory mucosal inflammatory conditions, we found elevated levels of certain inflammatory and counterregulatory cytokines in cerebrospinal fluid (CSF) (see Figure 20.1). Since inflammatory cytokines generally have short half-lives *in vivo*, determining inflammatory markers of longer half-lives in CSF will be more informative in ASD children.

Autonomic nerve fibers

Autonomic nerve fibers are distributed throughout both primary and secondary lymphoid organs as well as mucosal-associated lymphoid tissues. These fibers are associated with both smooth muscle and specific cellular elements of the immune system (lymphocytes, macrophages, mast cells, and so on). Autonomic nerve fibers release norepinephrine, VIP, CGRP, substance P, opioid peptides, and neuropeptide Y. These neurotransmitters in nerve fibers adjacent to the immune cells may establish a link between the CNS and the immune system. Stress-associated suppression of the immune system may be explained partly through the effects of autonomic nerve fibers transmitting signals from the CNS. It is likely that the immune system also affects the autonomic nerve fibers reciprocally. For example, certain cytokines appear to modulate release of these neurotransmitters from the autonomic nerve endings. Therefore, local production of various cytokines associated with gut inflammation can also influence neuroendocrine–immune interactions through autonomic nerve fibers. It is of interest that many ASD children with GI symptoms in early life tend to develop dysautonomic GI symptoms such as gut dysmotility and suffer from persistent constipation.

POTENTIAL UNDERLINING IMMUNE MECHANISMS ASSOCIATED WITH ASD

In previous sections, we have discussed the potential roles of innate immune abnormalities in CNS inflammation and CNS-mediated behaviors. The CNS has its own immune system, mainly composed of innate immune cells including constitutive parenchymal cells (microglial cells and astrocytes, that correspond to macrophages and fibroblasts in the periphery, respectively), and vascular endothelial cells. Microglial cells can function as APC and also produce a variety of inflammatory mediators including excitatory amino acids such as glutamate and reactive oxygen species (ROS).[31] Migration of activated immune cells and autoantibodies to the CNS can activate these innate immune cells. Inflammatory mediators produced in the peripheral organs could also activate the CNS inflammatory cells, leading to CNS inflammation. Thus innate immune abnormalities indicated in a subset of ASD children may predispose them to activation of the CNS innate immune cells. This could occur by various mechanisms including autoimmune reaction, microbial infection, inflammatory cytokines and mediators from the peripheral tissues, and through altered neurotransmission. In this section, we will discuss the potential underlining immune mechanisms that could lead to clinical features of autism with emphasis on activation of the CNS innate immune cells.

CNS autoimmunity

In a subset of ASD children, CNS autoimmunity may be the underlying etiology. Clustering of autoimmune disorders in the family,[32] and the presence of autoantibodies against neuronal cells,[33–35] support this assumption. Autoantibodies against serotonin receptors have also been reported[36,37] that may cause altered neurotransmission in the serotogenic nervous system.

A primary role for the immune system is well established in various CNS autoimmune disorders. In multiple sclerosis (MS), autoantigens in the CNS and the presence of autoreactive T cells are clearly demonstrated. In MS, autoreactive Th1 cells against CNS autoantigens trigger CNS inflammation, since activated T cells are able to penetrate the normal blood brain barrier and enter the CNS, and autoreactive T cells recognizing CNS antigens accumulate in the brain.[38,39] This will lead to activation of dormant CNS innate immune cells. Chronic inflammatory processes may also be partly carried out by PB macrophages that have migrated to the CNS along with constitutive CNS innate immune cells, leading to changes in CNS-mediated behaviors.[28]

However, as opposed to CNS autoimmune disorders like MS, the onset of autism is skewed to early childhood and the disease is not progressive, generally reaching the static phase before adulthood. CNS imaging studies seldom demonstrate demyelination, unlike in other CNS autoimmune disorders. The presence of autoantibodies against neuronal cells does not seem to correlate with the clinical features of autism. Moreover, these antibodies can also be detected in other neurodegerative disorders and even in a small fraction of normal children.[2] Autoantigens and autoreactive T cells against the brain which are specific for autism have not been identified, indicating that organ-specific autoimmunity is unlikely in a majority of ASD children.

Systemic autoimmune disorders can also cause altered CNS behaviors with some features of autistic behaviors. In rodent models of autoimmunity, cognitive impairment and progressive behavior changes have been reported.[40] In lupus-prone MRL/lpr mice with defect of Fas (CD95), a key cell surface receptor of one of the apoptotic pathways,[41] various neuroendocrine abnormalities have been reported. These include altered neurotransmission with increased dopamine levels in the paraventricular nucleus (PVN) and median eminence, decreased serotonin in the PVN with concurrent increase in serotonin in the hippocampus, and decreased norepinephrine levels in the prefrontal cortex.[42] Decreased CRH and augmented expression of vasopressin mRNA were also reported in this mouse model.[43] These changes are associated with neurodegeneration in this strain of mice.[44,45] The same genetic defect (FAS defect) of MRL mice can also be found in humans with autoimmune lymphoproliferative syndrome (ALPS). There is one case report of concurrent onset of autistic behavior with the onset of autoimmune hemolytic anemia in a FAS-defective ALPS patient.[46] Low dose of steroid apparently improved speech and other cognitive functions in this patient.[46]

On the other hand, we seldom detect underlying well-defined systemic autoimmunity in ASD children with autoimmune workup. As opposed to other CNS systemic autoimmune disorders, CNS inflammation may be less evident in ASD children,[2,30] despite the presence of elevated levels of certain inflammatory cytokines in a subset of ASD children (see Figure 20.1). These findings can be explained if the autoimmune or autoinflammatory phenomena have taken place in early life when counterregulatory immune mechanisms are not fully developed. With maturation of the immune system, such autoimmune phenomena could be better regulated or controlled by counterregulatory mechanisms such as tolerance induction and development of regulatory T cells.[19,21] This makes it difficult to detect evidence of CNS inflammation or autoimmunity. Aberrant innate immune abnormalities present in a subset of ASD children[25] could predispose these individuals to temporal activation of autoreactive T and B cells and resultant autoimmune phenomena in the window period. In summary, autistic behaviors reported in a variety of the CNS autoimmune disorders may be important clues for etiology of neuro-immune interactions. However, systemic autoimmune disorders as an underlying mechanism of autism are more likely to be found in only a limited number of ASD children.

Respiratory microbial infection and immune dysfunction

Many clinicians treating ASD children, including myself, report acute exacerbations of ASD concurrent with or following common respiratory illnesses. The behavioral changes may even be controlled by antibiosis in some ASD children. The possibilities explaining this observation include pathogen-triggered autoimmunity, abnormal effects of inflammatory cytokines produced by microbial infection on the CNS, and chronic viral infection with defective immune defense and subsequent dysregulated inflammatory responses. Pathogen-triggered autoimmunity could be due to production of autoantibodies and/or activation of autoreactive T cells secondary to cross-reactive Ags (molecular mimicry) and/or bystander effects (nonspecific activation of autoreactive cells due to inflammatory cytokines and other mediators). In general, activation of autoreactive T cells often causes irreversible tissue damage and progressive courses, as observed in MS. However, in most ASD children, apparent microbial-triggered exacerbation of autistic features are not progressive and appear to subside or reach the static stage with age. Thus activation of autoreactive T cells against the brain tissue may be less likely to have a major role in (apparent) microbial-triggered exacerbation of ASD.

One model of pathogen-triggered relatively self-limited CNS disease is post-infectious behavioral changes following group A streptococcal infection (post-strettpococcal CNS syndrome). Although its pathogenesis is not fully understood, it appears that group A streptococcal infection induces dysfunction of basal ganglia processes in genetically predisposed individuals. In addition to well-described chorea (Sydeham's chorea: SC) and other hyperkinetic movements (tics, dystonia, and myoclonus), post-streptococcal CNS syndrome is also accompanied by behavioral and emotional changes including obsessive compulsive disorder (OCD), anxiety, and depression.[47,48] This led to the creation of a new acronym, PANDAS (pediatric autoimmune neuropsychiatric disorders associated with streptococcal infections).[48–50] Since group A streptococci do not invade the CNS or produce neurotoxins, immune-mediated insults to the basal ganglia triggered by streptococcal infection appear to play a crucial role. As opposed to MS, PANDAS-associated symptoms are rarely fatal and somewhat self-limited with improvement of clinical symptoms in response to antibiosis.[51] However, a trial of penicillin prophylaxis for PANDAS in a small pilot study was inconclusive.[52] One favored hypothesis for PANDAS and SC is autoantibody production due to cross-reactivity of surface M protein (a major virulent protein) of group A streptococci with basal ganglia tissues. Some evidence suggests the presence of such cross-reactive antibodies,[53,54] but there is no defined molecular mimicry between group A streptococci and the brain tissue.

Although the cross-reactivity between neuronal cells and group A streptococcus is unclear, PANDAS patients have positive markers of rheumatoid fever. Murine IgM monoclonal antibody D8/17 was originally generated by immunizing mice with human B cells obtained from patients with rheumatic fever and has been used as a marker of this disease.[55] B cells binding to D8/17 were elevated in pediatric patients with SC, PANDAS, and Tourette's disorder as compared to age-matched controls.[56,57] Increased B cell binding to D8/17 was also reported in 17 pediatric autism patients,[58] leading to the speculation that certain behavioral changes in ASD children may be associated with group A streptococcal-induced immune reactivity to the basal ganglia. However, D8/17 reactive B cells were not elevated in adult patients with OCD, Tourette's disorder, or autism.[59] B cell epitopes recognized by D8/17 have not been identified and a role for B cells binding to D8/17 in the pathogenesis of post-streptoccccal CNS syndrome is unclear. Prospective studies of group A β-hemolytic streptococcal pharyngitis and OCD also confirmed significant association between these two entities with significantly elevated anti-DNAse B antibody.[51] Taken together, these findings indicate that a common microbial infection could have substantial impact on the CNS-mediated behaviors observed in children with common neuropsychiatric disorders.

A subset of ASD children share similar clinical features of PANDAS as described above. However, parents of ASD children report behavioral exacerbation and developmental regression following a variety of microbial infections and other insults to the immune system, such as vaccination. Given these results, we postulate that nonspecific effects of inflammatory mediators triggered by microbial infection or other stimulants may also have a role in PANDAS-like symptoms observed in ASD children. These proinflammatory mediators could affect CNS-mediated behaviors through interaction of the HPA axis and other mechanisms. In Tourette's syndrome patients with group A β-hemolytic streptococcal infection, increase in markers of immune activation (tryptophan metabolites, neopterin) has been reported.[49] These markers are often induced by inflammatory cytokines and similar conditions could happen in a subset of ASD children. We have also observed augmented production of proinflammatory cytokines in ASD children with LPS stimuli,[25] and others also reported increases in TNF-α production.[60] In summary, abnormalities of the cytokine network may have some relevance in (apparent) microbial-triggered ASD exacerbation and in that regard immunomodulating agents may have a therapeutic role in a subset of ASD children.[60–62]

A lack of appropriate immune responses causes failure of microbial clearance, leading to chronic infection. This could also lead to certain autoimmune conditions. Such conditions can also be induced by inoculation of a live viral vaccine. The role of the measles-mumps-rubella (MMR) vaccine in the development of autism is an exceedingly controversial issue. Following reports of temporal association of autistic regression and enterocolitis with MMR,[24,63] it was hypothesized that chronic measles infection is associated with autism enterocolitis in a subset of ASD children. However, so far epidemiological studies have failed to support this proposal,[35,64,65] and the evidence for measles virus-induced enterocolitis is not convincingly defined.[24,66] (Please see Chapter 21.) So far there are no data revealing direct evidence of chronic microbial infection in ASD children or the presence of markers for particular microbes specific for ASD. There are no well-documented immune mechanisms that can predispose a subset of ASD children to chronic microbial infection. Moreover, parents of ASD children also report temporal association of developmental regression and onset of other autistic features with not only MMR but also with other infant immunizations such as DTP. It remains to be seen whether any chronic microbial infection is associated with the etiology of ASD.

Gut microflora in association with autism

One striking finding in ASD children is frequent GI symptoms, especially in young children. Nonspecific colitis with ileal-lymphoid nodular hyperplasia has been reported in regressive autism[63] with colonic CD8 and TCR$\gamma\delta$ T cell infiltration with prominent epithelial cell damage.[67] The same group also reported epithelial IgG and complement deposition accompanied by infiltration of enterocytes and lymphocytes in epithelium and lamina propria in duodenal biopsies of 24 children with regression autism.[68] Others also reported GI abnormalities including esophagitis (69.4%), chronic gastritis (41.7%), and chronic duodenitis (66.7%) in 36 autism patients who underwent upper GI endoscopy secondary to various GI symptoms.[69] These results suggest that in children with ASD, GI symptoms are likely to reveal immunohistochemical changes in the gut mucosa, indicating the presence of immune-mediated GI inflammation.

In a subset of ASD children, exacerbation of autistic features is often preceded by insults to the GI mucosa such as recurrent and/or prolonged exposure to antibiotics and viral gastroenteritis. It was postulated that disruption of the gut flora might be associated with clinical deterioration due to colonization of neurotoxin-producing microbes. A trial of oral vancomycin in 11 children with regressive autism produced beneficial effects that lasted only a short while.[70] Candida overgrowth can occur following exposure to antibiotics and some ASD children have been tried on a yeast-free diet with concurrent use of antifungal medications with apparent clinical benefits, although lack of good prospective studies will not justify random use of antifungal medication in ASD children.

Antifungal medications and a yeast-free diet have been anecdotally described to induce improvement of chronic fatigue, poor concentration, impaired memory, GI distress, muscular/joint ache, vaginitis, and so on, in general population. Hypersensitive responses to fungal antigens as evidenced by marked delay type skin reactions and lymphocyte proliferative responses might be associated with the above-described symptoms (candida hypersensitivity syndrome). It was reported that a four-week course of nystatin was superior to placebo in a randomized, double blind, placebo-controlled study in 116 adult subjects with such complaints.[71] A combination of yeast-free diet plus nystatin appeared to be most effective in this study. These results indicate that fungal overgrowth and resultant immune reactions in the GI mucosa may exacerbate some autistic behaviors. However, a yeast-free diet is also an essentially wheat-free diet, since it avoids most fermented wheat products. Thus some of the effects of a yeast-free diet might be associated with avoidance of wheat proteins in ASD children who are intolerant to wheat proteins.

Dietary protein intolerance link to innate immune abnormalities

The clinical relevance of gut mucosal immune reactions to dietary proteins (DPs) has been controversial partly due to limited epidemiological data and poor understanding of the underlying mechanisms. Recent evidence indicates that IgE-mediated, immediate-type food allergy accounts for only a small portion of adverse reaction to DPs. Instead, cell-mediated immunity appears to play a vital role and TNF-α produced by T cells and other lineage cells may be closely associated with GI pathogenesis in patients with intolerance to cow's milk protein (CMP).[72–74] Cell-mediated immune reactions take place several hours and even one to two days following the intake of reactive DPs and this tendency may make diagnosis more challenging. Although such adverse reactions are seldom fatal, in extreme occasions, rapid increase in serum TNF-α could cause a shock-like syndrome.[73,75] Infants with CMP intolerance are reported to have increased intestinal membrane permeability as compared to control infants, reflecting damage to tight junctions of GI epithelium, with loss of intestinal integrity and increase in membrane permeability.[76] This abnormal intestinal permeability could persist beyond three years of age in some infants with severe CMP intolerance.[76] Similar increases in gut permeability suggesting the injury of tight junctions have also been reported in autistic children.[77]

Although digestive enzymes degrade most ingested proteins, a small proportion of DPs escape degradation and can be presented to the gut immune system. Even so, dietary antigens induce local and systemic tolerance with various mechanisms such as peripheral anergy, clonal deletion, and development of regulatory T cells.[19] However, activation of the gut mucosal immune system and an increase in DP exposure could occur with the stimuli of innate immunity through GI flora as described in the previous section. That is, changes in the intestinal microbial flora and production of PAMPs by pathogenic bacteria could activate innate immune responses and subsequently lead to broken tolerance. The most common PAMP produced by pathogenic microbes in the gut is an endotoxin. Endotoxin is a potent activator of innate immune cells through Toll-like receptor type 4 (TLR4).[78,79] Individuals with innate immune abnormalities may have a high risk of developing DPI early in life when the gut immune system is still immature and not fully equipped to mount counterregulatory mechanisms.

In ASD children, GI symptoms develop within the first one to two years of life and these symptoms include those commonly seen in patients with CMP intolerance, such as gastroesophageal reflux disease (GERD), colic, diarrhea, unformed stool, and bloating.[73] ASD children seldom reveal IgE positive antibodies against common DPs.[80] IgG antibodies against common DPs were also found in ASD children.[81] A recent report suggested possible cross-reactivity of milk protein-derived peptides with neuronal cells as a possible link between apparent DPI and changes in the CNS-mediated behavior.[81] However, IgG Ab levels agaist DPI do not seem to be associated with clinical features of DPI and this cross-sectional study did not address the relationship between IgG antibody levels and clinical features of ASD. Prospective longitudinal studies will be required to evaluate further a possible link between anti-DP IgG antibodies and ASD. Others also pointed out the effects of CMP and gliadin-derived morphine peptides in the gut and the CNS through their binding to opioid receptors.[82] It is also possible that these morphine peptides could influence inflammatory responses in the gut mucosa and the CNS.[83]

As summarized in the previous section, GI inflammation found in ASD children appears to be associated with cellular immune mechanisms similar to those seen in DPI infants.[73] Given the apparent beneficial effects of elimination diets such as a casein-free and gluten-free diet, some GI symptoms in ASD children could be caused by dysregulated immune reactivity to DPs. We have addressed this possibility by assessing cellular immune reactivity to DPI in ASD children, employing DPI children as positive controls.[80] Our results revealed significant cellular immune reactivity to common DPs in a number of ASD children, as observed in DPI children.[80] Autistic mononuclear cells produced a twofold increase of TNF-α and IFN-γ when stimulated by common DPs (CMP, soy protein, and gliadin, a major wheat protein) at high frequency (> 70–80%).[80] Moreover, most ASD children who produced excessive amounts of TNF-α with these DPs revealed resolution of GI symptoms and improvement of certain autistic features with implementation of appropriate elimination diets.[80] Thus, DPI against common DPs may play a role in GI inflammation in a number of ASD children and the proper elimination diet may be helpful in ASD children with evidence of DPI. One small open-pilot study indicated the beneficial effects of an elimination diet.[84] However, previous trials of the elimination diets at two centers assigned the ASD subjects randomly to the elimination diet without any screening measures and the results are mixed or inconclusive.[85,86]

The question arises as to why ASD children develop DPI so frequently when compared to typically developing children. Clinical features in some ASD children indicate the presence of innate immune abnormalities and our previous results support this hypothesis.[25] Interestingly, we have observed that production of TNF-α and IFN-γ against common DPs by ASD PBMCs positively correlated with their production of proinflammatory cytokines (TNF-α, IL-1β, and IL-6) with LPS.[80] Such a correlation was less evident in control DPI children than in ASD children. Thus we postulate that innate immune abnormalities frequently found in ASD children might make their gut immune system more easily activated by stimulants of innate immunity derived from GI flora, making them more vulnerable to sensitization by benign environmental factors, including DPs, than normal children. This may lead to the persistent production of various inflammatory mediators that subsequently affect the neuroendocrine system.[79] The constant activation of sensory nerve endings abundant in the gut mucosa may also affect the neuroendocrine system.

Recently, we have studied PB-derived macrophages from ASD children with evidence of innate immune abnormalities. Using these cells, we have assessed their responses against platelet activating factor (PAF) when cells were treated with medium only, LPS (0.1 μg/ml), or glutamate (500 mmol/L) along with

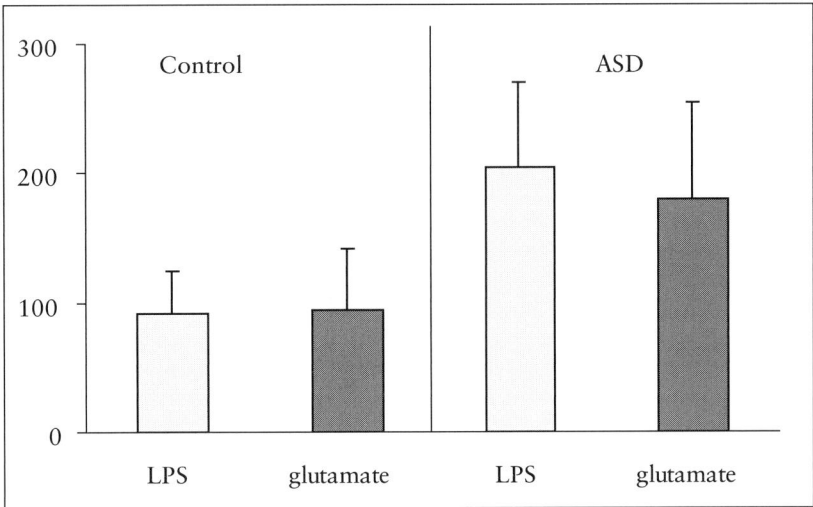

Figure 20.2 Changes in average peak intracellular Ca^{2+} concentrations with PAF using peripheral blood-derived macrophages obtained from controls ($n = 8$) and ASD children with innate immune abnormalities ($n = 8$). Cells were either treated with LPS (0.1 μg/ml) overnight or untreated prior to exposure to PAF (100 nM). Changes in $[Ca^{2+}]_i$ were detected by staining cells with Fura-2 AM and ratiometric imaging. Typically 20–30 cells in the same field were tested for their responses to PAF in each study subject. ASD macrophages revealed higher peak $[Ca^{2+}]_i$ in response to PAF following the treatment, while there was little change in PAF responses in control cells ($p < .005$ for LPS and $p < .05$ for glutamate by Mann-Whitney test).

cytokine production. Microglial cells were reported to become less responsive to PAF-like tissue macrophages.[87] However, our preliminary results indicate that treating cells with LPS and glutamate significantly increased the peak Ca^{2+} intracellular concentration in ASD PB-derived macrophages but not in control cells (see Figure 20.2). ASD macrophages also seem to produce more TNF-α and IL-6 than control cells in response to LPS (unpublished observation). These results indicate that once inflammatory changes take place in the GI tract, a chronic inflammatory condition may persist more easily in the gut mucosa and even in the CNS in ASD children with innate immune abnormalities. It remains to be seen how such abnormalities are associated with the clinical features of ASD.

CONCLUSIONS

A variety of immune abnormalities have been reported in ASD children. However, so far no definite immune markers specific for ASD have been identified. Since onset of ASD is skewed to an early age and the condition often becomes static or stabilized before reaching adulthood, immune parameters are likely to change with age, reflecting the complex effects of both genetic factors and exposure to various environmental factors. It is also unclear how these immune abnormalities could affect the development of ASD. Our results in two previous studies indicate that innate immune abnormalities in some ASD children could predispose them to dysregulated immune responses to common microbial infection and sensitization to benign environmental factors including DPs. However, it is unclear how such aberrant immune responses lead to the cognitive impairment and development of aberrant behaviors in children with ASD. Many potential mechanisms have been postulated but none of them are supported by definitive evidence. To address many unanswered questions, it is critical to assess promising immune and neuroendocrine parameters longitudinally in ASD children starting from a young age. It would be ideal if ASD children are subgrouped by objective immune and neuroendocrine markers in such prospective studies. These studies will be crucial to evaluate potential therapeutic effects of immunomodulating agents in subsets of ASD children.

ACKNOWLEDGEMENT

This study was partly supported by funding from Jonty Foundation, St Paul, MN, and UMDNJ Foundation, Newark, NJ.

REFERENCES

1. Gillberg C, Coleman M. *Biology of the Autistic Syndromes* (3rd ed). Clinics in Developmental Medicine No 153/4. London: Mac Keith Press, 2000.
2. Korvatska E, Ven de Water J, Anders TF, Gershwin ME. Genetic and immunologic considerations in autism. *Neurobiol Dis* 2002; 9: 102–25.
3. Ilan K, Xiao-Song H, Gershwin ME, Yehuda S. Immune factors in autism: a critical review. *J Autism Dev Disord* 2002; 32: 337–45.
4. Medzhitov R, Janeway C Jr. Innate immunity. *New Engl J Med* 2000; 343: 338–44.
5. Ulevitch RJ. Molecular mechanisms of innate immunity. *Immunol Res* 2000; 21: 49–54.
6. Wright SD. Toll, a new piece in the puzzle of innate immunity. *J Exp Med* 1999; 189: 605–9.
7. Dunn AJ, Wang J, Ando T. Effects of cytokines on cerebral neurotransmission: comparison with the effects of stress. *Adv Exp Med Biol* 1999; 461: 117–27.
8. Haddad JJ, Saadé NE, Safieh-Garabendian B. Cytokines and neuro-immune endocrine interactions: a role for the hypothalamic-pituitary-adrenal revolving axis. *J Neuroimmunol* 2002; 133: 1–19.
9. Mullington JM, Hinze-Selch D, Pollmacher T. Mediators of inflammation and their interaction with sleep: relevance for chronic fatigue syndrome and related conditions. *Ann NY Acad Sci* 2001; 933: 201–10.
10. Flavell, RA. The molecular basis of T cell differentiation. *Immunol Res* 1999; 19: 159–68.
11. Murphy KM, Reiner SL. The lineage decisions of helper T cells. *Nat Rev Immunol* 2002; 12: 933–44.
12. Rogge L. A genomic view of helper T cell subsets. *Ann NY Acad Sci* 2002; 974: 57–67.
13. Sewell DL, Reinke EK, Hogan LH et al. Immunoregulation of CNS autoimmunity by helminth and mycobaterial infections. *Immunol Lett* 2002; 82: 101–10.
14. Elias JA, Lee CG, Zheng T et al. New insights into the pathogenesis of asthma. *J Clin Invest* 2003; 111: 291–7.
15. Woodfolk JA, Platts-Mills TA. The immune response to intrinsic and extrinsic allergens: determinants of allergic disease. *Int Arch Allergy Immunol* 2002; 129: 277–85.
16. Bach JF. The effect of infections on susceptibility to autoimmune and allergic diseases. *N Engl J Med* 2002; 347: 911–20.
17. Gupta S, Aggarwal S, Rashanaravan B, Lee T. Th1- and Th2-like cytokines in $CD4^+$ and $CD8^+$ T cells in autism. *J Neuroimmunol* 1998; 85: 106–9.
18. Singh VK. Plasma increase of interleukin-12 and interferon-gamma. Pathologic significance in autism. *J Neuroimmunol* 1996; 66: 143–5.
19. Annacker O, Powrie F. Homeostasis of intestinal immune regulation. *Microbes Infect* 2002; 4: 567–74.
20. Shevack EM. CD4+ CD25+ suppressor T cells: more questions than answers. *Nat Rev Immunol* 2002; 2: 389–400.
21. Umetsu DT, McIntire JJ, Akbari O et al. Asthma: an epidemic of dysregulated immunity. *Nat Immunol* 2002; 3: 715–20.
22. Loustrinen L, Pirttilä T, Collin P. Celiac disease presenting with neurological disorders. *Eur Neurol* 1999; 42: 132–5.
23. Erb KJ, Wholleben G. Novel vaccine protecting against the development of allergic disorders: a double-edged sword? *Curr Opin Immunol* 2002; 14: 633–42.
24. Wakefield AJ, Anthony A, Murch SH et al. Enterocolitis in children with developmental disorders. *Am J Gastroenterol* 2000; 95: 2285–95.
25. Jyonouchi H, Sun S, Le H. Proinflammatory and regulatory cytokine production associated with innate and adaptive immune responses in children with autism spectrum disorders and developmental regression. *J Neuroimmunol* 2001; 20: 170–9.
26. Harbour-McMenamin D, Smith EM, Blalock JE. Bacterial lipopolysaccharide induction of leukocyte-derived corticotropin and endorphins. *Infect Immun* 1985; 48: 813–7.
27. Payne LC, Weignet DA, Blalock JE. Induction of pituitary sensitivity to interleukin-1: a new function for corticotropin-releasing hormone. *Biochem Biophys Res Cemm* 1994; 198: 480–4.
28. Minagar A, Shapshak P, Fujimura R et al. The role of macrophage/microglia and astrocytes in the pathogenesis of three neurologic disorders: HIV-associated dementia, Alzheimer disease, and multiple sclerosis. *J Neurol Sci* 2002; 202: 13–23.
29. Benveniste EN. Cytokines: influence on glial cell gene expression and function. In: *Neuroimmunodendrinology* 3rd ed (Blalock JE, ed). Basel: Karger, 1997: 31–75.
30. Zimmerman AW. Commentary: immunological treatments for autism. In search of reasons for promising approaches. *J Autism Dev Disord* 2000; 30: 481–4.
31. Bezzi P, Domercq M, Brambilla L et al. CXCR4-activated astrocyte glutamate release via TNFα: amplification by microglia triggers neurotoxicity. *Nature Neurosci* 2001; 4: 702–10.
32. Comi AM, Zimerman AW, Frye VH et al. Familial clustering of autoimmune disorders and evaluation of medical risk factors in autism. *J Chil Neurol* 1999; 14: 388–94.
33. Singh VK, Warren RP, Odell JD et al. Antibodies to myelin basic protein in children with autistic behavior. *Brain Behav Immunol* 1993; 7: 97–103.
34. Singh VK, Warren RP, Averett R, Chaziuddin M. Circulating autoantibodies to neuronal and glial filament proteins in autism. *Pediatr Neurol* 1997; 17: 88–90.
35. Krause I, He XS, Gershwin ME, Shoenfeld Y. Immune factors in autism: a critical review. *J Autism Dev Disord* 2002; 32: 337–45.
36. Todd RD, Ciaranello RD. Demonstration of inter- and intraspecies differences in serotonin binding sites by antibodies from an autistic child. *Proc Natl Acad Sci USA* 1985; 82: 612–6.
37. Singh VK, Singh EA, Warren RP. Hyperserotoninemia and serotonin receptor antibodies in children with autism but not mental retardation. *Biol Psychiatry* 1997; 41: 753–5.
38. Hickley WF, Hsu BL, Kimura H. T-lymphocyte entry into the central nervous system. *J Neurosci Res* 1991; 28: 254–60.
39. Schwartz M, Cohen IR. Autoimmunity can benefit self-maintenance. *Immunol Today* 2000; 21: 265–8.
40. Brey RL, Sakic B, Szechtman H, Denburg JA. Animal models for nervous system disease in systemic lupus erythematosus. *Ann NY Acad Sci* 1997; 823: 97–106.
41. Hussein MR, Haemel AK, Wood GS. Apoptosis and melanoma: molecular mechanisms. *J Pathol* 2003; 199: 275–88.
42. Sakic B, Lacosta S, Denburg JA, Szechtman H. Altered neurotransmission in brains of autoimmune mice: pharmacological and neurochemical evidence. *J Neuroimmunol* 2002; 129: 84–96.
43. Sakic B, Laflamme N, Crnic LS et al. Reduced corticotropin-releasing factor and enhanced vasopression gene expression in brains of mice with autoimmunity-induced behavioral dysfunction. *J Neuroimmunol* 1999; 96: 80–91.
44. Ballok DA, Millward JM, Sakic B. Neurodegeneration in autoimmune MRL-lpr mice as revealed by fluoro jade B staining. *Brain Res* 2003; 964: 200–10.
45. Sakic B, Szechtman H, Denburg JA et al. Progressive atrophy of pyramidal neuronal dendrites in autoimmune MRL-lpr mice. *J Neuroimmunol* 1998; 87: 162–70.
46. Shenoy S, Arnold S, Chatila T. Response to steroid therapy in autism secondary to autoimmune lymphoproliferative syndrome. *J Pediatr* 2000; 136: 576–7.
47. Dale RC. Autoimmunity and the basal ganglia: new insights into old diseases. *Q J Med* 2003; 96: 183–91.

48. Swedo SE, Leonard HL, Garvey M et al. Pediatric autoimmune neuropsychiatric disorders associated with streptococcal infections: clinical description of the first 50 cases. *Am J Psychiatry* 1998; **155**: 264–71.
49. Hoekstra PJ, Kallenberg CGM, Korf J, Minderaa RB. Is Tourette's syndrome an autoimmune disease? *Mol Psychiatry* 2002; **7**: 437–45.
50. Swedo SE. Pediatric autoimmune neuropsychiatric disorders associated with stretpoccal infections (PANDAS). *Mol Psychiatry* 2002; **2**: S24–5.
51. Murphy MI, Pichichero ME. Prospective identification and treatment of children with pediatric autoimmune neuropsychiatric disorder associated with group A streptococcal infection (PANDAS). *Arch Pediatr Adoles Med* 2002; **156**: 356–61.
52. Garvey MA, Perlmutter SJ, Allen AJ et al. A pilot study of penicillin prophylaxis for neuropsychiatric exacerbations triggered by streptococcal infections. *Sci Biol Psychiatry* 1999; **45**: 1564–71.
53. Husby G, van de Rijin I, Zabriskie JB et al. Antibodies reacting with cytoplasm of subthalamic and caudate nuclei neurons in chorea and acute rheumatic fever. *J Exp Med* 1976; **144**: 1094–110.
54. Church AJ, Cardoso F, Dale RC et al. Anti-basal ganglia antibodies in acute and persistent Sydenham's chorea. *Neurology* 2002; **50**: 227–31.
55. Gibofsky A, Khanna A, Suh E, Zabriske JB. The genetics of rheumatic fever: relationship to streptococcal infection and autoimmune disease. *J Rheumatol* 1991; **18**: S1–5.
56. Murphy TK, Goodman WK, Fudge MW et al. B lymphocyte antigen D8/17: a peripheral marker for childhood-onset obsessive-compulsive disorder and Tourette's syndrome? *Am J Psychiatry* 1997; **154**: 402–7.
57. Murphy TK, Benson N, Zaytoun A et al. Progress toward analysis of D8/17 binding to B cells in children with obsessive compulsive disorder and/or chronic tic disorder. *J Neuroimmunol* 2001; **120**: 146–51.
58. Hollander E, DelGiudice-Asch G, Simon L et al. B lymphocyte antigen D8/17 and repetitive behaviors in autism. *Am J Psychiatry* 1999; **156**: 317–20.
59. Eisen JL, Leonard HL, Swedo SE et al. The use of antibody D8/17 to identify B cells in adults with obsessive-compulsive disorder. *Psychiatry Res* 2001; **104**: 221–5.
60. Gupta S, Rimland B, Shilling PD. Pentoxifylline: brief review and rationale for its possible use in the treatment of autism. *J Child Neurol* 1996; **11**: 501–4.
61. Frielander RM. Apoptosis and caspases in neurodegenerative diseases. *N Engl J Med* 2003; **348**: 1365–75.
62. Gupta S, Aggarwal S, Heads C. Dysregulated immune system in children with autism: beneficial effects of intravenous immune globulin on autistic characteristics. *J Autism Dev Dis* 1996; **26**: 439–52.
63. Wakefield AJ, Murch SH, Anthony A et al. Ileal-lymphoid-nodular hyperplasia, non-specific colitis, and pervasive developmental disorder in children. *Lancet* 1998; **351**: 637–41.
64. Madsen KM, Hviid A, Vestergaard M et al. A population-based study of measles, mumps, and rubella vaccination and autism. *N Engl J Med* 2002; **347**: 1477–82.
65. Mäkelä A, Nuorti JP, Peltola H. Neurologic disorders after measles-mumps-rubella vaccination. *Pediatrics* 2002; **110**: 957–63.
66. Kawashima H, Mori T, Kahiwagi Y et al. Detection and sequencing of measles virus from peripheral mononuclear cells from patients with inflammatory bowel disease and autism. *Digest Dis Science* 2000; **45**: 723–9.
67. Furlano R, Anthony A, Day R et al. Colonic CD8 and γδ T-cell infiltration with epithelial damage in children with autism. *J Pediatr* 2001; **138**: 3663–72.
68. Torrente F, Ashwood P, Day R et al. Small intestinal enteropathy with epithelial IgG and complement deposition in children with regressive autism. *Mol Psychiatry* 2002; **7**: 375–82.
69. Horvath K, Papadimitriou JC, Rabsztyn A et al. Gastrointestinal abnormalities in children with autistic disorder. *J Pediatr* 1999; **135**: 559–63.
70. Sandler RH, Finegold SM, Bolte ER et al. Short-term benefit from oral vancomycin treatment of regressive-onset autism. *J Chil Neurol* 2000; **15**: 429–35.
71. Santelmann H, Laerum E, Roennevig J, Fagertun HE. Effectiveness of nystatin in polysymptomatic patients. A randomized, double-blind trial with nystatin versus placebo in general practice. *Family Practice* 2001; **18**: 258–65.
72. Benlounes N, Candalh C, Matarazzo P et al. The time-course of milk antigen-induced TNF-α secretion differs according to the clinical symptoms in children with cow's milk protein. *J Allergy Clin Immunol* 1999; **104**: 863–9.
73. Sampson HA, Anderson JA. Summary and recommendations: classification of gastrointestinal manifestations due to immunologic reactions to foods in infants and young children. *J Ped Gastroenterol Nutr* 2000; **30**: S87–94.
74. Sicherer SH. Food protein-induced enterocolitis syndrome: clinical perspectives. *J Ped Gastroenterol Nutr* 2000; **30**: S45–9.
75. Nowak-Wegrzyn A, Sampson HA, Wood RA, Sicherer SH. Food protein-induced enterocolitis syndrome caused by solid food proteins. *Pediatrics* 2003; **111**: 829–35.
76. Dupont C, Heyman M. Food protein-induced enterocolitis syndrome: laboratory perspectives. *J Ped Gastroenterol Nutr* 2000; **30**: S50–7.
77. D'Eufemia P, Celli M, Finocchiaro R et al. Abnormal intestinal permeability in children with autism. *Acta Pediatr* 1996; **85**: 1076–9.
78. Beutler B. TLR4 as the mammalian endotoxin sensor. *Curr Top Microbiol Immunol* 2002; **270**: 109–20.
79. Rivest S. Molecular insights on the cerebral innate immune system. *Brain Behav Immunol* 2003; **17**: 13–9.
80. Jyonouchi H, Sun S, Le H, Itokazu N. Innate immunity associated with inflammatory responses and cytokine production against common dietary proteins in patients with autism spectrum disorders. *Neuropsychobiol* 2002; **46**: 76–84.
81. Vojdani A, Campbell AW, Anyanwu E et al. Antibodies to neuron-specific antigens in children with autism: possible cross-reaction with encephalitogenic protein from milk, *Chlamydia penumoniae* and *streptococcus* group A. *J Neuroimmunol* 2002; **120**: 168–77.
82. Wakefield AJ, Puleston JM, Montgomery SM et al. Review article: the concept of entero-colonic encephalopahy, autism, and opioid receptor ligands. *Alim Pharmacol Ther* 2002; **16**: 663–74.
83. Robers TJ, Peterson PK. Opioid G protein-coupled receptors: signals at the crossroads of inflammation. *Trends Immunol* 2003; **24**: 116–21.
84. Lucarelli S, Frediani T, Zingoni AM et al. Food allergy and infantile autism. *Pamminerva Med* 1995; **37**: 137–41.
85. Knivsberg A, Richelt K, Høien T et al. Parents' observations after one year of dietary intervention for children with autistic syndrome. In: *Psychobiology of Autism: Current Research and Practice* (Shattock P, Linfoot G, eds). Sunderland: Autism Research Unit, University of Sunderland and Autism North, 1998: 13–24.
86. Whiteley P, Rogers J, Savery D et al. A gluten-free diet as an intervention for autism and associated spectrum disorders: preliminary findings. *Autism* 1999; **3**: 45–65.
87. Wang X, Bae JH, Kim SU, McLarnon JG. Platelet-activating factor induced Ca^{2+} signaling in human microglia. *Brain Res* 1999; **842**: 159–65.

21

The gut–brain axis in childhood developmental disorders: Viruses and vaccines

Andrew J Wakefield, Paul Ashwood, and Iain Collins

INTRODUCTION

This chapter is written from the perspective of the gastroenterologist. It seeks to summarize the evidence that viral exposure leading to an initial extracranial infection may be associated, indirectly or directly, with neuropsychiatric pathology. The focus is largely upon autism and gastrointestinal (GI) inflammation although recent reports suggest that the GI findings may be relevant to a broader spectrum of developmental disorders.[1,2]

Autism, like hepatic encephalopathy, is a behavioral syndrome that reflects cerebral dysfunction. Both may be the final common expression of a variety of different initiating insults, including primary genetic disorders, infection, toxic injury, and autoimmune disease. Can autism be caused by a viral infection and, if so, what is the pathogenetic chain of events that links exposure to neuropathology?

AUTISM AND VIRAL INFECTION

Clues to a possible infectious contribution to the etiology of autism come from the observation of a season-of-birth effect in different countries.[3–7] Volkmar and colleagues dismiss this but seem not to consider the possibility that such an effect may reflect an historical pattern of epidemic infectious exposure that has changed for more recent birth cohorts.[8] The possible role of vaccination in this context is discussed below.

Atypical exposures to common childhood infections and atypical outcomes from infections with *herpesviridae*, in particular, including herpes simplex,[9] cytomegalovirus,[10,11] and Epstein-Barr virus,[12] have been linked to autism. Measles, mumps, and rubella viruses, in their natural form, have been linked to childhood developmental disorders, including autism[13–16] and disintegrative disorder.[17] Measles-containing vaccines have been causally linked to developmental regression.[18] A study comparing exposure patterns of 183 children with autism and 355 sibling controls to the encephalitogenic viruses measles, mumps, rubella, and chickenpox found that 'total autistic symptomatology' was associated with prenatal exposure to measles and mumps, and early mumps postnatal infection, whereas prenatal rubella was associated with a 'partial autistic syndrome'.[13]

Sophisticated statistical modeling of the number of autism births compared with epidemics of measles, rubella, poliomyelitis, viral meningitis, and viral encephalitis revealed that children born during epidemics of measles and viral meningitis were at significantly greater risk of developing autism.[14]

A possible association between MMR vaccination and autistic regression in previously developmentally normal children has recently been reported.[19–21] The evidence for this link is controversial, reflecting the widely differing conclusions of basic and clinical science versus epidemiology. The basis for making such an association is best understood in the light of the clinical presentation and pathological findings in affected children.

GASTROINTESTINAL IMMUNOPATHOLOGY AND AUTISM

Our own studies of etiopathogenesis have been based upon the investigation of a cohort of children between the ages of three and 15 years referred for a GI opinion. The affected children had a history of normal early development followed by developmental regression (stagnation in a few) leading, in most, to a diagnosis of autism – often labeled as atypical in view of the associated regression. Behavioral and developmental regression frequently evolved through a variable hierarchy of changes in sleep pattern, loss of language and other communication skills including proto-declarative pointing, and increasing social isolation. Self-injurious behaviors were prominent in many. From early in their clinical deterioration, children were described as acquiring a glazed, distant look; many had been investigated for suspected hearing loss. Transient neurological problems were reported in some, including ataxias, gait disturbances, and loss of co-ordinated eating. Children who had established or started to establish continence often lost these skills. Loss of body temperature control and altered perception of temperature, taste, and pain, and excessive thirst were frequently reported.

The GI symptoms in affected children were of particular interest. These often started around the same time as the behavioral symptoms and included chronic constipation with overflow, frank diarrhea, pain, bloating, and esophageal reflux with nocturnal waking and distress. GI and behavioral symptoms were reported to be provoked by certain foods such as grains and dairy products, and withholding these foods often led to symptomatic improvements.

In prospective studies, GI symptoms in children with autism appear to be common,[22,23] but require careful attention since they are neither as florid as inflammatory bowel disease (IBD) nor, for obvious reasons, can they be readily articulated. A child in pain who is unable to communicate normally may be distressed, aggressive, and self injurious; our early empirical observations that bowel clearance or treatment of GI inflammation often abrogated these behavioral symptoms is a clue to their likely intestinal origin.

There is now compelling evidence that children with autism and GI symptoms have organic mucosal pathology.[19,24–27] Detailed analysis of over 150 affected children undergoing GI endoscopy and biopsy has identified ileo-colonic lymphoid nodular hyperplasia (LNH; see Figure 21.1a) – not a normal variant in children – and enterocolitis (see Figure 21.1b) as the two key pathologic features. Sabra and colleagues have presented preliminary evidence of similar findings in some children with attention deficit hyperactivity disorder (ADHD),[1,2] suggesting that GI pathology may be relevant to a broader spectrum of childhood developmental and behavioral disorders.

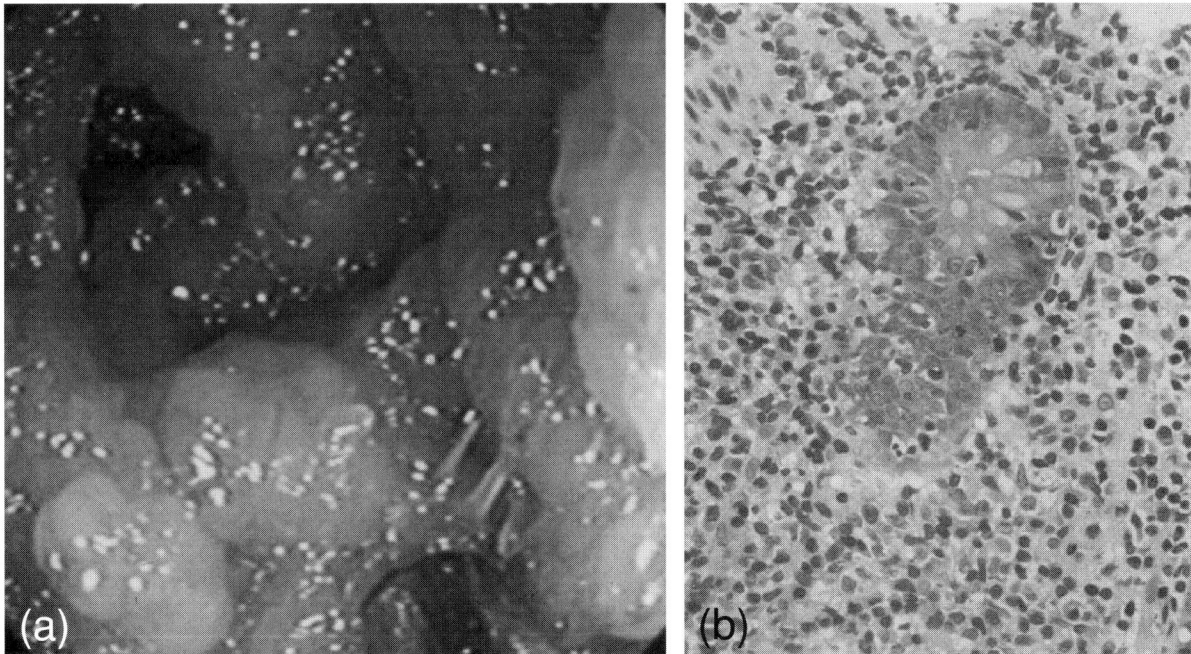

Figure 21.1 (a) Florid ileal lymphoid nodular hyperplasia in a child with autistic enterocolitis. (b) Focal active chronic colitis in an affected child associated with neutrophil infiltration of crypt epithelium (cryptitis).

The histological lesion consists of a patchy mild to moderate enterocolitis. Typical histological findings include infiltration of the lamina propria and crypt epithelium by acute and chronic inflammatory cells, with excess eosinophils and apoptotic debris within the upper lamina propria. Crypt abscess formation is seen in more advanced lesions, and mucosal regenerative changes are indicated by distorted crypt architecture.

Upper GI pathology is also present in these children at a surprisingly high rate. Horvath and colleagues have reported a high prevalence of upper GI pathology, including esophagitis, gastritis, and duodenitis with impaired brush-border hydrolase in affected children, data that concur with our own.[24]

In order to characterize the intestinal pathology further, extensive quantitative immunohistochemistry of the mucosal lesions in large and small intestine has been undertaken.[26,27] Comparison with appropriate controls, including colonic tissue from developmentally normal children with ileal LNH, Crohn's disease, or ulcerative colitis, and duodenal tissue from children with cerebral palsy or celiac disease, revealed a subtle but characteristic pathology. Briefly, the colonic lesion represents a novel lymphocytic colitis, with moderately dense infiltration of both T-cells and plasma cells, disproportionate to the inflammation seen on routine histological examination. In particular, both CD8$^+$ cells and γδ T-cells are present at high density, the latter in excess of all studied groups. Crypt cell proliferation was substantially increased and the epithelial basement membrane thicker than in either normal or disease control groups. Absence of colonic epithelial HLA-DR expression in autistic children suggested a T_H2-skewed mucosal immune response.

Studies of the corresponding small intestinal lesion in affected children also indicated a distinct cell-mediated immunopathology, in which lamina propria CD3$^+$ and CD8$^+$ T-cell density exceeded controls including celiac disease, and epithelial damage was prominent.[27] Specifically, IgG co-localized with complement C1q at the epithelial basolateral membrane, suggesting autoimmunity, and epithelial proliferation was grossly increased. This was not seen in either normal controls or in cerebral palsy. Similar findings of a CD8$^+$ predominant immunopathology have since been reported in gastric biopsies from affected children, where the lesion is distinct from *Helicobacter pylori* gastritis and focal Crohn's gastritis in children (submitted for publication).

The foregoing immunohistochemical findings of a pan-enteric mucosal immunopathology characterized by an excess of CD8$^+$ lymphocytes have recently been confirmed by flow cytometric analysis of mucosal lymphocyte populations in similarly affected children.[28,29] Flow cytometric analysis of CD3$^+$ lymphocyte intracellular cytokine profiles revealed extensive immunodysregulation, characterized by a significant excess of TNF-α, raised INF-γ, and a reduced counter-regulatory IL-10, in biopsies from duodenum, ileum, and colon. These changes are largely mirrored in the spontaneous peripheral blood CD3$^+$ lymphocyte cytokine profile of affected children, and in the induced cytokine production of these cells in response to lipopolysaccharide and phytohemagluttinin stimulation.[30,31]

It is likely that reported functional GI issues in many affected children, including impaired brush border enzyme activity,[24] dysbiosis,[32–34] and permeability changes,[35,36] are a reflection of underlying mucosal immunopathology.

SYSTEMIC IMMUNITY

Many affected children suffer from recurrent, prolonged infections, particularly of the upper respiratory tract, and there is a high incidence of dietary allergy, eczema, and adenotonsillar hypertrophy. Routine immunological investigation frequently reveals lymphopenia, affecting both CD4$^+$ and CD8$^+$ populations. Consistent with allergic predisposition, IgA is usually in the lower quartile of the normal range,[37] and a raised IgG1 and low IgG2 and 4 are common. Functionally, the majority of children assessed showed unresponsiveness for all common recall antigens on cutaneous delayed-hypersensitivity testing, in significant contrast to age-matched controls.[38] Similar findings of lymphopenia and systemic immune dysregulation have been reported by other groups.[39,40] A history of organ-specific autoimmunity in first-degree family members is common.[41]

Recently, we have examined the differentiation status of circulating CD8$^+$ lymphocytes, on the basis that in the presence of persistent virus infection, there is an over-representation of the CD38$^+$CD28$^-$CD27$^-$ phenotype, reflecting CD8$^+$ cell activation (CD38$^+$) with loss of costimulatory molecules (CD27$^-$CD28$^-$). The key findings in affected children included the observations that: there was no correlation between CD8$^+$CD38$^+$, CD8$^+$CD27$^-$, and CD8$^+$CD28$^-$ expression with age; and that within the CD8$^+$CD38$^+$ lymphocyte population there was a significant excess of CD27$^-$, CD28$^-$, and CD27$^-$28$^-$ cells compared with inflamed and non-inflamed developmentally normal controls (unpublished data).

SUMMARY

Within the autistic spectrum there is a group of children with what may be a primary intestinal pathology with autoimmune features (provisionally termed 'autistic enterocolitis'). Affected children have both systemic and mucosal immune dysregulation. The findings are consistent with a persistent viral pathogenesis. Autistic enterocolitis exhibits a striking overlap with human immunodeficiency virus (HIV) enteropathy, features of which include LNH in which the hyperplasic lymphoid follicles are a nidus of HIV infection, a diffuse increase in mucosal CD8+ lymphocytes in the colon and small intestine,[42,43] and a change in intestinal mucosal cytokine production. Specifically, upregulation of TNF-α and INF-γ, and downregulation of IL-10, have been reported in the GI mucosa from HIV-infected patients.[44]

ETIOLOGY

As with the great majority of cases of autism, the cause of the developmental disorder in these children is not known. However, in many children referred to us, parental reports suggest a temporal relationship with exposure to the measles-mumps-rubella (MMR) vaccine.

Anecdotal parental reports of UK and US children have suggested a role for the combined MMR vaccine rather than the monovalent measles vaccine in their child's regression, raising the possibility of a compound effect of the concurrent exposure. Certainly MV is capable of exhibiting interference phenomena[45–47] that may modify the immune response and increase the risk of persistent infection. Interference has also been reported in the MMR vaccine.[47,48] The possibility that polyvalent MMR might represent a compound risk for mucosal immunopathology is consistent with the observation that close temporal exposure to measles and mumps was a risk factor for later IBD.[49] Concurrent exposure to measles and rubella vaccines has been reported to increase the risk of acute gastrointestinal adverse events compared with the single vaccines given alone.[49] The findings of an intestinal pathology consistent with a viral etiology, and a temporal link with MMR vaccination, made it important to determine whether there was persistent viral RNA and protein within the reactive ileal lymphoid follicles, particularly as MV exhibits specific tropism for gut-associated lymphoid tissue.[50]

Analysis of ileal lymphoid tissues from affected children and developmentally normal pediatric controls was conducted with well-characterized specific antibodies against MV, mumps, rubella, HSV I and II, HIV, and adenovirus. A characteristic pattern of staining for MV was observed in the tissues of affected children, consistent with the follicular dendritic cell (FDC) matrix (see Figure 21.2a) as seen in HIV infection (see Figure 21.2b). Staining for other viruses was not seen. The difference between cases and controls for the presence of MV antigen was significant. Flow cytometric analysis of single cell suspensions derived from ileal lymphoid biopsies of affected children showed populations of MV+ lymphocytes and FDC. Mean percentage MV+ cell populations were significantly increased compared with developmentally normal controls. Serum IgG immunoreactivity for MV was significantly elevated in affected children compared with age-matched controls; however mumps, rubella, and CMV IgG antibody titers were not elevated.[51]

Further analysis of ileal lymphoid tissues was conducted using in-cell and TaqMan RT-PCR technologies.[52] Localization of the mRNA signal was performed using a specific follicular dendritic cell antibody. Of 91 affected children, 75 were positive for measles virus in their intestinal tissue, compared with five of 70 control patients. Measles virus was identified within FDC and some lymphocytes in foci of reactive follicular hyperplasia. Replication studies are underway.

In a series of studies of similarly affected children from the US, Singh and coworkers have identified quantitative and qualitative differences in the IgG antibody response to MV.[20,21,53] Anti-MV IgG antibody levels were significantly higher in the blood of affected children, compared with developmentally normal children of the same age and sibling controls. This was not the case for IgG antibodies against rubella virus and mumps virus. In addition, in immunoblotting studies there was a specific IgG antibody response in 80% of affected children to a 74 kD protein antigen from the MV hemagluttinin protein derived from the MMR vaccine that was not detected in any controls.

The data confirm an association between MV and GI pathology in some children with developmental disorder. The presence of the virus may reflect a bystander effect due to sequestration of MV in foci of inflammation, although this is unlikely. MV antigen was not detected in foci of colonic inflammation in the same children. In view of the presence of both MV antigen and genomic RNA in reactive lymphoid tissues, it is also unlikely that the observations indicate long-term trapping of viral antigen by FDC, as part of a normal immunological process.

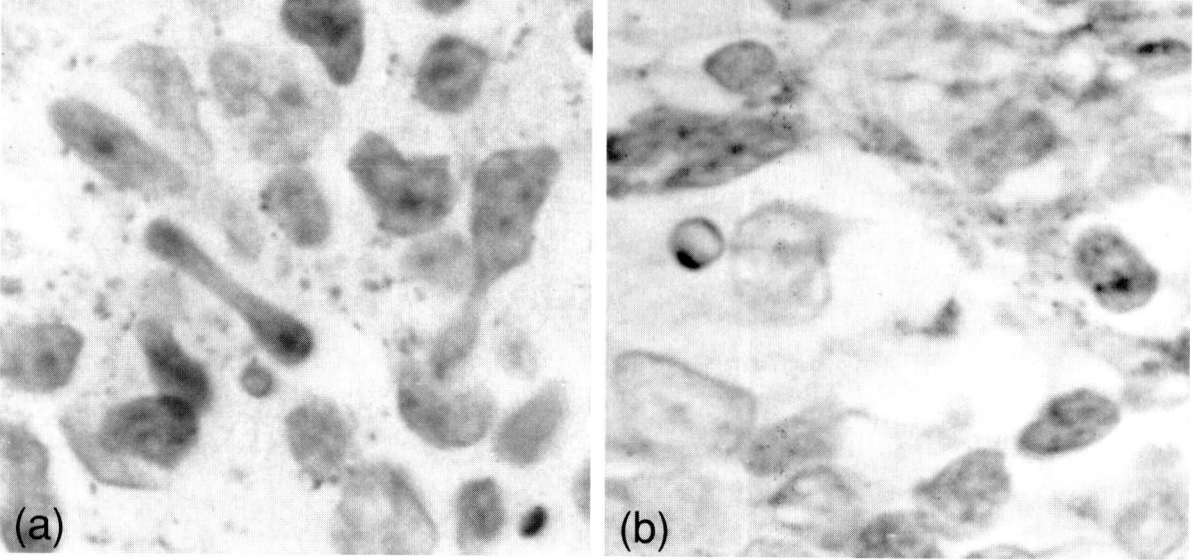

Figure 21.2 (a) Immunohistochemical staining of an ileal follicle center from a child with autistic enterocolitis with polyclonal anti-MV nucleocapsid protein antibody. Polyclonal control antibody and no antibody controls show no signal. The observed signal is consistent with the FDC matrix (original magnification ×1000).
(b) Immunohistochemical staining of an ileal follicle center from a patient with AIDS stained with monoclonal anti-HIV-1 capsid p24 protein antibody. Pattern of staining is identical to Figure 21.2a (original magnification ×1000).

THE GUT–BRAIN AXIS

Gut–brain interactions may operate through a variety of mechanisms including afferent neural pathways, synthesis and release of neurotransmitters from the intestine into the bloodstream, and egress of neuroactive compounds from the gut lumen. These interactions do not preclude the possibility that autoimmune pathology may operate concomitantly in the brain and GI tract, or that infectious agents may produce their effects through direct viral invasion, as reported for *H. simplex* and autism.[9] This chapter focuses on toxic gut–brain interactions that operate in situations where there is either inflammation of the intestine, or failure to exclude or eliminate in sufficient quantity neurotoxins derived from an inflamed or normal intestine.

The prototypic toxic gut–brain interaction occurs in hepatic encephalopathy, where impaired cognition, coma, and death may result from a failure of hepatic detoxification mechanisms. The intestine may be normal, but toxic byproducts of dietary and bacterial GI constituents are not degraded and eliminated by the diseased liver.[54] A key role for disturbances in endogenous opioid metabolism is becoming apparent in hepatic encephalopathy,[55] which, in a clinical setting, may be reversed in patients with celiac disease by the institution of a gluten-free diet, removing among other things a rich source of exorphins.[56]

Toxic gut–brain interactions are also seen where the liver and intestine are intact, but the neurotoxin from the intestinal lumen seemingly gains access to the developing brain in sufficient amounts to cause damage. Examples of this include phenylketonuria and autism following thalidomide or sodium valproate ingestion by a pregnant mother.[57–60]

A third toxic gut–brain interaction occurs where there is egress of luminal products from the intestine due to dysbiosis, increased intestinal permeability, and/or impaired enzymatic degradation within the small bowel brush border. Examples include D-lactic acidosis in short bowel syndrome, which is associated with a range of psychiatric and neurological sequelae following overgrowth of acid-resistant bacteria. Untreated celiac disease is associated with intestinal mucosal inflammation, increased intestinal permeability,[61] increased absorption and urinary excretion of dietary peptides,[62] autistic and psychotic behaviors,[63,64] and neurological complications.[65,66] This form of interaction may also be relevant in IBD. Patients with Crohn's disease have an increased risk of psychiatric and neurological problems,[67] which may pre-date the onset of intestinal symptoms.[68] A significant association has been shown between autistic spectrum disorder and perianal Crohn's disease in children.[69] In addition, both depression and anxiety have been shown to be associated with ulcerative colitis and Crohn's disease.[70]

AUTISTIC SPECTRUM DISORDERS AND OPIOID EXCESS

It has been proposed that some forms of autism may arise from the toxic effects of intestinal products on the developing brain or from inappropriate central activity of dietary-derived opioid peptides (exorphins) from the gut.[71–77] These include gliadmorphine and β-caseomorphine from the substrates wheat gliadin and bovine casein, respectively. Under normal circumstances, these dietary opioids are digested by brush border peptidases, such as dipeptidyl peptidase, but the presence of intestinal inflammation may facilitate the egress of these peptides, leading to systemic opioid excess. Once exorphins from the intestinal lumen become systemic, the potential exists for them to exert direct effects within the CNS. The confirmed presence of opioids of dietary origin in the urine of affected children,[78] and the clinical response of some children to exclusion of dietary opioid substrate,[79] is supportive of a toxic element to their encephalopathy.[1,2]

HYPOTHESIS

For the cohort of children with regressive autism and GI disease – a group that, we believe, may account for a large proportion of new diagnoses – we hypothesize that the root problem is in aberrant early immune programming, particularly within the mucosal immune system. Within the last decade there has been a substantial increase in allergies of all kinds, particularly dietary, which may be consequent upon recent dramatic changes in the pattern of infant environmental exposures. There are increasingly explicit links between mucosal infectious exposures and the establishment and maintenance of mucosal immune tolerance. The natural trajectory over time, from a T_H2 dominant fetal/neonatal immune response to a balanced T_H2/T_H1 responsiveness that probably reflects healthy immunological maturity,[80,81] may permit the generation of appropriate cytotoxicity in the face of viral exposures. Factors that modify this transition in T-helper cell effector function, including vaccines, toxins, or natural infections, may prolong T_H2 skewing,[82] and thus impair antiviral responses.

Inappropriate early conditioning of the mucosal immune system, for which the fecal flora plays an obligatory role,[83] may allow inappropriate persistence of agents which are home to gut-associated lymphoid tissue. The immunomodulatory nature of MV suggests that persistent expression within mucosal lymphoid tissue may affect mucosal tolerance mechanisms, in particular inducing T_H2-skewing through mechanisms including inhibition of dendritic cell IL-12 production.

The key to defining the child at risk, therefore, is an examination of the cofactors that may interfere with the appropriate T_H2–T_H1 transition prior to, or concomitant with, MMR exposure. One such factor may be mercury, for which the immunotoxicity (putting aside for now the associated neurotoxicity) of organic and inorganic derivatives is qualitatively similar. Is a synergistic adverse interaction between mercury and a live viral vaccine biologically plausible? The immunosuppressive and immunomodulatory effects associated with mercury exposure are accompanied by increased susceptibility to challenge by infectious agents. One of the best-characterized examples of T-helper cell functional polarity in response to infection is the murine model of *Leishmania major*. Murine susceptibility to *L. major* infection is dependent upon induction of a genetically restricted T_H2 response. Resistant animals, that exhibit a genetically restricted T_H1 response to *L. major*, are rendered susceptible by prior exposure to mercury.[84] In previously resistant animals, subtoxic doses of mercuric chloride induced an autoimmune syndrome characterized by the expansion of T_H2 cells, IL-4 production by splenocytes, and IgG1 and IgE production. This was accompanied by a nonhealing phenotype with increased footpad swelling and parasite burden. Methyl mercury enhanced the immune damage and chronicity of Coxsackie B3 myocarditis in mice, compared with mice infected without prior mercury exposure.[85] Similarly, mercuric chloride exposure significantly impaired macrophage-mediated resistance to generalized infection with *H. simplex* type-2 in a murine model.[86]

Mercury is only one of several immunomodulatory exposures that may potentially influence the infant response to live viral vaccines. Until recently, organic mercury – as thimerosal in bacterial and subunit vaccines – was present at levels that were far in excess of EPA guidelines on toxicity. In testing the correct hypothesis at the population level – a study yet to be conducted – factors such as prior mercury exposure will need to be taken into account and appropriate adjustments made. It may be, for example, that the rapidly expanded pattern of infant mercury exposure will, with the necessary adjustments, reduce statistical power to the extent that the studies become redundant.

Population-based studies, in contrast to molecular and immunological studies, have not found an association between MMR vaccination and autism. As pointed out by Madsen and colleagues,[87] and endorsed by others, epidemiological studies that have examined this relationship have been inadequate.[88–90] Madsen's group failed to disaggregate the relevant autism subset – one which they attempt to describe in the introduction to their paper – from the overall autism population. This is equivalent to considering hepatitis as a single outcome, irrespective of etiology, in a study designed to examine a possible causal relationship with a single, specific exposure that may account for only a minority of hepatitis cases. Recent analysis of the Centers for Disease Control and Prevention's (CDC) vaccine adverse events reporting system (VAERS) demonstrated a significant excess risk of autism following MMR vaccine compared with the mercury-containing DPT vaccine.[91] The latter had previously been associated with a significant risk for autism compared with the mercury-free DPT in a separate analysis of the VAERS database.[92]

If it is the case that MMR vaccine is causally related to this syndrome, it should not be assumed that the associated risk remains static within any given population over time. The rapid increase in the number of children with dietary allergy, itself associated with reduced CD8$^+$ cell numbers, prolonged viral infections, and familial autoimmunity,[37,83,93,94] suggests that the number of children who may be at risk of aberrant responses to infectious agents will have risen in the last decades. Potentially relevant overlap, in which ubiquitous infectious exposure is followed in a few children by probably autoimmune-mediated neuropsychiatric abnormality, occurs in the pediatric autoimmune neuropsychiatric disorders associated with streptococcal infection (PANDAS).[95,96] Propensity to autoimmunity, with its clear demographic links to socioeconomic privilege and developed-world upbringing, dominates as a risk factor, and population-based epidemiological studies would not have uncovered this association. The likely autoimmune basis of regressive autism suggests that any causal association with MMR vaccine would lead to a continuing upward trend in incidence after vaccine introduction – in developed-world but not developing-world populations, in parallel with other autoimmune lesions – rather than the reported epidemiological construct of a step-up-and-plateau model.[90]

REFERENCES

1. Sabra A, Bellanti JA, Colon AR. Ileal-lymphoid-nodular hyperplasia, non-specific colitis and pervasive developmental disorder in children. *Lancet* 1998; **352**: 234–5.
2. Sabra A, Hartman D, Zeligs BJ et al. Linkage of ileal-lymphoid-nodular hyperplasia (ILNH), food allergy and CNS developmental: evidence for a non-IgE association. *Ann Allergy Asthma Immunol* 1999; **82**: 81.
3. Barak Y, Ring A, Sulkes J et al. Season of birth and autistic disorder in Israel and the Middle East. *Am J Psychiatry* 1995; **152**: 798–800.
4. Barrlik BD. Monthly variation in birth of autistic children in North Carolina. *J Am Med Women's Assoc* 1981; **36**: 363–8.
5. Konstantareas M, Hauser P, Lennox C. Season of birth in infantile autism. *Child Psychiatr Hum Develop* 1986; **17**: 53–65.
6. Gillberg C. Do children with autism have March birthdays? *Acta Psychiatr Scand* 1990; **82**: 153–6.
7. Tanoue Y, Oda S, Asano F, Kawashima K. Epidemiology of infantile autism in southern Ibaraki, Japan: differences in prevalence in birth cohorts. *J Autism Dev Disord* 1988; **18**: 155–66.
8. Landau EC, Cicchetti DV, Klin A, Volkmar FR. Season of birth in autism: a fiction revisited. *Child Psychiatr Hum Dev* 1994; **25**: 31–43.
9. DeLong R, Bean C, Brown F. Acquired reversible autistic syndrome in acute encephalopathic illness in children. *Arch Neurol* 1981; **38**: 191–4.
10. Ivarsson SA, Bjerre I, Vegfors P, Ahlfors K. Autism as one of several disabilities in two children with congenital cytomegalovirus infection. *Neuropediatrics* 1990; **21**: 102–3.
11. Stubbs EG. Autistic symptoms in a child with congenital cytomegalovirus infection. *J Autism Child Schizophr* 1978; **8**: 37–43.
12. Shenoy S, Arnold S, Chatila T. Response to steroid therapy in autism secondary to autoimmune lympho-proliferative syndrome *J Pediatrics* 2000; **136**: 682–7.
13. Deykin EY, MacMahon B. Viral exposure and autism. *Am J Epidemiol* 1979; **109**: 628–38.
14. Ring A, Barak Y, Ticher A. Evidence for an infectious etiology in autism. *Pathophysiology* 1997; **4**: 1485–8.
15. Steiner CE, Guerreiro MM, Marques-De-Faria AP. Genetic and neurological evaluation in a sample of individuals with pervasive developmental disorders. *Arq Neuropsiquiatr* 2003; **61**: 176–80.
16. Chess S. Autism in children with congenital rubella. *J Autism Child Schizophr* 1971; **1**: 33–47.
17. Mouridsen SE, Rich B, Isager T. Epilepsy in disintegrative psychosis and infantile autism: a long-term validation study. *Dev Med Child Neurol* 1999; **41**: 110–4.
18. Weibel RE, Caserta V, Benor DE. Acute encephalopathy followed by permanent brain injury or death associated with further attenuated measles vaccines: a review of claims submitted to the national vaccine injury compensation program. *Paediatrics* 1998; **101**: 383–7.
19. Wakefield AJ, Murch SH, Anthony A et al. Ileal-lymphoid nodular hyperplasian non-specific colitis, and pervasive developmental disorder in children. *Lancet* 1998; **351**: 637–41.
20. Singh VK, Lin SX, Yang VC. Serological association of measles virus and human herpes virus-6 with brain autoantibodies in autism. *Clin Immunol Immunopathol* 1998; **89**: 105–8.
21. Singh VK, Jensen RL. Elevated levels of measles antibodies in children with autism. *Pediatric Neurol* 2003; **28**: 292–4.
22. Horvath K, Perman JA. Autistic disorder and gastrointestinal disease. *Curr Opin Pediatrics* 2002; **14**: 583–7.

23. Melmed RD, Schneider C, Fabes RA et al. Metabolic markers and gastrointestinal symptoms in children with autism and related disorders. *J Pediatr Gastroenterol Nutr* 2000; 31: S31–2.
24. Horvath K, Papadimitriou JC, Rabsztyn A et al. Gastrointestinal abnormalities in children with autistic disorder. *J Pediatr* 1999; 135: 559–63.
25. Wakefield AJ, Anthony A, Murch SH et al. Enterocolitis in children with developmental disorders. *Am J Gastroenterol* 2000; 95: 2285–95.
26. Furlano RI, Anthony A, Day R et al. Colonic CD8 and γδ T-cell infiltration with epithelial damage in children with autism. *J Pediatr* 2001; 138: 366–72.
27. Torrente F, Ashwood P, Day R et al. Small intestinal enteropathy with epithelial IgG and complement deposition in children with regressive autism. *Mol Psychiatry* 2002; 7: 375–82, 334.
28. Ashwood P, Murch SH, Anthony A et al. Mucosal and peripheral blood lymphocyte cytokine profiles in children with regressive autism and gastrointestinal symptoms: mucosal immune activation and reduced counter regulatory interleukin-10. *Gastroenterology* 2002; 122(Suppl): A617.
29. Ashwood P, Murch SH, Anthony A et al. Intestinal lymphocyte populations in children with regressive autism: evidence for extensive mucosal immunopathology. *J Clin Immunol* 2003; 23: 504–17.
30. Jyonouchi H, Sun S, Le H. Proinflammatory and regulatory cytokine production associated with innate and adaptive immune responses in children with autism spectrum disorders and developmental regression. *J Neuroimmunol* 2001; 120: 170–9.
31. Jyonouchi H, Sun S, Itokazu N. Innate immunity associated with inflammatory responses and cytokine production against common dietary proteins in patients with autism spectrum disorder. *Neuropsychobiology* 2002; 46: 76–84.
32. Sandler RH, Finegold SM, Bolte ER et al. Short-term benefit from oral vancomycin treatment of regressive-onset autism. *J Child Neurol* 2000; 15: 429–35.
33. Finegold SM, Molitoris D, Song Y et al. Gastrointestinal microflora studies in late-onset autism. *Clin Infect Dis* 2002; 35(Suppl 1): S6–16.
34. Rosseneu SLM, van Saene HKF, Heuschel R, Murch SH. Abnormal throat and gut flora in children with regressive autism. Presented to the International Meeting for Autism Research 2002.
35. D'Eufemia P, Celli M, Finocchiaro R et al. Abnormal intestinal permeability in children with autism. *Acta Paediatr* 1996; 85: 1076–9.
36. Horvath K, Zielke H, Collins J et al. Secretin improves intestinal permeability in autistic children. *J Pediatr Gastroenterol Nutr* 2000; 31: S30–1.
37. Ludviksson BR, Elriksson TH, Ardal B et al. Correlation between serum immunoglobulin A concentrations and allergic manifestations in infants. *J Pediatr* 1992; 121: 23–7.
38. Murch SH, Anthony A, Thompson M et al. Ileo-colonic lymphoid nodular hyperplasia is associated with immunodeficiency in children with developmental disorders. *Gut* 1999; 44: A127.
39. Warren RP, Singh VK, Averett RE et al. Immunogenetic studies in autism and related disorders. *Mol Clin Neuropathol* 1996; 28: 77–81.
40. Van Gent T, Heijnen CJ, Treffers PD. Autism and the immune system. *J Child Psychol Psychiatr* 1997; 38: 337–49.
41. Comi AM, Zimmerman AW, Frye VH et al. Familial clustering of autoimmune disorders and evaluation of medical risks in autism. *J Child Neurol* 1999; 14: 388–94.
42. Schneider T, Ullrich R, Zeitz M. The immunological aspects of human immunodeficiency virus infection in the gastrointestinal tract. *Sem Gastrointest Dis* 1996; 7: 19–29.
43. Zietz M. Mucosal immunodeficiency in HIV/SIV infection. *Pathobiology* 1998; 66: 151–7.
44. McGowan I, Radford-Smith G, Jewell DP. Cytokine gene expression in HIV-infected intestinal mucosa. *AIDS* 1994; 8: 1569–75.
45. Rima BK, Davidson WB, Martin SJ. The role of defective interfering particles in persistent infection of Vero cells by measles virus. *J Gen Virol* 1977; 35: 89–97.
46. Hirano A. Subacute sclerosing panencephalitis virus dominantly interferes with replication of wild-type measles virus in a mixed infection: implications for viral persistence. *J Virol* 1992; 66: 1891–8.
47. Minekawa Y, Ueda S, Yamanishi K et al. Studies on live rubella vaccine V. Quantitative aspects of interference between rubella, measles and mumps viruses in their trivalent vaccine. *Biken J* 1974; 17: 161–7.
48. Buynak EB, Weibel RE, Whitman JE et al. Combined live measles mumps rubella virus vaccines. *JAMA* 1969; 207: 2259–62.
49. Montgomery SM, Morris DL, Pounder RE, Wakefield AJ. Paramyxovirus infections in childhood and subsequent inflammatory bowel disease. *Gastroenterology* 1999; 116: 796–803.
50. Norrby E, Oxman MN. Measles virus. In: *Fields Virology* (Fields BN, Knipe D, eds). New York: Raven Press, 1990: 329–50.
51. Wakefield AJ, Anthony A, Schepelmann S et al. Persistent measles virus (MV) infection and immunodeficiency in children with autism, ileo-colonic lymphonodular hyperplasia and non-specific colitis. *Gastroenterology* 1998; 174: A430.
52. Uhlmann V, Martin CM, Sheils O et al. Potential viral pathogenic mechanism for new variant inflammatory bowel disease. *Mol Pathol* 2002; 55: 84–90.
53. Singh VK, Lin SX, Newell E, Nelson C. Abnormal measles-mumps-rubella antibodies and CNS autoimmunity in children with autism. *J Biomed Sci* 2002; 9: 359–64.
54. Butterworth RF. Complications of cirrhosis III. Hepatic encephalopathy. *J Hepatol* 2000; 32(Suppl 1): 171–80.
55. Wakefield AJ, Puleston JM, Montgomery SM et al. Review article: the concept of entero-colonic encephalopathy, autism and opioid receptor ligands. *Alimentary Pharmacol Therapeut* 2002; 16: 663–74.
56. Kaukinen K, Halme L, Collin P et al. Celiac disease in patients with severe liver disease: gluten-free diet may reverse hepatic failure. *Gastroenterology* 2002; 122: 881–8.
57. Miladi N, Larnaout A, Kaabachi N et al. Phenylketonuria: an underlying etiology of autistic syndrome. Case report. *J Child Neurol* 1992; 7: 22–3.
58. Stromland K, Nordin V, Miller M et al. Autism in thalidomide embryopathy: a population study. *Dev Med Child Neurol* 1994; 36: 351–6.
59. Moore SJ, Turnpenny P, Quinn A et al. A clinical study of 57 children with fetal anticonvulsant syndromes. *J Med Genet* 2000; 37: 489–97.
60. Williams G, King J, Cunningham M et al. Fetal valproate syndrome and autism: additional evidence of an association. *Dev Med Child Neurol* 2001; 43: 202–6.
61. Bjarnason I, Peters TJ, Veall N. Intestinal permeability defect in celiac disease. *Lancet* 1983; 1: 1284–5.
62. Reichelt WH, Stensrud J-EM, Reichelt KL. Peptide excretion in celiac disease. *J Paed Gastroenterol Nutrit* 1998; 26: 305–9.
63. Hallert C, Derefeldt T. Psychic disturbances in adult celiac disease. *Scand J Gastroenterol* 1982; 17: 17–9.
64. Asperger H. Der psychopathologie des coeliaki kranken kindes. *Ann Paediatr* 1961; 187: 346–51.
65. Cooke WT, Smith WT. Neurological disorders associated with adult celiac disease. *Brain* 1966; 89: 683–722.

66. Gobbi G, Bouquet F, Greco L et al. Celiac disease, epilepsy and cerebral calcifications. *Lancet* 1992; **340**: 439–43.
67. Engstrom I, Lindquist BL. Inflammatory bowel disease in children and adolescents: a somatic and psychiatric investigation. *Acta Paediar Scand* 1991; **86**: 640–7.
68. Tarter RE, Switala J, Carra J et al. Inflammatory bowel disease: psychiatric status of patients before and after disease onset. *Int J Psychiatry Med* 1987; **17**: 173–81.
69. Ericsson M, Grahnquist L, Hidebrand H et al. Perianal disease in paediatric Crohn's disease: prevalence and co-morbidity. *Gut* 2001; **49**(Suppl 3): A1600.
70. Kurina LM. Increased depression and anxiety in people with inflammatory bowel disease. *J Epidemiol Community Health* 2001; **55**: 716–20.
71. Kalat JW. Speculations on the similarities between autism and opioid addiction. *J Autism Child Schizophr* 1978; **8**: 477–9.
72. Dohan FC. More on celiac disease as a model for schizophrenia. *Biol Psychiatry* 1983; **18**: 561–4.
73. Panksepp J. A neurochemical theory of autism. *Trends Neurosci* 1979; **2**: 174–7.
74. Reichelt KL, Hole K, Hamberger A et al. Biologically active peptide-containing fractions in schizophrenia and childhood autism. *Adv Biochem Psychopharmacol* 1993; **28**: 627–43.
75. Shattock P, Kennedy A, Rowell F, Berney T. Role of neuropeptides in autism and their relationships with classical neurotransmitters. *Brain Dysfunct* 1991; **3**: 328–45.
76. Sun Z, Cade JR, Fregly MJ, Privette RM. β-casomorphin induces Fos-like immunoreactivity in discrete brain regions relevant to schizophrenia and autism. *Autism* 1999; **3**: 67–83.
77. Sun Z, Cade JR. A peptide found in schizophrenia and ASD causes behavioral changes in rats. *Autism* 1999; **3**: 85–95.
78. Reichelt, K. Analysis of neuroactive peptides with the urine of autistic patients. In: *Proceeding of the 49th Conference of Mass Spectrometry and Allied Topics*. Chicago, 2002: 27–31.
79. Knivsberg AM, Reichelt KL, Høien T, Nødland M. A randomised, controlled study of dietary intervention in autistic syndromes. *Nutr Neurosci* 2002; **5**: 251–61.
80. Holt PG, Sly PD, Björkstein B. Atopic vs infectious diseases in childhood: a question of balance? *Pediatr Allergy Immunol* 1997; **8**: 53–8.
81. Prescott S, Macaubas C, Smallacombe T et al. Development of allergen-specific T-cell memory in atopic and normal children. *Lancet* 1999; **353**: 196–200.
82. Rook GAW, Stanford JL. Give us this day our daily germs. *Immunol Today* 1998; **19**: 113–6.
83. Murch SH. The immunologic basis for intestinal food allergy. *Curr Opin Gastroenterol* 2000; **16**: 552–7.
84. Bagenstose LM, Mentink-Kane MM, Britingham A et al. Mercury enhances susceptibility to murine Leishaniasis. *Parasite Immunol* 2001; **23**: 633–40.
85. Ilback NG, Wesslen L, Fohlman Friman G. Effects of methyl mercury on cytokines, inflammation and virus clearance in a common infection (Coxsackie B3 myocarditis). *Toxicol Lett* 1996; **89**: 19–28.
86. Christensen MM, Ellermann-Eriksen S, Rungby J, Mogensen SC. Influence of mercuric chloride on resistance to generalized infection with herpes simplex virus type 2 in mice. *Toxicology* 1996; **114**: 57–66.
87. Madsen MK, Hviid A, Vestergaard M et al. A population-based study of measles mumps rubella vaccination and autism. *N Engl J Med* 2002; **347**: 1478–82.
88. Taylor B, Miller E, Lingam R et al. Measles, mumps, and rubella vaccination and bowel problems or developmental regression in children with autism: population study. *BMJ* 2002; **324**: 393–6.
89. Fombonne E, Chakrabarti S. No evidence for a new variant of measles-mumps-rubella-induced autism. *Pediatrics* 2001; **108**: E58.
90. Kaye JA, del Mar Melero-Montes M, Hershel J. Mumps, measles and rubella vaccine and the incidence of autism recorded by general practitioners: a time trend analysis. *BMJ* 2001; **322**: 0–2.
91. Geier MR, Geier DA. Pediatric MMR vaccination safety. *Int Pediatr* 2003; **18**: 203–8.
92. Geier MR, Geier DA. Neurodevelopmental disorders following thimerosal-containing vaccines: a brief communication. *Exp Biol Med* 2003; **228**: 660–4.
93. Jarvinen KM, Aro A, Juntunen-Backman K, Sumolainen H. Large numbers of CD19+/CD23+ B cells and small numbers of CD8+ T cells as early markers for cow's milk allergy (CMA). *Pediatr Allergy Immunol* 1998; **9**: 139–42.
94. Latcham F, Merino F, Winter C et al. Distinct immunological features of children with multiple food allergy. *JPGN* 2000; **31**: S328.
95. Trifiletti RR, Packard AM. Immune mechanisms in pediatric neuropsychiatric disorders. Tourette's syndrome, OCD, and Pandas. *Child Adolesc Psychiatry Clin N Amer* 1999; **8**: 767–75.
96. Garvey MA, Giedd J, Swedo SE. PANDAS: the search for environmental triggers of pediatric neuropsychiatric disorders. Lessons from rheumatic fever. *J Child Neurol* 1998; **13**: 413–23.

22

An animal model of neurodevelopmental damage: Neonatal Borna disease virus infection

Mikhail V Pletnikov, Steven A Rubin, Timothy H Moran, Michael W Vogel, and Kathryn M Carbone

ANIMAL MODELS OF DEVELOPMENTAL BEHAVIORAL DISORDERS

Experimental research of human developmental behavioral disorders (DBDs) is a difficult undertaking for obvious ethical reasons. Animal models can help us study the pathogenesis of developmental alterations and search for new pharmacological treatments. However, since DBDs such as schizophrenia and autism are unique human conditions, there is a tendency to negate the feasibility of developing animal models.[1,2] Indeed, animal models will always fall short of precisely mimicking human neuropsychiatric disorders. However, if we focus on more modest tasks, such as the mechanisms of abnormal brain maturation, we could address some of the important mysteries of these diseases.[1,3] The notion that a useful animal model does not need to mimic all features of complex syndromes is more productive than a call for the comprehensive and faithful reflection of all key symptoms of a disease. In this way, modeling key pathogenic events and/or processes is feasible and achievable.

There are different approaches to DBD models. According to the criteria proposed by Paul Willner, animal models can be classified into those with predictive validity, face validity, and construct validity.[4] Predictive validity is based on a model's ability to predict the effects of pharmacological drugs. Face validity is symptom similarity between the model and the human manifestation. Notably, the mechanisms involved in creating face validity may be quite different between the two species. Construct validity, on the other hand, is established on the basis of similarity with respect to the pathology (i.e., construct) underlying an overt deficit. This approach is based on the concept that the molecular and cellular mechanisms of a disease can be similar, if not the same, in animals and humans. Such homologous modeling fills an important niche in research into neurodevelopmental damage, as a tool for the mechanistic studies of pathophysiology and psychopharmacology.[2,5] Investigating the mechanisms of abnormal brain maturation in animals can advance our understanding of the pathological substrate of human psychiatric conditions.

Since a number of different etiologic agents are believed to cause DBDs, multiple animal models are probably needed in order to appreciate the complex pathogenic mechanisms. Current animal models of neurodevelopmental injury utilize various genetic approaches and physical and chemical insults to derail normal brain maturation.[6–11] Unfortunately, there are few animal models of neurodevelopmental injury using virus infections,[12,13] despite the fact that prenatal and early postnatal viral infections have been associated with a number of human psychiatric disorders, including schizophrenia and autism.[14–17] Effects of direct virus infection and effects of virus-induced immune response (i.e., cellular infiltration and/or soluble toxic factors) could be responsible for neural injury,[18,19] making viral models biologically plausible.

NEONATAL BORNA DISEASE VIRUS (BDV) INFECTION

In this chapter, we critically review neuroanatomical, behavioral, neurochemical, and immunological features of the animal model of early brain injury following persistent central nervous system (CNS) infection of neonatal rats with an experimental teratogen – an 8.9 kb, nonsegmented, negative-strand, round, enveloped RNA virus, Borna disease virus (BDV).[20,21]

Initially, neonatal BDV infection was described in the early 1980s.[22–24] Recently, interest in neonatal BDV infection has significantly grown, as many groups across the globe have recognized that this model may provide new insights into the pathogenesis of DBDs that have been associated with perinatal viral insult.[25] In addition, since neonatal BDV infection occurs with minimal signs of inflammatory reaction in the CNS, it allows for investigation of the direct effects of virus infection in the brain in the absence of a potentially confounding inflammatory response.[24]

In order to produce neonatal BDV infection, newborn rats are inoculated intracranially with the virus within 24 hours of birth. A few days post infection (p.i.), viral antigens and RNA can be found in the olfactory bulb, hippocampus, the frontal cortex, and the deep cerebellar nuclei.[26–30] At about three weeks p.i., viral antigens can be seen in neurons throughout the brain. At later time points (i.e., three to four weeks p.i.), viral antigens are also found in glial cells.[27,29] Since astrocytes become infected well after the early neural infection, it has been hypothesized that infection of astrocytes is a result of BDV release from infected neurons.[27] In contrast to neural and glial cells, no BDV infection has been demonstrated in microglia, supporting the finding that macrophage cell lines are resistant to BDV infection.[31]

In the late stages of infection, BDV spreads from the brain via anterograde axonal transport. Viral markers can be detected in the peripheral nerves of all tissues and organs. Consequently, ectodermal or epithelial tissues receiving nerve endings become infected with BDV.[26] Neonatally BDV-infected rats have been shown to excrete the virus in tears, saliva, and urine, and can potentially infect healthy rats housed in the same cage.[32]

Appearance and physical growth

Neonatally BDV-infected rats are smaller than uninfected animals. Both a reduced body weight and a smaller body length have been documented in BDV-infected rats.[28,33,34] A simultaneous and proportional BDV-induced decrease in the external parameters of development seems to indicate an overall inhibition in growth (i.e., growth retardation). While virus infections during prenatal and perinatal periods have been associated with growth inhibition in animals and humans,[35] the mechanisms of BDV-induced runting remain obscure. No detectable BDV-associated disturbances in the biosynthesis of growth hormone and insulin-like growth factor-1 have been found.[33] In addition to the effects of the virus infection per se, virus infection-associated malnourishment could also be responsible for growth retardation.[36] Although neonatally BDV-infected 10-week-old rats have been shown to consume a normal amount of food, when the amount of food was calculated in relation to body weight, neonatally BDV-infected rats actually consumed more food than control animals, suggesting that BDV-induced growth inhibition might result from undernutrition due to decreased absorption in the gastrointestinal tract, increased energy expenditure, or virus-induced alterations in cellular metabolism.[27] Since even a transient state of malnourishment during development can produce long-term neurobehavioral consequences,[36] a possible contribution of nutritional problems to growth retardation in BDV-infected rats is worth studying.

Brain pathology

Cerebellum

Neonatal BDV infection induces selective damage to the cerebellum. Early infection of Purkinje cells (PCs) on days three to five p.i.[27] leads to loss of these cells.[37–39] Although cerebellar granule cells remain uninfected, a loss of granule cells, though not quantitatively measured, has been suggested and might be due to diminished trophic support by infected PCs.[27,31,38] The mechanisms of neuronal loss in the cerebellum are obscure. A role of apoptosis in the death of PCs has not been unequivocally demonstrated,[28,38] and given the technical difficulties of demonstrating apoptosis of PCs,[40] different converging approaches may be needed better to elucidate the mechanisms of PC elimination. The fact that PCs are GABA neurons that contain high amounts of calcium-binding proteins (e.g., calbindin) may be of interest for further studies into the contribution of calcium-binding proteins to the mechanism of cellular resilience or vulnerability, a theme that has been discussed in HIV-related brain injury and Huntington disease.[41,42] In addition to the mechanisms of cell death due to direct viral infection, the role of soluble neurotoxins secreted by activated microglia cells and astrocytes is being intensively investigated (see below).

Hippocampus

Continuing degeneration of granule cells of the hippocampal dentate gyrus (DG) is a hallmark of BDV infection.[24] These degenerated neurons are replaced by astrocytes and microglia cells.[24,31] Preliminary quantitative analysis of BDV-associated loss of pyramidal neurons in one of the CA regions of the hippocampus (CA1) showed less dramatic, but clear, neuronal dropout.[43] Similar to the elimination of PCs, apoptosis has been implicated in degeneration of the DG.[31,38] In addition, BDV-induced decline in immunostaining for growth-associated protein (GAP-43) and synaptophysin (SYN) has been shown in the hippocampus, suggesting involvement of synaptic pathology.[30] Whether synaptic alterations are simply a byproduct of neuronal death or can occur independent of cell body injury remains to be explored.

Cortex

Neonatal BDV has been shown to be associated with thinning of the cortex.[30,39] Gonzalez-Dunia and colleagues have reported 30% shrinkage and a selective elimination of cortical cells with a diameter greater than 100 μm following neonatal infection with BDV.[30] Those findings have been confirmed by another group, who demonstrated a timespan of BDV-associated cortical thinning from 15% in 30-day-old rats to 32% in 120-day-old rats.[39] Apoptosis of pyramidal and/or GABA neurons as well as virus-induced degeneration of neuropil may be responsible for BDV-associated decrease in cortical volume.[31]

Other brain regions

Since BDV grossly affects brain regions with robust postnatal proliferation of neurons, such as the cerebellar cortex and hippocampus,[6] it remains unclear whether the virus can also cause neural injury/death in brain areas where cell division ceases before birth. There are several reasons to believe that this may be the case. BDV infects neurons and glial cells throughout the brain and, therefore, could induce cell death directly or indirectly in different parts of the brain. Also, since BDV infection is associated with dropout of PCs, neurons that do not divide postnatally, one could suggest that other types of nonproliferating neurons might be susceptible to BDV. For example, if the particular vulnerability of PCs is related to some yet-unknown features of GABA neurons such as calcium-binding proteins,[41,44] it is conceivable that other GABA neurons in the brain would also be susceptible to direct and/or indirect effects of BDV even if those neural cells no longer proliferate at the moment of infection. Curiously, there have been first observations that some neuronal loss may occur in deep cerebellar nuclei, ventral cochlear nucleus, and superior colliculus.[31] In addition, our unpublished quantitative analysis has indicated a neural loss in the striatum of BDV-infected Fischer344 rats when measured on day 120 p.i.

In summary, neonatal BDV infection causes selective developmental damage to the cortex, hippocampus, and cerebellum – the brain regions that continue to develop after birth, and may be sensitive to environmental insults.[6] The available data appear to indicate a possibility of neural loss in other brain regions, suggesting further quantifiable damage.

Role of the resident immune system

In contrast to many viral infections of the brain, neonatal BDV infection does not lead to widespread encephalitis.[18,22,23] Only mild and transient immune T-cell infiltrates have been found in the CNS of neonatally BDV-infected rats on days 22 and 33 p.i.[28,29,31] Nevertheless, neonatal BDV infection induces robust activation of astrocytes and microglia. The first signs of astrocytosis, evidenced by an increase in the number and size of cells expressing an astrocyte-specific marker, the glial fibrillary acidic protein (GFAP), can be found as early as three days p.i.[27]

Gliosis is a common marker of brain damage.[45] Soluble factors secreted by injured neurons are thought to stimulate the proliferation and activation of astrocytes and microglial cells in the brain.[19,46] In the case of neonatal BDV infection, direct BDV infection of astrocytes may also contribute to glial cell activation. The molecular mechanisms by which activated/infected astrocytes and microglia could lead to neuronal damage have been intensively studied. Using sensitive ribonuclease protection assays (RPA), several groups have shown a BDV-associated upregulation in expression of mRNA encoding numerous pro-inflammatory cytokines (e.g., IL-6, TNF-α, IL-1-α, and IL-1-β) in the brains of neonatally BDV-infected rats.[28,29,47] Regional localization of elevated expression of pro-inflammatory cytokine mRNAs coincided with the sites of major glial cell activation, supporting the hypothesis that astrocytes and microglia are a major source of cytokine production.

A sustained expression of chemokines IP-10 and RANTES, and reduced expression of the fractalkine gene, have been found in the brains of neonatally BDV-infected rats as early as two weeks p.i.[48,49] Interestingly, increased levels of mRNA encoding IP-10 were particularly conspicuous in the cerebellar astrocytes, especially the Bergman glia. It is likely that this may contribute to the death of PCs or act as an 'astrocyte alarm signal' of PC loss.[50] A marked increase of chemokine receptor mRNAs such as CCR5 and CX_3CR1 has been also found in BDV-infected rats. BDV-associated upregulation of CX_3CR1 has been shown to be mainly due to an increase in the number of CX_3CR1-expressing microglia.[48,49] Thus, cytokines and chemokines may be important participants in mediating viral insult, similar to the pathogenic role of soluble neurotoxins described for different neurodegenerative diseases.[19]

Postnatal brain development is strongly dependent on trophic support by neurotrophins, which play major roles in promoting neuronal proliferation, migration, and survival.[51] Several studies have shown that levels of mRNAs coding for neurotrophins and neurotrophin receptor genes are significantly altered following neonatal BDV infection.[28,38] Specifically, BDV infection was associated with diminished expression of mRNAs for the neurotrophin receptors BDNF and NT-3 and a related reduction in BDNF, NT-3, and NGF mRNA levels in the rat hippocampus by two weeks p.i. Such reductions in neurotrophin levels may contribute to abnormal brain maturation.

Another potential contribution of activated/infected astrocytes to neural injury following BDV infection can be related to decreased re-uptake of glutamate and ensuing glutamate excitotoxicity.[52] This mechanism may become more important when increased expression of cytokines and chemokines subsides.[28,29]

Direct effects of BDV infection

Until recently, few studies have examined the direct effects of BDV on neuronal cells. A recent report has demonstrated that the rat pheochromocytoma cell line PC12 becomes resistant to NGF-induced neuronal differentiation upon infection with BDV.[53] This effect can be linked to BDV-induced perturbations in the signal transduction cascade triggered by NGF, and most notably a chronic activation of the mitogen-activated protein kinase ERK1/2. Interestingly, a selective blockade of the ERK1/2 signaling cascade has been found to prevent BDV replication.[54] These findings support the hypothesis that BDV-associated neurodevelopmental damage may be a result of lower responsiveness of BDV-infected neurons to the effects of neurotrophic factors.

Direct effects of viral replication in neurons, effects of soluble factors secreted by resident immune cells, glutamate excitotoxicity, and a decreased production of neurotrophic factors could all contribute to cellular injury in the brains of neonatally BDV-infected rats.

Neurochemical changes

Since virally-damaged brain regions receive substantial monoamine innervation, there have been attempts to evaluate the effects of virus infection on the development of brain monoamine systems. Pletnikov and coworkers have measured concentrations of norepinephrine (NE), dopamine (DA) and its metabolite 3,4-dihydroxyphenylacetic acid (DOPAC), and serotonin (5-HT) and its metabolite 5-hydroxyindole-3-acetic acid (5-HIAA) in the frontal cortex, cerebellum, hippocampus, hypothalamus, and striatum following neonatal BDV infection at various time points p.i.[55] Both NE and 5-HT concentrations were significantly affected by neonatal BDV infection. The cortical and cerebellar levels of NE and 5-HT were significantly greater in BDV-infected rats than control animals on days 60 and 90 p.i. In the hippocampus, neonatally BDV-infected rats had lower 5-HT levels on day eight p.i. and significantly elevated levels on day 21 p.i. and onwards. Neither striatal levels of 5-HT nor hypothalamic levels of 5-HT and NE were affected by neonatal BDV infection, suggesting that monoamine systems in prenatally maturing brain regions are less sensitive to the effects of BDV. These data demonstrate significant and specific alterations in monoamine systems in neonatally BDV-infected rats.[55]

In addition to measurements of tissue concentrations that primarily reflect the status of presynaptically stored neurotransmitters, effects of neonatal BDV infection on the density of pre- and postsynaptic DA and 5-HT receptors have been studied.[56,57] Neonatal BDV increased the density of 5-HT transporter (5-HTT) sites in cortical regions and hippocampus but did not change the density of 5-HTT sites in the striatum. Neonatal BDV infection also significantly increased the density of $5-HT_{1a}$ receptors in the hippocampal CA1 field and the density of $5-HT_{2a}$ receptors in the cortex. The status of monoamine receptors has been further evaluated by pharmacologically targeting specific subtypes of 5-HT receptors in BDV-infected rats at postnatal day (PND) 60 and 120. A selective agonist of $5-HT_{1a}$ receptors, 8-OH-DPAT (0.1 and 0.5 mg/kg, intraperitoneally) did not alter novelty-induced hyperactivity in BDV-infected Lewis rats, while acute injections of a selective 5-HT re-uptake inhibitor, fluoxetine (1 and 5 mg/kg, ip) significantly and dose-dependently decreased novelty-induced hyperactivity in BDV-infected Lewis rats. No effects on hyperactivity in BDV-infected rats were seen after ip injections of ketanserin, an antagonist of $5-HT_{2a/2b}$ receptors (Pletnikov, unpublished observations).

Neurochemical and pharmacological studies showed a seemingly paradoxical profile of alterations in monoamine neurotransmission, namely increased presynaptic concentrations of 5-HT and upregulation of postsynaptic 5-HT receptors along with enhanced responses to compounds stimulating 5-HT neurotransmission.[56] In order to evaluate further the status of 5-HT neurotransmission in BDV-infected rats, development of their monoamine systems has been examined by studying a temporal correlation between alterations in DA and 5-HT tissue concentrations and the density of post- and presynaptic DA and 5-HT receptors. A significant virus-associated increase in the density of 5-HT$_{1a}$ receptors in the hippocampus (CA1 field and dentate gyrus) and 5-HT$_{2a}$ receptors in the cortex was found on day 14 p.i., whereas a BDV-associated increase in 5-HT concentrations in the same brain areas was not observed until after day 30 p.i.[43] Thus, BDV-induced upregulation of postsynaptic 5-HT receptors precedes an elevation of 5-HT. Such neurochemical data have been corroborated in behavioral experiments. In particular, a nonselective agonist of 5-HT receptors, quipazine, dose-dependently increased stereotypic behavior (e.g., paws treading) in BDV-infected rats yet had marginal effects on control animals, suggesting elevated sensitivity of 5-HT receptors to compounds stimulating 5-HT neurotransmission.[43] Our pilot experiments also addressed a putative structural basis for the increased density of postsynaptic 5-HT receptors. We found that BDV infection led to a 35% decline in the number of pyramidal neurons in the CA1 field on day 14 p.i., while the density of 5-HT$_{1a}$ receptors on pyramidal neurons in BDV-infected rats was greater than that in uninfected animals. These results suggest that virus infection may increase the number of postsynaptic receptors on remaining hippocampal pyramidal neurons.[43] To summarize, BDV may produce a decrease in 5-HT neurotransmission by affecting the release and/or axonal transport of the neurotransmitter. This suggestion is consistent with the notion that BDV may use the synaptic apparatus to spread within the CNS.[30,58]

Hormonal effects

Despite the known role of hormones in the postnatal development of the brain,[59] the effects of neonatal BDV infection on hormonal systems have been poorly studied. A lack of virus-associated changes in levels of growth hormone and insulin-like growth factor-1 and an absence of histological alterations in the adrenal glands in neonatally BDV-infected rats have been reported.[31,33] On the other hand, indirect evidence for an interaction between effects of BDV and hormones comes from one group that evaluated neurobehavioral abnormalities in BDV-infected tree shrews. Specifically, BDV-associated neurological and behavioral symptoms have been found to be sex-dependent, suggesting a role for sex hormones in mediating viral insult.[60] The lack of knowledge in this area calls for additional studies focusing on the role of hormonal systems in BDV-induced damage.

Behavioral alterations

Virus-associated structural and neurochemical alterations may underlie sensorimotor deficits, emotional disturbances, cognitive abnormalities, and altered social behaviors observed in infected rats.

Sensorimotor deficits

Neonatal BDV infection produces various impairments in motor and postural skills. While no evidence of gross ataxia and a normal swimming speed have been documented in BDV-infected rats,[61] there are several sensorimotor alterations, of which some could be explained by developmental damage to the cerebellum.[34]

Neonatally infected rats demonstrate mild gait ataxia, hind paw spasticity, and a decreased grip ability.[28] In addition, BDV-infected rats show deficient negative geotropism, fore and hind limb placing and grasping. The related ability to hold on to and move along a suspended bar is also impaired by the virus infection. Attenuated responses to the acoustic startle stimuli and impaired habituation of the acoustic startle are also observed.[34] Thus, BDV-induced abnormal development of the cerebellum is associated with selective deficits in sensorimotor and postural skills in rats.

Emotional disturbances

An early report has demonstrated that compared to control rats, BDV-infected Wistar rats show hyperactivity in the open field and a greater number of transitions in the white–black box paradigm, suggesting decreased anxiety.[62] BDV-associated emotional disturbances were assessed further in a series of experiments on Lewis rats tested at different time points after infection. BDV-infected rats exhibit hyperreactivity to novelty and aversive environments compared to control animals.[28,63] The neurobiological basis of emotional alterations in BDV-infected rats remains unclear and may be explained by BDV-associated damage to the cerebellum, hippocampus, and cortex. In addition, virus replication in neurons located in the other parts of the limbic system (e.g., the central nucleus of amygdala) could be responsible for disturbed emotionality in infected rats.[64]

Cognitive abnormalities

The hippocampus plays a major role in the brain mechanisms of learning and memory.[65] Thus, an association between BDV-induced hippocampal injury and learning and memory processes has been a focus of several studies.

Dittrich and colleagues have reported BDV-associated deficient performance in the Y-maze and hole board tests, suggesting abnormalities in spatial learning and memory in infected Wistar rats.[62] Spatial learning and memory in BDV-infected Lewis rats have been further assessed using the Morris water maze (MWM).[66] In the MWM, neonatally BDV-infected rats performed significantly worse than control rats.[61] Importantly, there was a correlation between loss of granule cells in the hippocampus and worsening of performance in the MWM in BDV-infected rats, indicating a pathogenic link between degenerating dentate gyrus and deteriorating spatial learning in infected animals.[61] The contextual fear-conditioning paradigm has also been used for examining the function of the limbic system in BDV-infected rats. Neonatal BDV infection produced attenuation of conditional responses in rats to the context that was previously paired with an aversive experience (e.g., loud noise), suggesting abnormalities in contextual conditioning. Notably, not all conditional responses were uniformly affected in BDV-infected rats. For example, conditioned defecation response to the context was spared, indicating that some components of the brain system mediating fear conditioning may be unaltered by the virus infection.[67] The observed deficits in learning and memory may be related to BDV-associated developmental injury to the hippocampus.

Social behavior deficits

Since BDV affects the brain regions that are involved in the neuronal mechanisms of social activity in rats (e.g., cortex and cerebellum),[68] in a series of experiments, Pletnikov and colleagues have assessed social behaviors of young and adult BDV-infected rats.[63] In the intruder–resident test, compared to control animals BDV-infected rats exhibited attenuated play activity and play solicitation. Although deficient in play, BDV-infected rats demonstrated elevated social nonplay interaction, suggesting specific defects in some forms of social behaviors.[63] Interestingly, abnormal play activity and play solicitation in BDV-infected animals was amenable to behavioral treatments. For example, improvements in play activity in BDV-infected rats resulted after repeated interactions with normal rats.

Abnormal social interaction in BDV-infected rats tested as adults has also been found (Pletnikov, unpublished data). In the open field test, far fewer social interactions were observed between BDV-infected and uninfected rats compared to normal levels. Social interactions were further reduced when BDV-infected rats were placed with each other. These data indicate attenuated social activity in young and adult BDV-infected rats. In order to gain more information about which particular components of social interaction are affected by BDV, different social responses have been assessed in BDV-infected rats following their exposure to uninfected and BDV-infected rats using the intruder–resident paradigm. BDV-infected rats have been shown to be unable to respond properly to social signals (e.g., postures) emitted by a healthy partner. Specifically, as intruders, BDV-infected rats did not react to threatening postures of resident rats. In contrast, control intruders promptly reacted with defensive freezing behavior when confronted by residents. Importantly, the lack of proper responses to threatening stimuli is unlikely to be due to nonspecific diminished fear in BDV-infected rats since BDV-infected animals showed elevated fear responses towards aversive nonsocial stimuli. Thus, abnormalities in social interaction in BDV-infected rats could be a result of virus-induced deficiency in the processing of social stimuli (Pletnikov, unpublished data).

In summary, neonatal BDV infection produces a number of distinct behavioral abnormalities that can be attributed to regional developmental brain damage and selective neurochemical and molecular alterations in infected rats. The possibility of relating brain pathology to behavioral deficits in the BDV model opens new perspectives for studying the mechanisms by which virus infections can lead to behavioral disorders.

Effects of genetic background

One of the unique features of BDV infection in general, and neonatal BDV infection in particular, includes species- and strain-dependence.[69,70] For example, neonatal BDV infection leads to different brain pathology, behavioral deficits, and responses to pharmacological treatments in rat strains with different vulnerability to environmental insults.[39,56] Compared to Lewis rats, Fisher344 rats were found to be more vulnerable to neonatal BDV infection with greater thinning of the cortex, more profound alterations in the monoamine brain systems, and, as a result, a broader spectrum of behavioral deficits. Moreover, different responses to pharmacological treatments have been found in BDV-infected rats of the two strains.[39,56]

Studies on different mouse strains after BDV infection have also revealed effects of genetic background on the type and degree of neurological manifestations.

Staeheli and his collaborators have shown variable outcomes of neurobehavioral disease among newborn mice of different strains.[71] Mice of the MRL strain were most susceptible to BDV, while BALB/c and C57BL/6 mice exhibited minimal, if any, neurological symptoms following neonatal BDV infection.

Further demonstrations of an impact of the genetic background on the severity of BDV-associated developmental abnormalities have come from studies of BDV infection in newborn gerbils, where severe neurological disease and death of infected animals occurs without significant signs of CNS inflammation or neuronal damage.[72] Importantly, during the asymptomatic phase of the disease, virus replication was predominantly detected in the cerebral cortex and hippocampus. In contrast, the symptomatic phase of disease was associated with virus replication in the lower brain stem and cerebellum. These observations suggested that replication of the virus and its effects on neuronal cells could be responsible for ensuing neurological disorders.

Another potential influence of the host on disease outcome can include host species/strain-specific selection of unique virus mutants with greater or lesser virulence. For example, recent investigations by Nishino and her coworkers have demonstrated that serial passage of BDV through mouse brain results in the selection of a virus population possessing greater virulence for rats. Interestingly, this mouse-passaged strain differed from the parental strain by only a few changes at the nucleotide level.[73]

Thus, the BDV model is a valuable system for studying the role of the genetic background–environment interaction in the causation of variable brain and behavioral pathology and different responses to therapy.

VIRAL ANIMAL MODELS OF NEUROPSYCHIATRIC DISEASES

For more than a decade, neonatal BDV infection has been a valuable animal model for exploring the mechanisms of viral neuropathogenesis and has significantly advanced our understanding of the mechanisms of abnormal brain and behavior development. The results of BDV research also have a widespread application as scientists in the area continue to develop new animal models that may mirror selective DBDs and the underlying pathogenic processes. For example, in a series of elegant behavioral tests, Sauder and colleagues have used β2 microglobulin knockout C57BL/10J mice that lack mature, functional CD8+ T cells and show asymptomatic, persistent BDV infection in the absence of inflammation. The authors correlated the abnormal MWM performance of these BDV-infected mice with altered chemokine levels. These studies showed that BDV infection can disturb the function of the mammalian CNS without causing overt neuronal loss and that selective BDV-induced disturbances in chemokine production might be responsible for selective behavioral alterations.[74]

New insights from BDV animal model studies are particularly relevant to the longlasting debates about possible BDV infection in humans where neither overt inflammation nor visible brain damage have been documented.[75] In this context, animal models with virus-induced functional (e.g., neurochemical or neuroimmune) rather than structural alterations may serve to recapitulate possible BDV-associated syndromes in patients where the existence of BDV infection seems to have been demonstrated, but the clinical pictures are not consistent with the existing animal models.[75]

REFERENCES

1. Ellenbroek BA, Cools AR. Animal models with construct validity for schizophrenia. *Behav Pharmacol* 1990; **1**: 469–90.
2. Kilts CD. The changing roles and targets for animal models of schizophrenia. *Biol Psychiatry* 2001; **50**: 845–55.
3. Geyer MA, Braff DL. Startle habituation and sensorimotor gating in schizophrenia and related animal models. *Schizophr Bull* 1987; **13**: 643–68.
4. Willner P. Animal models of depression: validity and applications. *Adv Biochem Psychopharmacol* 1995; **49**: 19–41.
5. Lipska BK, Weinberger DR. To model a psychiatric disorder in animals: schizophrenia as a reality test. *Neuropsychopharmacology* 2000; **23**: 223–39.
6. Altman J. Morphological and behavioral markers of environmentally induced retardation of brain development: an animal model. *Env Health Perspectives* 1987; **74**: 153–68.
7. Sanberg PR, Moran TH, Coyle JT. Microencephaly: cortical hypoplasia induced by methylazoxymethanol. In: *Animal Models of Dementia* (Coyle JT, ed). New York: Alan R Liss Inc, 1987: 253–78.
8. Bachevalier J. Medial temporal lobe structures and autism: a review of clinical and experimental findings. *Neuropsychologia* 1994; **32**: 627–48.
9. Ferguson SA. Neuroanatomical and functional alterations resulting from early postnatal cerebellar insults in rodents. *Pharmacol Biochem Behav* 1996; **55**: 663–71.
10. Lijam N, Paylor R, McDonald MP et al. Social interaction and sensorimotor gating abnormalities in mice lacking Dvl1. *Cell* 1997; **90**: 895–905.
11. Gainetdinov RR, Mohn AR, Caron MG. Genetic animal models: focus on schizophrenia. *Trends Neurosci* 2001; **24**: 527–33.
12. Pearce BD. Schizophrenia and viral infection during neurodevelopment: a focus on mechanisms. *Mol Psychiatry* 2001; **6**: 634–46.
13. Shi L, Fatemi SH, Sidwell RW, Patterson PH. Maternal influenza infection causes marked behavioral and pharmacological changes in the offspring. *J Neurosci* 2003; **23**: 297–302.

14. DeLisi LE. Is there a viral or immune dysfunction etiology to schizophrenia? Re-evaluation a decade later. *Schizophr Res* 1986; **22**: 1–4.
15. van Gent T, Heijnen CJ, Treffers PD. Autism and the immune system. *J Child Psychol Psychiatry* 1997; **38**: 337–49.
16. Yolken RH, Karlsson H, Yee F et al. Endogenous retroviruses and schizophrenia. *Brain Res Rev* 2000; **31**: 93–9.
17. Carbone KM. Borna disease virus and human disease. *Clin Microbiol Rev* 2001; **14**: 513–27.
18. Johnson RT. *Viral Infections of the Nervous System*. Philadelphia: Lippincott-Raven, 1998.
19. Rausch DM, Stover ES. Neuroscience research in AIDS. *Progress Neuropsychopharmacol Biol Psychiatry* 2001; **25**: 231–57.
20. Briese T, Schneemann A, Lewis AJ et al. Genomic organization of Borna disease virus. *Proc Natl Acad Sci USA* 1994; **91**: 4362–6.
21. Cubitt B, de la Torre JC. Borna disease virus (BDV), a nonsegmented RNA virus, replicates in the nuclei of infected cells where infectious BDV ribonucleoproteins are present. *J Virol* 1994; **68**: 1371–81.
22. Narayan O, Herzog S, Frese K et al. Behavioral disease in rats caused by immunopathological responses to persistent borna virus in the brain. *Science* 1983; **220**: 1401–3.
23. Hirano N, Kao M, Ludwig H. Persistent, tolerant or subacute infection in Borna disease virus-infected rats. *J Gen Virol* 1983; **64**: 1521–30.
24. Carbone KM, Park SW, Rubin SA et al. Borna disease: association with a maturation defect in the cellular immune response. *J Virol* 1991; **65**: 6154–64.
25. Ciaranello AL, Ciaranello RD. The neurobiology of infantile autism. *Ann Rev Neurosci* 1995; **18**: 101–28.
26. Gosztonyi G, Ludwig H. Borna disease – neuropathology and pathogenesis. *Curr Topics Microbiol Immunol* 1995; **190**: 39–73.
27. Bautista JR, Rubin SA, Moran TH et al. Developmental injury to the cerebellum following perinatal Borna disease virus infection. *Dev Brain Res* 1995; **90**: 45–53.
28. Hornig M, Weissenbock H, Horscroft N, Lipkin WI. An infection-based model of neurodevelopmental damage. *Proc Natl Acad Sci USA* 1999; **96**: 12102–7.
29. Sauder C, de la Torre JC. Cytokine expression in the rat central nervous system following perinatal Borna disease virus infection. *J Neuroimmunol* 1999; **96**: 29–45.
30. Gonzalez-Dunia D, Watanabe M, Syan S et al. Synaptic pathology in Borna disease virus persistent infection. *J Virol* 2000; **74**: 3441–8.
31. Weissenbock H, Hornig M, Hickey WF, Lipkin WI. Microglial activation and neuronal apoptosis in Bornavirus infected neonatal Lewis rats. *Brain Pathol* 2000; **10**: 260–72.
32. Morales JA, Herzog S, Kompter C et al. Axonal transport of Borna disease virus along olfactory pathways in spontaneously and experimentally infected rats. *Med Microbiol Immunol (Berlin)* 1988; **177**: 51–68.
33. Bautista JR, Schwartz GJ, de la Torre JC et al. Early and persistent abnormalities in rats with neonatally acquired Borna disease virus infection. *Brain Res Bull* 1994; **34**: 31–6.
34. Pletnikov M, Rubin S, Carbone K et al. Neonatal Borna disease virus infection (BDV)-induced damage to the cerebellum is associated with sensorimotor deficits in developing Lewis rats. *Dev Brain Res* 2001; **126**: 1–12.
35. Han VK. Pathophysiology, cellular and molecular mechanisms of foetal growth retardation. *Equine Veterinary J* 1993; **14**(Suppl.): 12–6.
36. Levitsky DA, Strupp BJ. Malnutrition and the brain: changing concepts, changing concerns. *J Nutrition* 1995; **125**: 2212S–20S.
37. Eisenman LM, Brothers R, Tran MH et al. Neonatal Borna disease virus infection in the rat causes a loss of Purkinje cells in the cerebellum. *J Neurovirol* 1999; **5**: 181–9.
38. Zocher M, Czub S, Schulte-Monting J et al. Alterations in neurotrophin and neurotrophin receptor gene expression patterns in the rat central nervous system following perinatal Borna disease virus infection. *J Neurovirol* 2000; **6**: 462–77.
39. Pletnikov MV, Rubin SA, Vogel MW et al. Effects of genetic background on neonatal Borna disease virus infection-induced neurodevelopmental damage. I. Brain pathology and behavioral deficits. *Brain Res* 2002; **944**: 97–107.
40. Norman DJ, Feng L, Cheng SS et al. The lurcher gene induces apoptotic death in cerebellar Purkinje cells. *Development* 1995; **121**: 1183–93.
41. Masliah E, Ge N, Achim CL, Wiley CA. Differential vulnerability of calbindin-immunoreactive neurons in HIV encephalitis. *J Neuropathol Exp Neurol* 1995; **54**: 350–7.
42. Mitchell IJ, Cooper AJ, Griffiths MR. The selective vulnerability of striatopallidal neurons. *Progress Neurobiol* 1999; **59**: 691–719.
43. Dietz D, Vogel M, Rubin S et al. Developmental alterations in serotoninergic neurotransmission in Borna disease virus (BDV)-infected rats: a multidisciplinary analysis. *J Neurovirol* 2004; **10**: 267–77.
44. Baimbridge KG, Celio MR, Rogers JH. Calcium-binding proteins in the nervous system. *Trends Neurosci* 1992; **15**: 303–8.
45. Messing A, Brenner M. GFAP: functional implications gleaned from studies of genetically engineered mice. *Glia* 2003; **43**: 87–90.
46. Becher B, Prat A, Antel JP. Brain-immune connection: immunoregulatory properties of CNS-resident cells. *Glia* 2000; **29**: 293–304.
47. Plata-Salaman CR, Ilyin SE, Gayle D et al. Persistent Borna disease virus infection of neonatal rats causes brain regional changes of mRNAs for cytokines, cytokine receptor components and neuropeptides. *Brain Res Bull* 1999; **49**: 441–51.
48. Sauder C, Hallensleben W, Pagenstecher A et al. Chemokine gene expression in astrocytes of Borna disease virus-infected rats and mice in the absence of inflammation. *J Virol* 2000; **74**: 9267–80.
49. Rauer M, Pagenstecher A, Schulte-Monting J, Sauder C. Upregulation of chemokine receptor gene expression in brains of Borna disease virus (BDV)-infected rats in the absence and presence of inflammation. *J Neurovirol* 2002; **8**: 168–79.
50. Asensio VC, Campbell IL. Chemokines in the CNS: plurifunctional mediators in diverse states. *Trends Neurosci* 1999; **22**: 504–12.
51. Levi-Montalcini R, Skaper SD, Dal Toso R et al. Nerve growth factor: from neurotrophin to neurokine. *Trends Neurosci* 1996; **19**: 514–20.
52. Billaud JN, Ly C, Phillips TR, de la Torre JC. Borna disease virus persistence causes inhibition of glutamate uptake by feline primary cortical astrocytes. *J Virol* 2000; **74**: 10438–46.
53. Hans A, Syan S, Crosio C et al. Borna disease virus persistent infection activates mitogen-activated protein kinase and blocks neuronal differentiation of pc12 cells. *J Biol Chemistry* 2001; **276**: 7258–65.
54. Planz O, Pleschka S, Ludwig S. MEK-specific inhibitor U0126 blocks spread of Borna disease virus in cultured cells. *J Virol* 2001; **75**: 4871–7.
55. Pletnikov M, Rubin S, Schwartz G et al. Effects of neonatal rat Borna disease virus (BDV) infection on the postnatal development of brain monoaminergic systems. *Dev Brain Res* 2000; **119**: 179–85.
56. Pletnikov MV, Moran TH, Carbone KM. Borna disease virus infection of the neonatal rat: developmental brain injury model

of autism spectrum disorders. *Frontiers Biosci* 2002; **7**: 593–607.
57. Pletnikov MV, Rubin SA, Vogel MW et al. Effects of genetic background on neonatal Borna disease virus infection-induced neurodevelopmental damage. II. Neurochemical alterations and responses to pharmacological treatments. *Brain Res* 2002; **944**: 108–23.
58. Carbone KM, Duchala CS, Griffin JW et al. Pathogenesis of Borna disease in rats: evidence that intra-axonal spread is the major route for virus dissemination and the determinant for disease incubation. *J Virol* 1987; **61**: 3431–40.
59. McEwen BS. Steroid hormone actions on the brain: when is the genome involved? *Hormones Behav* 1994; **28**: 396–405.
60. Sprankel H, Richarz K, Ludwig H, Rott R. Behavior alterations in tree shrews (*Tupaia glis*) induced by Borna disease virus. *Med Microbiol Immunol (Berlin)* 1978; **165**: 1–18.
61. Rubin SA, Sylves P, Vogel MW et al. Borna disease virus-induced hippocampal dentate gyrus damage is associated with spatial learning and memory deficits. *Brain Res Bull* 1999; **48**: 23–30.
62. Dittrich W, Bode L, Ludwig H et al. Learning deficiencies in Borna disease virus-infected but clinically healthy rats. *Biol Psychiatry* 1989; **20**: 818–28.
63. Pletnikov M, Rubin S, Schwartz G et al. Persistent neonatal Borna disease virus (BDV) infection of the brain causes chronic emotional abnormalities in adult rats. *Physiol Behav* 1999; **66**: 823–31.
64. Fanselow MS. Contextual fear, gestalt memories, and the hippocampus. *Behav Brain Res* 2000; **110**: 73–81.
65. Rolls E. Memory systems in the brain. *Ann Rev Psychology* 2000; **51**: 599–630.
66. Eichenbaum H, Stewart C, Morris RG. Hippocampal representation in place learning. *J Neurosci* 1990; **10**: 3531–42.
67. Panksepp J, Siviy S, Normansell L. The psychobiology of play: theoretical and methodological perspectives. *Neurosci Biobehav Rev* 1984; **8**: 465–92.
68. Pletnikov M, Rubin S, Vasudevan K et al. Developmental brain injury associated with abnormal play behavior in neonatally Borna disease virus-infected Lewis rats: a model of autism. *Behav Brain Res* 1999; **100**: 43–50.
69. Herzog S, Frese K, Rott R. Studies on the genetic control of resistance of black hooded rats to Borna disease. *J Gen Virol* 1991; **72**: 535–40.
70. Rubin SA, Waltrip RW II, Bautista JR, Carbone KM. Borna disease virus in mice: host-specific differences in disease expression. *J Virol* 1993; **67**: 548–52.
71. Hallensleben W, Schwemmle M, Hausmann J et al. Borna disease virus-induced neurological disorder in mice: infection of neonates results in immunopathology. *J Virol* 1998; **72**: 4379–86.
72. Watanabe M, Byeong-Jae L, Kamitani W et al. Neurological diseases and viral dynamics in the brains of neonatally Borna disease virus-infected gerbils. *Virology* 2001; **282**: 65–76.
73. Nishino Y, Kobasa D, Rubin SA et al. Enhanced neurovirulence of Borna disease virus variants associated with nucleotide changes in the glycoprotein and L polymerase genes. *J Virol* 2002; **76**: 8650–8.
74. Sauder C, Wolfer DP, Lipp HP et al. Learning deficits in mice with persistent Borna disease virus infection of the CNS associated with elevated chemokine expression. *Behav Brain Res* 2001; **120**: 189–201.
75. Ludwig H, Bode L. Borna disease virus: new aspects on infection, disease, diagnosis and epidemiology. *Rev Sci Technol* 2001; **19**: 259–88.

23

Inflammatory perinatal brain damage: Observations, experiments, explanations

Dorothee B Bartels and Olaf Dammann

INTRODUCTION

Over recent years, a plethora of evidence has accumulated in support of the hypothesis that antenatal maternal infection and a subsequent fetal inflammatory response are associated with an increased risk for neonatal brain white matter damage.[1–5] This chapter is an update on this topic, based on observational and experimental studies. We also offer some speculations regarding possible biological explanations for these findings.

OBSERVATIONS

The association between antenatal infection of the brain by organisms such as *Toxoplasma gondii*, rubella, or cytomegalovirus and fetal brain damage is well known. In essence, a maternal infection during pregnancy is transmitted to the fetus and directly damages the fetal brain.

In the early 1970s, perinatal neuroepidemiologists started to investigate a potential role for remote infection (outside the fetus's central nervous system) and perinatal brain damage.[6,7] Since then, multiple studies have confirmed neonatal sepsis as one risk factor,[8–10] thereby supporting the concept of infection-related perinatal brain damage without the brain itself being infected.[1]

In the following three sections, we review data on the association of potential remote infectious mechanisms and outcome defined by pathology, neonatal neuroimaging, and clinical examination.

Outcome defined postmortem

A limited number of histological studies have been published. Investigators found a fivefold increased risk for perinatal telencephalic leucoencephalopathy among infants with postmortem bacteremia in one study,[6] and a 30-fold increased risk in another.[7] Studies that revealed no association between maternal infection and white matter injury in infants <32 weeks[11] or all gestational ages[12] did not take into account the potential confounder of intrauterine growth restriction, which was present twice as often in cases as in controls.

Immunohistochemical staining revealed increased numbers of cells positive for tumor necrosis factor-α (TNF-α)[13] and other cytokines[14–18] in the brains of preterm infants with white matter damage compared to controls. The presence of β-amyloid precursor protein, a marker of neuronal damage and activated astrocytes,[19] in brains with white matter damage but not in controls[19,20] supports the hypothesis that white matter damage involves damage not only to glial, but also to neuronal cells.[21] Indeed, cortical and deep gray matter neurons stain positive for the pro-inflammatory cytokines TNF-α and interleukin-1β in the brains of infants who died with macroscopic evidence of white matter damage.[18]

Outcome defined by neonatal neuroimaging

The best currently-established neuroimaging modality in neonatology is cerebral ultrasound.[22] Ultrasound abnormalities of the white matter can be hyperechoic (echodensities), representing an early expression of white matter damage[23,24] and sometimes already identified before birth,[25] or hypoechoic (echolucencies), a later expression of white matter damage.[23]

Chorioamnionitis was associated with echodensities in some[26] but not all studies.[27] This inconsistency might result from the supposedly heterogeneous natural history of intraparenchymal echodensities, which are currently interpreted as either an indicator of parenchymal involvement after intraventricular hemorrhage, or an early stage of periventricular leucomalacia.[24]

The prevalence of echolucencies was increased more than threefold in one study of 753 infants born between 24 and 32 weeks after intrauterine infection combined with premature rupture of membranes.[28] Pooled data from multiple studies yielded odds ratios of 1.6 (95% confidence interval 1.0–2.5) for histologic chorioamnionitis and 2.6 (1.7–3.9) for clinical chorioamnionitis and echolucency.[4] In one study, chorioamnionitis of unspecified definition was associated with a (univariably estimated) sixfold risk increase for echolucency.[29]

Not all studies show an association between histologic chorioamnionitis and echolucency.[30,31] However, among infants with histologic chorioamnionitis who were born within one hour of membrane rupture, fetal vasculitis (defined as the presence of polymorphonuclear leukocytes in the walls of chorionic and umbilical cord vessels) was associated with an 11-fold increase in the risk of late echolucency – defined as an echolucency first identified on the 21st postnatal day (median).[30] This suggests that a fetal inflammatory response to chorioamnionitis, present long before the membranes ruptured, might contribute to the pathogenesis of white matter damage. The hypothesis that fetal exposure to longstanding infection and/or inflammation contributes to an increased risk of white matter damage is supported by the finding that prenatal cultures of the upper vagina and cervix were more likely to grow bacteria or candida in women whose infants subsequently had sonographic echolucencies.[27] Thus bacterial vaginosis could constitute a chronic inflammatory stimulus that increases the risk of a gestational intrauterine infection, a fetal inflammatory response, echolucencies, and eventually its consequence, cerebral palsy (CP) in preterm infants.[32]

Elevated cytokine levels in the amniotic fluid[31–33] and umbilical cord[34–37] are associated with an increased risk for abnormalities in the white matter identified by neonatal imaging. Infants with elevated interleukin-6 serum levels in cordocentesis specimens are twice as likely as infants with lower levels to have severe neonatal morbidity, including intraventricular hemorrhage and white matter damage.[38] One report that infants with white matter damage have lower median amniotic fluid pro-inflammatory cytokine levels than controls is limited by a very small sample size ($n = 33$).[39]

One study has reported an association between increased levels of circulation markers of infection/inflammation and white matter abnormalities on neonatal magnetic resonance images (MRI) of the brain.[35] In this most intriguing paper, investigators not only looked at cytokine levels, but also at CD45R0+ white blood cells. Indeed, the proportion of these cells, interpreted as indicators of prenatal fetal contact with an antigen, was significantly higher among babies with white matter abnormalities on MRI compared to controls.

Outcome defined by clinical examination

Chorioamnionitis appears to be associated with an increased risk of white matter damage and its longterm clinical correlate cerebral palsy in preterm infants.[40] In a pooled analysis, the odds ratio was 1.9 (1.5–2.5) for clinical and 1.5 (0.9–2.5) for histologic chorioamnionitis.[4] In one recent study, not included in this meta-analysis, the corresponding univariable risk estimates were 1.8 (0.9–36) and 3.6 (1.2–12).[41] However, these results are not easily interpreted due to small numbers, heterogeneity of groups, and the absence of control for confounders in a multivariable fashion. A recent publication shows an absence of association between histologic chorioamnionitis and cerebral palsy in preterm infants.[42] This is most likely due to the exclusion of infants at highest (birth within three hours of admission) and lowest (preeclampsia) risk of antenatal infection, which is equivalent to an exclusion of those who smoke more than two packs daily and lifelong nonsmokers from a study on smoking as a risk factor for lung cancer.

In one recent set of analyses, investigators found that fetal, but not maternal, placental inflammatory characteristics were associated with neurologic impairment, predominantly among infants whose placentas had chorionic plate thrombi.[43,44] One explanation would be that a fetal systemic inflammatory response might increase the risk of chorionic plate thrombosis, probably via such mechanisms as upregulation of adhesion molecules, increased concentrations of procoagulants, and endothelial dysfunction.[45]

The prediction of cerebral palsy from the presence of umbilical cord inflammation,[46] amniotic fluid pro-inflammatory cytokines,[14,46] and matrix metalloproteinase-8,[47] an enzyme that degrades components of the extracellular matrix, further supports the concept that a fetal inflammatory response is associated with longterm neurologic disability.

EXPERIMENTS

From the previous section we conclude that an inflammatory response is present in the placenta, the systemic circulation, and the brain of preterm newborns with brain white matter damage. This section is devoted to experimental animal models of perinatal infection. Although the focus of this discussion is neuroinflammation, it does not exclude models that lead to brain damage.

Maternal infection

Some,[48,49] but not all,[50] recently developed rabbit models showed that antenatal bacterial infection of pregnant animals can cause white matter damage in their offspring. In an extension of earlier findings in rats,[51] more recently developed rat models show fetal neuroinflammation as a consequence of infection at the maternal systemic level.[52,53]

Fetal systemic infection

Early studies in newborn kittens had shown that intraperitoneal injection of bacterial endotoxins causes brain white matter damage.[54] In newborn dogs, subcutaneous administration of E. coli endotoxin causes periventricular white matter necrosis and a generalized inflammatory reaction in both gray and white matter.[55] While it is already well known that systemic infection can cause brain damage in mature animals (piglets),[56] it has now been demonstrated that a systemic infectious challenge is followed by brain damage in animal fetuses (sheep).[57,58] In a comparative study, endotoxemia led to selective white matter damage and inflammation, while asphyxia produced lesions in both white and subcortical grey matter in association with microglial activation.[58]

Brain infection

Some investigators have injected the stimulus that mimics infection (bacterial lipopolysaccharide, LPS) directly into the brain. In one study, unilateral injection was followed by ipsilateral cystic damage and bilateral ventriculomegaly.[59] These investigators also found that Toll-like receptor 4, the receptor for LPS, was present only on microglial cells. Moreover, only the supernatant from LPS-stimulated microglial cells resulted in a significant reduction of mature oligodendrocytes in a coculture model.

Finally, some investigators have created two-hit models.[60–63] Generally speaking, the concept of preconditioning can be viewed as the alteration of susceptibility to a potentially damaging insult by prior exposure to another or even the same insult. While a full discussion of this topic is far beyond the scope of this chapter, it should be mentioned that exposure to an infectious stimulus appears to increase the damage potential of subsequent experimental hypoxia-ischemia.[62,63]

An excellent overview of animal models of white matter damage after exposure to bacterial, viral, or lipopolysaccharide challenge has most recently been provided by Hagberg and colleagues.[64] Obviously, it is extremely difficult to create an animal model of antenatal subclinical infection and fetal brain damage. Among the critical issues are the choice of animal species and within-species differences between strains, the timing (early or late antenatal or postnatal) and localization (intraperitoneal, intracervical, intra-amniotic, intracerebral) of stimulus administration, infectious versus inflammatory stimuli, issues of fetal mortality, and avoidance of fetal death by antibiotic therapy.

EXPLANATIONS

A theory has been proposed that explains the observed association between prematurity and brain damage[65] by suggesting that antenatal infection is a cause of both preterm birth and brain damage.[66,67] This concept is now well supported by observations that antenatal infection/inflammation is associated with preterm birth[68–70] and perinatal brain damage (vida supra), and by experiments that show that infection/inflammation can cause preterm delivery[71,72] and perinatal brain damage (vida supra).

We have subsequently expanded this concept by proposing that antenatal intrauterine infection results in a systemic fetal inflammatory response which might be even more harmful for the fetal brain than infection per se.[2,30] Cytokines, chemokines, and growth factors are potential mediators of this association by virtue of their increased levels in amniotic fluid, placenta, fetal circulation, and the fetal brain.[67,73] A white cell invasion of the central nervous system might be an integral part of this scenario, providing the link between fetal systemic and neuroinflammatory responses.[74] Kadhim and coworkers have found increased levels of interleukin-2 (IL-2) in the brains of infants with white matter damage.[17] Since they were not able to find concomitantly increased levels of producer cells (lymphocytes), they interpret their finding as support for the hypothesis that the IL-2 seen inside the brain might originate from outside the brain.[75] Indeed, IL-2 is not produced by microglial cells upon LPS challenge.[76] However, microglial cells do express IL-2 receptors[77] and elevated levels of IL-2 in the systemic circulation might spill over into the brain and help trigger microglia activation.

If the intracerebral production/presence of cytokines was indeed harmful, how would the damage occur? Obviously, perinatal brain injury is not exclusively necrotic, but also has an apoptotic (programmed cell death) component.[78] While necrosis is one likely explanation for the focal white matter damage frequently called cystic periventricular leukomalacia, apoptosis might slow down or even interrupt oligodendrocyte development.[79] Thus, it might be one explanation for the generalized white matter paucity seen in cases of ventriculomegaly due to hydrocephalus ex vacuo.[80]

Some students of perinatal brain damage have proposed that the neuroinflammation component of white matter damage pathogenesis might not only be a consequence of infection, but also of hypoxia-ischemia.[81] While it is eminently clear that hypoxia-ischemia does induce brain inflammation,[82] this does not preclude a direct damaging effect of circulating markers of inflammation on developing glial and/or neuronal cells. Moreover, it is unlikely that a localized ischemic insult in the brain elicits a systemic inflammatory response characterized by sepsis-like concentrations of pro-inflammatory cytokines in the fetal/neonatal circulation, measurable in the amniotic fluid days before birth (vida supra). In light of histological differences seen in experimental animal models of inflammatory WMD and ischemic WMD,[64] attempts should be made to identify these WMD-subtypes in postmortem studies in humans.

Even adult stroke is associated with (and sometimes preceded by) systemic inflammation, which makes it possible that the causal pathway leads from inflammation to ischemia, not vice versa. We have recently summarized and discussed the interesting phenomena adult stroke and perinatal brain damage have in common.[83] Agents with potential for modifying parts of the fetal neuroinflammatory response might be candidates for the development of protective therapies.[84–86] Nevertheless, further research is needed to identify those mothers and fetuses who are at highest risk and would therefore benefit most from such a potentially harmful intervention.

REFERENCES

1. Dammann O, Leviton A. Infection remote from the brain, neonatal white matter damage, and cerebral palsy in the preterm infant. *Semin Pediatr Neurol* 1998; 5: 190–201.
2. Dammann O, Leviton A. Role of the fetus in perinatal infection and neonatal brain damage. *Curr Opin Pediatr* 2000; 12: 99–104.
3. Toti P, De Felice C. Chorioamnionitis and fetal/neonatal brain injury. *Biol Neonate* 2001; 79: 201–4.
4. Wu YW. Systematic review of chorioamnionitis and cerebral palsy. *Ment Retard Dev Disabil Res Rev* 2002; 8: 25–9.
5. Willoughby RE Jr, Nelson KB. Chorioamnionitis and brain injury. *Clin Perinatol* 2002; 29: 603–21.
6. Leviton A, Gilles FH. An epidemiologic study of perinatal telencephalic leucoencephalopathy in an autopsy population. *J Neurol Sci* 1973; 18: 53–66.
7. Leviton A, Gilles F, Neff R, Yaney P. Multivariate analysis of risk of perinatal telencephalic leucoencephalopathy. *Am J Epidemiol* 1976; 104: 621–6.
8. Faix RG, Donn SM. Association of septic shock caused by early-onset group B streptococcal sepsis and periventricular leukomalacia in the preterm infant. *Pediatrics* 1985; 76: 415–9.
9. Vermeulen GM, Bruinse HW, Gerards LJ, de Vries LS. Perinatal risk factors for cranial ultrasound abnormalities in neonates born after spontaneous labour before 34 weeks. *Eur J Obstet Gynecol Reprod Biol* 2001; 94: 290–5.
10. Wheater M, Rennie JM. Perinatal infection is an important risk factor for cerebral palsy in very-low-birthweight infants. *Dev Med Child Neurol* 2000; 42: 364–7.
11. Murphy DJ, Squier MV, Hope PL et al. Clinical associations and time of onset of cerebral white matter damage in very preterm babies. *Arch Dis Child Fetal Neonatal Ed* 1996; 75: F27–32.
12. Gaffney G, Squier MV, Johnson A et al. Clinical associations of prenatal ischaemic white matter injury. *Arch Dis Child* 1994; 70: F101–6.
13. Deguchi K, Mizuguchi M, Takashima S. Immunohistochemical expression of tumor necrosis factor alpha in neonatal leukomalacia. *Pediatr Neurol* 1996; 14: 13–6.
14. Yoon BH, Romero R, Kim CJ et al. High expression of tumor necrosis factor-alpha and interleukin-6 in periventricular leukomalacia. *Am J Obstet Gynecol* 1997; 177: 406–11.
15. Deguchi K, Oguchi K, Takashima S. Characteristic neuropathology of leukomalacia in extremely low birth weight infants. *Pediatr Neurol* 1997; 16: 296–300.
16. Kadhim H, Tabarki B, Verellen G et al. Inflammatory cytokines in the pathogenesis of periventricular leukomalacia. *Neurology* 2001; 56: 1278–84.
17. Kadhim H et al. Interleukin-2 in the pathogenesis of perinatal white matter damage. *Neurology* 2002; 58: 1125–8.
18. Kadhim H, Tabarki B, De Prez C, Sebire G. Cytokine immunoreactivity in cortical and subcortical neurons in periventricular leukomalacia: are cytokines implicated in neuronal dysfunction in cerebral palsy? *Acta Neuropathol (Berlin)* 2003; 105: 209–16.
19. Arai Y, Deguchi K, Mizuguchi M, Takashima S. Expression of beta-amyloid precursor protein in axons of periventricular leukomalacia brains. *Pediatr Neurol* 1995; 13: 161–3.
20. Hirayama A, Okoshi Y, Hachiya Y et al. Early immunohistochemical detection of axonal damage and glial activation in extremely immature brains with periventricular leukomalacia. *Clin Neuropathol* 2001; 20: 87–91.
21. Dammann O, Hagberg H, Leviton A. Is periventricular leukomalacia an axonopathy as well as an oligopathy? *Pediatric Res* 2001; 49: 453–7.
22. De Vries LS, Groenendaal F. Neuroimaging in the preterm infant. *Ment Retard Dev Disabil Res Rev* 2002; 8: 273–80.
23. De Vries LS, Eken P, Dubowitz LM. The spectrum of leukomalacia using cranial ultrasound. *Behav Brain Res* 1992; 49: 1–6.
24. Dammann O, Leviton A. Duration of transient hyperechoic images of white matter in very-low-birthweight infants: a proposed classification. *Dev Med Child Neurol* 1997; 39: 2–5.
25. Yamamoto N, Utsu M, Serizawa M et al. Neonatal periventricular leukomalacia preceded by fetal periventricular echodensity. *Fetal Diagn Ther* 2000; 15: 198–208.
26. O'Shea TM, Kothadia JM, Roberts DD, Dillard RG. Perinatal events and the risk of intraparenchymal echodensity in very-low-birthweight neonates. *Paediatr Perinat Epidemiol* 1998; 12: 408–21.

27. Spinillo A, Capuzzo E, Stronati M et al. Obstetric risk factors for periventricular leukomalacia among preterm infants. *Br J Obstet Gynaecol* 1998; **105**: 865–71.
28. Zupan V, Gonzalez P, Lacaze-Masmonteil T et al. Periventricular leukomalacia: risk factors revisited. *Dev Med Child Neurol* 1996; **38**: 1061–7.
29. Resch B, Vollaard E, Maurer U et al. Risk factors and determinants of neurodevelopmental outcome in cystic periventricular leucomalacia. *Eur J Pediatr* 2000; **159**: 663–70.
30. Leviton A, Paneth N, Reuss ML et al. Maternal infection, fetal inflammatory response, and brain damage in very low birth-weight infants. *Pediatr Res* 1999; **46**: 566–75.
31. Martinez E, Figueroa R, Garry D et al. Elevated amniotic fluid interleukin-6 as a predictor of neonatal periventricular leukomalacia and intraventricular hemorrhage. *J Mat Fet Invest* 1998; **8**: 101–7.
32. Dammann O, Leviton A. Does prepregnancy bacterial vaginosis increase a mother's risk of having a preterm infant with cerebral palsy? *Dev Med Child Neurol* 1997; **39**: 836–40.
33. Yoon BH, Romero R, Jun JK et al. Amniotic fluid inflammatory cytokines (interleukin-6, interleukin-1beta, and tumor necrosis factor-alpha), neonatal brain white matter lesions, and cerebral palsy. *Am J Obstet Gynecol* 1997; **177**: 825–30.
34. Yoon BH, Romero R, Yang SH et al. Interleukin-6 concentrations in umbilical cord plasma are elevated in neonates with white matter lesions associated with periventricular leukomalacia. *Am J Obstet Gynecol* 1996; **174**: 1433–40.
35. Duggan PJ, Maalouf EF, Watts TL et al. Intrauterine T-cell activation and increased proinflammatory cytokine concentrations in preterm infants with cerebral lesions. *Lancet* 2001; **358**: 1699–700.
36. Minagawa K, Tsuji Y, Ueda H et al. Possible correlation between high levels of IL-18 in the cord blood of pre-term infants and neonatal development of periventricular leukomalacia and cerebral palsy. *Cytokine* 2002; **17**: 164–70.
37. Tauscher MK, Berg D, Brockmann M et al. Association of histologic chorioamnionitis, increased levels of cord blood cytokines, and intracerebral hemorrhage in preterm neonates. *Biol Neonate* 2003; **83**: 166–70.
38. Gomez R, Romero R, Ghezzi F et al. The fetal inflammatory response syndrome. *Am J Obstet Gynecol* 1998; **179**: 194–202.
39. Baud O, Emilie D, Pelletier E et al. Amniotic fluid concentrations of interleukin-1beta, interleukin-6 and TNF-alpha in chorioamnionitis before 32 weeks of gestation: histologic associations and neonatal outcome. *Br J Obstet Gynaecol* 1999; **106**: 72–7.
40. Hagberg H, Wennerholm UB, Savman K. Sequelae of chorioamnionitis. *Curr Opin Infect Dis* 2002; **15**: 301–6.
41. Jacobsson B, Hagberg G, Hagberg B et al. Cerebral palsy in preterm infants: a population-based case-control study of antenatal and intrapartal risk factors. *Acta Paediatr* 2002; **91**: 946–51.
42. Grether JK, Nelson KB, Walsh E et al. Intrauterine exposure to infection and risk of cerebral palsy in very preterm infants. *Arch Pediatr Adolesc Med* 2003; **157**: 26–32.
43. Redline RW, Wilson-Costello D, Borawski E et al. Placental lesions associated with neurologic impairment and cerebral palsy in very-low-birthweight infants. *Arch Pathol Lab Med* 1998; **122**: 1091–8.
44. Redline RW, Wilson-Costello D, Borawski E et al. The relationship between placental and other perinatal risk factors for neurologic impairment in very low birth weight children. *Pediatr Res* 2000; **47**: 721–6.
45. Vallance P, Collier J, Bhagat K. Infection, inflammation, and infarction: does acute endothelial dysfunction provide a link? *Lancet* 1997; **349**: 1391–2.
46. Yoon BH, Romero R, Park JS et al. Fetal exposure to an intra-amniotic inflammation and the development of cerebral palsy at the age of three years. *Am J Obstet Gynecol* 2000; **182**: 675–81.
47. Moon JB, Kim JC, Yoon BH et al. Amniotic fluid matrix metalloproteinase-8 and the development of cerebral palsy. *J Perinat Med* 2002; **30**: 301–6.
48. Debillon T, Gras-Leguen C, Verielle V et al. Intrauterine infection induces periventricular white matter cell death in rabbits. *Pediatr Res* 2000; **47**: 736–42.
49. Yoon BH, Kim CJ, Romero R et al. Experimentally induced intrauterine infection causes fetal brain white matter lesions in rabbits. *Am J Obstet Gynecol* 1997; **177**: 797–802.
50. Gibbs RS, Davies JK, McDuffie RS Jr et al. Chronic intrauterine infection and inflammation in the preterm rabbit, despite antibiotic therapy. *Am J Obstet Gynecol* 2002; **186**: 234–9.
51. Ornoy A, Altshuler G. Maternal endotoxemia, fetal anomalies, and central nervous system damage: a rat model of a human problem. *Am J Obstet Gynecol* 1976; **124**: 196–204.
52. Cai Z, Pan ZL, Pang Y et al. Cytokine induction in fetal rat brains and brain injury in neonatal rats after maternal lipopolysaccharide administration. *Pediatr Res* 2000; **47**: 64–72.
53. Bell MJ, Hallenbeck JM. Effects of intrauterine inflammation on developing rat brain. *J Neurosci Res* 2002; **70**: 570–9.
54. Gilles FH, Leviton A, Kerr CS. Endotoxin leucoencephalopathy in the telencephalon of the newborn kitten. *J Neurol Sci* 1976; **27**: 183–91.
55. Young RSK, Yagel SK, Towfighi J. Systemic and neuropathologic effects of *E. coli* endotoxin in newborn dogs. *Pediatr Res* 1983; **17**: 349–53.
56. Bogdanski R, Blobner M, Becker I et al. Cerebral histopathology following portal venous infusion of bacteria in a chronic porcine model. *Anesthesiology* 2000; **93**: 793–804.
57. Duncan JR, Cock ML, Scheerlinck JP et al. White matter injury after repeated endotoxin exposure in the preterm ovine fetus. *Pediatr Res* 2002; **52**: 941–9.
58. Mallard C, Welin AK, Peebles D et al. White matter injury following systemic endotoxemia or asphyxia in the fetal sheep. *Neurochem Res* 2003; **28**: 215–23.
59. Lehnardt S, Lachance C, Patrizi S et al. The toll-like receptor TLR4 is necessary for lipopolysaccharide-induced oligodendrocyte injury in the CNS. *J Neurosci* 2002; **22**: 2478–86.
60. Tasaki K, Ruetzler CA, Ohtsuki T et al. Lipopolysaccharide pretreatment induces resistance against subsequent focal cerebral ischemic damage in spontaneously hypertensive rats. *Brain Res* 1997; **748**: 267–70.
61. Ahmed SH, He YY, Nassief A et al. Effects of lipopolysaccharide priming on acute ischemic brain injury. *Stroke* 2000; **31**: 193–9.
62. Eklind S, Mallard C, Leverin AL et al. Bacterial endotoxin sensitizes the immature brain to hypoxic-ischaemic injury. *Eur J Neurosci* 2001; **13**: 1101–6.
63. Coumans AB, Middelanis JS, Garnier Y et al. Intracisternal application of endotoxin enhances the susceptibility to subsequent hypoxic-ischemic brain damage in neonatal rats. *Pediatr Res* 2003; **53**: 770–5.
64. Hagberg H, Peebles D, Mallard C. Models of white matter injury: comparison of infectious, hypoxic-ischemic, and excitotoxic insults. *Ment Retard Dev Disabil Res Rev* 2002; **8**: 30–8.
65. Hagberg B, Hagberg G, Beckung E, Uvebrant P. Changing panorama of cerebral palsy in Sweden. VIII. Prevalence and origin in the birth year period 1991–94. *Acta Paediatr* 2001; **90**: 271–7.
66. Leviton A, Paneth N. White matter damage in preterm newborns – an epidemiologic perspective. *Early Hum Dev* 1990; **24**: 1–22.

67. Leviton A. Preterm birth and cerebral palsy: is tumor necrosis factor the missing link? *Dev Med Child Neurol* 1993; **35**: 553–8.
68. The collaborative perinatal project of the National Institute of Neurological and Communicative Disorders and Stroke. In: *The First Year of Life* (Hardy JB, Drage JS, Jackson EC, eds). Baltimore: John Hopkins University Press, 1979: 78–92.
69. Goldenberg RL, Hauth JC, Andrews WW. Intrauterine infection and preterm delivery. *N Engl J Med* 2000; **342**: 1500–7.
70. Gonçalves LF, Chaiworapongsa T, Romero R. Intrauterine infection and prematurity. *Ment Retard Dev Disabil Res Rev* 2002; **8**: 3–13.
71. Romero R, Mazor M, Tartakovsky B. Systemic administration of interleukin-1 induces preterm parturition in mice. *Am J Obstet Gynecol* 1991; **165**: 969–71.
72. Gravett MG, Witkin SS, Haluska GJ et al. An experimental model for intraamniotic infection and preterm labor in rhesus monkeys. *Am J Obstet Gynecol* 1994; **171**: 1660–7.
73. Dammann O, Leviton A. Maternal intrauterine infection, cytokines, and brain damage in the preterm newborn. *Pediatr Res* 1997; **42**: 1–8.
74. Dammann O, Durum S, Leviton A. Do white cells matter in white matter damage? *Trends Neurosci* 2001; **24**: 320–4.
75. Kadhim H, Sebire G. Immune mechanisms in the pathogenesis of cerebral palsy: implication of proinflammatory cytokines and T lymphocytes. *Eur J Paediatr Neurol* 2002; **6**: 139–42.
76. Du ZY, Li XY. Cytokine and nitric oxide production by rat microglia stimulated with lipopolysaccharides in vitro. *Zhongguo Yao Li Xue Bao* 1998; **19**: 257–60.
77. Sawada M, Suzumura A, Marunouchi T. Induction of functional interleukin-2 receptor in mouse microglia. *J Neurochem* 1995; **64**: 1973–9.
78. Mazarakis ND, Edwards AD, Mehmet H. Apoptosis in neural development and disease. *Arch Dis Child Fetal Neonatal Ed* 1997; **77**: F165–70.
79. Pang Y, Cai Z, Rhodes PG. Disturbance of oligodendrocyte development, hypomyelination and white matter injury in the neonatal rat brain after intracerebral injection of lipopolysaccharide. *Brain Res Dev Brain Res* 2003; **140**: 205–14.
80. Leviton, A Gilles F. Ventriculomegaly, delayed myelination, white matter hypoplasia, and 'periventricular' leukomalacia: how are they related? *Pediatr Neurol* 1996; **15**: 127–36.
81. Rezaie P, Dean A. Periventricular leukomalacia, inflammation and white matter lesions within the developing nervous system. *Neuropathology* 2002; **22**: 106–32.
82. Danton GH, Dietrich WD. Inflammatory mechanisms after ischemia and stroke. *J Neuropathol Exp Neurol* 2003; **62**: 127–36.
83. Leviton A et al. Adult stroke and perinatal brain damage: like grandparent, like grandchild? *Neuropediatrics* 2002; **33**: 281–7.
84. Dammann O, Leviton A. Brain damage in preterm newborns: might enhancement of developmentally-regulated endogenous protection open a door for prevention? *Pediatrics* 1999; **104**: 541–50.
85. Dammann O, Leviton A. Brain damage in preterm newborns: biologic response modification as a strategy to reduce disabilities. *J Pediatr* 2000; **136**: 433–8.
86. Dammann O, Leviton A. Possible strategies to protect the preterm brain against the fetal inflammatory response. *Dev Med Child Neurol Suppl* 2001; **86**: 20–2.

24

Mumps virus and CNS disease

Steven A Rubin and Mikhail Pletnikov

INTRODUCTION

Mumps is an acute, communicable viral disease that is transmitted by direct contact or via respiratory droplets. Mumps virus infection often results in viremia with dissemination of virus to a number of organ systems, including the central nervous system (CNS), producing a variety of acute inflammatory reactions. Mumps morbidity has affected populations worldwide for thousands of years. The contagious epidemic illness was described by Hippocrates in the 5th century BC in his *Book of Epidemics* wherein a number of clinical manifestations were depicted; however it wasn't until 1790 that central nervous system (CNS) involvement was recognized in association with mumps.[1] Later studies would prove mumps virus a highly neurotropic agent, invading the CNS in approximately 50% of cases.[2] In fact, in the pre-vaccine modern day era, mumps virus was recognized as the leading cause of virus-induced aseptic meningitis and encephalitis in North America and Europe. Mumps virus continues to be one of the most frequent viral etiologies of acute childhood encephalitis in countries lacking high vaccine coverage.[3] Although usually benign and self-limited, mumps virus infection of the CNS can lead to permanent neurological damage.

VIRUS PROPERTIES

Mumps virus is a member of the *Paramyxoviridae* family, subfamily *Paramyxovirinae*, genus *Rubulavirus*. The virus consists of a helical ribonucleocapsid core surrounded by a host cell-derived lipid envelope and ranges in size from 100 to 600 nm. The virus genome is a nonsegmented, single-stranded RNA macromolecule of negative polarity containing 15,384 nucleotides. The gene order is 3′ N-P-M-F-SH-HN-L 5′ representing the genes for the nucleoprotein, phosphoprotein, matrix protein, fusion protein, small hydrophobic protein, hemagglutinin-neuraminidase protein, and polymerase, respectively.[4] Each gene is translated into a single protein except for the P gene from which mRNAs are transcribed encoding the phosphoprotein and two non-structural proteins, V and I.[5,6] The N, P, and L proteins associate with the viral RNA genome forming the ribonucleocapsid, of which the L protein is the RNA-dependant RNA polymerase.[7–9] Surrounding the ribonucleocapsid and forming the luminal side of the viral envelope is the M protein, which is believed to be responsible for the alignment of the ribonucleocapsid during virus assembly.[10] The F and HN glycoproteins are present on the outer surface of the viral host-derived envelope. The F glycoprotein is responsible for fusion of viral and cellular membranes whereas the HN glycoprotein promotes viral attachment to and release from its cellular receptor, N-acetyl neuraminic acid (sialic acid).[11,12] The functions of the SH, V, and I proteins are less clear. The SH protein has only been identified in infected cells and may or may not be present in the intact virion.[13] The V and I proteins are, by inference from other members of the *Paramyxoviridae* family, probably involved in the regulation of gene transcription and translation.[14,15]

The replicative cycle of paramyxoviruses has been described in detail.[16] Replication begins with the binding and fusion of the viral and host cell lipid membranes, allowing the viral ribonucleocapsid to enter the host cell cytoplasm. Here, the genomic viral RNA is transcribed by the viral RNA-dependent RNA polymerase into monocistronic mRNAs, which are translated by the host cell. As intracellular levels of viral proteins reach a threshold, the activity of the viral polymerase switches to synthesizing full-length antisense genomic RNA, which is transcribed into negative sense progeny RNA. Virion assembly begins in the cell cytoplasm with the binding of the N proteins to the genomic RNA followed by the binding of the P and L protein complex.[17] This encapsidation process is believed to be initiated by specific leader and trailer sequences of the viral genome.[18] The ribonucleocapsid is then brought to the cellular cytoplasmic membrane, an event presumably mediated by the M protein,[10] whereby the virion picks up its lipid envelope containing the HN and F viral glycoproteins as it exits the cell, usually resulting in cell lysis.

TRANSMISSION AND EPIDEMIOLOGY

Humans are the only natural host for mumps virus infection; there is no known animal reservoir. Mumps virus is transmitted by oropharyngeal secretions via direct contact, respiratory droplet, or fomites entering the nose or mouth. Primary replication occurs in the nasal mucosa or upper respiratory mucosal epithelium. Often, a transient plasma viremia can develop allowing the virus to disseminate throughout the body, including the CNS, resulting in a wide variety of inflammatory reactions and complications (Box 24.1).[19] The development of viremia probably accounts for the two- to four-week incubation period prior to presentation of clinical symptoms. Notably, mumps virus can infect T-lymphocytes, which may allow the virus to spread despite rapid development of a humoral immune response.[20–22] The virus is shed in the saliva over a period spanning three to five days before and after the appearance of clinical symptoms. The virus can also be present in breast milk and urine, although transmission via these routes has not been established.

Mumps is endemic worldwide with outbreaks occurring every two to five years in unvaccinated populations.[23,24] Although highly transmissible, mumps is less contagious than measles or varicella, with secondary attack rates of approximately 30%.[25] Historically, mumps was most commonly seen in winter months and the highest incidence rates were reported between five and nine years of age. However, within the past decade there has been a gradual shift in the typical age of infection towards the 10- to 19-year-old group and seasonality is no longer evident.[26,27]

The most frequent clinical manifestation of mumps is parotitis, occurring in approximately 95% of all

---

Box 24.1 Symptoms and complications of mumps reported in the medical literature[19]

Albuminuria	Hemiplegia		Papilledema
Appendicitis	Hepatitis		Parotitis
Arthritis	Hydrocephalus		Pericarditis
Ataxia	Hypertension		Phlebitis
Basophilism	Keratitis		Pleurisy
Blindness	Labyrinthitis		Pneumonia
Cerebellitis	Landry's paralysis		Polyneuritis
Cerebral diplegia	Laryngeal edema		Presternal edema
Choreo-athetosis	Mastitis		Prostatitis
Choroiditis	Meningitis		Pulmonary infarction
Coma	Mental disorder		Retinitis
Congenital defects/fetal death	Mesencephalic syndrome		Scleritis
Deafness	Myelitis/neuromyelitis		Serositis
Diabetes mellitus	Myocarditis		Sialadenitis
Encephalitis	Nephritis		Subarachnoid hemorrhage
Endocardial fibroelastosis	Ocular paralysis		Sublinguitis
Endocarditis	Oophoritis		Submandibular adenitis
Epididymo-orchitis	Optic atrophy		Thrombocytopenia purpura
Facial paralysis	Optic neuritis		Thyroiditis
Glaucoma	Orchitis		Uveitis
Guillain-Barre syndrome	Pancreatitis		

symptomatic cases. While parotitis typically precedes other clinical manifestations, parotid involvement is not an obligatory step in the infection, thus involvement of other tissues and organs can occur in the total absence of detectable salivary gland swelling. Serious mumps morbidity is primarily due to complications of meningitis and encephalitis. The case fatality rate for mumps is between 1.6 and 3.8 per 10,000.[28] Prior to widespread vaccine use, mumps virus accounted for up to half of all reported encephalitis cases in unvaccinated populations.[29] Following the licensure of a live virus mumps vaccine in 1967, the number of cases of mumps in the United States decreased by more than 99%.[30]

Considering the high vaccine coverage, unexpectedly numerous cases of mumps have been reported in vaccinated subjects. While in some cases this can be attributed to primary or secondary vaccine failure, in others, insufficient attenuation of the vaccine and retention of virus virulence has been cited.[31-34] Consequently, there is now a greater focus on the safety of the vaccine itself. One of the most serious vaccine-related adverse events is aseptic meningitis. The risk for aseptic meningitis varies by vaccine strain. While no increased risk for meningitis was found following vaccination with the Jeryl Lynn strain, the only mumps vaccine strain used in the USA, the risk associated with the Urabe-AM9 or Hoshino vaccine strains ranged from 15.6–38.1 and greater risks were associated with the Leningrad-3 strain.[35-37] While use of higher-risk vaccine strains has been discontinued in most developed countries and replaced with the Jeryl Lynn strain, other countries continue to use these vaccines due to their lower costs, citing risk/benefit ratios.[38-41]

CNS DISEASE AND PATHOGENESIS

The CNS is a frequent target of mumps virus following viremia in humans. The mechanism by which the virus invades the human CNS has been inferred from animal studies. Following intraperitoneal or intravenous inoculation of laboratory animals, a transient viremia develops allowing for virus entry into the choroid plexus, infecting choroidal and ventricular ependymal cells (Figure 24.1a and 24.1b).[22,42] This then serves as a potential source for further viral spread in the brain, leading to a variety of neuropathological outcomes including meningitis, encephalitis, and hydrocephalus.[42-44] Not only are these complications of mumps virus infection known in humans,[45-48] but in some animal models the severity of the neuropathological outcomes has been shown to correlate with the known human neurovirulence potential of the mumps virus strains used,[42,49] demonstrating the value of animal models in studying mumps virus pathogenesis.

Notably, the majority of cases of mumps virus infection of the CNS are asymptomatic, demonstrable

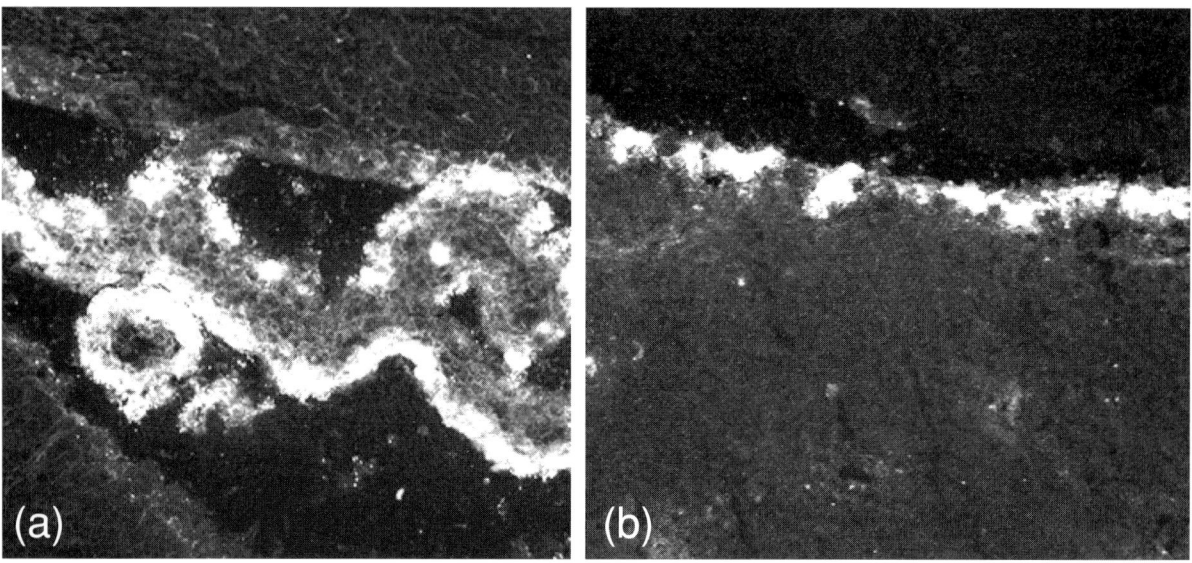

Figure 24.1 Mumps virus antigen expression in (a) the choroid plexus and (b) ependymal cell lining of the lateral ventricle in a four-day-old rat inoculated with mumps virus at birth.

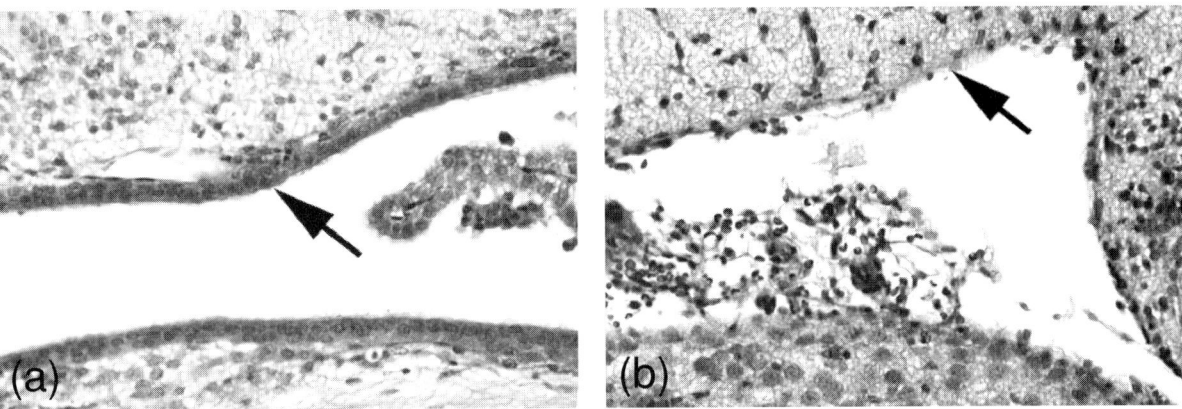

Figure 24.2 Hematoxylin and eosin stained sagittal sections of rat brain. Arrow shows (a) presence of ependymal cells lining the ventricle in the uninfected rat whereas (b) the ventricle in the infected rat brain is virtually stripped of these cells.

only by the finding of cerebrospinal fluid (CSF) pleocytosis.[2,50,51] Of the neurological manifestations of mumps in humans, meningitis is the most common, diagnosed in approximately one in 10 cases[2,48,52] Mumps meningitis is generally a benign condition with complete recovery in three to four days. Encephalitis, on the other hand, is a serious but more rare complication, occurring in 2.6 per 1000 cases with a mortality of 1.4%.[53-54] There are two pathological mechanisms of mumps encephalitis, one resulting from direct viral invasion, and the other an immune-mediated inflammatory disease involving demyelination of the white matter of the CNS (i.e., postinfectious encephalitis). Of these, the latter mechanism appears to be more frequent. Clinical features of encephalitis include ataxia, paresis, paralysis of one or more limbs, spasticity, cranial nerve palsies, personality changes, impaired consciousness, coma, and respiratory failure.[25,45,55-58] Despite the severity of symptoms, the prognosis for complete recovery is excellent, usually resolving over a period of one to two weeks. Changes typical of encephalitis have been reported upon autopsy and include edema and congestion throughout the brain with hemorrhages, lymphocytic infiltration, perivascular gliosis, and demyelination. Findings in the spinal cord include early degenerative changes in the anterior horn cells and perineuronal edema.[57]

Hydrocephalus is a rare complication in humans and the precise cause is not well understood. Animal studies suggest that damage to and loss of virus-infected ventricular ependymal cells (Figure 24.2) leads to accumulation of debris blocking egress of CSF through the aqueduct of Sylvius, resulting in the development of hydrocephalus (Figure 24.3).[59-61] A similar mechanism is believed to be responsible for mumps virus hydrocephalus in humans.[46,48] Indeed, ependymal cell debris has been found in the CSF of humans presenting with mumps virus CNS infection.[62] However, hydrocephalus has also been observed prior to, or in the total absence of, aqueductal stenosis,[63-66] suggesting that stenosis of the aqueduct could be a secondary consequence of external compression by surrounding edematous tissue in already hydrocephalic animals and not causally related to the pathogenesis of hydrocephalus.

Other rare neurological manifestations of mumps virus infection of the CNS include cerebellar ataxia,[67] transverse myelitis,[68,69] and Guillain-Barre syndrome.[70] The most frequent permanent neurological deficit associated with virus CNS invasion is unilateral deafness. Deafness is believed to be the result of direct damage to the cochlea and cochlea neurons, which become infected by the perilymph, which freely communicates with the CSF.[71-74] Although typically seen in patients presenting with encephalitis, there is no known etiological association between encephalitis and deafness.[72]

NEUROLOGICAL DEFICITS

The overwhelming majority of reports of behavioral changes associated with mumps virus infection, including personality changes, emotional lability, aggressiveness, impaired consciousness, delirium, irritability, convulsions, ataxia, and so on, are associated with development of encephalitis.[26,45,55-58] These

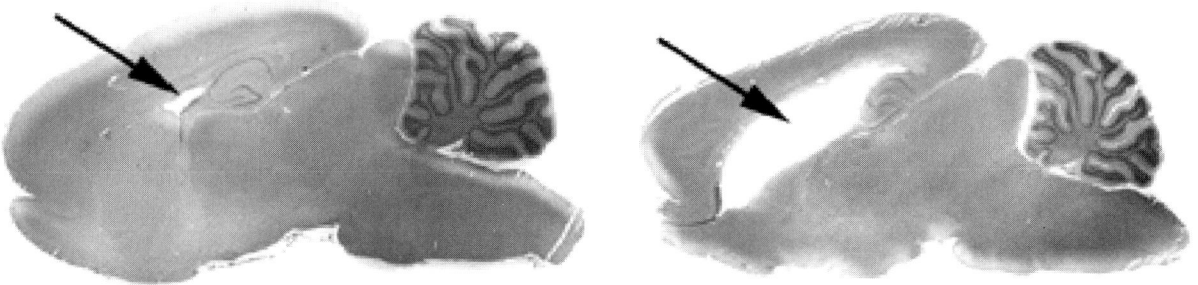

Figure 24.3 Midline sagittal section through uninfected (left) and mumps virus infected (right) rat brain. Note enlarged lateral ventricle (hydrocephalus) in the mumps virus-infected rat.

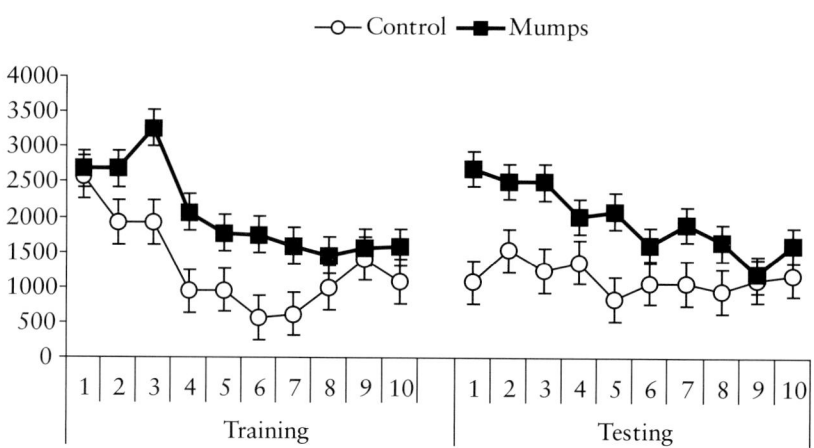

Figure 24.4 Effects of neonatal mumps infection on habituation of the acoustic startle response in 90-day-old rats. Rats were tested in an acoustic startle chamber (San Diego Instruments, San Diego, CA) following a standard three-day procedure. The first day consisted of an acclimatization period where rats were placed in the startle chamber for five minutes with no presentation of background noise or startle stimuli. A training session (left panel) was performed on the second day wherein the acclimatization period was repeated but was then immediately followed by 10 consecutive presentations of startle stimuli (108 dB) separated by 15-second intervening periods of background noise (65dB) (x axis). Upon completion of the training session, rats were returned to their home cage. The testing session (right panel) was performed on the third day and consisted of a repetition of the training session. The amplitudes of the rats' startle responses were recorded and mean startle amplitudes for control (open circles) and mumps-infected animals (solid squares) are presented. Compared to control rats, mumps-infected animals exhibited significantly greater startle responses throughout the training and testing sessions, suggesting increased sensitization to the startle response. Although presentations of startle stimuli led to the within-session habituation of the startle response in the both groups, only the control animals demonstrated the phenomenon of long-term habituation of the startle response, as indicated by comparing the amplitude of the startle response on the first presentation during the training session to that during the testing session. In contrast, the mumps-infected rats responded similarly to the first startle stimuli during both sessions, indicating lack of long-term habituation of the startle response.

manifestations are usually transient and upon resolution of encephalitis, behaviors typically return to normal. However, there is evidence for chronic mumps virus CNS infection, which has been associated with encephalitis sequelae including mental deterioration and other neurological deficits.[3,75-77] It is important to note, however, that diagnoses of chronic mumps virus CNS infection are based on persistent CSF pleocytosis and intrathecal antibody synthesis.[76,78-80] While this may suggest continued antigenic stimulation by a persistent mumps infection, prolonged CSF pleocytosis and intrathecal synthesis of antibody to mumps virus have also been found in cases where there is otherwise no indication of an ongoing infection.[80,81] Thus, in the absence of immunocytopathologic and virologic studies, it is not clear whether mumps virus can persistently infect the CNS and lead to lasting neuropsychiatric abnormalities.

Animal studies, on the other hand, have clearly implicated mumps as an etiologic agent of permanent neurobehavioral deficits. In rats inoculated intracranially with neurovirulent mumps virus strains, sensitization of the startle response and impaired long-term habituation of the startle response are evident (Figure 24.4). These abnormalities are reflective of either anxiety or of learning and memory deficits, both of which could be related to hydrocephalus-associated hippocampal damage. The exact mechanisms are yet to be elucidated.

REFERENCES

1. Hamilton R. An account of a distemper by the common people of England vulgarly called the mumps. *London Med J* 1790; **11**: 190–211.
2. Bang HO, Bang J. Involvement of the central nervous system in mumps. *Acta Med Scand* 1943; **113**: 487–505.
3. Aygun AD, Kabakus N, Celik I et al. Long-term neurological outcome of acute encephalitis. *J Trop Pediatr* 2001; **47**: 243–7.
4. Elango N, Varsanyi TM, Kovamees J, Norrby E. Molecular cloning and characterization of six genes, determination of gene order and intergenic sequences and leader sequence of mumps virus. *J Gen Virol* 1988; **69**: 2893–900.
5. Elliott GD, Yeo RP, Afzal MA et al. Strain-variable editing during transcription of the P gene of mumps virus may lead to the generation of non-structural proteins NS1 (V) and NS2. *J Gen Virol* 1990; **71**: 1555–60.
6. Paterson RG, Lamb RA. RNA editing by G-nucleotide insertion in mumps virus P-gene mRNA transcripts. *J Virol* 1990; **64**: 4137–45.
7. McCarthy M, Johnson RT. A comparison of the structural polypeptides of five strains of mumps virus. *J Gen Virol* 1980; **46**: 15–27.
8. Okazaki K, Tanabayashi K, Takeuchi K et al. Molecular cloning and sequence analysis of the mumps virus gene encoding the L protein and the trailer sequence. *Virology* 1992; **188**: 926–30.
9. Orvell C. Structural polypeptides of mumps virus. *J Gen Virol* 1978; **41**: 527–39.
10. Matsumoto T. Assembly of paramyxoviruses. *Microbiol Immunol* 1982; **26**: 285–320.
11. Jensik SC, Silver S. Polypeptides of mumps virus. *J Virol* 1976; **17**: 363–73.
12. Orvell C. Immunological properties of purified mumps virus glycoproteins. *J Gen Virol* 1978; **41**: 517–26.
13. Takeuchi K, Tanabayashi K, Hishiyama M, Yamada A. The mumps virus SH protein is a membrane protein and not essential for virus growth. *Virology* 1996; **225**: 156–62.
14. Curran J, Marq JB, Kolakofsky D. The Sendai virus nonstructural C proteins specifically inhibit viral mRNA synthesis. *Virology* 1992; **189**: 647–56.
15. Horikami SM, Hector RE, Smallwood S, Moyer SA. The Sendai virus C protein binds the L polymerase protein to inhibit viral RNA synthesis. *Virology* 1997; **235**: 261–70.
16. Lamb RA, Kolakofsky D. Paramyxoviridae: the viruses and their replication. In: *Fields Virology* (Knipe DM, Howley PM, eds). Philadelphia: Lippincott Williams and Wilkins, 2001: 1305–40.
17. Kingsbury DW, Hsu CH, Murti KG. Intracellular metabolism of sendai virus nucleocapside. *Virology* 1978; **91**: 86–94.
18. Blumberg BM, Kolakofsky D. Intracellular vesicular stomatitis virus leader RNAs are found in nucleocapsid structures. *J Virol* 1981; **40**: 568–76.
19. Hyatt HW. Complications of mumps. *G P* 1962; **25**: 124–6.
20. Fleischer B, Kreth HW. Mumps virus replication in human lymphoid cell lines and in peripheral blood lymphocytes: preference for T cells. *Infect Immun* 1982; **35**: 25–31.
21. Ukkonen P, Granstrom ML, Penttinen K. Mumps-specific immunoglobulin M and G antibodies in natural mumps infection as measured by enzyme-linked immunosorbent assay. *J Med Virol* 1981; **8**: 131–42.
22. Wolinsky JS, Klassen T, Baringer JR. Persistance of neuroadapted mumps virus in brains of newborn hamsters after intraperitoneal inoculation. *J Infect Dis* 1976; **133**: 260–7.
23. Centers for Disease Control and Prevention. Mumps surveillance 1973. *Morbid Mortal Weekly Rep* 1974; **23**: 431.
24. Centers for Disease Control and Prevention. Summary of notifiable diseases, United States, 1991. *Morbid Mortal Weekly Rep* 1991; **40**: 3.
25. Hope-Simpson RE. Infectiousness of communicable diseases in the household (measles, chickenpox, and mumps). *Lancet* 1952; **2**: 549–54.
26. Centers for Disease Control and Prevention. Summary of notifiable diseases, United States, 1996. *Morbid Mortal Weekly Report* 1996; **45**: 1–88.
27. van Loon FPL, Holmes SJ, Sirotkin BI et al. Mumps surveillance – United States, 1988–1993. *Morbid Mortal Weekly Rep* 1995; **44**: 1–14.
28. Centers for Disease Control and Prevention. Mumps surveillance report. *Morbid Mortal Weekly Rep* 1972; **21**: 1–12.
29. Centers for Disease Control and Prevention. Mumps – United States. *Morbid Mortal Weekly Rep* 1978; **27**: 379–81.
30. Centers for Disease Control and Prevention. Summary of notifiable diseases, United States, 1998. *Morbid Mortal Weekly Rep* 1999; **47**: ii–92.
31. Colville A, Pugh S, Miller E. Withdrawal of a mumps vaccine. *Eur J Pediatr* 1994; **153**: 467–8.
32. da Cunha SS, Rodrigues LC, Barreto ML, Dourado I. Outbreak of aseptic meningitis and mumps after mass vaccination with MMR vaccine using the Leningrad-Zagreb mumps strain. *Vaccine* 2002; **20**: 1106–12.
33. Dourado I, Cunha S, Teixeira MG et al. Outbreak of aseptic meningitis associated with mass vaccination with a urabe-containing measles-mumps-rubella vaccine: implications for immunization programs. *Am J Epidemiol* 2000; **151**: 524–30.
34. Furesz J. Safety of live mumps virus vaccines. *J Med Virol* 2002; **67**: 299–300.

35. Cizman M, Mozetic M, Radescek-Rakar R et al. Aseptic meningitis after vaccination against measles and mumps. *Pediatr Infect Dis J* 1989; **8**: 302–8.
36. Farrington P, Pugh S, Colville A et al. A new method for active surveillance of adverse events from diphtheria/tetanus/pertussis and measles/mumps/rubella vaccines. *Lancet* 1995; **345**: 567–9.
37. Ki M, Park T, Yi SG et al. Risk analysis of aseptic meningitis after measles-mumps-rubella vaccination in Korean children by using a case-crossover design. *Am J Epidemiol* 2003; **157**: 158–65.
38. da Silveira CM, Kmetzsch CI, Mohrdieck R et al. The risk of aseptic meningitis associated with the Leningrad-Zagreb mumps vaccine strain following mass vaccination with measles-mumps-rubella vaccine, Rio Grande do Sul, Brazil, 1997. *Int J Epidemiol* 2002; **31**: 978–82.
39. Fullerton KE, Reef SE. Commentary: ongoing debate over the safety of the different mumps vaccine strains impacts mumps disease control. *Int J Epidemiol* 2002; **31**: 983–4.
40. Galazka AM, Robertson SE, Kraigher A. Mumps and mumps vaccine: a global review. *Bull World Health Organ* 1999; **77**: 3–14.
41. Ueda K, Miyazaki C, Hidaka Y et al. Aseptic meningitis caused by measles-mumps-rubella vaccine in Japan. *Lancet* 1995; **346**: 701–2.
42. Saika S, Kidokoro M, Ohkawa T et al. Pathogenicity of mumps virus in the marmoset. *J Med Virol* 2002; **66**: 115–22.
43. Johnson RT. Mumps virus encephalitis in the hamster: studies of the inflammatory response and neuropathic infection of neurons. *J Neuropathol Exp Neurol* 1968; **27**: 80–95.
44. Rubin SA, Pletnikov M, Carbone KM. Comparison of the neurovirulence of a vaccine and a wild-type mumps virus strain in the developing rat brain. *J Virol* 1998; **72**: 8037–42.
45. Koskiniemi M, Donner M, Pettay O. Clinical appearance and outcome in mumps encephalitis in children. *Acta Paediatr Scand* 1983; **72**: 603–9.
46. Ogata H, Oka K, Mitsudome A. Hydrocephalus due to acute aqueductal stenosis following mumps infection: report of a case and review of the literature. *Brain Dev* 1992; **14**: 417–9.
47. Russell RR, Donald JC. The neurological complications of mumps. *BMJ* 1958; **2**: 27–35.
48. Timmons GD, Johnson KP. Aqueductal stenosis and hydrocephalus after mumps encephalitis. *N Eng J Med* 1970; **283**: 1505–7.
49. Rubin SA, Pletnikov M, Taffs R et al. Evaluation of a neonatal rat model for prediction of mumps virus neurovirulence in humans. *J Virol* 2000; **74**: 5382–4.
50. Brown JW, Kirkland HB, Hein GE. Central nervous system involvement during mumps. *Am J Med Sci* 1948; **215**: 434–41.
51. Finkelstein H. Meningo-encephalitis in mumps. *JAMA* 1938; **3**: 17–9.
52. Immunization Practices Advisory Committee. Mumps prevention. *Morbid Mortal Weekly Rep* 1989; **38**: 397–400.
53. Baum SG, Litman N. Mumps virus. In: *Principles and Practise of Infectious Diseases* (Mandell GL, Douglas RG, Bennett JE, eds). Philadelphia: Churchill Livingstone, 2000: 1776–81.
54. Modlin JF, Orenstein WA, Brandling-Bennett AD. Current status of mumps in the United States. *J Infect Dis* 1975; **132**: 106–9.
55. Koyama S, Morita K, Yamaguchi S et al. An adult case of mumps brain stem encephalitis. *Internal Med* 2000; **39**: 499–502.
56. Leonberg SC. Nervous system affections caused by the mumps virus. *Neurol Neurocir Psiquiatr* 1977; **18**: 485–93.
57. Miller HG, Stanton JB, Gibbons JL. Para-infectious encephalomyelitis and related syndromes. A critical review of the neurological complications of certain specific fevers. *Quart J Med* 1956; **25**: 427–505.
58. Nussinovitch M, Volovitz B, Varasano I. Complications of mumps requiring hospitalization in children. *Eur J Pediatr* 1995; **154**: 732–4.
59. Johnson RT, Johnson KP, Edmonds CJ. Virus-induced hydrocephalus: development of aqueductal stenosis in hamsters after mumps infection. *Science* 1967; **157**: 1066–7.
60. Johnson RT, Johnson KP. Hydrocephalus following viral infection: the pathology of aqueductal stenosis developing after experimental mumps virus infection. *J Neuropathol Exp Neurol* 1968; **27**: 591–606.
61. Johnson RT, Johnson KP. Hydrocephalus as a sequela of experimental myxovirus infections. *Exp Mol Pathol* 1969; **10**: 68–80.
62. Herndon RM, Johnson RT, Davis LE, Descalzi LR. Ependymitis in mumps virus meningitis: electron microscopical studies of cerebrospinal fluid. *Arch Neurol* 1974; **30**: 475–9.
63. Johnson KP, Johnson RT. Granular ependymitis: occurrence in myxovirus infected rodents and prevalence in man. *Am J Path* 1972; **67**: 511–26.
64. Takano T, Mekata Y, Yamano T, Shimada M. Early ependymal changes in experimental hydrocephalus after mumps virus inoculation in hamsters. *Acta Neuropathol* 1993; **85**: 521–5.
65. Takano T, Takikita S, Shimada M. Experimental mumps virus-induced hydrocephalus: viral neurotropism and neuronal maturity. *NeuroReport* 1999; **10**: 2215–21.
66. Wolinsky JS, Baringer JR, Margolis G, Kilham L. Ultrstructure of mumps virus replication in newborn hamster central nervous system. *Lab Investig* 1974; **31**: 403–12.
67. Cohen HA, Ashkenazi A, Nussinovitch M et al. Mumps-associated acute cerebellar ataxia. *Am J Dis Child* 1992; **146**: 930–1.
68. Nussinovitch M, Brand N, Frydman M, Varsano I. Transverse myelitis following mumps in children. *Acta Paediatr* 1992; **81**: 183–4.
69. Venketasubramanian N. Transverse myelitis following mumps in an adult – a case report with MRI correlation. *Acta Neurol Scand* 1997; **96**: 328–30.
70. Ghosh S. Guillain-Barre syndrome complicating mumps. *Lancet* 1967; **1**: 895.
71. Hall R, Richards H. Hearing loss due to mumps. *Arch Dis Child* 1987; **62**: 189–91.
72. McKenna M. Measles, mumps, and sensorineural hearing loss. *Ann NY Acad Sci* 1997; **830**: 291–8.
73. Smith GA, Guessen R. Inner ear pathologic features following mumps infection. *Arch Otolaryngal* 1976; **102**: 108–11.
74. Westmore GA, Pickard BH, Stern H. Isolation of mumps virus from the inner ear after sudden deafness. *BMJ* 1979; **1**: 14–5.
75. Ito M, Go T, Okuno T, Mikawa H. Chronic mumps virus encephalitis. *Pediatr Neurol* 1991; **7**: 467–70.
76. Julkunen I, Lehtokoski-Lehtiniemi E, Koskiniemi M, Vaheri A. Elevated mumps antibody titers in the cerebrospinal fluid suggesting chronic mumps virus infection in the central nervous system. *Pediatr Infect Dis* 1985; **4**: 99.
77. Vaheri A, Kabakus N, Koskiniemi M. Chronic encephalomyelitis with specific intrathecal mumps antibodies. *Lancet* 1982; **2**: 685–8.
78. Fryden A, Link H, Moller E. Demonstration of CSF lymphocytes sensitized against mumps virus antigens in mumps meningitis. *Acta Neurol Scand* 1978; **57**: 396–404.
79. Link H, Laurenzi MA, Fryden A. Viral antibodies in oligoclonal and polyclonal IgG synthesized within the central nervous system over the course of mumps meningitis. *J Neuroimmunol* 1981; **1**: 287–98.
80. Vandvik B, Norrby E, Steen-Johnson J, Stensvold K. Mumps meningitis: prolonged pleocytosis and occurrence of mumps virus-specific oligoclonal IgG in the cerebrospinal fluid. *Eur Neurol* 1978; **17**: 13–22.
81. Vandvik B, Nilsen RE, Vartdal F, Norrby E. Mumps meningitis: specific and non-specific antibody responses in the central nervous system. *Acta Neurol Scand* 1982; **65**: 468–87.

25

Chlamydia pneumoniae as a potential etiologic agent in sporadic Alzheimer's disease

Hérve C Gérard, Kristin L Wildt, Ute Dreses-Werringloer, Judith A Whittum-Hudson, and Alan P Hudson

INTRODUCTION

Alzheimer's disease (AD) is a neurodegenerative disorder that currently affects more than four million people in the United States and perhaps 15 million individuals worldwide.[1,2] The disease is associated with atrophy/death of neurons in specific brain regions and occurs in two forms: an early-onset form that is primarily genetically determined, and a far more common late-onset form that is not. In its early stages, the disease manifests itself in the form of minor memory loss and progresses to major cognitive dysfunction. This latter may take the form of behavioral disorders, loss of orientation, language difficulties, and/or other attributes.[3,4] The rate of progression to cognitive dysfunction varies among affected individuals but can be two decades or more; death in late-onset AD patients occurs from secondary causes, not from the disease itself. The incidence of sporadic AD increases with increasing age, and it is currently thought to be the most significant single cause of senile dementia.[1,5] Indeed, as many as half the total cases of dementia in the elderly may be attributable to AD. Essentially the only risk factor identified and generally accepted as valid for late-onset disease is possession of the *APOE* ε4 allele on chromosome 19, although how this gene product engenders the neuropathology characteristic of AD is poorly understood at present.[6] Not all patients expressing the ε4 allele develop AD, but its presence appears to increase risk for the disease; the allele is also associated with earlier disease onset and rapid progression to cognitive dysfunction.

The etiology underlying the well-described neuropathology observed in AD patients is not well understood. Neuritic senile plaques (NSP) are comprised of deposits of β-amyloid peptide (Aβ), and these appear to be critical in neuronal degeneration.[3,7] Indeed, the dominant hypothesis guiding Alzheimer's research focuses specifically on the role of NSP in disease genesis,[8,9] although some authors have recently questioned the general utility of the so-called 'amyloid cascade hypothesis' as a paradigm for the field.[10] In the early-onset, familial form of the disease, mutations in the amyloid precursor protein gene (*βAPP*) are associated with increased Aβ deposition and early onset of symptoms.[11] Mutations in the genes encoding presenilin-1 (*PS-1*) and presenilin-2 (*PS-2*) also lead to increased Aβ deposition in early-onset patients.[7] However, the similar neuropathology observed in late-onset disease cannot be attributed to these or other known mutations. Neurofibrillary tangles (NFT) also appear to be important in the neuropathogenesis of AD, and these are comprised of modified tau protein. This protein is a standard component of the neuronal cytoskeleton, and data indicate that its abnormal deposition in NFT results from various aberrant post-translational modifications of the protein.[12,13]

The neuropathologies characteristic of both early- and late-onset AD are similar but, as indicated above, the processes initiating that pathology remain to be elucidated for late-onset disease.[14] Neurologic diseases, of course, can be caused by infectious agents, and infection with organisms that do not target the nervous system specifically can and often do engender neuropathologic effects.[15,16] In light of this, a number of groups have investigated potential associations between various viruses and late-onset AD, but none has been generally accepted. Measles virus, lentiviruses, adenovirus, and several others have been studied and dismissed as agents associated with the disease.[17,18] Interestingly, recent studies have identified *Herpes simplex* virus type 1 (HSV-1) infection as a risk factor for development of AD in people expressing *APOE* ε4.[19,20] A number of bacterial species have also been investigated and dismissed, including *Chlamydia trachomatis* and *Coxiella burnettii*.[21] Prions and other unconventional agents have been considered, as have the potential influences of factors such as diet and acute or extended exposure to aluminum in disease genesis, but no relationship has been established or agreed upon. However, one recent report argued that these or other environmental factors may potentiate the brain inflammation that is characteristic of sporadic AD.[22] Several years ago, we described a potential relationship between infection with the bacterial pathogen *Chlamydia pneumoniae* and the genesis of late-onset disease.[23] In this chapter, we review currently available data regarding that association.

CHLAMYDIA PNEUMONIAE

Chlamydia pneumoniae is an obligate intracellular bacterial pathogen of the respiratory tract, and initial acquisition of the organism thus occurs via the oral and nasal mucosa.[24,25] *C. pneumoniae* is an important etiologic agent in acute respiratory infections, including community-acquired pneumonia, sinusitis, and bronchitis. Moreover, a number of studies have implicated infection with this organism in more severe, chronic pulmonary pathologies, including sarcoidosis and chronic obstructive pulmonary disease.[25–28] Epidemiologic analyses have demonstrated that the prevalence of infection with *C. pneumoniae* is high in essentially all adult populations studied, and that it increases with increasing age.[27,29,30] In developed nations where population densities are usually relatively low, children under the age of five to 10 rarely show anti-*C. pneumoniae* antibodies, but incidence rises sharply thereafter. In crowded conditions, childhood infection with *C. pneumoniae* is more common than in less densely populated regions.[31] Serum antibody titers against *C. pneumoniae* peak in the sixth to seventh decades in most population groups examined; for example, in one study in Seattle males 60 years and older showed a prevalence rate of 70%.[27,31] Virtually all studies indicate that most individuals are infected with *C. pneumoniae* during their lifetime, and that multiple re-infections are common.

Over the last decade, infection with *C. pneumoniae* has been implicated in a large number of unexpected nonpulmonary clinical entities, including atherosclerosis, inflammatory arthritis, giant cell (temporal) arteritis, and others.[32–36] In relation to atherosclerosis, elegant *in vitro* studies have demonstrated that *C. pneumoniae* infection of monocytes induces foam cell formation and accumulation of cholesteryl esters if LDL is present in the growth medium,[37] providing a biochemical mechanism supporting a direct role for the organism in atherogenesis. Moreover, a correlation exists between serum anti-*C. pneumoniae* antibody titers and coronary artery disease; the bacterium has been identified by several methods in atheromatous plaques.[38] In all anatomic contexts infection with any chlamydial species, including *Chlamydia pneumoniae*, is always associated with a strong inflammatory reaction.[39–41] Importantly, infection with *Chlamydia pneumoniae* has been associated with diseases of the nervous system, most notably multiple sclerosis;[42,43] some reports have also indicated a relationship with cerebrovascular disease.[44,45] While these and other associations between infection with *Chlamydia pneumoniae* and various chronic diseases are highly controversial, they remain a focus of interest and active investigation.

C. PNEUMONIAE AND LATE-ONSET AD

The initial evidence for an association between *C. pneumoniae* and sporadic AD was derived from polymerase chain reaction (PCR)-based assays targeting chromosomal sequences of *C. pneumoniae* in DNA preparations from frozen brain autopsy tissues of 19 AD and 19 roughly age- and sex-matched non-AD control individuals.[23] Samples from hippocampus, temporal cortex, and other brain regions displaying characteristic neuropathology were PCR-positive for the organism in 17/19 AD patients in multiple repeated and independently-targeted assays, while only a single sample from an age-matched, non-AD control individual was weakly positive (but repeatable). More recently, frozen tissue samples from temporal cortex, hippocampus, and other brain regions from nine additional AD patients and several controls were screened; again, multiple PCR assays independently targeting several *C. pneumoniae* genes were all negative for control samples but positive for each of the AD patients (HCG, APH, unpublished observations). PCR screening assays have been extended to frozen brain tissue samples from patients with Parkinson's disease and additional non-AD controls. DNA samples from temporal cortex and hippocampus were assayed from three non-AD/non-Parkinson's control individuals, three patients with Parkinson's disease, and two patients with both Parkinson's and AD. In multiple PCR assays targeting the *C. pneumo-*

niae 16S rRNA gene, the gene encoding the major outer membrane protein (MOMP), and others, each control sample was negative, as were all samples from the Parkinson's patients; however, samples from the two patients with both Parkinson's and AD were PCR-positive for *C. pneumoniae* (HCG, APH, unpublished observations). Along the same lines, in our original study three non-AD control brain samples assessed by PCR for *C. pneumoniae* DNA were derived from patients with multiple sclerosis, and all were negative.[23] Thus, although the sample number assayed so far is somewhat limited, PCR-positivity for the organism appears to be specific to AD brain samples and not samples from normal individuals or those with other neurologic diseases. Moreover, the various samples analyzed to date using PCR-based methods were drawn from widely diverse geographic regions in the United States and Canada, indicating that the presence of *Chlamydia pneumoniae* in the AD brain is not specific to any one particular region.

In our initial studies, two monoclonal antibodies (mAb) were employed for immunohistochemical analyses of tissues from affected AD brain regions and congruent regions from non-AD control brains. These were a genus-specific mAb targeting the lipopolysaccharide (LPS) of *Chlamydiae* and a *C. pneumoniae*-specific anti-MOMP mAb. These studies gave staining in perivascular regions of small blood vessels, and in astroglia- and microglia-like cells not in the immediate vicinity of vessels; sections from non-AD control brain tissues showed no labeling at all. These non-neuronal cell types were confirmed to be host cells harboring *C. pneumoniae* via double immunolabeling, using the antichlamydial LPS mAb and an antiglial fibrillary acidic protein mAb for astroglia; an anti-inducible nitric oxide synthase (iNOS) Ab in combination with the anti-MOMP mAb confirmed activated microglia as host cells (Figure 25.1). The chlamydia-infected cells surrounding blood vessels in the AD brain were confirmed to be pericytes via labeling with the anti-iNOS and anti-MOMP Ab, as well as a mAb targeting CD68.[23] In more recent studies employing the neuron-specific MAP-2 mAb in combination with a mAb targeting the chlamydial LPS, we demonstrated that neurons in affected AD brain regions are also infected with *C. pneumoniae* (Figure 25.2; KLW, APH, manuscript in preparation).

Direct visualization of the organism in the AD brain was a critical issue in the initial study. Analysis of several brain tissue samples from PCR-positive AD patients and PCR-negative controls by electron microscopy demonstrated that areas of the hippocampus, temporal cortex, and/or other regions of AD brains with NFT and NSP contained objects that resembled *C. pneumoniae*, as well as structures that appeared to be more or less normal chlamydial inclusions, when compared to those from standard electron microscopic studies of the organism.[46] Nothing similar was identified in the non-AD control brains. Immunoelectron microscopy using the mAb targeting the *C. pneumoniae* MOMP confirmed the objects resembling chlamydia as authentic *C. pneumoniae*. Parallel examination of brain tissue sections from PCR-negative patients showed no labeling.[23]

An issue of some importance in the initial studies was to define the geographic relationship between *C. pneumoniae*-infected host cells and NSP/NFT. The PHF-1 (paired helical filaments of tau) mAb has been used extensively to identify neuritic pathology in AD brain tissues. Staining of consecutive brain tissue sections with the PHF-1 and anti-MOMP mAb demonstrated the presence of *C. pneumoniae*-infected glial cells in the immediate vicinity of NFT in the AD brain. Similarly performed immunolabeling of brain areas showing little or no neuropathology in AD brains showed few or no cells harboring *C. pneumoniae*, and no infected cells were identified in any non-AD brain examined.[23] Thus, these studies strongly indicated that *C. pneumoniae*-infected cells, primarily astroglia and microglia, in the late-onset AD brain are concentrated in regions of characteristic neuropathology.

We understood that the case for an etiologic or exacerbatory role for *C. pneumoniae* in sporadic AD would be strengthened significantly if the organism could be shown to be viable in the brain. Standard reverse transcription-PCR analyses of RNA prepared from affected brain regions of AD patients demonstrated the presence of several different mRNAs from the organism, suggesting both viability and metabolic activity (HCG, APH unpublished observations).[23] Standard laboratory culture of *C. pneumoniae* was also attempted, first using a human monocyte cell line (THP-1), and later HEp-2 cells, as an *in vitro* host with homogenates of AD patient and control brains. Cultures from AD but not control brain materials were positive by microscopy; the apparent culture positivity for the organism was confirmed by subsequent immunohistochemistry with the anti-MOMP mAb. *C. pneumoniae* within infected THP-1 cells were also visualized by electron microscopy.[23] Strain differentiation in *C. pneumoniae* is not currently well-defined, but some information can be obtained from DNA sequence determination of the *omp1* gene, which encodes the MOMP of the organism. In recent studies, we have cloned and sequenced this gene in *C. pneumoniae* cultured directly from several different AD patient samples. Initial analysis of

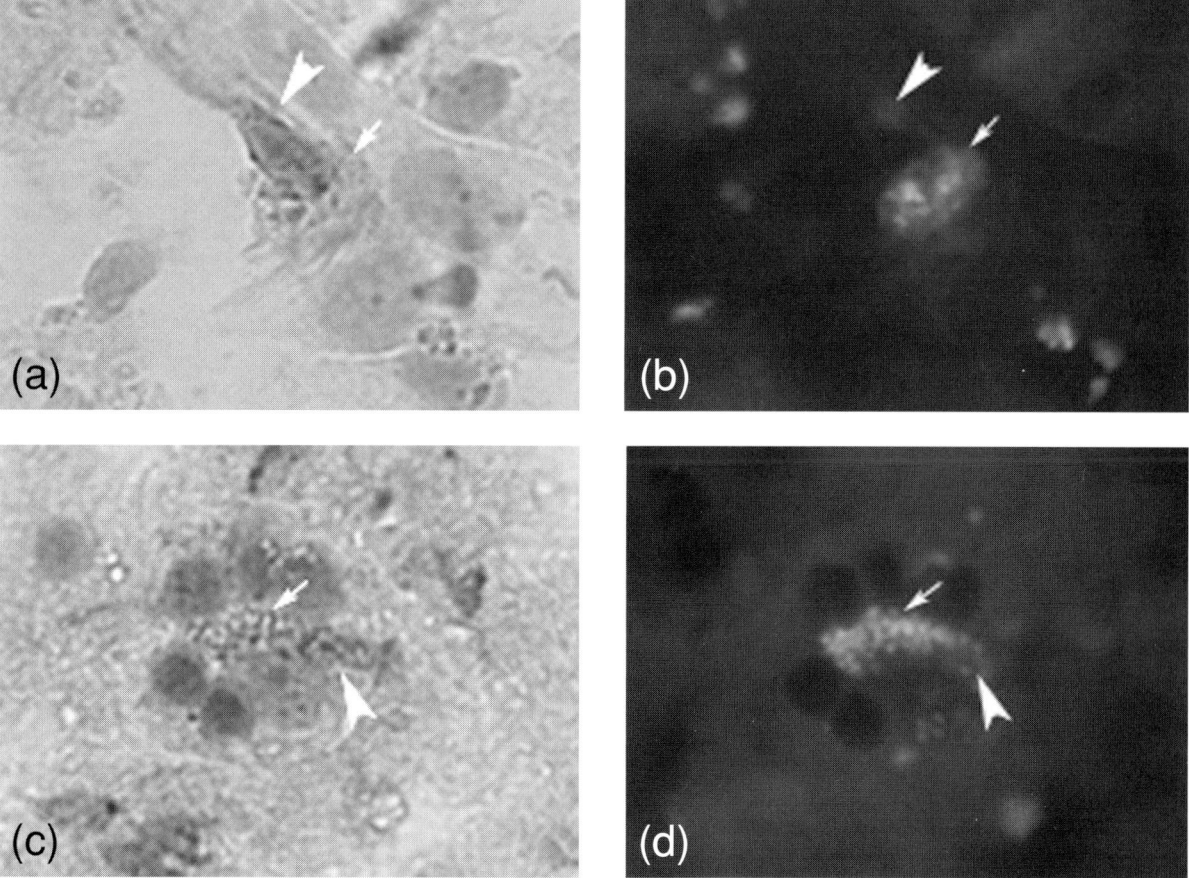

Figure 25.1 Double immunostaining to demonstrate infection of astrocytes (panels a and b) and microglia (panels c and d) by *Chlamydia pneumoniae* in the temporal cortex of an AD brain. Staining in panels (a) and (c) was done using anti-inducible nitric oxide synthase and anti-glial fibrillary acid protein monoclonal antibodies, respectively, to identify microglia and astrocytes (indicated with arrow heads on all panels). Staining in panels (b) and (d) was done using the anti-chlamydial LPS monoclonal antibody to highlight chlamydial inclusions (indicated with small arrows on all panels). Staining was done as given in Balin et al.[23] Magnification ×600 in all panels.

the sequence information suggests differences at both the nucleotide (silent change) and amino acid sequence levels in the brain-derived strains compared to the standard strains in the databases (e.g., www.stdgen.lanl.gov). Much more analysis of these *omp1* sequences, and sequencing of other genomic regions, must be done before it is clear whether we have identified a neurotropic strain of the organism in the AD brain.

Chlamydia pneumoniae is a respiratory pathogen known to disseminate widely from its site of primary infection; the vehicle for dissemination has been shown to be the monocyte/macrophage.[47,48] A question of significant interest therefore centers on how this organism might breach the blood brain barrier to reach the central nervous system. Recent studies from one of our collaborating laboratories have addressed this issue. Those workers reasoned that *C. pneumoniae* infection of vascular endothelial cells might alter the blood brain barrier in such a manner as to permit access for the organism. In one study, western blotting and immunohistochemical analyses were employed to show that infection of human microvascular endothelial cells in culture elicited increased expression of a number of relevant proteins, including N-cadherin and β-catenin;[49] interestingly, expression of occludin, a protein associated with tight junctions, was attenuated in the *C. pneumoniae*-infected cells. A

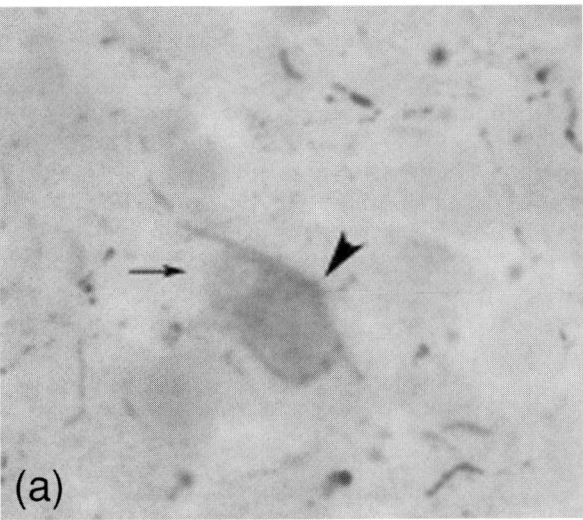 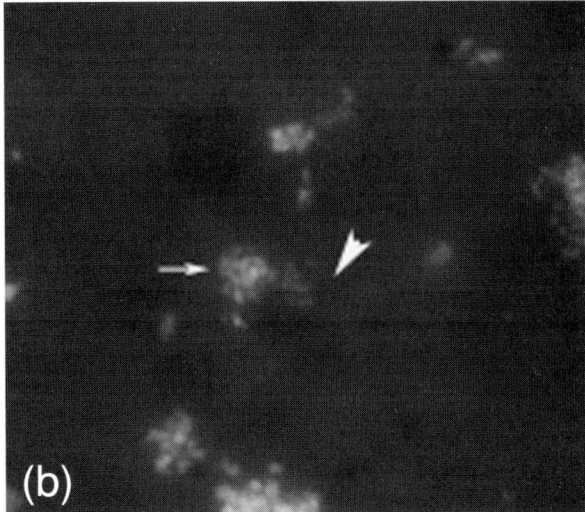

Figure 25.2 Double immunostaining to demonstrate infection of neurons by *Chlamydia pneumoniae* in the temporal cortex of an AD brain. Staining was done using the neuron-specific MAP-2 monoclonal antibody (panel a) to identify the cell type (indicated with arrow heads on both panels) and the anti-chlamydial LPS monoclonal antibody (panel b) to highlight chlamydial inclusions (indicated with small arrows on both panels). Staining was done as given in Balin et al.[23] Magnification ×600 in both panels.

subsequent report from the same group indicated that infection of human microvascular endothelial cells from the brain promotes passage of monocytic cells through that cell layer; expression was argued to be stimulated by upregulation of various adhesion molecules, including VCAM-1, ICAM-1, and others;[50] MAC-1 and other molecules expressed by monocytic cells were also increased in these experiments. Thus, these studies suggest that access to the central nervous system from the vascular system for *C. pneumoniae* may be a process strongly influenced, and perhaps partly governed, by the organism itself.

Studies from other laboratories

Since publication of the initial study, a number of groups have tried to replicate the PCR-based aspects of the studies outlined above, with variable success (Table 25.1). A group in Seattle could not identify *C. pneumoniae* in paraffin-embedded brain tissues from 12 confirmed and 13 suspected late-onset AD patients using either PCR or immunohistochemical analyses.[51] In a similar study from Germany, the organism could not be identified in any of 20 paraffin-embedded AD brain samples, again via either immunohistochemical analysis or PCR-based screening.[52] Similar results were recently obtained by a group in England.[53] In a fourth study, a California group assessed multiple samples from each of 15 confirmed AD and five non-AD control brains by PCR; in this study, each sample was assayed independently several times;[54] samples were prepared from frozen brain tissues, and culture of the organism from some samples was attempted. Cultures were negative for all samples attempted, but a few weak positives were obtained in the PCR screening. In all these studies, the authors concluded that the presence of *C. pneumoniae* in the AD brain could not be confirmed, or that the association between organism and the late-onset AD brain was not strong.

Recovery of high quality template for PCR amplification from paraffin-embedded or otherwise fixed tissue is often unreliable, and this probably explains in large part the negative results from some studies; only frozen brain tissue samples were used in our studies and in the California study.[54] However, it is difficult to understand why the embedded tissue samples used in two of the studies were negative in immunohistochemical analyses, since a Dutch group reported success in identifying *C. pneumoniae* by this method in 11 of 12 paraffin-embedded AD brain samples;[55] all control samples were negative in this study, including those from individuals with other neurologic diseases. In our own work, the negative immunohistochemical studies, and in the positive Dutch study, the same mAb targeting the organism's

Table 25.1 Published attempts to identify *C. pneumoniae* in the Alzheimer's brain

Patient samples	Source	Results[a]	Reference
19 AD/19 control	Frozen	PCR+ 17/19 AD, 1/19 control IHC+ 6/6 AD, 0/6 control EM+ 10/10 AD, 0/6 control IEM+ 10/10 AD, 0/7 control Culture+ 2/2 AD, 0/2 control	23
12 AD/7 possible AD/6 control	Paraffin	PCR+ 0/25 IHC+ 0/25	51
20 AD	Paraffin	PCR+ 0/20 IHC+ 0/20	52
15 AD/5 control	Frozen	PCR+ 2 weak AD and 1 weak control culture+ 0/3 (2 AD/1 control)	54
12 AD/16 control	Paraffin	IHC+ 11/12 AD, 3/16 controls	55
21 AD/10 control	Frozen	PCR+ 18/21 AD[b] 0/10 controls	56
19 AD/2 control[c]	Frozen	PCR+ 0/19 AD, 0/2 controls IHC+ 0/19 AD, 0/2 controls	53

[a] PCR, polymerase chain reaction assay; IHC, immunohistochemical analysis; EM, electron microscopic analysis; IEM, immunoelectron microscopic analysis.
[b] Positive in at least one of 10 repetitions of PCR reaction.
[c] Some AD samples supplied for these studies were from the original 1998 study.[23]

MOMP or LPS were employed, suggesting differences in technique in obtaining congruently positive results. Another report provides useful insight into the mixed positive and negative PCR data from the California study above.[56] This latter study employed replicate PCR assays and probit regression analyses to show that DNA prepared from up to 85% of the frozen AD brain samples analyzed were PCR-positive for *C. pneumoniae* if enough replicates were performed; multiply-assayed controls were always PCR-negative. These data suggest that the overall load of *C. pneumoniae* in the AD brain, and probably elsewhere as well, can be low, in turn indicating that identification of chlamydial DNA in such source materials requires both careful template preparation and repetitive analyses.

APOE ε4, sporadic AD, and *C. pneumoniae*

Five allele types have been identified at the *APOE* locus on chromosome 19, two of which (ε1, ε5) are rare and three of which (ε2, ε3, ε4) are relatively common. The product of this gene has long been known to be critically important for cholesterol transport and homeostasis.[57,58] Interestingly, possession of the ε4 allele at *APOE* has been associated with multiple sclerosis as well as late-onset AD.[43] In patients with the former disease, presence of the gene product is currently thought to be related to relatively rapid progression to disability, rather than to increased risk for disease genesis;[59] how the ε4 gene product might modulate disease course in multiple sclerosis remains to be elucidated. Possession of the ε4 allele type is, of course, the single well-established and accepted risk factor for development of late-onset AD.[60–62] Not all individuals bearing this allele develop AD, but its presence increases risk for disease development several-fold, as well as promoting earlier onset and more rapid neurodegeneration. As in the case of multiple sclerosis, precisely how the product of the ε4 allele promotes AD-related neuropathology is not understood, although several hypotheses have been advanced. These include interaction with the neuronal cytoskeleton via tau[63,64] and promotion of Aβ formation.[65] Some data suggest that variant expression of *APOE*, rather than the detailed structure of the ε4 gene product itself compared to ε2 or ε3, may contribute to development of AD.[66] Other data suggest that the effect of the ε4 gene product in engendering the neuropathology of AD may obtain directly at the level of cholesterol metabolism.[67]

We explored the possiblity that the *APOE* ε4 gene product is associated in some manner with the pathobiology of *C. pneumoniae*. In initial studies, that possible relationship was examined in a different, non-AD context. Specifically, we chose to investigate the frequency of ε4 in patients with synovial infection by *C. pneumoniae*, since the organism had been identified in the joints of some patients with inflammatory arthritis.[34] DNA prepared from synovial tissue biopsies of a large cohort of relatively young (average age 43) nondemented patients was screened by PCR for DNA from *C. trachomatis*, *C. pneumoniae*, and other bacteria, and *APOE* genotype was defined for patients in each of four groups: those PCR-positive for *C. trachomatis* only, *C. pneumoniae* only, other bacteria only, or no bacteria. *APOE* expression in synovial tissue from these patients was confirmed by RT-PCR. Such genotyping demonstrated that patients PCR-negative in all assays, and those PCR-positive in the *C. trachomatis*-only and non-*Chlamydia* directed assays, showed distributions of the three most common *APOE* allele types (ε2, ε3, ε4) which mirrored those of the general population. However, 68% of patients with synovial *C. pneumoniae* DNA had a copy of ε4, a rate four to five times that of the general population.[68] This observation strongly suggests a role for this gene product in the pathobiology of the organism, strengthening the association between *C. pneumoniae* and development of late-onset AD.

We have also suggested that these data may mean that possession of the *APOE* ε4 allele is a surrogate marker for risk of late-onset AD, and a direct marker for the pathobiology of *C. pneumoniae*.

Interestingly, another group has suggested a relationship among possession of the ε4 allele, infection with HSV-1, and late-onset AD.[20] Precisely how the ε4 gene product promotes AD-related (or other) pathogenesis by *C. pneumoniae*, HSV-1, or any other micro-organism, is not at all clear. It is possible that potential host cells for *C. pneumoniae* which express the allele take up the organism more efficiently than do ε4-lacking cells, and initial experiments in our laboratory indicate that this is indeed the case (manuscript in preparation). Infection of ε4-bearing cells may also allow more rapid passage through the organism's biphasic developmental cycle or more efficient production of new elementary bodies, the extracellular, infectious form of the organism at the end of that cycle. Regardless, it is clear that expression of the ε4 allele is related both to pathogenesis by *C. pneumoniae* and development of sporadic AD, and elucidation of the details of that relationship will be important in understanding disease genesis.

SUMMARY

The idea that the development and/or maintenance of pathogenesis in some idiopathic chronic diseases may involve an infectious component certainly is not new. Rather, interest in this notion has peaked and receded a number of times during the 20th century. Beginning with the demonstration of *Helicobacter pylori* as an etiologic agent for ulcers a decade or more ago, however, the notion that microbial pathogens can play an initiating and/or exacerbatory role in such diseases has garnered renewed interest.[69] Studies along this line have indicated associations between *C. trachomatis* infection and cervical cancer,[70] infection by *Nocardia asteroides* and Parkinson's disease,[71] early prenatal infection with *Toxoplasma gondii* and later development of schizophrenia,[72] infection with human herpes virus 6 and multiple sclerosis,[73] and several others. The possible relationship between infection with *C. pneumoniae* and development of late-onset AD outlined in this chapter must be viewed in this context.

The experimental observations briefly summarized here from our initial studies and others argue that *C. pneumoniae* is present and viable in the AD brain, and that the organism is found primarily in regions of characteristic AD-related neuropathology. While much work remains to be done, including providing an explanation for the failure to identify the organism in AD brain samples published by other groups, these results demonstrate the proximity of a known and important bacterial pathogen to regions of standard AD-related neuropathology. It is important that the organism was identified only in AD brain materials, and not in congruent brain samples from various relevant control patients or in samples from patients with other neurological diseases. However, the number of samples assayed from patients with multiple sclerosis, Parkinson's disease, or other neurologic conditions both in this laboratory and others so far is relatively limited and must be expanded. It will also be critically important for other laboratories to replicate the PCR, immunohistochemistry, EM, and IEM observations in larger AD and control patient populations.

Assuming that *C. pneumoniae* is present in the late-onset AD brain but not those of normal individuals or patients with other neurologic diseases, such an association does not constitute a demonstration that the organism causes the disease. *C. pneumoniae* is an extremely capable opportunistic pathogen, and it is possible that it takes up residence in the AD brain in infected individuals only after the initiation of the neuropathologic process by some other means. As mentioned, *C. pneumoniae*, like all species of this genus, is well known to cause inflammation at sites of residence,[40] and data from many studies indicate that inflammation is an important clinical aspect of sporadic AD.[74,75] Indeed, treatment of AD patients with anti-inflammatory drugs has been shown to provide significant benefits.[76] This observation, in turn, suggests that the inflammation which characterizes the AD brain is an important component of neuropathogenesis. Thus, whether *C. pneumoniae* actually initiates the neurodegeneration process in late-onset AD or not, it seems probable that AD-related brain inflammation is attributable at least in part to the presence of *C. pneumoniae*. It is therefore reasonable to suggest that infection with *C. pneumoniae* is a risk factor for development of sporadic AD, even if it does not turn out to be the etiologic agent ultimately responsible for disease genesis.[77]

ACKNOWLEDGMENTS

The writing of this chapter was supported by NIH grants AR-47186 (HCG), AI-44493 (JAW-H) and AI-44055 (APH).

REFERENCES

1. Keefover RW. The clinical epidemiology of Alzheimer's disease. *Neurol Clinic* 1996; **14**: 337–51.
2. Clark CM, Karlawish JH. Alzheimer's disease: current concepts and emerging diagnostic and therapeutic strategies. *Ann Internal Med* 2003; **138**: 400–10.
3. Schellenberg GD. Genetic dissection of Alzheimer disease, a heterogeneous disorder. *Proc Natl Acad Sci USA* 1995; **92**: 8552–9.
4. Tanzi RE, Bertram L. New frontiers in Alzheimer's disease genetics. *Neuron* 2001; **32**: 181–4.
5. Breteler MM, Claus JJ, Van Duijn CM et al. Epidemiology of Alzheimer's disease. *Epidemiol Rev* 1992; **14**: 59–82.
6. Blacker D, Haines JL, Rodes L et al. APOE-4 and age at onset of Alzheimer's disease – the NIMH Genetics Initiative. *Neurology* 1997; **48**: 139–47.
7. Scheuner D, Eckman C, Jensen M et al. Secreted amyloid β-protein similar to that in the senile plaques of Alzheimer's disease is increased *in vivo* by the presenilin 1 and 2 mutations linked to familial Alzheimer's disease. *Nature Med* 1996; **2**: 864–70.
8. Hardy JA, Higgins GA. Alzheimer's disease: the amyloid cascade hypothesis. *Science* 1992; **256**: 184–5.
9. Sommer B. Alzheimer's disease and the amyloid cascade hypothesis: ten years on. *Curr Opin Pharmacol* 2002; **2**: 87–92.
10. Bishop GM, Robinson SR. The amyloid hypothesis: let sleeping dognas lie? *Neurobiol Aging* 2002; **23**: 1101–5.
11. Yankner BA. New clues to Alzheimer's disease: unraveling the roles of amyloid and tau. *Nature Med* 1996; **2**: 850–2.
12. Goedert M. Tau protein and the neurofibrillary pathology of Alzheimer's disease. *Trends Neurosci* 1993; **16**: 460–5.
13. Alonso AC, Grundke-Iqbal I, Iqbal K. Alzheimer's disease hyperphosphorylated tau sequesters normal tau into tangles of filaments and disassembles microtubules. *Nature Med* 1996; **2**: 783–7.
14. Lippa CF, Saunders AM, Smith TW et al. Familial and sporadic Alzheimer's disease: neuropathology cannot exclude a final common pathway. *Neurology* 1996; **46**: 406–12.
15. Bolton CF, Yound GB, Zochodne DW. The neurological consequences of sepsis. *Ann Neurol* 1993; **33**: 94–100.
16. Johnson RT. Emerging viral infections. *Arch Neurol* 1996; **53**: 18–22.
17. Pogo BG, Casals J, Elizan TS. A study of viral genomes and antigens in brains of patients with Alzheimer's disease. *Brain* 1987; **110**: 907–15.
18. Friedland RP, May C, Dahlberg J. The viral hypothesis of Alzheimer's disease. Absence of antibodies to lentiviruses. *Arch Neurol* 1990; **47**: 177–8.
19. Itzhaki R, Lin WR, Shang D et al. Herpes simplex virus type 1 in brain and risk of Alzheimer's disease. *Lancet* 1997; **349**: 241–4.
20. Itzhaki RF, Dobson CB, Lin WR, Wozniak MA. Association of HSV-1 and apolipoprotein E-varepsilon4 in Alzheimer's disease. *J Neuropathol* 2001; **7**: 570–1.
21. Renvoize EB, Awad IO, Hambling MH. A sero-epidemiological study of conventional infectious agents in Alzheimer's disease. *Age and Ageing* 1987; **16**: 311–4.
22. Grant WB, Campbell A, Itzhaki RF, Savory J. The significance of environmental factors in the etiology of Alzheimer's disease. *J Alzheimer's Dis* 2002; **4**: 179–89.
23. Balin BJ, Gerard HC, Arking EJ et al. Identification and localization of *Chlamydia pneumoniae* in the Alzheimer's brain. *Med Microbiol Immunol* 1998; **187**: 23–42.
24. Grayston JT, Campbell LA, Kuo CC et al. A new respiratory tract pathogen: *Chlamydia pneumoniae* strain TWAR. *J Infect Dis* 1990; **161**: 618–25.

25. Grayston JT. *Chlamydia pneumoniae*, strain TWAR pneumonia. *Ann Rev Med* 1992; **43**: 317–23.
26. Hahn DL, Dodge RW, Golubjatnikov R. Association of *Chlamydia pneumoniae* (strain TWAR) infection with wheezing, asthmatic bronchitis, adult-onset asthma. *J Amer Med Assoc* 1991; **266**: 225–30.
27. Grayston JT, Aldous MB, Easton A et al. Evidence that *Chlamydia pneumoniae* causes pneumonia and bronchitis. *J Infect Dis* 1993; **168**: 1231–5.
28. Clementsen P, Permin H, Norn S. *Chlamydia pneumoniae* infection and its role in asthma and chronic obstructive pulmonary disease. *J Invest Allergol Clin Immunol* 2002; **12**: 73–9.
29. Miyashita N, Niki Y, Nakajima M et al. Prevalence of asymptomatic infection with *Chlamydia pneumoniae* in subjectively healthy adults. *Chest* 2001; **119**: 1416–9.
30. Ferrari M, Poli A, Olivieri M et al. Respiratory symptoms, asthma, atopy, and *Chlamydia pneumoniae* IgG antibodies in a general population sample of young adults. *Infection* 2002; **30**: 203–7.
31. Leinonen M. Pathogenetic mechanisms and epidemiology of *Chlamydia pneumoniae*. *Eur Heart J* 1993; **14**: 57–61.
32. Gran JT, Hjetland R, Andreassen AH. Pneumonia, myocarditis and reactive arthritis due to *Chlamydia pneumoniae*. *Scand J Rheumatol* 1993; **22**: 43–4.
33. Campbell LA, O'Brien ER, Cappuccio AL et al. Detection of *Chlamydia pneumoniae* TWAR in human coronary atherectomy tissues. *J Infect Dis* 1995; **172**: 585–8.
34. Schumacher HR, Gérard HC, Arayssi TK et al. *Chlamydia pneumoniae* is present in synovial tissue of arthritis patients with lower prevalence than that of *C. trachomatis*. *Arthritis and Rheumatism* 1999; **42**: 1889–93.
35. Wagner AD, Gérard HC, Fresemann T et al. Detection of *Chlamydia pneumoniae* in giant cell vasculitis and correlation with the topographical arrangement of tissue-infiltrating dendritic cells. *Arthritis and Rheumatism* 2000; **43**: 1543–51.
36. Kalayoglu MV, Libby P, Byrne GI. *Chlamydia pneumoniae* as an emerging risk factor in cardiovascular disease. *J Amer Med Assoc* 2002; **288**: 2724–31.
37. Kalayoglu MV, Byrne GI. Induction of macrophage foam cell formation by *Chlamydia pneumoniae*. *J Infect Dis* 1998; **177**: 725–9.
38. Mahony JB, Coombes BK. *Chlamydia pneumoniae* and atherosclerosis: does the evidence support a causal or contributory role? *FEMS Microbiol Lett* 2001; **197**: 1–9.
39. Rosenfeld ME, Blessing E, Lin TM et al. *Chlamydia*, inflammation, and atherogenesis. *J Infect Dis* 2000; **181**(Suppl 3): S492–7.
40. Campbell LA, Kuo CC. *Chlamydia pneumoniae* pathogenesis. *J Med Microbiol* 2002; **51**: 623–5.
41. Stephens RS. The cellular paradigm of chlamydial pathogenesis. *Trends Microbiol* 2003; **11**: 44–51.
42. Sriram S, Stratton CW, Yao S et al. *Chlamydia pneumoniae* infection of the central nervous system in multiple sclerosis. *Ann Neurol* 1999; **46**: 6–14.
43. Swanborg RH, Whittum-Hudson JA, Hudson AP. Infectious agents and multiple sclerosis – are human herpes virus 6 and *Chlamydia pneumoniae* involved? *J Neuroimmunol* 2003; **136**: 1–8.
44. Koskiniemi M, Gencay M, Salonen O et al. *Chlamydia pneumoniae* associated with central nervous system infections. *Eur Neurol* 1996; **36**: 160–3.
45. Wimmer ML, Sandmann-Strupp R, Saikku P, Haberl RL. Association of chlamydial infection with cerebrovascular disease. *Stroke* 1996; **27**: 2207–10.
46. Miyashita N, Kanamoto Y, Matsumoto A. The morphology of *Chlamydia pneumoniae*. *J Med Microbiol* 1993; **38**: 418–25.
47. Moazed TC, Kuo CC, Patton DL et al. Experimental rabbit models of *Chlamydia pneumoniae* infection. *Am J Pathol* 1996; **148**: 667–76.
48. Moazed TC, Kuo CC, Grayston JT, Campbell LA. Evidence of systemic dissemination of *Chlamydia pneumoniae* via macrophages in the mouse. *J Infect Dis* 1998; **177**: 1322–5.
49. MacIntyre A, Hammond CJ, Little CS et al. *Chlamydia pneumoniae* infection alters the junctional complex proteins of human brain microvascular endothelial cells. *FEMS Microbiol Lett* 2002; **217**: 167–72.
50. MacIntyre A, Abramov R, Hammond CJ et al. *Chlamydia pneumoniae* infection promotes the transmigration of monocytes through human brain endothelial cells. *J Neurosci Res* 2003; **71**: 740–50.
51. Nochlin D, Shaw CM, Campbell LA, Kuo CC. Failure to detect *Chlamydia pneumoniae* in brain tissues of Alzheimer's disease. *Neurology* 1999; **53**: 1888.
52. Gieffers J, Reusche E, Solbach W, Maass M. Failure to detect *Chlamydia pneumoniae* in brain sections of Alzheimer's disease patients. *J Clin Microbiol* 2000; **38**: 881–2.
53. Taylor GS, Vipond IG, Paul ID et al. Failure to correlate *C. pneumoniae* with late-onset Alzheimer's disease. *Neurology* 2002; **59**: 142–3.
54. Ring RH, Lyons JM. Failure to detect *Chlamydia pneumoniae* in the late-onset Alzheimer's brain. *J Clin Microbiol* 2000; **38**: 2591–4.
55. Ossewarde JM, Gielis-Proper SK, Meijer A et al. *Chlamydia pneumoniae* antigens are present in the brains of Alzheimer patients but not the brains of patients with other dementias. In: *Chlamydia Research* (Saikku P, ed). Bologna: Societa Editrice Esculapio, 2000: 284.
56. Mahony J, Woulfe J, Munoz D et al. *Chlamydia pneumoniae* in the Alzheimer's brain – is DNA detection hampered by low copy number? In: *Chlamydia Research* (Saikku P, ed). Bologna: Societa Editrice Esculapio, 2000: 275.
57. Mahley RW. Apolipoprotein E: cholesterol transport protein with expanding role in cell biology. *Science* 1998; **240**: 622–30.
58. Strittmatter WJ. Apolipoprotein E and Alzheimer's disease: signal transduction mechanisms. *Biochem Soc Symp* 2001; **67**: 101–9.
59. Fazekas F, Strasser-Fuchs S, Kollegger H et al. Apolipoprotein E epsilon 4 is associated with rapid progression of multiple sclerosis. *Neurology* 2001; **57**: 853–7.
60. Roses AD. Apolipoprotein E alleles as risk factor in Alzheimer's disease. *Ann Rev Med* 1996; **47**: 387–400.
61. Deary IJ, Whiteman MC, Pattie A et al. Cognitive change and the *APOE* epsilon 4 allele. *Nature* 2002; **418**: 932.
62. Bennett DA, Wilson RS, Schneider JA. Apolipoprotein E epsilon 4 allele, AD pathology, and the clinical expression of Alzheimer's disease. *Neurology* 2003; **60**: 246–52.
63. Lovestone S, Anderton B, Betts J et al. Apolipoprotein E gene and Alzheimer's disease: is *tau* the link? *Biochem Soc Symp* 2001; **67**: 111–20.
64. Huang Y, Liu XQ, Wyss-Coray T et al. Apolipoprotein E fragments present in Alzheimer's disease brains induce neurofibrillary tangle-like intracellular inclusions in neurons. *Proc Natl Acad Sci USA* 2001; **98**: 8838–43.
65. Hartman RE, Laurer H, Longhi L et al. Apolipoprotein E4 influences amyloid deposition but not cell loss after traumatic brain injury in a mouse model of Alzheimer's disease. *Neuroscience* 2002; **22**: 10083–7.
66. Laws SM, Hone E, Gandy S, Martins RN. Expanding the association between the *APOE* gene and risk of Alzheimer's disease: possible roles for *APOE* promoter polymorphisms and

alterations in *APOE* transcription. *J Neurochem* 2003; **84**: 1215–36.
67. Puglielli L, Tanzi RE, Kovacs DM. Alzheimer's disease: the cholesterol connection. *Nature Neurosci* 2003; **6**: 345–51.
68. Gérard HC, Wang GF, Balin BJ et al. Frequency of apolipoprotein E (*APOE*) allele types in patients with *Chlamydia*-associated arthritis and other arthritides. *Microbial Pathogenesis* 1999; **26**: 35–43.
69. Zimmer C. Do chronic diseases have an infectious root? *Science* 2001; **293**: 1974–7.
70. Anttila R, Saikku P, Koskela P et al. Serotypes of *Chlamydia trachomatis* and risk for development of cervical squamous cell carcinoma. *J Am Med Assoc* 2001; **285**: 47–51.
71. Kohbata S, Beaman BL. L-dopa-responsive movement disorder caused by *Nocardia asteroides* localized in the brains of mice. *Infection and Immunity* 1991; **59**: 181–91.
72. Yolken RH, Bachmann S, Ruslanova I et al. Antibodies to *Toxoplasma gondii* in individuals with first-episode schizophrenia. *Clin Infect Dis* 2001; **32**: 842–4.
73. Tejada-Simon MV, Zang YCQ, Hong J et al. Detection of viral DNA and immune responses to the human herpesvirus 6 101-kilodalton virion protein in patients with multiple sclerosis and controls. *J Virol* 2002; **76**: 6147–54.
74. Aisen PS. Inflammation and Alzheimer's disease. *Mol Chem Neuropathol* 1996; **28**: 83–8.
75. Hoozemans JJ, Veerhuis R, Rozemuller AJ, Eikelenboom P. The pathological cascade of Alzheimer's disease: the role of inflammation and its therapeutic implications. *Drugs Today* 2002; **38**: 429–43.
76. Breitner JC. The role of anti-inflammatory drugs in the prevention and treatment of Alzheimer's disease. *Ann Rev Med* 1996; **47**: 401–11.
77. Balin BJ, Appelt DM. Role of infection in Alzheimer's disease. *J Amer Osteopathic Assoc* 2000; **101**(Suppl 12): S1–6.

26

Psychiatric and neurological complications of HIV infection and AIDS

Diane M P Lawrence, Lynnae Schwartz and Eugene O Major

INTRODUCTION

Worldwide, an estimated 40 million people are infected with HIV, including 2.5 million children under the age of 15 years, with five million new infections and three million deaths related to HIV occurring in 2003.[1] The devastating economic and social impact of this pandemic has been particularly severe in sub-Saharan Africa, where one in five adults is infected. Unfortunately, the epidemic continues to expand internationally in countries with large populations, limited resources, low awareness, and/or minimal prevention and education programs, including Eastern Europe, India, and China.

Approximately 700,000 children were newly infected with HIV in 2003 (14% of all new cases). The majority of HIV-1 infected children acquire their infection vertically as the virus is passed from mother to fetus. Antiretroviral therapy given to pregnant women has substantially reduced prenatal transmission in the United States,[2,3] but prenatal and perinatal medications are not administered to the majority of HIV positive women and their infants worldwide. In addition, a new epidemic of HIV-1 infection is evolving among sexually active adolescents: one-third of the people with AIDS worldwide are between the ages of 15 and 24,[1] and HIV was identified as the seventh leading cause of death in this age group in the United States.[4] This development is of great concern because an awareness of diagnosis may not be reached until young adulthood, allowing for substantial viral transmission.

Psychiatric and neurological complications associated with HIV infection are well described in both adult and pediatric AIDS patients. The link between these diagnoses and HIV is not a direct one, but instead involves opportunistic infection, neuroinflammation, neuronal dysfunction, and/or neurodegeneration. Neurological and psychiatric symptoms generally improve if therapy, especially highly active antiretroviral therapy (HAART), is successful in reducing the systemic viral load and restoring immune function.[5–9] This improvement is partially due to the reduced incidence of opportunistic infections affecting the CNS.[8,10] Unfortunately, control of viral load may not be sufficient to prevent neurological and psychiatric complications; even for patients taking HAART, the incidence of HIV-1 encephalopathy has continued to increase in long-term survivors.[10] The reasons for this are not yet fully understood, but possible factors include the fact that not all antiretroviral agents efficiently cross the blood brain barrier, and for those that do, there may be distinct neurotoxicity associated with treatment.[11] Viral sequestration within the CNS may also be a factor; a latent infection that is not affected by drug therapy can be reactivated under particular circumstances, providing an additional source of virus in the brain.

In recent years, it has become apparent that the factors directly responsible for HIV-1-associated neurological dysfunction are primarily cellular and viral toxins, rather than HIV-1 itself. Effective future measures to prevent or treat the neurologic and psychiatric sequalae of HIV-1 infection will depend upon gaining an improved understanding of how infection triggers these inflammatory and cellular responses.

PSYCHIATRIC DISORDERS ASSOCIATED WITH HIV-1 INFECTION

After infection with HIV-1, many years may pass before the virus causes enough damage to produce the clinical symptoms of immunosuppression known as

AIDS. There is wide variation in the prevalence of psychiatric disorders in HIV-infected patients, depending on the criteria for evaluation, the stage of infection or disease, and the factors associated with the patient risk group (e.g., gender, age, drug use, nutrition, and socioeconomic status).[12] Aside from cognitive disorders such as dementia, which will be described in the next section, there is no specific psychiatric syndrome associated with HIV infection. However, mood disorders such as anxiety and major depression are common in both adults and children. For example, the prevalence of depression among HIV-infected adults ranges from 15–40%, which is higher than in the general population,[13-15] and in HIV-infected children the prevalence is 12–44%.[16-18] In recent years there has been an increase in psychiatric hospitalizations in children infected with HIV.[19] In adults, one study described an 'AIDS-lethargy' organic personality disorder in 34% of infected individuals, characterized by apathy, tiredness, and lack of emotional participation.[20] Other reports showed new-onset psychosis, unrelated to drug abuse, occurring in a small proportion of HIV-positive patients.[21-23] The true incidence of neuropsychiatric disorders in HIV-1 may be underestimated in the world literature when compared to studies limited to well-educated, middle-class Caucasian men.[24]

Mood and psychotic disorders associated with AIDS may not arise specifically from HIV infection, however, as anxiety, depression, or post-traumatic stress disorder could be the result of distress associated with an AIDS diagnosis and its implications.[23] Alternatively, people with underlying psychiatric disorders may be more at risk for acquiring HIV-1 as a consequence of diminished judgement, drug abuse, homelessness, or engaging in high-risk sexual behaviors.[25] Once the infection is established, these patients may not adhere to treatment regimens, increasing their likelihood of progressing to AIDS and developing neurological complications.

In many patients, AIDS-related immunosuppression leads to opportunistic infections (Table 26.1), which may have their own psychiatric consequences,[26-28] although since the introduction of HAART, the incidence of opportunistic infections has dropped in adults.[8] Finally, there is evidence that antiretroviral treatment itself may occasionally induce psychosis, or other psychiatric or neurological disturbances.[11,29,30]

Among HIV-infected children, several studies have found an increased incidence of anxiety, affective disorders, depression, and hyperactivity disorders,[18] but this remains somewhat controversial. A recent report found that rates of psychiatric hospitalizations among children and adolescents with HIV were almost three times higher than that reported for the general pediatric population, with depression or behavior disorder as the most frequent diagnosis.[19] A recent review[31] notes that HIV-infected preschool patients experience more subjective stress than their uninfected peers,[32] perhaps related to chronic illness, family and social stressors, neurocognitive and growth delays, and negative life events in general. Negative life events have also been shown to increase immune suppression in a cohort of children followed longitudinally through the Pediatric AIDS Clinical Trials Late Outcomes Study.[33] The importance of social and family context in the diagnosis and treatment of HIV-infected children with psychiatric issues has been emphasized.[34]

One important issue in the pediatric literature is the impact of environment, maternal substance abuse, and parental depression upon the HIV-infected child's neurocognitive development and behavior, compared to uninfected siblings and peers. The literature is somewhat conflicted but, in general, it appears that parental HIV status in itself does not affect psychological status, whereas parental injection drug use and depression both have a negative impact on behavior.[35] Children of depressed or medically ill intravenous drug-using parents may be particularly at risk for depression and anxiety disorders.[36] Despite a high prevalence of emotional and behavioral problems in HIV-infected children, a recent study found that biological or environmental factors are linked to these problems, but neither the infection itself nor prenatal drug exposure appear to be directly involved.[37]

In summary, there are multiple factors involved in HIV-associated psychiatric disease, making the viral etiology of these disorders unclear. In the remaining sections, we will describe clinical and basic science studies of AIDS dementia complex in adults and progressive encephalopathy in children, neurologic syndromes more definitively linked to HIV-1 infection. We will also attempt to define what is currently understood about the viral and biological basis for these syndromes.

NEUROLOGICAL FACTORS LINKED TO HIV-1 INFECTION

Shortly after the appearance of the AIDS pandemic, cognitive deficits and dementia were recognized as frequent neurological complications of HIV infection, as were motor abnormalities, vacuolar myelopathy, and peripheral neuropathy.[38] Neurological symptoms may be the initial manifestation of AIDS in some patients, and clinical observations suggest that more than half of all current AIDS patients will experience some form of neurological abnormality.[39,40]

Table 26.1 Opportunistic brain infections linked to AIDS

Etiological agent	Neurological correlates
Viral infections	
JC virus	Progressive multifocal leucoencephalopathy
Cytomegalovirus	Encephalitis, radiculmyelitis, peripheral neuritis, retinitis
Varicella zoster virus	Shingles, progressive encephalitis, seizures, necrotizing vasculitis
Human *Herpes simplex* virus 1/2	Temporal encephalitis, meningoencephalitic syndrome
Epstein-Barr virus	CNS lymphoma, encephalomyelitis (rare)
Human herpes virus 6	Retinitis, myelopathy, encephalitis
Bacterial infections	
Mycobacterium tuberculosis	Meningitis, encephalitis
Mycobacterium avium intracellulare	Meningitis, encephalitis, cranial nerve palsy
Treponema pallidum	Neurosyphilus, encephalitis
Bartonella hemselae	Meningitis, encephalitis
Listeria monocytogenes	Meningitis, encephalitis
Nocardia asteroides	Meningitis, cerebral abscess
Parasitic infections	
Toxoplasma gondii	Encephalitis, meningitis
Trypanosoma cruzi	Chagas' disease, encephalitis, meningitis
Fungal infections	
Cryptococcus neoformans	Meningitis, encephalitis, vision deficits
Coccidioides immitis	Meningitis, encephalitis, myelitis, radiculitis, cerebral abscess
Histoplasma capsulatum	Meningitis, encephalitis, seizures
Candida albicans	Meningitis, encephalitis, brain abscess
Aspergillus	Meningitis, meningomyelitis, encephalitis, brain abscess
Blastomyces	Meningitis, encephalitis, brain abscess

Many factors other than HIV may contribute to these symptoms, particularly CNS lymphoma or opportunistic brain infections (shown in Table 26.1) which result from HIV-1-induced immunosuppression.[27,28] However, for patients without these conditions, a disorder called AIDS subacute encephalopathy has been proposed (currently termed AIDS dementia complex, ADC, or HIV-associated dementia, HAD), defined as a diffuse neurologic impairment occurring primarily in the later stages of AIDS.[41] ADC may be the principal manifestation of AIDS in up to 20% of cases, and the initial presentation in up to 10% of cases;[42] interestingly, the prevalence was found to be highest in children and elderly adults. A significant association between neurological compromise and mortality has been observed in the context of HIV infection in adults[43,44] as well as children.[45,46]

Early manifestations of ADC in adults may be subtle and not diagnosed at the time of initial neurological assessment.[41,47] Routine mental status examination can be normal in early stages, or may show slow but accurate verbal and motor processing. Often the initial deficits are only apparent when compared to the patient's previous abilities. Additional signs and symptoms include loss of concentration, frequent forgetting, and difficulty following a conversation. Early motor symptoms include loss of balance, weakness of the legs, tremor, and loss of fine motor coordination. Generalized convulsive seizures may also occur, with or without co-existing opportunistic brain infection. Early behavioral changes include apathy, social withdrawal, and irritability, all of which may be organic, or caused by reactive depression. In general this disorder has been classified as a subcortical dementia,[48,49] similar to that observed in advanced Parkinson's disease patients but distinct from the cortical dementia in Alzheimer's disease.

In advanced stages of the disease, patients show moderate to severe degrees of dementia, with global cognitive and motor dysfunction prior to death.[41,47] Neurological examination at these later stages shows more definite mental deficits, impaired information processing, and slow responses, as well as pronounced fine and gross motor abnormalities including tremor, myoclonus, frank seizures, paraparesis, or quadriparesis. Some individuals reach a mute or vegetative stage, where they may be conscious but unable to respond to stimuli. Painful peripheral neuropathy is very common and sometimes difficult to alleviate, resulting in diminished quality of life.

The first reports of vertically transmitted pediatric HIV-1 infection described CNS complications,[50–52] often as part of the initial clinical presentation. Although dementia is rarely seen in infected children, a triad of abnormalities comprising a progressive encephalopathy (PE) was described, with:

1) Brain atrophy or impaired brain growth
2) Motor dysfunction progressing to severe spasticity or rigidity
3) Severe neurodevelopmental delays, with either loss of or failure to gain developmental milestones.[53]

It has been suggested that these features of PE are the result of toxic inflammatory molecules that stimulate glutamate neurotoxicity, and it is possible that neurons in the developing brain are more susceptible to HIV-related injury than those in the adult.[54]

The term 'HIV-related CNS compromise' has been used to describe pediatric patients with cognitive functioning within normal limits overall, but who have declining psychometric scores on serial tests, or deficits in selective areas of neurocognitive function.[55] Mild neurocognitive deficits may limit school performance, as well as the potential for independence into late adolescence and young adulthood for long-term survivors. Language deficits are a major characteristic of neurobehavioral dysfunction in pediatric HIV disease.[56] Expressive language is more impaired than receptive,[57] and may be tied to impairments in expressive behaviors which may affect school performance and social interactions.[58]

NEUROPSYCHOLOGICAL FINDINGS

In addition to neurological examination, neuropsychological testing is a cornerstone in the diagnosis of cognitive decline and dementia associated with HIV-1, particularly in the early, asymptomatic phase of AIDS.[59] Cognitive manifestations of HIV-associated dementia are particularly characterized by deficits in attention, concentration, and processing speed,[49] and these deficits often precede evidence of clinical CNS dysfunction as measured by neurological examination or imaging. Decline in psychomotor speed is frequently the first evidence of AIDS dementia,[60] and it reliably predicts HIV dementia, according to the Multicenter AIDS Cohort Study (MACS).[61] Overall, cognitive impairment has been found to be an accurate predictor of postmortem brain pathology, or HIV encephalopathy.[62]

There is considerable variation in the batteries of neuropsychological tests used to diagnose cognitive decline in HIV-1 infected individuals, and the results are quite variable. Prior to the establishment of criteria defining mild neurocognitive disorder, dementia, and delirium, estimates of the prevalence of dementia ranged between 6.5% and 66% of symptomatic seropositive patients.[59,63] In asymptomatic infected patients, some studies have shown evidence of subtle cognitive dysfunction with minimal impact on activities of daily living. In one study of asymptomatic patients, the median rate of impairment was 35%, higher than the 12% in seronegative controls.[64] However, other studies have shown no neurological impairment in asymptomatic HIV-infected patients.[65–67]

To be useful, standard psychometric batteries must be altered and validated for different patient cohorts, particularly to address different ages, languages, cultures, and education levels. The World Health Organization has created a neuropsychological battery for use in a multicultural study comparing clinical manifestations of HIV-associated dementia across different socio-cultural and geographic contexts.[68] Scales that sensitively measure cognitive decline, behavioral alterations, and impairment of activities of daily living are particularly important for objective evaluation of both the onset of disease and the impact of antiretroviral therapy.[59,69]

The American Academy of Neurology AIDS Task Force has provided recommendations for nomenclature and case definitions of the neurological manifestations of HIV-1 for research purposes, including some definitions for neuropsychological alterations.[70] Cognitive alterations are classified as either HIV-1-associated dementia complex, or HIV-1-associated minor cognitive/motor disorder, depending on the severity. The Memorial Sloan Kettering Staging of the AIDS dementia complex was developed in 1988 to standardize neurological testing criteria by rating the degree of functional impairment in mobility and activities of daily life. Definitions of each stage included normal function (stage 0) and subclinical with normal daily function but mild neurological signs (stage 0.5), up to an end-stage, nearly vegetative state (stage IV). This structured scale has been useful for the clinical study of patients without requiring special expertise in neuropsychological testing,[71,72] and has provided more consistent estimates of the prevalence of HIV-1 associated neurological impairments.

In order better to understand the factors in the progression of HIV-associated dementia as defined by the American Academy of Neurology, the Dana Consortium on Therapy for HIV Dementia and Related Cognitive Disorders was initiated in 1994 with the goal of developing a computerized, standardized algorithm to consistently diagnose both HIV-1 dementia and minor cognitive/motor disorder.[73] More recently, the Memorial Sloan Kettering scale was modified for a multicenter longitudinal study of the Northeast AIDS Dementia (NEAD) Consortium.[74] To distinguish better between HIV-1 dementia and minor cognitive/motor disorder, a neuropsychological battery to test for verbal memory, visual memory, constructional skills, psychomotor skills, motor coordination, and timed gait was added. The modified scale was found to have excellent inter-rater reliability,[74] and is therefore expected to be useful in future multicenter clinical trials.

A classification system for the evaluation of CNS disease in HIV-1 infected children has been proposed by the neurobehavioral team at the HIV and AIDS Malignancy Branch of the National Cancer Institute, in an effort to develop a consistent and objective system upon which to base treatment and standardize neurobehavioral research efforts.[55] Specific criteria are given for the diagnosis of encephalopathy and CNS compromise. Briefly, a diagnosis of HIV-related encephalopathy is made upon the presence of one or more of the following criteria: loss of previously acquired skill, significant drop in cognitive test scores, cognitive test scores in the borderline or delayed range with functional deficits, a significantly abnormal neurological exam, or significant improvement with antiretroviral treatment. Subtypes of encephalopathy are also suggested: acute (inflammation, irritability, insomnia, frank psychosis, motor disturbances such as rigidity), subacute (loss of previously acquired skills, decline in raw and standard score on psychometric tests, new neurologic abnormalities), plateau (no acquisition of new skills or slowed rate of development compared to previous rate, resulting in significant drop in standard scores on psychometric tests), and static (delayed or arrested development that does not decline, slower than normal development in the delayed range, or stability of neuropsychologic functioning for at least one year after a significant decline).[55]

NEUROPATHOLOGY AND BIOLOGICAL BASIS FOR HIV-1 ASSOCIATED DEMENTIA

Although chronic neuronal dysfunction and/or apoptosis ultimately leads to the cognitive and motor dysfunction associated with HIV-1 infection, the exact mechanisms by which infection causes neuronal damage are complex and incompletely understood.[75] HIV-1 does not productively infect neurons; in addition, the specific subpopulations of neurons affected by HIV-1, and their locations in the brain, are highly variable among patients,[76] as is the level and location of viral gene product and pattern of virus mutation in the brain. These factors may explain the variability in symptoms and inconsistent clinical correlation between viral load and neurologic impairment.[77]

Evidence of neuropathology in some form has been observed in a majority of adult AIDS patients, with a higher incidence observed in pediatric cases.[78,79] The hallmarks of HIV-1-associated neuropathology include:

1) The formation of microglial nodules and multinucleated giant cells in central white matter and deep gray matter, suggestive of virus-induced fusion of microglia and/or macrophages
2) Astrogliosis, indicative of astrocyte activation and damage
3) The loss of specific neuron subpopulations, particularly those involved in cognition (hippocampus) and motor function (basal ganglia, spinal cord)
4) The loss of synaptic connections
5) The loss of myelin, which indicates damage to oligodendrocytes
6) The presence of HIV-1 DNA in the CSF.[80–82]

Collectively these features are called HIV-1-associated encephalitis (HIVE). Although severe HAD is typically observed during the late stages of infection, mild to moderate neuropsychological, neurophysiological, and neuroanatomical abnormalities in the context of HIVE can occur well before the end stages of AIDS,[83] suggesting that HIV-1 encephalopathy is a gradual process which may begin early in the course of infection.

Neuropathology and neuroimaging

Neuroimaging has an important role in the detection and differential diagnosis of neuropathologic findings seen in HIV-1 infected patients. In adults, pathologic changes occur in the basal ganglia, thalamus, subcortical white matter, and spinal cord. Metabolic, functional, and perfusion studies may be abnormal prior to the development of clinical neurologic disease, whereas imaging studies in advanced neuroAIDS may show white matter atrophy with ventricular enlargement, advanced leukoencephalopathy including progressive multifocal leukoencephalopathy (PML), and myelopathy of the thoracic cord.[84] Secondary complications that may be identified with the help of imaging include tuberculosis, toxoplasmosis, CNS lymphoma, invasive fungal infections with abscess formation, and other opportunistic bacterial, mycobacterial, viral, and spirochetal infections. Neuropathology in pediatric patients that can be detected by imaging includes calcification of the basal ganglia, microcephaly with significant cortical atrophy, cerebral vasculopathy with vasculitis, calcification, and/or aneurysmal dilatation of vessels, in addition to the changes seen in adult brains, with the exception of PML which has rarely been reported.[85] There may be a predilection in pediatric patients for basal ganglia involvement with calcifications, greater than that noted in adults.

Neuroimaging techniques include computed tomography (CT) with or without contrast, magnetic resonance acquisition of T2- and T1-weighted images, enhanced with gadolinium (Gd)-based contrast as needed, positron emission tomography (PET), functional MRI (fMRI), magnetic resonance spectroscopy (MRS) or proton magnetic resonance spectroscopy (^{1}H-MRS), magnetization transfer ratio (MTR) histogram analysis, volumetric magnetic resonance, and single-photon emission computed tomography (SPECT). Table 26.2 shows the specific applications of these techniques for neurological examination of HIV-1 infected patients.

Cellular involvement and neurotoxicity

In the brain, the principal cells that support productive HIV-1 infection are activated macrophages and microglial cells, as shown by several studies using immunohistochemistry, *in situ* hybridization, and *in situ* PCR.[88,97–103] The infected monocytes carrying virus into the brain parenchyma have been described as perivascular macrophages, which are readily apparent upon histopathological examination. HIV-1 proteins have been identified in macrophages and microglial cells pathologically described as multinucleated giant cells, and in microglial nodules which are found mainly in the basal ganglia.[80,82] The numbers of infected macrophages in the brains of patients with HIV-1-associated dementia, as well as the total amounts of virus production within the brain tissues, are highly variable. However, the amount of virus and the numbers of infected cells are generally too low to explain the extent of pathology observed, suggesting that the brain's responses to HIV-1 infection contribute to the process of HIV-1 encephalitis, to a greater degree than viral replication and virus-mediated cell lysis.[75,80–82]

Macrophages and microglia activated by infection secrete potentially neurotoxic cellular products, including nitrous oxide (iNOS), platelet activating factor, quinolinic acid, arachidonic acid metabolites, and pro-inflammatory cytokines such as TNF-α and IL-1β. These factors and others have been implicated in HIV neuropathology because they are upregulated in AIDS brain tissues,[80,82] and may be directly neurotoxic, or indirectly involved by inducing neuronal apoptosis. They may also act by damaging or overstimulating other cell types in the CNS critical for neuronal function, such as astrocytes.[104–106] Uninfected macrophages and microglia can also be activated by these products, thus amplifying the pathophysiologic cascade.

Infected cells also release the viral structural proteins gp120 and gp41, as well as the nonstructural proteins nef and tat, all of which are associated with CNS pathology. The gp120 glycoprotein molecule shed from the surface of infected cells can damage neurons.[107,108] For several years it was believed that this damage was a direct effect of gp120 on the neurons, but recent evidence indicates that gp120-mediated neurotoxicity depends on the presence of other cells, either macrophages, microglia, or astrocytes, suggesting an indirect mechanism involving toxic intermediates.[108] These observations suggest that HIV-1 causes damage in the nervous system primarily by indirect mechanisms, through the production of toxic cell-derived factors or the secretion of viral proteins.

It is also becoming clear that infection and/or damage to astrocytes plays a significant role in HIV-1-associated encephalopathy.[109,110] Astrocytes are the predominant cell type in the brain, and provide critical metabolic and synapse-associated functions that keep neurons alive and functioning normally. Although astrocytes lack the CD4 receptor, there is definitive evidence that HIV-1 can affect and sometimes infect astrocytes. HIV-1 mRNA and DNA has been detected in brain astrocytes in human autopsy material,[109,111–114] and infection of human astrocytes in culture has been demonstrated using both native virus, pseudotyped virus, and transfection of infectious HIV-1 clones.[115–117] Histopathologic and cell culture studies suggest that pediatric or fetal astrocytes may be more susceptible to HIV-1 infection than adult astrocytes.[111,113] Astrocyte infection appears to be noncytopathic, transient, and restricted, producing

Table 26.2 Neuroimaging techniques for differential diagnosis of HIV-related neuropathology

Technique	Indication	Studies or reviews in HIV-1 (+) patients
CT	Initial examination mass lesions, calcifications, ventricular size, cortical atrophy, leukomalacia, cerebral edema.	86
MRI	Better detection of white matter disease, meningeal pathology, posterior fossa lesions, other mass lesions; T1-weighted image for anatomy, parenchymal lesions; T2-weighted image for edema, hemorrhage	87
SPECT	Differentiation primary CNS lymphoma from other lesions; cortical perfusion defects; neuronal degeneration; abnormal energy metabolism; alterations in acetylcholine metabolism	88,89
MRS and ¹H-MRS	*In vivo* metabolism, differential diagnosis lymphoma from other mass lesion, inflammatory versus noninflammatory processes	90,91
MTR	Combine with volumetric MR imaging for early detection neurodegeneration	92
fMRI	*In vivo* measurement regional cerebral blood volume and blood flow as indicator of regional activation	93,94
PET	*In vivo* measurement metabolic and neurotransmitter mediated processes; correlation with motor and cognitive impairments	95,96

relatively little viral progeny and diminishing to a latent stage.[116] The restriction has been characterized by the diminished production and/or function of certain viral proteins.[111,116,118,119] Proviral DNA in astrocytes can be reactivated to make more virus in the presence of inflammatory cytokines found in the infected brain.[115,120]

One critical function of astrocytes is to maintain appropriate levels of synaptic glutamate by transporter-mediated high-affinity uptake and exocytosis-like release of glutamate.[121] Astrocytes that are infected or exposed to HIV-1 proteins gp120 or tat may contribute to neuronal loss and CNS dysfunction by alterations in extracellular glutamate processing.[122–125] Decreased glutamate uptake or excessive release by astrocytes may lead to the accumulation of excitotoxic concentrations of extracellular glutamate at neuronal synapses, which in turn can cause neuronal apoptosis and loss.[126] A fivefold increase in CSF glutamate levels has been found in HIV-1+ patients compared to controls, and this increase correlated with the degree of dementia.[127]

In addition, astrocyte function and/or survival may be affected by viral proteins or toxic products secreted from infected and/or activated macrophages, and astrocytes themselves can be stimulated to produce toxic inflammatory mediators. For example, HIV-1 can activate the astrocytic complement system, a cascade of inflammatory events that can help eliminate virus but also may participate in neuropathology.[128,129] The viral tat protein, as well as inflammatory cytokines, stimulates astrocytes to produce the inflammatory β chemokine monocyte chemoattractant protein (MCP)-1.[130,131] This chemokine production would attract additional monocytes into the brain, and is known to be elevated in the CSF of AIDS dementia patients.[130,132] Astrocytes exposed to HIV-1, gp120, or tat become impaired in their ability to transport glutamate, which would be expected to contribute to neurotoxicity. Thus, astrocytes appear to participate in HIV-1 neuropathology in several ways, including failure to maintain glutamate homeostasis, harboring latent infection, producing inflammatory factors, and recruiting infected and/or activated monocytes into the brain.

INFLAMMATORY CYTOKINES AND CHEMOKINES IN THE DISEASED BRAIN

While profound deficiency of cellular immunity is the hallmark of AIDS, it is clear that inflammatory responses from activated monocytes and lymphocytes occur during HIV-1 infection, and are implicated in the neurological consequences of AIDS. Increased levels of pro-inflammatory cytokines such as IL-1, IFN-γ, and especially TNF-α, anti-inflammatory cytokines including TGF-β and IL-6, and soluble cytokine receptors are found in the CSF of AIDS patients.[133,134] Importantly, the levels of cytokine production in the CNS correlate with the severity of neurologic symptoms.[133,134] Activated macrophages are most likely the predominant source of pro-inflammatory cytokines in the CNS, but astrocytes, neurons, and endothelial cells, particularly when stimulated by activated macrophages or HIV-1-Tat protein, also have the capacity for cytokine production.[82,133,134]

The cytokines TNF-α and IL-1β enhance HIV-1 replication through increased production and viral DNA binding of the NFκB transcription factor in macrophages.[134] These same cytokines can activate HIV-1 replication in microglia[135] and in latently infected astrocytes,[115] and stimulate macrophages and microglia to produce the cellular toxins described earlier.[82,133] TNF-α can affect astrocytes by stimulating the production of other cytokines and chemokines,[133] and can inhibit the ability of astrocytes to buffer extracellular glutamate.[123,136] Cytokines such as TNF-α and IL-1 in the brain can adversely affect oligodendrocyte function and pituitary hormone secretion, as well as induce fever, nausea, and loss of appetite, explaining some of the more general symptoms associated with HIV-1-associated dementia.[133] IFN-γ can stimulate macrophage production of quinolinic acid, which as described above can overstimulate and destroy neurons via glutamate receptor activation.[80] Thus, in addition to promoting the survival of the virus, cytokines in the HIV-1-infected brain serve as messengers between various cell types to amplify the production of molecules that are toxic to neurons.

Chemokine production is also considered to be a significant factor in HIV-1 encephalitis. Chemokines, a family of small cytokines typically produced by damaged or infected cells, work in a gradient fashion to attract and activate particular subsets of cells from the immune system to the site of damage. Cells expressing receptors that recognize a specific chemokine respond to low concentrations, and move in the direction of increasing concentrations of the chemokine until the source is reached. Some chemokine receptors are coreceptors for HIV-1, so the reported production of certain chemokines, such as SDF-1, RANTES, and MIP-1α,[132,137] may be beneficial as blockers of viral entry but may also be toxic to neurons.[108] Levels of fractalkine production in the CSF are associated with the magnitude of cognitive impairment in AIDS patients,[138] but it is unclear if this chemokine has a damaging or protective role in response to infection.[139–141] Chemokines also help responding cells enter the brain more efficiently by increasing adhesion molecule expression.

As described in the previous section, several studies have shown a specific upregulation of MCP-1 in the CSF of HIV-1 dementia patients[130,132] and in cultured astrocytes and microglia exposed to the HIV-1 regulatory protein Tat.[130,142] This response may be inhibited by neuropeptides such as opioids.[143] TNF-α is known to induce MCP-1 production, and may play a role in the upregulation observed in HIV-1 dementia.[132] Production of other chemokines, such as macrophage inhibitory protein (MIP)-1α, MIP-1β, or RANTES, has also been detected in the CSF of HIV-1 dementia patients.[132] In HIV-1 encephalopathy, it is likely that these chemokines contribute to pathogenesis by bringing into the brain increased numbers of infected and/or activated monocytes, another source of both viral and cellular toxins that affect neuronal function and survival.[130] In addition, resident brain cells, including neurons, express chemokine receptors and it is possible that chemokines act directly on neurons either to provide protection or to induce cell death.[108,144]

A study of simian immunodeficiency virus in macaques provided definitive evidence that the level of MCP-1 in the CSF is a strong predictor of encephalitis.[145] Infected monkeys that later developed either moderate or severe encephalitis showed significantly higher CSF:plasma ratios of MCP-1 than monkeys that did not develop encephalitis. The MCP-1 increase occurred well before the onset of symptoms or lesions. If MCP-1 or other inflammatory molecules have the same predictive power in humans, this finding might lead to earlier treatment with antiviral drugs that access the brain, which would reduce the incidence of HIV-1-associated encephalopathy and/or dementia. In addition, knowing which specific molecules are responsible for specific neurological symptoms could lead to the development of selective anti-inflammatory treatments that would stop the neurotoxic processes induced by brain infection.

TREATMENT ISSUES

The advent of antiretroviral therapy provided great hope for prolonging the lives of HIV-1-infected patients, and for reducing the immunosuppression responsible for the susceptibility to opportunistic infections that are often the direct cause of death in AIDS patients. HAART, a combination of at least three anti-HIV-1 drugs including protease inhibitors and reverse transcriptase inhibitors, has been most successful in restoring lymphocyte function and suppressing viral replication to nearly undetectable levels within weeks of treatment initiation.

Indeed, early studies examining neurological function with antiretroviral treatment supported that optimism. For example, the use of antiretroviral medications preserved or improved neurological function in a large cohort of infected patients.[6] In other studies, HAART therapy was associated with partial reversal of cognitive deficits and white matter spectroscopic abnormalities in HIV-infected patients[9] and reduced incidence of HIV-1-associated dementia by nearly 50%, compared to earlier cohorts of patients taking only one or two anti-HIV-1 drugs.[7,8] Another longitudinal study of homosexual and bisexual men found evidence that HAART was associated with improved psychomotor processing speed and a 50% reduction in neuropsychological impairment; however, more than one-third of all participants continued to demonstrate impairment by the end of study, and 9% who were unimpaired in the beginning developed deficits despite HAART and good viral suppression.[146] Unfortunately, the occurrence of less severe cognitive deficits and neuropathology in postmortem tissue has not changed.[147,148]

In the first antiretroviral pediatric treatment trial, continuous intravenous administration of zidovudine (AZT) was shown to be of significant benefit in children presenting with encephalopathy prior to treatment, as documented by improved verbal and performance IQ scores.[5] This outcome led to early optimism that successful control of viral load with restoration of functional immune status might limit, if not reverse, the neurocognitive deficits associated with pediatric HIV infection. Although it is true that HAART has been associated with a dramatic decrease in the number of severely encephalopathic children, some continue to have cognitive decline despite control of viral load and stabilized immune status.[149]

Taken together, these longitudinal studies suggest that, although successful in some patients, systemic therapeutic approaches are not likely to eradicate the neurological consequences of HIV-1 infection. For those who do have access to HAART and can tolerate treatment, lowered systemic viral load may lead to less viral trafficking into the CNS, and less CNS inflammation. Blocking viral entry into the CNS is critical for the prevention of HIV-1-associated neurological disorders, but unfortunately entry may occur with primary infection, prior to diagnosis of HIV-1 infection,[150] and systemic HIV-1 infection is resistant to therapy in 20–50% of patients.[151]

In order to develop better treatment options for HIV-1-associated encephalopathy, it is critical to understand that this disease is not a simple case of virus-induced cell damage, but rather a chain of events that leads to neuronal dysfunction. In other words, eliminating virus may not stop the process of HIV-1-induced cell damage in the brain mediated by inflammation, glutamate neurotoxicity, and apoptosis. As described in the previous section, numerous inflammatory or toxic factors produced by activated glia contribute to cognitive and/or motor impairment via microglia–astrocyte–neuron interactions. However, it is unclear how this complex array of responses induces specific neuropathology. As depicted in Figure 26.1, similar inflammatory responses may play a significant role in other neurodegenerative diseases, including Alzheimer's disease, Parkinson's disease, Huntington's disease, amyotrophic lateral sclerosis (ALS), and even prion disease.[152–158] Complicating the treatment options is the fact that some inflammatory responses may also be neuroprotective; cytokines, chemokines, and even complement activation all have dual roles in the CNS.[82,129,159] It is thus important for any treatment to maintain the beneficial functions of both neurons and glial cells.

One possible treatment may be the NMDA-blocking drug memantine, which appears to block glutamate damage to neurons[160] and has recently gained FDA approval for the treatment of Alzheimer's disease. Memantine seems to have fewer psychomimetic side effects than other NMDA antagonists, so it is possible that this drug will be useful in treating various neurological diseases involving glutamate,[161] including ADC. Another strong candidate drug is minocycline, a drug that directly inhibits both

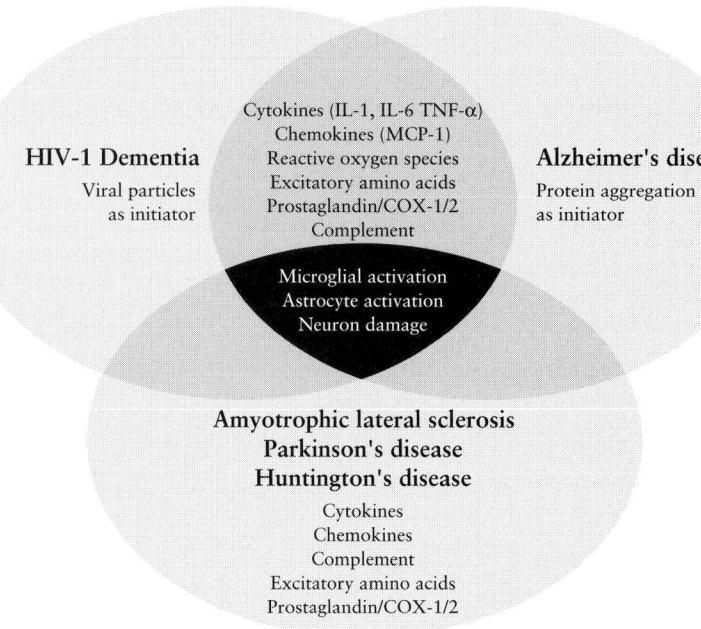

Figure 26.1 Mechanisms of glial inflammation in HIV-1 dementia and other neurodegenerative disorders.

caspase-independent and -dependent mitochondrial cell death pathways, and seems to provide neuroprotection in animal models of Huntington's disease, Parkinson's disease, and ALS.[162–164] This drug may also hold promise for treatment of dementia and AIDS-related neuropathology. The complexity of glial regulation, particularly during the development of disease, presents a wide range of possible approaches to developing therapeutic interventions for multiple chronic neurodegenerative diseases including the AIDS dementia complex.

REFERENCES

1. UNAIDS. Joint United Nations Programme on HIV/AIDS. *AIDS Epidemic Update 2003*. 2003: Geneva.
2. Connor EM, Sperling RS, Gelber R et al. Reduction of maternal-infant transmission of human immunodeficiency virus type 1 with zidovudine treatment. Pediatric AIDS Clinical Trials Group Protocol 076 Study Group. *N Engl J Med* 1994; **331**: 1173–80.
3. Cooper ER, Charurat M, Mofenson L et al. Combination antiretroviral strategies for the treatment of pregnant HIV-1-infected women and prevention of perinatal HIV-1 transmission. *J Acquir Immune Defic Syndr* 2002; **29**: 484–94.
4. Centers for Disease Control and Prevention. Trends in HIV-related sexual risk behaviors among high school students – selected US cities, 1991–1997. *Morbid Mortal Weekly Rep* 1999; **48**: 440–3.
5. Pizzo PA, Eddy J, Falloon J et al. Effect of continuous intravenous infusion of zidovudine (AZT) in children with symptomatic HIV infection. *N Engl J Med* 1988; **319**: 889–96.
6. Price RW, Yiannoutsos CT, Clifford DB et al. Neurological outcomes in late HIV infection: adverse impact of neurological impairment on survival and protective effect of antiviral therapy. AIDS Clinical Trial Group and Neurological AIDS Research Consortium study team. *AIDS* 1999; **13**: 1677–85.
7. Maschke M, Kastrup O, Esser S et al. Incidence and prevalence of neurological disorders associated with HIV since the introduction of highly active antiretroviral therapy (HAART). *J Neurol Neurosurg Psychiatry* 2000; **69**: 376–80.
8. Sacktor N, Lyles RH, Skolasky R et al. HIV-associated neurologic disease incidence changes: Multicenter AIDS Cohort Study, 1990–1998. *Neurology* 2001; **56**: 257–60.
9. Stankoff B, Tourbah A, Suarez S et al. Clinical and spectroscopic improvement in HIV-associated cognitive impairment. *Neurology* 2001; **56**: 112–5.
10. Neuenburg JK, Brodt HR, Herndier BG et al. HIV-related neuropathology, 1985 to 1999: rising prevalence of HIV encephalopathy in the era of highly active antiretroviral therapy. *J Acquir Immune Defic Syndr* 2002; **31**: 171–7.
11. Langford TD, Letendre SL, Larrea GJ, Masliah E. Changing patterns in the neuropathogenesis of HIV during the HAART era. *Brain Pathol* 2003; **13**: 195–210.
12. Koutsilieri E, Scheller C, Sopper S et al. Psychiatric complications in human immunodeficiency virus infection. *J Neurovirol* 2002; **8**(Suppl 2): 129–33.
13. Brown GR, Rundell JR, McManis SE et al. Prevalence of psychiatric disorders in early stages of HIV infection. *Psychosom Med* 1992; **54**: 588–601.
14. Blazer DG, Kessler RC, McGonagle KA, Swartz MS. The prevalence and distribution of major depression in a national community sample: the National Comorbidity Survey. *Am J Psychiatry* 1994; **151**: 979–86.
15. Treisman G, Fishman M, Schwartz J et al. Mood disorders in HIV infection. *Depress Anxiety* 1998; **7**: 178–87.
16. Bose S, Moss HA, Brouwers P et al. Psychologic adjustment of human immunodeficiency virus-infected school-age children. *J Dev Behav Pediatr* 1994; **15**: S26–33.
17. Tardieu M, Mayaux MJ, Seibel N et al. Cognitive assessment of school-age children infected with maternally transmitted human immunodeficiency virus type 1. *J Pediatr* 1995; **126**: 375–9.

18. Pao M, Lyon M, D'Angelo LJ et al. Psychiatric diagnoses in adolescents seropositive for the human immunodeficiency virus. *Arch Pediatr Adolesc Med* 2000; **154**: 240–4.
19. Ganghan DM, Hughes MD, Oleske JM et al. Psychiatric hospitalizations among children and youths with human immunodeficiency virus infection. *Pediatrics* 2004; **113**: e544–51.
20. Diederich N, Karenberg A, Peters UH. [Psychopathologic pictures in HIV infection: AIDS lethargy and AIDS dementia]. *Fortschr Neurol Psychiatr* 1988; **56**: 173–85.
21. Harris MJ, Jeste DV, Gleghorn A, Sewell DD. New-onset psychosis in HIV-infected patients. *J Clin Psychiatry* 1991; **52**: 369–76.
22. Sewell DD, Jeste DV, Atkinson JH et al. HIV-associated psychosis: a study of 20 cases. San Diego HIV Neurobehavioral Research Center Group. *Am J Psychiatry* 1994; **151**: 237–42.
23. Alciati A, Fusi A, D'Arminio Monforte A et al. New-onset delusions and hallucinations in patients infected with HIV. *J Psychiatry Neurosci* 2001; **26**: 229–34.
24. Maj M, Janssen R, Starace F et al. WHO neuropsychiatric AIDS study, cross-sectional phase I. Study design and psychiatric findings. *Arch Gen Psychiatry* 1994; **51**: 39–49.
25. Lyon DE. Human immunodeficiency virus (HIV) disease in persons with severe mental illnesses. *Issues Ment Health Nurs* 2001; **22**: 109–19.
26. Cohen BA, Berger JR. Neurologic opportunistic infections in AIDS. In: *The Neurology of AIDS* (Gendelman HE, Lipton SA, Epstein L, Swindells S, eds). New York: Chapman & Hall, 1998: 303–32.
27. Clifford DB. Opportunistic viral infections in the setting of human immunodeficiency virus. *Semin Neurol* 1999; **19**: 185–92.
28. Roullet E. Opportunistic infections of the central nervous system during HIV-1 infection (emphasis on cytomegalovirus disease). *J Neurol* 1999; **246**: 237–43.
29. Wise ME, Mistry K, Reid S. Drug points: neuropsychiatric complications of nevirapine treatment. *BMJ* 2002; **324**: 879.
30. Foster R, Olajide D, Everall IP. Antiretroviral therapy-induced psychosis: case report and brief review of the literature. *HIV Med* 2003; **4**: 139–44.
31. Brown LK, Lourie KJ, Pao M. Children and adolescents living with HIV and AIDS: a review. *J Child Psychol Psychiatry* 2000; **41**: 81–96.
32. Trad PV, Kentros M, Solomon GE, Greenblatt ER. Assessment and psychotherapeutic intervention for an HIV-infected preschool child. *J Am Acad Child Adolesc Psychiatry* 1994; **33**: 1338–45.
33. Howland LC, Gortmaker SL, Mofenson LM et al. Effects of negative life events on immune suppression in children and youth infected with human immunodeficiency virus type 1. *Pediatrics* 2000; **106**: 540–6.
34. Stolar A, Fernandez F. Psychiatric perspective of pediatric human immunodeficiency virus infection. *South Med J* 1997; **90**: 1007–16.
35. Pilowsky DJ, Zybert PA, Hsieh PW et al. Children of HIV-positive drug-using parents. *J Am Acad Child Adolesc Psychiatry* 2003; **42**: 950–6.
36. Pilowsky DJ, Knowlton AR, Latkin CA et al. Children of injection drug users: impact of parental HIV status, AIDS, and depression. *J Urban Health* 2001; **78**: 327–39.
37. Mellins CA, Smith R, O'Driscoll P et al. High rates of behavioral problems in perinatally HIV-infected children are not linked to HIV disease. *Pediatrics* 2003; **111**: 384–93.
38. Snider WD, Simpson DM, Nielsen S et al. Neurological complications of acquired immune deficiency syndrome: analysis of 50 patients. *Ann Neurol* 1983; **14**: 403–18.
39. Price RW, Brew B, Sidtis J et al. The brain in AIDS: central nervous system HIV-1 infection and AIDS dementia complex. *Science* 1988; **239**: 586–92.
40. Lanska DJ. Epidemiology of human immunodeficiency virus infection and associated neurologic illness. *Semin Neurol* 1999; **19**: 105–11.
41. Navia BA, Jordan BD, Price RW. The AIDS dementia complex: I. Clinical features. *Ann Neurol* 1986; **19**: 517–24.
42. Janssen RS, Nwanyanwu OC, Selik RM, Stehr-Green JK. Epidemiology of human immunodeficiency virus encephalopathy in the United States. *Neurology* 1992; **42**: 1472–6.
43. Mayeux R, Stern Y, Tang MX et al. Mortality risks in gay men with human immunodeficiency virus infection and cognitive impairment. *Neurology* 1993; **43**: 176–82.
44. Price RW. Neurological complications of HIV infection. *Lancet* 1996; **348**: 445–52.
45. Fragoso YD, Mendez V, Adams AP et al. Neurological manifestations of AIDS: a review of fifty cases in Santos, Sao Paolo, Brazil. *Rev Paul Med* 1998; **116**: 1715–20.
46. Bobat R, Coovadia H, Moodley D, Coutsoudis A. Mortality in a cohort of children born to HIV-1 infected women from Durban, South Africa. *S Afr Med J* 1999; **89**: 646–8.
47. Navia BA, Price RW. Clinical and biologic features of the AIDS dementia complex. In: *The Neurology of AIDS* (Gendelman HE, Lipton SA, Epstein L, Swindells S, eds). New York: Chapman & Hall, 1998: 229–40.
48. Price RW, Sidtis JJ, Brew BJ. AIDS dementia complex and HIV-1 infection: a view from the clinic. *Brain Pathol* 1991; **1**: 155–62.
49. Berger JR, Arendt G. HIV dementia: the role of the basal ganglia and dopaminergic systems. *J Psychopharmacol* 2000; **14**: 214–21.
50. Belman AL, Ultmann MH, Horoupian D et al. Neurological complications in infants and children with acquired immune deficiency syndrome. *Ann Neurol* 1985; **18**: 560–6.
51. Epstein LG, Sharer LR, Joshi VV et al. Progressive encephalopathy in children with acquired immune deficiency syndrome. *Ann Neurol* 1985; **17**: 488–96.
52. Epstein LG, Sharer LR, Oleske JM et al. Neurologic manifestations of human immunodeficiency virus infection in children. *Pediatrics* 1986; **78**: 678–87.
53. Mintz M, Epstein LG. Neurologic manifestations of pediatric acquired immunodeficiency syndrome: clinical features and therapeutic approaches. *Semin Neurol* 1992; **12**: 51–6.
54. Epstein LG, Gelbard HA. HIV-1-induced neuronal injury in the developing brain. *J Leukoc Biol* 1999; **65**: 453–7.
55. Wolters P, Brouwers P. Neurodevelopmental function and assessment of children with HIV-1 infection. In: *Handbook of Pediatric HIV Care* (Zeichner S, Read S, eds). Philadelphia: Lippincott, Williams & Wilkins, 1999: 210–27.
56. Brouwers P, van Engelen M, Lalonde F et al. Abnormally increased semantic priming in children with symptomatic HIV-1 disease: evidence for impaired development of semantics? *J Int Neuropsychol Soc* 2001; **7**: 491–501.
57. Wolters PL, Brouwers P, Civitello L, Moss HA. Receptive and expressive language function of children with symptomatic HIV infection and relationship with disease parameters: a longitudinal 24-month follow-up study. *AIDS* 1997; **11**: 1135–44.
58. Wolters PL, Brouwers P. Evaluation of neurodevelopmental deficits in children with HIV infection. In: *The Neurology of AIDS* (Gendelman HE, Lipton SA, Epstein L, Swindells S, eds). New York: Chapman and Hall, 1998: 425–42.
59. Grant I, Heaton RK, Atkinson JH. Neurocognitive disorders in HIV-1 infection. HNRC Group. HIV Neurobehavioral Research Center. *Curr Top Microbiol Immunol* 1995; **202**: 11–32.

60. Arendt G, Hefter H, Elsing C et al. Motor dysfunction in HIV-infected patients without clinically detectable central-nervous deficit. *J Neurol* 1990; 237: 362–8.
61. Sacktor NC, Bacellar H, Hoover DR et al. Psychomotor slowing in HIV infection: a predictor of dementia, AIDS and death. *J Neurovirol* 1996; 2: 404–10.
62. Cherner M, Masliah E, Ellis RJ et al. Neurocognitive dysfunction predicts postmortem findings of HIV encephalitis. *Neurology* 2002; 59: 1563–7.
63. Maj M, Satz P, Janssen R et al. WHO neuropsychiatric AIDS study, cross-sectional phase II. Neuropsychological and neurological findings. *Arch Gen Psychiatry* 1994; 51: 51–61.
64. White DA, Heaton RK, Monsch AU. Neuropsychological studies of asymptomatic human immunodeficiency virus-type-1 infected individuals. The HNRC Group. HIV Neurobehavioral Research Center. *J Int Neuropsychol Soc* 1995; 1: 304–15.
65. Janssen RS, Saykin AJ, Cannon L et al. Neurological and neuropsychological manifestations of HIV-1 infection: association with AIDS-related complex but not asymptomatic HIV-1 infection. *Ann Neurol* 1989; 26: 592–600.
66. McArthur JC, Cohen BA, Selnes OA et al. Low prevalence of neurological and neuropsychological abnormalities in otherwise healthy HIV-1-infected individuals: results from the multicenter AIDS Cohort Study. *Ann Neurol* 1989; 26: 601–11.
67. Selnes OA, Miller E, McArthur J et al. HIV-1 infection: no evidence of cognitive decline during the asymptomatic stages. The Multicenter AIDS Cohort Study. *Neurology* 1990; 40: 204–8.
68. Maj M, Janssen R, Satz P et al. The World Health Organization's cross-cultural study on neuropsychiatric aspects of infection with the human immunodeficiency virus 1 (HIV-1). Preparation and pilot phase. *Br J Psychiatry* 1991; 159: 351–6.
69. Schifitto G, Kieburtz K, McDermott MP et al. Clinical trials in HIV-associated cognitive impairment: cognitive and functional outcomes. *Neurology* 2001; 56: 415–8.
70. Janssen RS, Cornblath DR, Epstein LG et al. Nomenclature and research case definitions for neurologic manifestations of human immunodeficiency virus-type 1 (HIV-1) infection. Report of a Working Group of the American Academy of Neurology AIDS Task Force. *Neurology* 1991; 41: 778–85.
71. Price RW, Brew B. Management of the neurologic complications of HIV infection and AIDS. *Infect Dis Clin North Am* 1988; 2: 359–72.
72. Bouwman FH, Skolasky RL, Hes D et al. Variable progression of HIV-associated dementia. *Neurology* 1998; 50: 1814–20.
73. Dana Consortium. Clinical confirmation of the American Academy of Neurology algorithm for HIV-1-associated cognitive/motor disorder. Report from the Dana Consortium on Therapy for HIV Dementia and Related Cognitive Disorders. *Neurology* 1996; 47: 1247–53.
74. Marder K, Albert SM, McDermott MP et al. Inter-rater reliability of a clinical staging of HIV-associated cognitive impairment. *Neurology* 2003; 60: 1467–73.
75. Kaul M, Garden GA, Lipton SA. Pathways to neuronal injury and apoptosis in HIV-associated dementia. *Nature* 2001; 410: 988–94.
76. Wiley CA, Soontornniyomkij V, Radhakrishnan L et al. Distribution of brain HIV load in AIDS. *Brain Pathol* 1998; 8: 277–84.
77. Glass JD, Fedor H, Wesselingh SL, McArthur JC. Immunocytochemical quantitation of human immunodeficiency virus in the brain: correlations with dementia. *Ann Neurol* 1995; 38: 755–62.
78. Budka H, Wiley CA, Kleihues P et al. HIV-associated disease of the nervous system: review of nomenclature and proposal for neuropathology-based terminology. *Brain Pathol* 1991; 1: 143–52.
79. Simpson DM. Human immunodeficiency virus-associated dementia: review of pathogenesis, prophylaxis, and treatment studies of zidovudine therapy. *Clin Infect Dis* 1999; 29: 19–34.
80. Gendelman HE, Lipton SA, Tardieu M et al. The neuropathogenesis of HIV-1 infection. *J Leukoc Biol* 1994; 56: 389–98.
81. Bell JE. The neuropathology of adult HIV infection. *Rev Neurol (Paris)* 1998; 154: 816–29.
82. Nath A. Pathobiology of human immunodeficiency virus dementia. *Semin Neurol* 1999; 19: 113–27.
83. Heaton RK, Grant I, Butters N et al. The HNRC 500 – neuropsychology of HIV infection at different disease stages. HIV Neurobehavioral Research Center. *J Int Neuropsychol Soc* 1995; 1: 231–51.
84. Gonzales RG, Ruiz A, Tracey I, McConnell J. Structural, functional, and molecular neuroimaging in AIDS. In: *The Neurology of AIDS* (Gendelman HE, Lipton SA, Epstein L, Swindells S, eds). New York: Chapman & Hall, 1998: 333–52.
85. Berger JR, Scott G, Albrecht J et al. Progressive multifocal leukoencephalopathy in HIV-1-infected children. *AIDS* 1992; 6: 837–41.
86. Weisberg LA, Garcia C, Stazio A. Computerized tomographic diagnostic aspects of acquired immunodeficiency syndrome. *Comput Med Imaging Graph* 1988; 12: 225–36.
87. Avison MJ, Nath A, Berger JR. Understanding pathogenesis and treatment of HIV dementia: a role for magnetic resonance? *Trends Neurosci* 2002; 25: 468–73.
88. Meyerhoff DJ, Weiner MW, Fein G. Deep gray matter structures in HIV infection: a proton MR spectroscopic study. *AJNR Am J Neuroradiol* 1996; 17: 973–8.
89. Ernst T, Itti E, Itti L, Chang L. Changes in cerebral metabolism are detected prior to perfusion changes in early HIV-CMC: a coregistered (1)H MRS and SPECT study. *J Magn Reson Imaging* 2000; 12: 859–65.
90. Moller HE, Vermathen P, Lentschig MG et al. Metabolic characterization of AIDS dementia complex by spectroscopic imaging. *J Magn Reson Imaging* 1999; 9: 10–18.
91. Lee PL, Yiannoutsos CT, Ernst T et al. A multi-center 1H MRS study of the AIDS dementia complex: validation and preliminary analysis. *J Magn Reson Imaging* 2003; 17: 625–33.
92. Ge Y, Kolson DL, Babb JS et al. Whole brain imaging of HIV-infected patients: quantitative analysis of magnetization transfer ratio histogram and fractional brain volume. *AJNR Am J Neuroradiol* 2003; 24: 82–7.
93. Ernst T, Chang L, Jovicich J et al. Abnormal brain activation on functional MRI in cognitively asymptomatic HIV patients. *Neurology* 2002; 59: 1343–9.
94. Ernst T, Chang L, Arnold S. Increased glial metabolites predict increased working memory network activation in HIV brain injury. *Neuroimage* 2003; 19: 1686–93.
95. Wiseman MB, Sanchez JA, Buechel C et al. Patterns of relative cerebral blood flow in minor cognitive motor disorder in human immunodeficiency virus infection. *J Neuropsychiatry Clin Neurosci* 1999; 11: 222–33.
96. von Giesen HJ, Antke C, Hefter H et al. Potential time course of human immunodeficiency virus type 1-associated minor motor deficits: electrophysiologic and positron emission tomography findings. *Arch Neurol* 2000; 57: 1601–7.
97. Wiley CA, Schrier RD, Nelson JA et al. Cellular localization of human immunodeficiency virus infection within the brains of acquired immune deficiency syndrome patients. *Proc Natl Acad Sci USA* 1986; 83: 7089–93.
98. Nuovo GJ, Gallery F, MacConnell P, Braun A. In situ detection of polymerase chain reaction-amplified HIV-1 nucleic acids

and tumor necrosis factor-alpha RNA in the central nervous system. *Am J Pathol* 1994; **144**: 659–66.
99. Bagasra O, Lavi E, Bobroski L et al. Cellular reservoirs of HIV-1 in the central nervous system of infected individuals: identification by the combination of in situ polymerase chain reaction and immunohistochemistry. *Aids* 1996; **10**: 573–85.
100. Takahashi K, Wesselingh SL, Griffin DE et al. Localization of HIV-1 in human brain using polymerase chain reaction/in situ hybridization and immunocytochemistry. *Ann Neurol* 1996; **39**: 705–11.
101. Wiley CA. Polymerase chain reaction in situ hybridization – opening Pandora's box? *Ann Neurol* 1996; **39**: 691–2.
102. An SF, Groves M, Giometto B et al. Detection and localisation of HIV-1 DNA and RNA in fixed adult AIDS brain by polymerase chain reaction/in situ hybridisation technique. *Acta Neuropathol (Berl)* 1999; **98**: 481–7.
103. Wang TH, Donaldson YK, Brettle RP et al. Identification of shared populations of human immunodeficiency virus type 1 infecting microglia and tissue macrophages outside the central nervous system. *J Virol* 2001; **75**: 11686–99.
104. Lipton SA. AIDS-related dementia and calcium homeostasis. *Ann NY Acad Sci* 1994; **747**: 205–24.
105. Garden GA. Microglia in human immunodeficiency virus-associated neurodegeneration. *Glia* 2002; **40**: 240–51.
106. Garden GA, Budd SL, Tsai E et al. Caspase cascades in human immunodeficiency virus-associated neurodegeneration. *J Neurosci* 2002; **22**: 4015–24.
107. Dreyer EB, Kaiser PK, Offermann JT, Lipton SA. HIV-1 coat protein neurotoxicity prevented by calcium channel antagonists. *Science* 1990; **248**: 364–7.
108. Kaul M, Lipton SA. Chemokines and activated macrophages in HIV gp120-induced neuronal apoptosis. *Proc Natl Acad Sci USA* 1999; **96**: 8212–6.
109. Brack-Werner R. Astrocytes: HIV cellular reservoirs and important participants in neuropathogenesis. *AIDS* 1999; **13**: 1–22.
110. Thompson KA, McArthur JC, Wesselingh SL. Correlation between neurological progression and astrocyte apoptosis in HIV-associated dementia. *Ann Neurol* 2001; **49**: 745–52.
111. Saito Y, Sharer LR, Epstein LG et al. Overexpression of nef as a marker for restricted HIV-1 infection of astrocytes in postmortem pediatric central nervous tissues. *Neurology* 1994; **44**: 474–81.
112. Sharer LR, Saito Y, Epstein LG, Blumberg BM. Detection of HIV-1 DNA in pediatric AIDS brain tissue by two-step ISPCR. *Adv Neuroimmunol* 1994; **4**: 283–5.
113. Tornatore C, Chandra R, Berger JR, Major EO. HIV-1 infection of subcortical astrocytes in the pediatric central nervous system. *Neurology* 1994; **44**: 481–7.
114. Trillo-Pazos G, Diamanturos A, Rislove L et al. Detection of HIV-1 DNA in microglia/macrophages, astrocytes and neurons isolated from brain tissue with HIV-1 encephalitis by laser capture microdissection. *Brain Pathol* 2003; **13**: 144–54.
115. Tornatore C, Nath A, Amemiya K, Major EO. Persistent human immunodeficiency virus type 1 infection in human fetal glial cells reactivated by T-cell factor(s) or by the cytokines tumor necrosis factor alpha and interleukin-1 beta. *J Virol* 1991; **65**: 6094–100.
116. Tornatore C, Meyers K, Atwood W et al. Temporal patterns of human immunodeficiency virus type 1 transcripts in human fetal astrocytes. *J Virol* 1994; **68**: 93–102.
117. Canki M, Thai JN, Chao W et al. Highly productive infection with pseudotyped human immunodeficiency virus type 1 (HIV-1) indicates no intracellular restrictions to HIV-1 replication in primary human astrocytes. *J Virol* 2001; **75**: 7925–33.
118. Gorry PR, Howard JL, Churchill MJ et al. Diminished production of human immunodeficiency virus type 1 in astrocytes results from inefficient translation of gag, env, and nef mRNAs despite efficient expression of Tat and Rev. *J Virol* 1999; **73**: 352–61.
119. Ludwig E, Silberstein FC, van Empel J et al. Diminished rev-mediated stimulation of human immunodeficiency virus type 1 protein synthesis is a hallmark of human astrocytes. *J Virol* 1999; **73**: 8279–89.
120. Atwood WJ, Tornatore CS, Traub R et al. Stimulation of HIV type 1 gene expression and induction of NF-kappa B (p50/p65)-binding activity in tumor necrosis factor alpha-treated human fetal glial cells. *AIDS Res Hum Retroviruses* 1994; **10**: 1207–11.
121. Bezzi P, Volterra A. The active role of astrocytes in synaptic transmission. *Cell Mol Life Sci* 1999; **56**: 1–100.
122. Patton HK, Zhou ZH, Bubien JK et al. gp120-induced alterations of human astrocyte function: Na^+/H^+ exchange, K^+ conductance, and glutamate flux. *Am J Physiol Cell Physiol* 2000; **279**: C700–8.
123. Bezzi P, Domercq M, Brambilla L et al. CXCR4-activated astrocyte glutamate release via TNFalpha: amplification by microglia triggers neurotoxicity. *Nat Neurosci* 2001; **4**: 702–10.
124. Koller H, Schaal H, Freund M et al. HIV-1 protein Tat reduces the glutamate-induced intracellular Ca^{2+} increase in cultured cortical astrocytes. *Eur J Neurosci* 2001; **14**: 1793–9.
125. Wang Z, Pekarskaya O, Bencheikh M et al. Reduced expression of glutamate transporter EAAT2 and impaired glutamate transport in human primary astrocytes exposed to HIV-1 or gp120. *Virology* 2003; **312**: 60–73.
126. Lipton SA, Rosenberg PA. Excitatory amino acids as a final common pathway for neurologic disorders. *N Engl J Med* 1994; **330**: 613–22.
127. Ferrarese C, Aliprandi A, Tremolizzo L et al. Increased glutamate in CSF and plasma of patients with HIV dementia. *Neurology* 2001; **57**: 671–5.
128. Speth C, Stockl G, Mohsenipour I et al. Human immunodeficiency virus type 1 induces expression of complement factors in human astrocytes. *J Virol* 2001; **75**: 2604–15.
129. Speth C, Stoiber H, Dierich MP. Complement in different stages of HIV infection and pathogenesis. *Int Arch Allergy Immunol* 2003; **130**: 247–57.
130. Conant K, Garzino-Demo A, Nath A et al. Induction of monocyte chemoattractant protein-1 in HIV-1 Tat-stimulated astrocytes and elevation in AIDS dementia. *Proc Natl Acad Sci USA* 1998; **95**: 3117–21.
131. McManus CM, Weidenheim K, Woodman SE et al. Chemokine and chemokine-receptor expression in human glial elements: induction by the HIV protein, Tat, and chemokine autoregulation. *Am J Pathol* 2000; **156**: 1441–53.
132. Kelder W, McArthur JC, Nance-Sproson T et al. Beta-chemokines MCP-1 and RANTES are selectively increased in cerebrospinal fluid of patients with human immunodeficiency virus-associated dementia. *Ann Neurol* 1998; **44**: 831–5.
133. Yoshioka M, Bradley WG, Shapshak P et al. Role of immune activation and cytokine expression in HIV-1-associated neurologic diseases. *Adv Neuroimmunol* 1995; **5**: 335–58.
134. Griffin DE. Cytokines in the brain during viral infection: clues to HIV-associated dementia. *J Clin Invest* 1997; **100**: 2948–51.
135. Janabi N, Di Stefano M, Wallon C et al. Induction of human immunodeficiency virus type 1 replication in human glial cells after proinflammatory cytokines stimulation: effect of IFNgamma, IL1beta, and TNFalpha on differentiation and chemokine production in glial cells. *Glia* 1998; **23**: 304–15.
136. Fine SM, Angel RA, Perry SW et al. Tumor necrosis factor alpha inhibits glutamate uptake by primary human astrocytes.

Implications for pathogenesis of HIV-1 dementia. *J Biol Chem* 1996; **271**: 15303–6.
137. Rostasy K, Egles C, Chauhan A et al. SDF-1alpha is expressed in astrocytes and neurons in the AIDS dementia complex: an in vivo and in vitro study. *J Neuropathol Exp Neurol* 2003; **62**: 617–26.
138. Erichsen D, Lopez AL, Peng H et al. Neuronal injury regulates fractalkine: relevance for HIV-1 associated dementia. *J Neuroimmunol* 2003; **138**: 144–55.
139. Tong N, Perry SW, Zhang Q et al. Neuronal fractalkine expression in HIV-1 encephalitis: roles for macrophage recruitment and neuroprotection in the central nervous system. *J Immunol* 2000; **164**: 1333–9.
140. Cotter R, Williams C, Ryan L et al. Fractalkine (CX3CL1) and brain inflammation: implications for HIV-1-associated dementia. *J Neurovirol* 2002; **8**: 585–98.
141. Mizuno T, Kawanokuchi J, Numata K, Suzumura A. Production and neuroprotective functions of fractalkine in the central nervous system. *Brain Res* 2003; **979**: 65–70.
142. McManus C, Berman JW, Brett FM et al. MCP-1, MCP-2 and MCP-3 expression in multiple sclerosis lesions: an immunohistochemical and in situ hybridization study. *J Neuroimmunol* 1998; **86**: 20–9.
143. Sheng WS, Hu S, Lokensgard JR, Peterson PK. U50,488 inhibits HIV-1 Tat-induced monocyte chemoattractant protein-1 (CCL2) production by human astrocytes. *Biochem Pharmacol* 2003; **65**: 9–14.
144. Miller RJ, Meucci O. AIDS and the brain: is there a chemokine connection? *Trends Neurosci* 1999; **22**: 471–9.
145. Zink MC, Coleman GD, Mankowski JL et al. Increased macrophage chemoattractant protein-1 in cerebrospinal fluid precedes and predicts simian immunodeficiency virus encephalitis. *J Infect Dis* 2001; **184**: 1015–21.
146. Ferrando SJ, Rabkin JG, van Gorp W et al. Longitudinal improvement in psychomotor processing speed is associated with potent combination antiretroviral therapy in HIV-1 infection. *J Neuropsychiatry Clin Neurosci* 2003; **15**: 208–14.
147. Masliah E, DeTeresa RM, Mallory ME, Hansen LA. Changes in pathological findings at autopsy in AIDS cases for the last 15 years. *AIDS* 2000; **14**: 69–74.
148. Sacktor N, McDermott MP, Marder K et al. HIV-associated cognitive impairment before and after the advent of combination therapy. *J Neurovirol* 2002; **8**: 136–42.
149. Tamula MA, Wolters PL, Walsek C et al. Cognitive decline with immunologic and virologic stability in four children with human immunodeficiency virus disease. *Pediatrics* 2003; **112**: 679–84.
150. Major EO, Rausch D, Marra C, Clifford D. HIV-associated dementia. *Science* 2000; **288**: 440–2.
151. Powderly WG. Current approaches to treatment for HIV-1 infection. *J Neurovirol* 2000; **6**(Suppl 1): S8–13.
152. Almer G, Guegan C, Teismann P et al. Increased expression of the pro-inflammatory enzyme cyclooxygenase-2 in amyotrophic lateral sclerosis. *Ann Neurol* 2001; **49**: 176–85.
153. McGeer PL, McGeer EG. Inflammation, autotoxicity and Alzheimer disease. *Neurobiol Aging* 2001; **22**: 799–809.
154. Almer G, Teismann P, Stevic Z et al. Increased levels of the pro-inflammatory prostaglandin PGE2 in CSF from ALS patients. *Neurology* 2002; **58**: 1277–9.
155. Bamberger ME, Landreth GE. Inflammation, apoptosis, and Alzheimer's disease. *Neuroscientist* 2002; **8**: 276–83.
156. Eikelenboom P, Bate C, Van Gool WA et al. Neuroinflammation in Alzheimer's disease and prion disease. *Glia* 2002; **40**: 232–9.
157. Maier CM, Chan PH. Role of superoxide dismutases in oxidative damage and neurodegenerative disorders. *Neuroscientist* 2002; **8**: 323–34.
158. Hunot S, Hirsch EC. Neuroinflammatory processes in Parkinson's disease. *Ann Neurol* 2003; **53**(Suppl 3): S49–58; discussion S58–60.
159. Meucci O, Miller RJ. gp120-induced neurotoxicity in hippocampal pyramidal neuron cultures: protective action of TGF-beta1. *J Neurosci* 1996; **16**: 4080–8.
160. Rogawski MA, Wenk GL. The neuropharmacological basis for the use of memantine in the treatment of Alzheimer's disease. *CNS Drug Rev* 2003; **9**: 275–308.
161. Le DA, Lipton SA. Potential and current use of N-methyl-D-aspartate (NMDA) receptor antagonists in diseases of aging. *Drugs Aging* 2001; **18**: 717–24.
162. Kriz J, Nguyen MD, Julien JP. Minocycline slows disease progression in a mouse model of amyotrophic lateral sclerosis. *Neurobiol Dis* 2002; **10**: 268–78.
163. Thomas M, Le WD, Jankovic J. Minocycline and other tetracycline derivatives: a neuroprotective strategy in Parkinson's disease and Huntington's disease. *Clin Neuropharmacol* 2003; **26**: 18–23.
164. Wang X, Zhu S, Drozda M et al. Minocycline inhibits caspase-independent and -dependent mitochondrial cell death pathways in models of Huntington's disease. *Proc Natl Acad Sci USA* 2003; **100**: 10483–7.

27

Autoimmune component in anorexia and bulimia nervosa

Serguëi O Fetissov

INTRODUCTION

Anorexia nervosa (AN) and bulimia nervosa (BN) are two officially recognized eating disorders that affect about 3% of women over their lifetime.[1,2] They may also occur in men, although in lower proportions (1 vs. 10–30 in women). Both illnesses usually make their debut at a young age, are characterized by hyperactivity, exaggerated concern about body shape and weight, and often occur in the same patients.[3] AN is manifested by an aversion to food and amenorrhea with decrease in food intake often underlying life-threatening weight loss (restrictive type of AN), whereas BN includes large uncontrolled eating episodes normally without significant change in body weight. When BN is accompanied by AN, hyperphagia is followed by voluntary vomiting or use of laxatives (binge-purging type of AN) resulting in a malnourished condition and loss of weight. The mortality rate in AN is estimated around 2–10% over a period of 5–10 years for both males and females; suicide accounts for almost half of the deaths.[4] Mortality in BN is considerably lower than in AN.[5]

For the purpose of this chapter, it is important to emphasize that both AN and BN have for a long time been recognized as hypothalamic disorders of unknown etiology.[6,7] In fact, it has been stressed that the main symptoms of AN, such as low basal metabolic rate, amenorrhea, weight loss, bradycardia, low blood pressure, poikilothermia, and some degree of diabetes insipidus can all be reproduced by selective lesions of hypothalamic nuclei in experimental animals. Accordingly, studies investigating the activity of hypophyseotropic factors such as corticotrophin releasing factor (CRH) and luteinizing hormone releasing hormone (LHRH) in anorexia revealed a decreased ability to stimulate secretion of anterior pituitary hormones.[8] However, in spite of convincing data pointing to a hypothalamic origin of AN, its etiology is still unclear and complicated by the presence of psychological factors. Suitable animal models of AN, which could reproduce this human disease and may help to uncover underlying neurochemical mechanisms, have not been identified.

Another recent approach to understanding eating disorders is based on the finding that neuropeptides and monoamines are the main molecules responsible for neurochemical mechanisms that regulate appetite, body weight, and other homeostatic functions which occur primarily in the hypothalamus.[9,10] A modern model of energy metabolism regulation consists of a central integrative role for some hypothalamic neurons which can be responsible for the maintenance of the body weight set-point.[11] These neurons include those in the paraventricular nucleus[12] and in the lateral hypothalamic area.[13] Thus, peripheral hormones such as leptin, insulin, and ghrelin are relayed in the hypothalamic arcuate nucleus, bringing information about the metabolic status to these integratory neurons. The autonomic nervous system also sends its afferents to the hypothalamic neurons via the nucleus of the tractus solitarius and other hindbrain nuclei. Both the arcuate and the ascending hindbrain systems contain neuropeptides but monoamines such as noradrenaline and serotonin are confined to the hindbrain neurons.

In a search for possible pathogenic mechanisms of appetite deregulation, one may hypothesize that one or several peptidergic or monoaminergic brain systems involved in the regulation of appetite could be potentially targeted by autoantibodies (autoAbs) in patients with eating disorders. This hypothesis was explored to some extent by several investigators,[14,15] and more recently autoAbs against α-melanocyte-stimulating hormone (α-MSH), adrenocorticotropic hormone (ACTH), and LHRH were identified in AN and BN patients.[16] Since α-MSH, ACTH, and LHRH are neuropeptides critically involved in neuroendocrine mechanisms responsible for appetite control, stress response, and reproductive function, this finding opens a new perspective on the origin of AN and BN.

It is important to emphasize, however, that the finding of autoimmunity does not necessarily signify an autoimmune disease or an implication of autoantibodies in the main pathological process. Also, the finding of autoAbs against neuropeptides in apparently normal control subjects points to some underestimated interactions between the nervous and immune systems which may exert some important physiological functions. In fact, evidence for an antihormonal response by the immune system was collected more than 60 years ago,[17] but remained largely unexplored. Therefore, in the future, it will be of importance to study the mechanisms of origin of these antipeptide autoAbs, their possible mechanisms of interference with normal neuronal and hormonal messengers, and their relevance to eating disorders. Nevertheless, more frequent occurrence of autoAbs in patients with eating disorders than in controls suggests that these three identified autoAbs (against α-MSH, ACTH, and LHRH) may be involved in the pathogenesis of AN and BN and possible mechanisms of their action will be discussed below in more detail.

AUTOANTIBODIES AGAINST α-MSH

Cleavage of the precursor molecule proopiomelanocortin (POMC) yields α-MSH, ACTH, and several other biologically active peptides. This process is site-specific, giving different combinations of cleaved peptides in different locations in which the POMC gene is expressed; this may also depend on the local activity of endopeptidases. The highest synthesis of α-MSH occurs in the intermediate pituitary lobe melanotrophes as well as in the brain arcuate nucleus and some peripheral sites. α-MSH fibers innervate the hypothalamus extensively, suggesting active participation of α-MSH in homeostatic regulation. Accordingly, binding of α-MSH as well as ACTH in the brain was shown to be concentrated primarily in the hypothalamus.[18] α-MSH acts on melanocortin (MC) receptors, which are seven transmembrane G-protein-coupled receptors, and stimulates adenylyl cyclase. It should be noted that α-MSH shares receptors with ACTH with the exception of the MC2 receptor which is specific for ACTH and is expressed in the adrenal cortical cells.

Based on the distribution of melanocortin receptors[19] and clinical sequelae of AN, the possible sites where α-MSH autoAbs may interfere with normal functioning of α-MSH-mediated signaling include both peripheral tissues and the central nervous system. More than half of AN/BN patients have autoAbs which bind to pituitary melanotrophes; however, only part of them could bind to the α-MSH-producing cells in the arcuate nucleus. One explanation for this discrepancy could be a very high concentration of α-MSH in the melanotrophes, so that some sera with relatively low affinity for α-MSH autoAbs will have an undetectable binding to the arcuate α-MSH-producing neurons with a normally low α-MSH content. Whether this difference in binding has functional significance remains to be established, but it could be suggested that lower affinity autoAbs can preferentially affect the peripheral effects of α-MSH.

The peripheral effects of α-MSH are mainly assigned to increasing pigmentation via action on the MC1 receptors in melanocytes, due to dispersion of melanophores. This effect of α-MSH is antagonized by melanin-concentrating hormone (MCH), a hormone which decreases pigmentation by concentrating the melanophores within melanocytes. The amino acid sequence of a fragment of MCH precursor molecule is homologous to α-MSH,[20] and is also targeted by α-MSH autoAbs as revealed on hypothalamic slices.[16] Although a change of skin pigmentation has clear significance in some lower vertebrates, the functional importance of this action in humans is not clear. Nevertheless melanocytes appear to play an important function in maintaining skin and hair homeostasis in humans.[21] Hence, yellow palms, a symptom which is constantly found in AN patients, can be of possible relevance to circulating α-MSH autoAbs. α-MSH normally stimulates production of a brown pigment eumelanin and an increase of a yellow pigment phaeomelanin occurs when α-MSH action on melanocytes is antagonized by agouti protein.[22] In half of AN patients, dry scaly skin and fine lightly pigmented lanugo-type hair are also observed. Therefore, α-MSH autoAbs may be in part responsible for skin and hair defects found in AN patients.

Other effects of α-MSH include anti-inflammatory and immunomodulatory actions,[23] mediated via MC receptors expressed in leukocytes, macrophages, and T- and B-lymphocytes,[24–27] as well as via the central nervous system.[28,29] Possible relevance of these α-MSH anti-inflammatory and immunomodulatory effects to the clinical characteristics of AN is reflected by the peculiar state of the immune system in AN patients. In fact, the functional condition of the immune system in AN patients is surprisingly well preserved, with subtle deviations from healthy controls, a phenomenon studied in detail by several investigators.[30–33] Usually, conditions of malnutrition which are not associated with AN are accompanied by inhibition of normal function of the immune system, an effect regulated in the central nervous system,[34] with an important contribution from circulating cytokines such as leptin.[35] Consequently, starved subjects are susceptible to infections. This situation does not occur in AN patients, at least until the very late stage of cachexia, suggesting a dissociation between the nervous and immune systems.[36] Alterations in cellular immunity found in AN are minimal and represented by a decrease in the CD4/CD8 ratio.[37] Although a decrease in the CD4/CD8 ratio can be a mere reflection of malnutrition,[38] the significance of this change with regard to autoimmunity in AN is noteworthy since a relative increase in CD8 may indicate an ongoing autoimmune process.[39] Thus, whether α-MSH autoAbs in AN patients can contribute to dissociation between the normally co-ordinated functioning of the nervous and immune systems is worth investigation.

The presence of α-MSH autoAbs may also interfere with normal functioning of the hypothalamo-pituitary-gonadal axis. A stimulatory effect of α-MSH on LHRH, luteinizing hormone (LH), and prolactin was reported,[40] and interestingly, injection of α-MSH antiserum in lactating rats severely attenuated suckling-induced rise in serum prolactin.[41] Since around one-half of AN patients develop amenorrhea together with anorexia and a comparable number of AN patients display binding of sera to melanotrophes, it is possible that α-MSH autoAbs may directly interfere with the hypothalamo-pituitary-gonadal axis.

Other peripheral effects of α-MSH that could be compromised in AN may include its effect on bone turnover,[42,43] lipolysis and leptin secretion in adipocyte,[44,45] and insulin secretion by pancreatic cells.[46]

From the functional point of view, which provides a new hypothesis on the origin of feeding disturbances in AN and BN, the most important site where α-MSH autoAbs are relevant to anorexia or bulimia appears to be the central nervous system. This hypothesis will be discussed below.

AUTOANTIBODIES AGAINST ACTH

ACTH is the main secretagogue for adrenal corticosteroids, representing an essential component of the hypothalamo-pituitary-adrenal (HPA) axis. Besides its main production site in the anterior pituitary, ACTH synthesis has also been found in the POMC neurons of the hypothalamic arcuate nucleus,[47] and in the leukocytes.[48]

A clear selective binding of AN sera to the anterior pituitary corticotrophes was not as frequent as binding to melanotrophes. This is somewhat surprising, because the α-MSH molecule represents the first 13 amino acids of the ACTH (see Figure 27.1). However, it was also surprising that an adsorption test was sometimes more efficient with ACTH than with α-MSH to block binding of AN sera to the melanotrophes. These discrepancies can be understood only when the actual site of binding of autoantibodies to these two molecules is determined. As discussed above for α-MSH autoAbs, ACTH autoAbs may act in some central and peripheral sites according to the distribution of melanocortin receptors.

Abnormality of the HPA axis in AN is a well-known phenomenon which has been studied extensively but is still not completely understood. In fact, AN patients display a high–normal or elevated plasma cortisol concentration; however, they do not exhibit symptoms of hypercortisolism.[49] Thus, peripheral resistance to cortisol has been proposed,[50] and the hypothesis that AN is a compensatory reaction to overcome cortisol resistance has been offered.[51] In fact, AN patients are often restless and engage in physical activity which normally increases cortisol concentration.[52] However, this change in physical activity could be a result of a central mechanism of adaptation to stress and starvation[53] rather than an unconscious or conscious willingness to feel better. Moreover, hypercorticosolism may contribute to the depressive state[54,55] often found in AN/BN patients.[56] Thus, the present consensus is that the primary defect of the HPA in AN is located in the hypothalamus. This consensus is based on data showing that the ACTH response to CRH is blunted in AN, and because in the cerebrospinal fluid, CRH levels are high[57,58] but ACTH levels are low.[59] Since ACTH is also known to stimulate dehydroepiandrosterone (DHEA) secretion in the adrenal cortex,[60] the low DHEA and its sulfate levels found in AN can also be related to insufficient ACTH activity.

Thus, the presence of ACTH autoAbs in AN patients is consistent with the theory of an HPA defect, and explains the blunted ACTH response to CRH. Elevated cortisol concentrations in AN may also be related to circulating ACTH autoAbs, since elevated cortisol levels were found in both of two control subjects who displayed α-MSH/ACTH autoAbs.[16] The mechanism of this connection is not clear but one can suggest that autoAbs can prevent degradation of ACTH by endopeptidases and prolong the action of ACTH on its receptors following

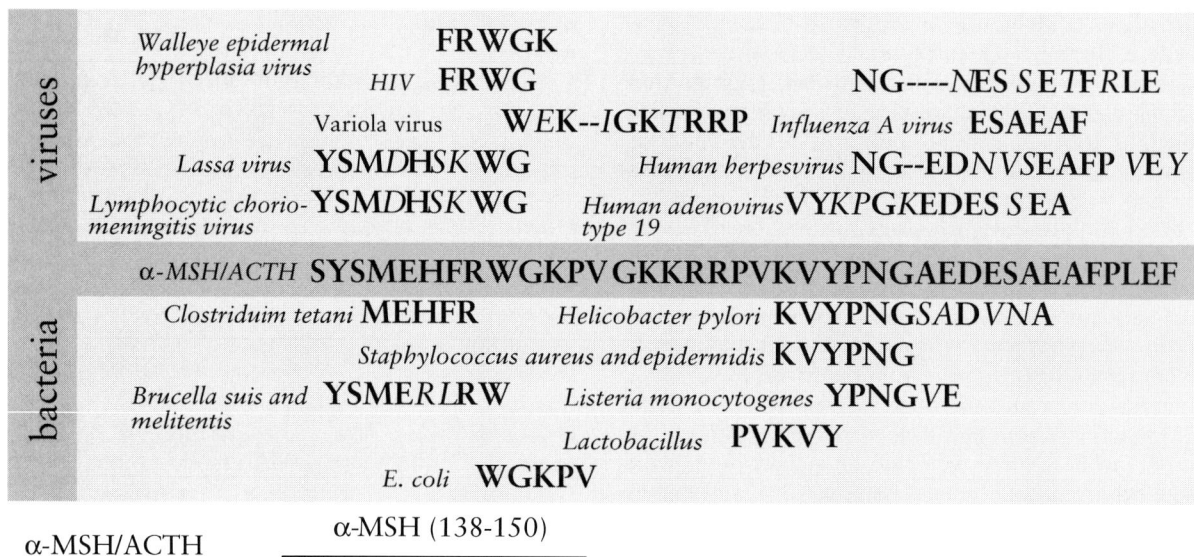

Figure 27.1 Several bacteria and viruses have proteins which display homology of amino acid sequences with α-MSH and ACTH.

binding. The presence of α-MSH autoAbs can also add to malfunction of the HPA axis since α-MSH concentration is increased in response to stress,[61] and α-MSH was shown to stimulate cortisol secretion via increasing CRH release.[62] ACTH deficiency and hypocorticosolism were reported in a patient with anticorticotrophe autoAbs, providing another example of a possible autoimmune attack on the HPA axis.[63]

HYPOTHESIS: CENTRAL ACTION OF α-MSH AND ACTH AUTOANTIBODIES ALTERS APPETITE IN AN AND BN

Since AN is a CNS disease and its primary site of pathology is suggested to be in the hypothalamus, possible mechanisms of interference of α-MSH and ACTH autoAbs with the hypothalamic circuitries involved in the regulation of appetite must be considered. The arcuate nucleus of the hypothalamus is an important brain area for appetite control. It contains neuropeptide Y (NPY) and POMC neurons, which are accessible to peripheral hormones and therefore can also be reached by circulating autoAbs. Since both α-MSH and ACTH are releasable molecules, their interaction with autoAbs should occur in the brain extracellular space where different scenarios are possible.

The first possibility is that autoAbs can attenuate neurotransmission on MC receptors by binding the corresponding peptide. In the arcuate nucleus, both POMC and NPY neurons express melanocortin MC3 receptors.[64] Such a possibility is supported by the efficacy of blocking peptidergic neurotransmission via administration of commercial antipeptide Abs, including anti α-MSH Abs, into the brain.[29,65] Another example of circulating autoAbs against pituitary hormones is prolactin autoAbs, which appear to be protective in hyperprolactinemia in patients with systemic lupus erythematosus.[66] Thus, if effective in this way, an increase in α-MSH and ACTH release induced by stress or other stimuli will be partly neutralized by α-MSH and ACTH autoAbs, resulting in blunted response by MC receptor-expressing cells.

The second possibility is that antigen–Ab complexes of the α-MSH and ACTH peptides and their corresponding Abs can still bind to MC receptors, with resulting activation of the MC receptor-mediated intracellular pathway. In these peptide–antipeptide immune complexes, peptides can be protected from degradation by endopeptidases and may induce prolonged activation of MC receptor-expressing cells. An interesting observation found in AN is a decreased activity of prolyl endopeptidase, an enzyme responsible for degradation of several neuropeptides including α-MSH.[67] Thus, if α-MSH and ACTH are protected from degradation, this may result in a chronic activation of MC receptor-expressing cells.

Another possibility which may follow the formation of peptide–Ab immune complexes bound to MC receptors is activation of the complement system and cell-mediated immunity. These processes should ultimately lead to complement-mediated neuronal damage. In future studies using animal models of AN, it will be important to determine whether neurons are in fact attacked by the immune system and, if so, what type of neurons are targeted. In addition to lesion function, the complement system is also responsible for the elimination of immune complexes from circulation.

Thus, if one or several mechanisms of interference of autoAbs with normal MC transmission take place in AN, this may compromise normal regulation of feeding circuitry. Detection of α-MSH autoAbs in subjects without apparent eating disorders, however, suggests that the presence of these autoAbs does not automatically imply a dysregulation of central control of appetite and anorexia. It suggests that other disease-triggering factors exist which enable α-MSH and ACTH autoAbs to interfere with brain mechanisms of appetite. One of these factors could be a voluntary starvation which is known to produce a major effect on the neurochemistry of arcuate neurons, and is possibly mediated with an important contribution from the MC system. Another factor which can possibly trigger anorexia is related to a change in permeability of the blood brain barrier (BBB). Normally, central neurons cannot be reached by bloodstream macromolecules, but several conditions are known to increase BBB permeability and therefore may allow access of α-MSH, ACTH, and LHRH autoAbs to diverse groups of appetite regulatory neurons. Stress, trauma, and infection are known to increase BBB permeability and may possibly trigger AN in subjects with circulating α-MSH and ACTH autoAbs. Interestingly, α-MSH itself was shown to cross the BBB by a nonsaturable process and was able to increase BBB permeability to other molecules using this process to enter the brain.[68]

If autoAbs can cross the BBB, they can interfere with normal transmission on the MC4 receptor, another MC receptor involved in the regulation of appetite. As mentioned above, α-MSH autoAbs can also bind to MCH precursors. MCH-precursor-derived peptides were shown to mimic α-MSH signaling via MC1 receptors.[69] MCH-expressing neurons are located in the lateral hypothalamic area and project to the cortex and brainstem. MCH in CNS is known for its appetite stimulatory role and therefore its precursor molecule can also be a potential target for α-MSH autoAbs in AN. Another putative central mechanism of anorexia induced by α-MSH autoAbs can be related to a normally antagonizing effect of α-MSH on CRH-induced anorexia.[70]

Since the central regulation of appetite and food intake is a very complex and redundant mechanism, it is difficult to suggest all neurochemical mechanisms underlying the behavioral outcome based on the action of α-MSH and ACTH autoAbs. For instance, the neurotransmitter NPY, which potently stimulates appetite in ad libitum food conditions, decreases food intake when administered to starved, stressed, and hyperactive rats.[71] Thus, depending on the type of neurons primarily targeted by autoAbs and their functional state, it could be suggested that disruption in circuitries formed by these diverse neurons may produce binge eating behavior or resistance to food ingestion or alternating between both, which would ultimately constitute an eating disorder.

LHRH AUTOANTIBODIES

A small percentage of AN patients were found to have LHRH autoAbs. This is an intriguing finding because one-fifth of AN patients develop amenorrhea before significant weight loss. About one-half of AN patients develop amenorrhea concomitant with decrease in food intake, while other AN patients develop amenorrhea later when critical decrease of body weight occurs. Persistence of amenorrhea in AN patients was the reason to call AN a starvation-amenorrhea syndrome.[6] It is now generally accepted that the primary reason for amenorrhea is the impaired release of LHRH from hypothalamic neurons, resulting in insufficient stimulation of pituitary LH and FSH secretion.[72] Although LHRH autoAbs could explain LHRH functional deficiency in AN by preventing the normal stimulatory effect of LHRH on pituitary gonadotrophes, the presence of a small percentage of these autoAbs contradicts the validity of this hypothesis. Alternatively, some messengers such as NPY, which is increased strongly in the arcuate neurons during starvation, is known to inhibit reproductive function[73] and, as discussed above, α-MSH autoAbs can also play a role in inhibiting the hypothalamo-pituitary-gonadal axis. An experimental approach is needed to understand possible involvement of LHRH autoAbs in starvation-amenorrhea syndrome.

ORIGIN OF α-MSH, ACTH, AND LHRH AUTOANTIBODIES

With regard to the origins of α-MSH, ACTH, and LHRH autoAbs, we presently cannot speculate further than the mechanisms of involvement of these autoAbs in eating disorders. This situation is not unique for these antipeptide Abs; it also exists for a number of CNS and other autoimmune diseases where the exact origin of autoAbs has not as yet been identified.[74] According to the concept of an immune mechanism of chemical homeostasis,[75] endogenous substances including hormones may induce an autoimmune response following their increased secretion and direct binding to their receptors on lymphocytes. This concept is very interesting with regard to the origin of antipeptide autoAbs in AN/BN patients. Whether and how a presumably adaptive mechanism becomes pathogenic should be investigated. However, for many autoimmune diseases one of the main hypotheses on the origin of autoAbs depends on the concept of molecular mimicry.[76] The response of the immune system against antigens of infectious organisms can by happenstance also be directed against selfproteins if they appear to have identical structures to the pathogens. So far, however, no strong link between AN and infectious diseases has been reported, but it could be that some viral or microbial infections noticed by the immune system may have occurred long before the onset of AN. Alternatively, formation of immune system memory against some unexpected epitopes can be associated with active immunization. A link between possible streptococcal infection and AN has been proposed based on the more frequent occurrence of lymphocyte B marker D8/17 in AN patients with possible PANDAS (pediatric autoimmune neuropsychiatric disorders associated with streptococcus).[77] This marker was originally described as being selective for rheumatic fever,[78] but later it was also found in several neuropsychiatric conditions termed PANDAS.[79] The significance of the D8/17 marker in neuropsychiatric disorders needs to be clarified, since it was found to be equally prevalent in healthy controls and patients with obsessive-compulsive disorder,[80] and there is no significant association of D8/17 with preceding streptococcal infection.[81]

To test the possibility of applying the concept of molecular mimicry to the origin of α-MSH, ACTH, and LHRH autoAbs, the amino acid sequences for α-MSH, ACTH, and LHRH have been 'blasted' against the protein databases of viruses and bacteria at the National Center for Biotechnology Information (Bethesda, MD, www.ncbi.nlm.nih.gov) to search for homology. Figure 27.1 illustrates the results of this search, in which common human pathogens appeared to have homology in their proteins with α-MSH and ACTH. Among the viruses, influenza A virus NS1 protein displayed homology of six amino acids with ACTH and could be of interest due to its common occurrence. Although HIV does not seem of importance for the origin of autoAbs, some evidence exists that HIV-infected individuals have better prognosis if they have higher α-MSH plasma concentration.[82] Therefore, if they develop Abs which can cross react with α-MSH, it may worsen the disease. In bacteria, *E. coli* and *Clostridium tetani* both showed a five amino acid homology to α-MSH, and *Helicobacter*, *Staphylococcus*, and *Lactobacillus* also showed some homology to ACTH and could be of potential interest. Interestingly, in a study of 32 patients with eating disorders 18% of AN, 18% of BN, and 25% of AN/BN patients were tested positive for *Helicobacter pylori*.[83] LHRH sequence also was found to have homology with several viral and bacterial proteins (Figure 27.2), such as human herpes virus, and again *E. coli*, *Helicobacter*, and *Lactobacillus*. Together with *Streptococcus* these microorganisms can potentially be common immunogens in the human population.

It is not known if the immune system can develop memory associated with specific fragments of these microorganisms homologous to neuropeptides. Moreover, if this memory exists, the factors which trigger the immune system to activate antibody production are also unknown. Since the onset of AN usually occurs in 14-year-old girls, one can suggest that increased secretion of α-MSH, ACTH, and LHRH associated with hormonal changes of puberty or with stress can trigger an activation of the immune system. In this regard it is noteworthy that secretion of both pituitary α-MSH and prolactin are mainly regulated by dopamine neurons from the mediobasal hypothalamus.

Although autoAbs against α-MSH, ACTH, and LHRH have not been previously described, a number of natural autoAbs exist which react with structural and releasable substances,[84–87] and may represent the first line of defense against pathogens.[88,89] Occurrence of natural autoAbs was also studied in bulimic patients and a decrease in IgG reacting against dopamine and/or serotonin was found to be lower in bulimics than in controls.[14] Whether autoAbs against α-MSH, ACTH, and LHRH also belong to the repertoire of natural autoAbs as a part of the innate immune system remains to be clarified. One study has described an increase in AN sera binding to human putamen homogenates, but the nature of a possible antigen was not explored.[15] AN and BN also have strong genetic links,[90,91] but which genes are implicated is not yet known. Since AN patients are susceptible to other autoimmune disorders such as type 1 diabetes,[92] a possible genetic background for this increased autoimmunity should be explored.

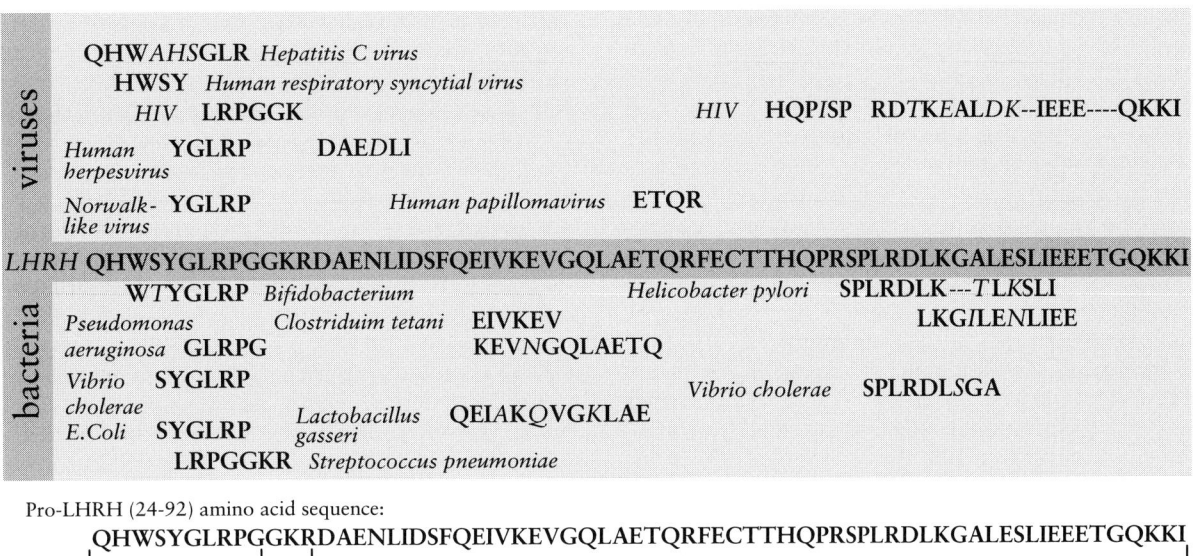

Figure 27.2 Several bacteria and viruses have proteins which display homology of amino acid sequences with LHRH.

CONCLUSION

Although the presence of α-MSH and ACTH autoAbs can explain many symptoms and endocrine findings in AN and BN patients, more research and different approaches are needed to confirm the importance of these autoAbs in the development of eating disorders.

Moreover, our preliminary studies indicate that α-MSH and ACTH autoAbs found in AN and BN are in fact not specific for AN and BN but may also occur in other stress-related neuropsychiatric disorders.[93] However, this finding should not prompt us to underestimate the pathophysiological significance of these autoAbs. Rather, it suggests that autoAbs can be responsible for the malfunctioning HPA axis, which, when combined with different genetic backgrounds and psychophysiological factors, can precipitate into several distinct neuropsychiatric disorders. Also, since control of appetite is a function precisely regulated in the brain, and which together with adaptation to stress involves the melanocortin system, a derangement of the stress axis should always be accompanied by changes in food intake. At present, these statements are hypothetical and the significance of the autoimmune component in the etiology and pathogenesis of AN and BN still needs to be clarified.

ACKNOWLEDGMENTS

To Carola Förster and Tomas Hökfelt, Karolinska Institutet. This study was supported by the Swedish MRC (04X-2887), Marianne and Marcus Wallenberg's Foundation, Knut and Alice Wallenberg's Foundation, Torsten and Ragnar Söderberg's Foundations, an Unrestricted Bristol-Myers Squibb Neuroscience Grant, and the Wenner-Gren Foundations.

REFERENCES

1. Walsh BT, Devlin MJ. Eating disorders: progress and problems. *Science* 1998; **280**: 1387–90.
2. Fairburn CG, Harrison PJ. Eating disorders. *Lancet* 2003; **361**: 407–16.
3. Kaye WH, Klump KL, Frank GK, Strober M. Anorexia and bulimia nervosa. *Annu Rev Med* 2000; **51**: 299–313.
4. Theander S. Outcome and prognosis in anorexia nervosa and bulimia: some results of previous investigations, compared with those of a Swedish long-term study. *J Psychiatr Res* 1985; **19**: 493–508.
5. Quadflieg N, Fichter MM. The course and outcome of bulimia nervosa. *Eur Child Adolesc Psychiatry* 2003; **12**(Suppl 1): I99–109.
6. Vande Wiele RL. Anorexia nervosa and the hypothalamus. *Hosp Pract* 1977; **12**: 45–51.
7. Stoving RK, Hangaard J, Hansen-Nord M, Hagen C. A review of endocrine changes in anorexia nervosa. *J Psychiatr Res* 1999; **33**: 139–52.

8. Wilson JD, Foster DW, Wilson JD et al. *Williams Textbook of Endocrinology*. Philadelphia PA: WB Saunders Company, 1992.
9. Meguid MM, Fetissov SO, Varma M et al. Hypothalamic dopamine and serotonin in the regulation of food intake. *Nutrition* 2000; **16**: 843–57.
10. Schwartz MW, Woods SC, Porte D Jr et al. Central nervous system control of food intake. *Nature* 2000; **404**: 661–71.
11. Keesey RE, Hirvonen MD. Body weight set-points: determination and adjustment. *J Nutr* 1997; **127**: 1875S–83S.
12. Sawchenko PE, Brown ER, Chan RK et al. The paraventricular nucleus of the hypothalamus and the functional neuroanatomy of visceromotor responses to stress. *Prog Brain Res* 1996; **107**: 201–22.
13. Elias CF, Saper CB, Maratos-Flier E et al. Chemically defined projections linking the mediobasal hypothalamus and the lateral hypothalamic area. *J Comp Neurol* 1998; **402**: 442–59.
14. Corcos M, Atger F, Levy-Soussan P et al. Bulimia nervosa and autoimmunity. *Psychiatry Res* 1999; **87**: 77–82.
15. Harel Z, Hallett J, Riggs S et al. Antibodies against human putamen in adolescents with anorexia nervosa. *Int J Eat Disord* 2001; **29**: 463–9.
16. Fetissov SO, Hallman J, Oreland L et al. Autoantibodies against α-MSH, ACTH, and LHRH in anorexia and bulimia nervosa patients. *Proc Natl Acad Sci USA* 2002; **99**: 17155–60.
17. Collip JB, Selye H, Thomson DL. The antihormones. *Biol Rev* 1940; **15**.
18. Tatro JB. Melanotropin receptors in the brain are differentially distributed and recognize both corticotropin and alpha-melanocyte stimulating hormone. *Brain Res* 1990; **536**: 124–32.
19. MacNeil D, Howard A, Guan X et al. The role of melanocortins in body weight regulation: opportunities for the treatment of obesity. *Eur J Pharmacol* 2002; **450**: 93–109.
20. Bittencourt JC, Presse F, Arias C et al. The melanin-concentrating hormone system of the rat brain: an immuno- and hybridization histochemical characterization. *J Comp Neurol* 1992; **319**: 218–45.
21. Tsatmali M, Ancans J, Thody AJ. Melanocyte function and its control by melanocortin peptides. *J Histochem Cytochem* 2002; **50**: 125–33.
22. Lu D, Willard D, Patel IR et al. Agouti protein is an antagonist of the melanocyte-stimulating-hormone receptor. *Nature* 1994; **371**: 799–802.
23. Catania A, Airaghi L, Colombo G, Lipton JM. Alpha-melanocyte-stimulating hormone in normal human physiology and disease states. *Trends Endocrinol Metab* 2000; **11**: 304–8.
24. Johnson HM, Smith EM, Torres BA, Blalock JE. Regulation of the in vitro antibody response by neuroendocrine hormones. *Proc Natl Acad Sci USA* 1982; **79**: 4171–4.
25. Clarke BL, Bost KL. Differential expression of functional adrenocorticotropic hormone receptors by subpopulations of lymphocytes. *J Immunol* 1989; **143**: 464–9.
26. Bhardwaj R, Becher E, Mahnke K et al. Evidence for the differential expression of the functional alpha-melanocyte-stimulating hormone receptor MC-1 on human monocytes. *J Immunol* 1997; **158**: 3378–84.
27. Namba K, Kitaichi N, Nishida T, Taylor AW. Induction of regulatory T cells by the immunomodulating cytokines alpha-melanocyte-stimulating hormone and transforming growth factor-beta2. *J Leukoc Biol* 2002; **72**: 946–52.
28. Lipton JM, Zhao H, Ichiyama T et al. Mechanisms of antiinflammatory action of alpha-MSH peptides. In vivo and in vitro evidence. *Ann NY Acad Sci* 1999; **885**: 173–82.
29. Papadopoulos AD, Wardlaw SL. Endogenous alpha-MSH modulates the hypothalamic-pituitary-adrenal response to the cytokine interleukin-1beta. *J Neuroendocrinol* 1999; **11**: 315–9.
30. Staurenghi AH, Masera RG, Prolo P et al. Hypothalamic-pituitary-adrenal axis function, psychopathological traits, and natural killer (NK) cell activity in anorexia nervosa. *Psychoneuroendocrinology* 1997; **22**: 575–90.
31. Monteleone P, Maes M, Fabrazzo M et al. Immunoendocrine findings in patients with eating disorders. *Neuropsychobiology* 1999; **40**: 115–20.
32. Marcos A. Eating disorders: a situation of malnutrition with peculiar changes in the immune system. *Eur J Clin Nutr* 2000; **54**(Suppl 1): S61–4.
33. Brambilla F, Monti D, Franceschi C. Plasma concentrations of interleukin-1-beta, interleukin-6 and tumor necrosis factor-alpha, and of their soluble receptors and receptor antagonist in anorexia nervosa. *Psychiatry Res* 2001; **103**: 107–14.
34. Plata-Salaman CR. Central nervous system mechanisms contributing to the cachexia-anorexia syndrome. *Nutrition* 2000; **16**: 1009–12.
35. Matarese G, La Cava A, Sanna V et al. Balancing susceptibility to infection and autoimmunity: a role for leptin? *Trends Immunol* 2002; **23**: 182–7.
36. Brambilla F. Social stress in anorexia nervosa: a review of immuno-endocrine relationships. *Physiol Behav* 2001; **73**: 365–9.
37. Marcos A, Varela P, Santacruz I et al. Nutritional status and immunocompetence in eating disorders. A comparative study. *Eur J Clin Nutr* 1993; **47**: 787–93.
38. Chandra RK. Nutrition and immunology: from the clinic to cellular biology and back again. *Proc Nutr Soc* 1999; **58**: 681–3.
39. Neumann H, Medana IM, Bauer J, Lassmann H. Cytotoxic T lymphocytes in autoimmune and degenerative CNS diseases. *Trends Neurosci* 2002; **25**: 313–9.
40. Schioth HB, Watanobe H. Melanocortins and reproduction. *Brain Res Rev* 2002; **38**: 340–50.
41. Hill JB, Lacy ER, Nagy GM et al. Does alpha-melanocyte-stimulating hormone from the pars intermedia regulate suckling-induced prolactin release? Supportive evidence from morphological and functional studies. *Endocrinology* 1993; **133**: 2991–7.
42. Stenstrom A, Hansson LI, Thorngren KG. Influence of alpha-MSH and ACTH on cortical bone remodelling in hypophysectomized rats. *Experientia* 1979; **35**: 132–3.
43. Cornish J, Callon KE, Mountjoy KG et al. Alpha-melanocyte-stimulating hormone is a novel regulator of bone. *Am J Physiol Endocrinol Metab* 2003; **284**: E1181–90.
44. Boston BA, Cone RD. Characterization of melanocortin receptor subtype expression in murine adipose tissues and in the 3T3-L1 cell line. *Endocrinology* 1996; **137**: 2043–50.
45. Norman D, Isidori AM, Frajese V et al. ACTH and alpha-MSH inhibit leptin expression and secretion in 3T3-L1 adipocytes: model for a central-peripheral melanocortin-leptin pathway. *Mol Cell Endocrinol* 2003; **200**: 99–109.
46. Shimizu H, Tanaka Y, Sato N, Mori M. Alpha-melanocyte-stimulating hormone (MSH) inhibits insulin secretion in HIT-T 15 cells. *Peptides* 1995; **16**: 605–8.
47. Guy J, Leclerc R, Vaudry H, Pelletier G. Identification of a second category of alpha-melanocyte-stimulating hormone (alpha-MSH) neurons in the rat hypothalamus. *Brain Res* 1980; **199**: 135–46.
48. Blalock JE. Proopiomelanocortin and the immune-neuroendocrine connection. *Ann NY Acad Sci* 1999; **885**: 161–72.
49. Kaye WH. Neuropeptide abnormalities in anorexia nervosa. *Psychiatry Res* 1996; **62**: 65–74.
50. Gold PW, Gwirtsman H, Avgerinos PC et al. Abnormal hypothalamic-pituitary-adrenal function in anorexia nervosa. Pathophysiologic mechanisms in underweight and weight-corrected patients. *N Engl J Med* 1986; **314**: 1335–42.
51. Wheatland R. Alternative treatment considerations in anorexia nervosa. *Med Hypotheses* 2002; **59**: 710–5.

52. Davis C, Katzman DK, Kaptein S et al. The prevalence of high-level exercise in the eating disorders: etiological implications. *Compr Psychiatry* 1997; **38**: 321–6.
53. Kas MJ, Van Dijk G, Scheurink AJ, Adan RA. Agouti-related protein prevents self-starvation. *Mol Psychiatry* 2003; **8**: 235–40.
54. Belanoff JK, Rothschild AJ, Cassidy F et al. An open label trial of C-1073 (mifepristone) for psychotic major depression. *Biol Psychiatry* 2002; **52**: 386–92.
55. Gold PW, Drevets WC, Charney DS. New insights into the role of cortisol and the glucocorticoid receptor in severe depression. *Biol Psychiatry* 2002; **52**: 381–5.
56. O'Brien KM, Vincent NK. Psychiatric comorbidity in anorexia and bulimia nervosa: nature, prevalence, and causal relationships. *Clin Psychol Rev* 2003; **23**: 57–74.
57. Hotta M, Shibasaki T, Masuda A et al. The responses of plasma adrenocorticotropin and cortisol to corticotropin-releasing hormone (CRH) and cerebrospinal fluid immunoreactive CRH in anorexia nervosa patients. *J Clin Endocrinol Metab* 1986; **62**: 319–24.
58. Kaye WH, Gwirtsman HE, George DT et al. Elevated cerebrospinal fluid levels of immunoreactive corticotropin-releasing hormone in anorexia nervosa: relation to state of nutrition, adrenal function, and intensity of depression. *J Clin Endocrinol Metab* 1987; **64**: 203–8.
59. Gwirtsman HE, Kaye WH, George DT et al. Central and peripheral ACTH and cortisol levels in anorexia nervosa and bulimia. *Arch Gen Psychiatry* 1989; **46**: 61–9.
60. O'Connell Y, McKenna TJ, Cunningham SK. Effects of pro-opiomelanocortin-derived peptides on adrenal steroidogenesis in guinea-pig adrenal cells in vitro. *J Steroid Biochem Mol Biol* 1993; **44**: 77–83.
61. Kjaer A, Knigge U, Bach FW, Warberg J. Stress-induced secretion of pro-opiomelanocortin-derived peptides in rats: relative importance of the anterior and intermediate pituitary lobes. *Neuroendocrinology* 1995; **61**: 167–72.
62. Vecsernyes M, Biro E, Gardi J et al. Involvement of endogenous corticotropin-releasing factor in mediation of neuroendocrine and behavioral effects to alpha-melanocyte-stimulating hormone. *Endocr Res* 2000; **26**: 347–56.
63. Sauter NP, Toni R, McLaughlin CD et al. Isolated adrenocorticotropin deficiency associated with an autoantibody to a corticotroph antigen that is not adrenocorticotropin or other proopiomelanocortin-derived peptides. *J Clin Endocrinol Metab* 1990; **70**: 1391–7.
64. Bagnol D, Lu XY, Kaelin CB et al. Anatomy of an endogenous antagonist: relationship between Agouti-related protein and proopiomelanocortin in brain. *J Neurosci* 1999; **19**: 21–7.
65. Goodman CB, Heyliger S, Emilien B et al. Chronic exposure to antibodies directed against anti-opiate peptides alter delta-opioid receptor levels. *Peptides* 1999; **20**: 1419–24.
66. Leanos-Miranda A, Pascoe-Lira D, Chavez-Rueda KA, Blanco-Favela F. Persistence of macroprolactinemia due to antiprolactin autoantibody before, during, and after pregnancy in a woman with systemic lupus erythematosus. *J Clin Endocrinol Metab* 2001; **86**: 2619–24.
67. Maes M, Monteleone P, Bencivenga R et al. Lower serum activity of prolyl endopeptidase in anorexia and bulimia nervosa. *Psychoneuroendocrinology* 2001; **26**: 17–26.
68. Banks WA, Kastin AJ. Permeability of the blood-brain barrier to melanocortins. *Peptides* 1995; **16**: 1157–61.
69. Hintermann E, Tanner H, Talke-Messerer C et al. Interaction of melanin-concentrating hormone (MCH), neuropeptide E-I (NEI), neuropeptide G-E (NGE), and alpha-MSH with melanocortin and MCH receptors on mouse B16 melanoma cells. *J Recept Signal Transduct Res* 2001; **21**: 93–116.
70. Oohara M, Negishi M, Shimizu H et al. Alpha-melanocyte stimulating hormone (MSH) antagonizes anorexia by corticotropin releasing factor (CRF). *Life Sci* 1993; **53**: 1473–7.
71. Kas M, Bruijnzeel A, Haanstra J et al. A stressful event dissociates food stimulating systems in hypothalamic neurons; implications for obesity and anorexia nervosa. *Eur Neuropsychopharmacol* 2002; **12**(Suppl. 3): S90–1.
72. Devlin MJ, Walsh BT, Katz JL et al. Hypothalamic-pituitary-gonadal function in anorexia nervosa and bulimia. *Psychiatry Res* 1989; **28**: 11–24.
73. Sainsbury A, Schwarzer C, Couzens M et al. Y4 receptor knockout rescues fertility in ob/ob mice. *Genes Dev* 2002; **16**: 1077–88.
74. Whitney KD, McNamara JO. Autoimmunity and neurological disease: antibody modulation of synaptic transmission. *Ann Rev Neurosci* 1999; **22**: 175–95.
75. Bykova A, Baker E. The concept of an immune mechanism of chemical homeostasis and its importance in biology and medicine. *Nat Immun* 1998; **16**: 198–206.
76. Oldstone MB. Molecular mimicry and immune-mediated diseases. *Faseb J* 1998; **12**: 1255–65.
77. Sokol MS, Ward PE, Tamiya H et al. D8/17 expression on B lymphocytes in anorexia nervosa. *Am J Psychiatry* 2002; **159**: 1430–2.
78. Khanna AK, Buskirk DR, Williams RC Jr et al. Presence of a non-HLA B cell antigen in rheumatic fever patients and their families as defined by a monoclonal antibody. *J Clin Invest* 1989; **83**: 1710–6.
79. Swedo SE, Leonard HL, Mittleman BB et al. Identification of children with pediatric autoimmune neuropsychiatric disorders associated with streptococcal infections by a marker associated with rheumatic fever. *Am J Psychiatry* 1997; **154**: 110–2.
80. Eisen JL, Leonard HL, Swedo SE et al. The use of antibody D8/17 to identify B cells in adults with obsessive-compulsive disorder. *Psychiatry Res* 2001; **104**: 221–5.
81. Murphy TK, Benson N, Zaytoun A et al. Progress toward analysis of D8/17 binding to B cells in children with obsessive compulsive disorder and/or chronic tic disorder. *J Neuroimmunol* 2001; **120**: 146–51.
82. Airaghi L, Capra R, Pravettoni G et al. Elevated concentrations of plasma alpha-melanocyte stimulating hormone are associated with reduced disease progression in HIV-infected patients. *J Lab Clin Med* 1999; **133**: 309–15.
83. Hill KK, Hill DB, Humphries LL et al. A role for *Helicobacter pylori* in the gastrointestinal complaints of eating disorder patients? *Int J Eat Disord* 1999; **25**: 109–12.
84. Martin WJ, Martin SE. Thymus reactive IgM autoantibodies in normal mouse sera. *Nature* 1975; **254**: 716–8.
85. Sela BA, Wang JL, Edelman GM. Antibodies reactive with cell surface carbohydrates. *Proc Natl Acad Sci USA* 1975; **72**: 1127–31.
86. Guilbert B, Dighiero G, Avrameas S. Naturally occurring antibodies against nine common antigens in human sera. I. Detection, isolation and characterization. *J Immunol* 1982; **128**: 2779–87.
87. Dighiero G, Rose NR. Critical self-epitopes are key to the understanding of self-tolerance and autoimmunity. *Immunol Today* 1999; **20**: 423–8.
88. Bouvet JP, Dighiero G. From natural polyreactive autoantibodies to la carte monoreactive antibodies to infectious agents: is it a small world after all? *Infect Immun* 1998; **66**: 1–4.
89. Nielsen CH, Leslie RG, Jepsen BS et al. Natural autoantibodies and complement promote the uptake of a self antigen, human thyroglobulin, by B cells and the proliferation of thyroglobulin-reactive CD4(+) T cells in healthy individuals. *Eur J Immunol* 2001; **31**: 2660–8.

90. Grice DE, Halmi KA, Fichter MM et al. Evidence for a susceptibility gene for anorexia nervosa on chromosome 1. *Am J Hum Genet* 2002; **70**: 787–92.
91. Bulik CM, Devlin B, Bacanu SA et al. Significant linkage on chromosome 10p in families with bulimia nervosa. *Am J Hum Genet* 2003; **72**: 200–7.
92. Nielsen S, Borner H, Kabel M. Anorexia nervosa/bulimia in diabetes mellitus. A review and a presentation of five cases. *Acta Psychiatr Scand* 1987; **75**: 464–73.
93. Fetissov SO, Hallman H, Oreland L, Hökfelt T. Autoantibody binding profile to the brain and pituitary in neuropsychiatric disorders. European Neuropsychopharmacology 2003; **13**(Suppl. 4).

28

Infectious etiology of adult schizotypal personality: A paradigm and the evidence

Ricardo A Machón, Matti O Huttunen, and Sarnoff A Mednick

INTRODUCTION

This chapter will explore the potential infectious etiology of psychiatric disorders, especially schizotypal personality disorder. These findings will be examined in the context of the neurodevelopmental hypothesis of mental disorders. The evidence for the proposed paradigm points to a disruption of normal brain development during a critical prenatal period which increases the risk for adult schizophrenia spectrum disorders.

The possible infectious etiology of psychotic disorders was first proposed by Perfect in 1787.[1] He speculated on whether a case of insanity might be caused by influenza. Later, Kraepelin would note that infections during the years of development might be causally connected to dementia praecox.[2] Bleuler also recommended that additional research was necessary to study the potential involvement of an infectious process in schizophrenia.[3]

Interest in the possible etiology by infectious agents of psychiatric disorders was quickened by the discovery during the early decades of the 20th century that a spirochete was the cause of general paresis, the terminal stage of neurosyphilis. In 1926, Menninger published a report describing a series of 175 post-influenza psychoses following the great 1918 influenza pandemic.[4] He noted that a third of these resembled dementia praecox. Additionally, the cases of encephalitis lethargica (Von Economo's disease), presumably of viral etiology, which were discovered in the 1920s frequently presented as schizophrenia.[5]

The infectious hypothesis gained indirect support when Tramer first noted a seasonal effect for schizophrenia.[6] His sample of 3,100 cases comprised all patients admitted to a Swiss hospital during the years 1876–1927. He observed a modest increase (15%) in schizophrenic patients born in December through March. Other earlier studies conducted in the 1930s in Europe and the USA produced similar findings.[7–9] These earlier studies, marked by poor sampling and inadequate controls, went unnoticed and largely ignored.

Beginning in the late 1960s, a series of methodologically superior studies were published seeking to replicate the earlier seasonality findings. A series of convergent studies drawn from the northern and southern hemispheres and equatorial areas essentially replicated the basic finding of winter and early spring births of later-diagnosed schizophrenics.[10–17] In general the findings have been fairly robust and consistent; the effects appear to be modest in that the studies tend to show only a 5–15% excess of winter and early spring births among persons who are later diagnosed with schizophrenia. Influenza infection has been suspected of being etiologically involved since its seasonal peak also coincides with winter and the early spring months. Additionally, prenatal exposure has been linked with adverse CNS outcomes.[18,19] Torrey and Peterson proposed a formal virus hypothesis of the etiology of schizophrenia in a seminal article published in 1976.[20] The seasonality of schizophrenia findings have played a critical role, along with clinical, neuroimaging, and postmortem studies, in the advancement of a neurodevelopmental hypothesis of mental disorders.[1]

NEURODEVELOPMENT OF SCHIZOPHRENIA SPECTRUM DISORDERS

There now exists a solid body of evidence that schizophrenia and other major mental disorders may have, as one of their bases, an underlying neurodevelopmental etiology.[21–24] Specifically, the evidence suggests that at least one form of schizophrenia is due to a disruption of normal brain development during a critical prenatal risk period in the second trimester. Disturbances occurring during active development of certain critical brain areas (the mesolimbic system, the thalamus, and the entorhinal regions) may produce incomplete or inappropriate migration; incorrect positioning; failures of connection, misconnections, or all of the above.[25] Disruptions in these neural processes, in turn, may increase the probability of adult schizophrenia spectrum disorders as well as other major psychiatric disorders. Psychiatric epidemiological studies examining the association between prenatal exposure to influenza (or infection) and adult schizophrenia have played a major role in helping define this critical period of gestation.[1]

Some of the previous work suggests that the critical period may lie in the sixth month of gestation.[26–30] We have also completed a study indicating that a sixth-month, documented maternal infection is associated with cognitive deficit (poor habituation) in the offspring at a postnatal age of six months.[31] Our Helsinki maternal influenza studies also show that the timing of the exposure may be critical. While prenatal exposure in the fifth month is a risk factor for adult major affective disorder (mainly unipolar depression), exposure in the sixth month is a risk factor for adult schizophrenia,[32] as well as schizotypal personality.[33] Differential behavioral outcomes have also been noted in rats exposed to infection at various stages of neural development. Rubin and colleagues reported that exposure to a Borna disease virus at day 1 vs. day 15 yields different, deviant behavioral outcomes.[34] 'Unlike rats infected with Borna disease on postnatal day 1, postnatal day 15 inoculated rats did not show signs of cerebellar hypoplasia or hyperactivity. Thus the risk of BDV-induced damage to specific brain regions and their associated behaviors appears, in part, dependent upon the brain's developmental stage at the time of BDV infection.'

We have suggested that the basic genetic disorder of the schizophrenia spectrum is expressed as a severe form of disruption of neural development during a critical period in the sixth month of gestation. A teratogenic agent, such as influenza infection, an earthquake, or other stressor, disturbing the development of the fetus during the sixth month critical period may mimic the effects of this genetically-caused neurodevelopmental disruption, thereby increasing the risk for disorders of the schizophrenia spectrum.[24,35] We propose that the phenotypic manifestation of the basic genetic-neurodevelopmental disorder consists of characteristics approximated by the DSM-IV diagnosis of schizotypal personality disorder (SPD).[36] This model is based, in part, on the work of Paul Meehl, who first suggested that a schizotaxic disturbance in neural functioning predisposes to schizophrenia.[37] Decompensation to schizophrenia may result from the vulnerable individual being exposed to negative environments or other adventitious processes. From these considerations one would therefore predict an increase in SPD characteristics among individuals who have suffered a neurodevelopmental disruption in the sixth month of gestation, be it genetic or teratogenic in origin.

INFLUENZA AND SCHIZOTYPAL PERSONALITY

Peter Venables conducted a study examining the relation between influenza exposure during gestation and scores on a schizotypy scale administered to 17-year-olds as part of the Mauritius Study.[38] The schizotypy scale has a two-factor structure; Factor 1 (anhedonia) represents the more negative symptoms of schizotypy and Factor 2 (schizophrenism) represents the positive symptoms of schizotypy.

Venables reported that those exposed to maternal influenza as fetuses evidenced significantly elevated schizophrenism scale scores. When Venables examined the relationship by month of exposure, he noted a significant increase in schizophrenism scores among those exposed to the influenza epidemic in the fifth month of gestation. No significant elevation was noted for the anhedonia factor.

We have recently published a report in which we examined a database containing Minnesota Multiphasic Personality Inventory (MMPI) data for all male conscripts in Finland.[33] We identified individuals who, as fetuses, were exposed to the severe influenza epidemic (the 'Hong Kong flu') of 1969. We also identified a group of controls born during a relatively low year for infectious epidemics (1971); for these two groups, we compared the pattern of MMPI scale scores, indicative of SPD characteristics. A significantly higher proportion of sixth-month exposed index subjects (39%) had elevated schizotypal personality characteristics scale scores as compared to their controls (26%; $p < .003$). Further analyses revealed that these differences were accounted for by those exposed to the influenza epidemic in week 23 (51% vs. 24%) of the sixth month ($p < .005$). These results are summarized in Figure 28.1. Exploratory analyses for the other months did not reveal any significant differences. These findings replicated those of Venables.[38]

Venables reported a significant increase in positive schizotypy scores among those exposed to influenza during their fifth month of gestation (calculated on a

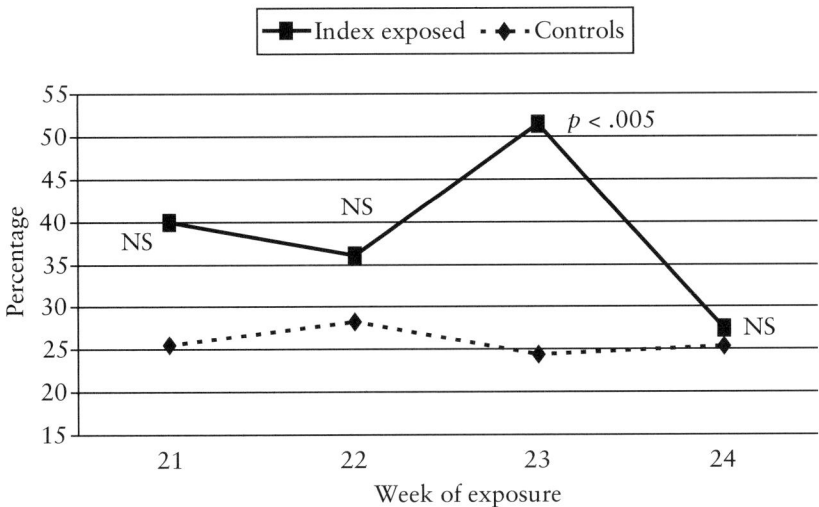

Figure 28.1 Scores in the upper quartile on SPD profile scale for weeks 21–24.

nine-month pregnancy);[38] we report a significant number of high scores of schizotypal personality characteristics among those exposed to influenza during their sixth month of gestation (calculated on a 40-week or 10-month pregnancy). Both reference points, however, correspond to the same relative gestational period – likely exposure to influenza five months prior to the birth of the fetus.

Our recent findings[33] and those of Venables[38] point to the relationship between positive features of schizotypy and prenatal influenza. We have previously reported that among patients with schizophrenia, those exposed to influenza in the second trimester had significantly higher levels of positive symptoms (delusions of jealousy, delusions of reference, and suspiciousness) as compared to schizophrenics exposed in the first or third trimester or controls.[32] There is compelling evidence suggesting that 'schizotypal personality is related to schizophrenia in terms of common phenomenological, outcome and treatment response characteristics'.[39] This may suggest that maternal exposure to second-trimester influenza increases the risk for some specific personality organization (positive features of schizotypy), which then places the individual at increased risk for later decompensation for schizophrenia depending on additional psychosocial and neuromaturational factors.

EARTHQUAKE AND SCHIZOTYPAL PERSONALITY

On 28 July 1976, a 7.9 (Richter scale) earthquake struck Tangshan, in the People's Republic of China. The epicenter of the quake was five miles east-by-northeast of Tangshan. The devastating effects of the quake included widespread destruction of houses and disruption of basic services. Countless numbers of Tangshan residents were injured; an estimated 240,000 people were killed. This catastrophic event (unpredictable and uncontrollable) represents a natural quasi-experiment since all Tangshan women who were pregnant were stressed by the quake at the same instant. In a series of analyses recently completed, we assessed symptoms of schizotypal personality disorder in a group of 18-year-old high school students whose mothers were exposed to the Tangshan earthquake, a non-viral stressor, at various stages of pregnancy (the index group). Their controls, born a year later, were not subjected to the earthquake (the control group).

One aim of this study was to try to replicate, in an independent sample, our earlier findings implicating the sixth month, and in particular the 23rd week of gestation, in later schizotypal personality characteristics.[33] We employed Raine's Schizotypy Personality Questionnaire-B (SPQ-B) to assess schizotypy.[40,41] The SPQ-B, which yields a total score and three subscale scores (cognitive perceptual disturbance; interpersonal deficit; and disorganization), has been translated and validated in a Chinese population.[42]

It was hypothesized that those exposed to the 1976 Tangshan earthquake in their sixth month (weeks 21–24) of gestation (the index group), would obtain higher mean scores on the SPQ-B than their controls born in the same month of the year but who were not exposed to the earthquake. We further predicted that among those index subjects exposed in the sixth month, those who were in their 23rd week of gestation would show the highest SPQ-B scores as compared to their controls.

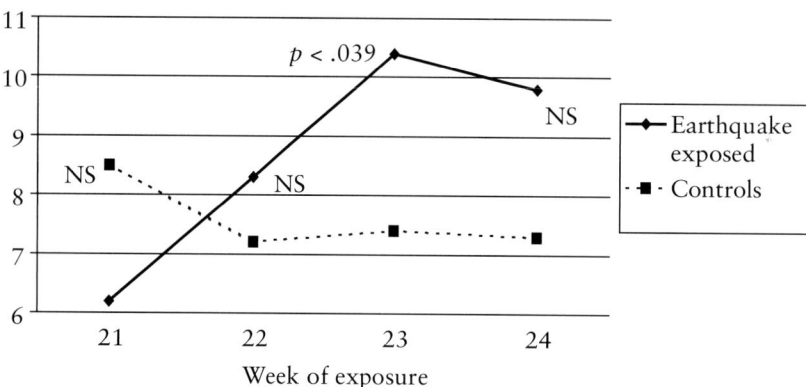

Figure 28.2 Mean SPQ-B total scale scores for earthquake exposed (index) subjects and controls by week of exposure in the sixth month.

The results indicated that index subjects exposed in their sixth month of gestation (weeks 21–24 combined) showed a statistically significant higher mean SPQ-B total scale score than their sixth month controls [$t(97.7) = 2.04$, $p < .04$]. Index subjects exposed in their sixth month also showed a statistically significant higher mean SPQ-B subscale cognitive perceptual score than their sixth month controls [$t(95.8) = 2.0$, $p < .049$]. Index subjects exposed in the sixth month and controls did not differ in their mean SPQ-B subscale interpersonal deficits score [$t(122) = 1.1$, $p > .05$]. There was a trend for index subjects exposed in their sixth month to show higher mean SPQ-B subscale disorganization scores than controls but these differences did not reach statistical significance [$t(122) = 1.8$, $p < .07$].

Based on our recent findings implicating the 23rd week in the sixth month of gestation as being relevant to schizotypal personality characteristics,[33] we then tested whether the observed differences in the sixth month were attributable to differences in the 23rd week of gestation. As predicted, those index subjects exposed in their 23rd week of gestation showed significantly higher mean SPQ-B total scale scores than their 23rd week controls [$t(39) = 2.1$, $p < .039$]. These results are presented in Figure 28.2. There was a trend for index subjects exposed in their 23rd week of gestation to show higher SPQ-B subscale cognitive perceptual scores than controls but these differences did not reach statistical significance [$t(39) = 1.6$, $p < .10$]. These results are presented in Figure 28.3. Index subjects exposed in the 23rd week did not differ in SPQ-B subscale interpersonal deficits score (3.2) from their sixth month controls [2.5; $t(39) = 1.2$, $p > .05$]. Index subjects exposed in their 23rd week of gestation exhibited significantly higher SPQ-B subscale disorganization scores (3.1) than controls [1.9; $t(39) = 2.3$, $p < .028$]. These results are presented in Figure 28.4.

Index subjects exposed in the 21st, 22nd, or 24th weeks of gestation did not differ from controls on either the SPQ-B total scale or the three SPQ-B subscales. We also compared the exposed index group scores with their corresponding controls on SPQ-B total scale and the three SPQ-B subscales for the other nine months of gestation (1–5 and 7–10) for which we had no hypothesis, adjusting the alpha level for

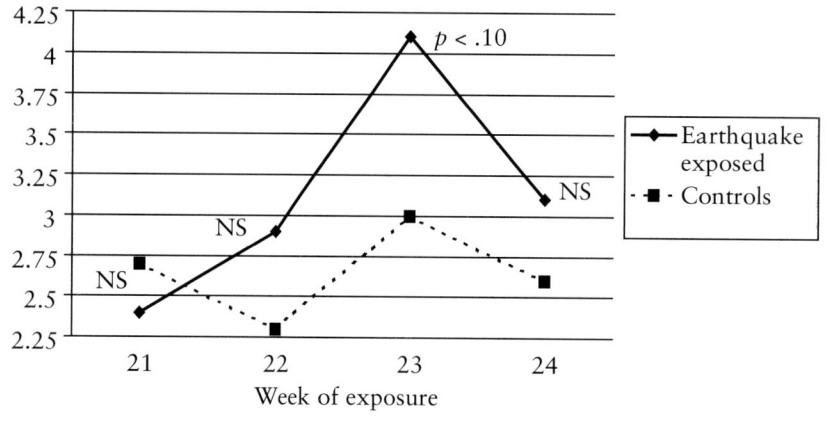

Figure 28.3 Mean SPQ-B cognitive perceptual subscale scores for earthquake exposed (index) subjects and controls by week of exposure in the sixth month.

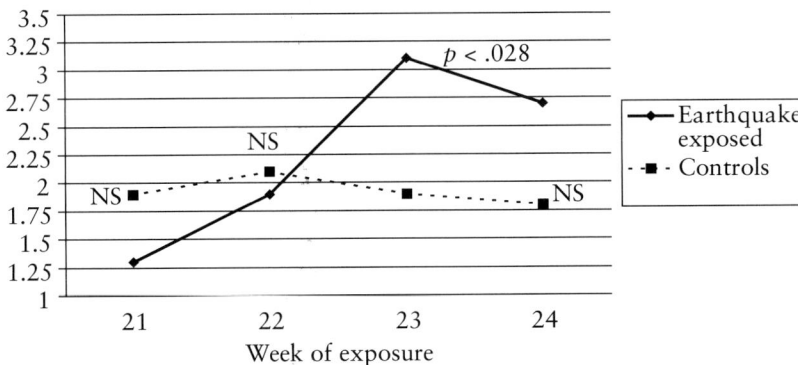

Figure 28.4 Mean SPQ-B disorganization subscale scores for earthquake exposed (index) subjects and controls by week of exposure in the sixth month.

these analyses with a Bonferroni correction set at .0055. No significant differences were noted.

POLIOVIRUS AND SCHIZOPHRENIA

Are there other viruses whose epidemiology supports the genesis of schizophrenia spectrum disorders? Several lines of evidence point to the potential causal relationship between polio and schizophrenia. A decrease in the incidence of schizophrenia in many countries followed the introduction of polio vaccination.[43] The winter seasonality of schizophrenic births could be explained by fetal exposure to poliovirus during the second trimester of gestation; this exposure would have occurred during the summer months when polio epidemics are most prevalent.[43] Additionally, geographic variation in the seasonality of poliomyelitis epidemics parallels the seasonality of births of individuals who are later diagnosed with schizophrenia.[14] Further convergent evidence is suggested from the latency of the effect of poliovirus. Following decades after a primary infection, a post-polio syndrome has been described. The brain areas affected by this syndrome parallel those of the schizophrenia disorder.[44]

Suvisaari and colleagues examined the relationship between prenatal exposure to poliovirus infection and adult schizophrenia.[45] They identified all Finnish patients ($n = 13{,}559$) born between 1951 and 1969 with discharge diagnoses of schizophrenia. They also obtained archival information on the monthly number of cases of paralytic poliomyelitis for each province in Finland. They found that exposure to poliovirus infection five months before birth increased the risk for the later development of schizophrenia. Without seasonality in the model, they observed stronger effects covering the whole of the second trimester, thus suggesting that exposure to poliovirus infection may explain some of the seasonality in births of individuals who as adults are diagnosed with schizophrenia.

SYNTHESIS

The pattern of results from Venables' Mauritius study,[38] our study of Finnish male conscripts,[33] and our recent China earthquake study support a neurodevelopmental basis for mental disorders, particularly schizotypal personality. This hypothesis suggests that disturbances at certain critical periods of neurodevelopment increase the risk for schizophrenia, major affective disorder, and perhaps the schizophrenia-spectrum, schizotypal personality disorder as well. Previous studies have pointed to the second trimester and in particular the sixth month as the critical period for disturbance. The results of the China earthquake study supported our primary aim of replicating our recent findings from Finland,[33] which showed that the window of vulnerability might lie in the 23rd week of gestation for increasing the risk for later, adult schizotypal personality. What might be the etiological significance of the 23rd week of gestation? What is the likely mechanism of the pathogenesis of schizophrenia spectrum disorders? Which is more critical: the type of stressor or disruptor of neurodevelopment or the timing in the neurodevelopmental process?

POSSIBLE SIGNIFICANCE OF 23RD WEEK

Both the China earthquake study and the Finnish male conscript study suggest that fetal neural maldevelopment in the 23rd week of gestation may increase risk for adult schizotypal personality characteristics. This could open new lines of inquiry. But there are two potential problems with this suggestion:

1) The gestational age of the subjects at the time of the earthquake was estimated from their date of birth. Some relative error in these estimates may be introduced by pre- and post-term births.
2) If we could appeal to a literature providing precise information on the areas or circuits of the

human brain which are developing rapidly in the 23rd week of gestation, we would be in a position to make interesting hypotheses regarding which brain areas are involved in the etiology of SPD and what this may portend for disturbed function. But such precision does not exist in the neurodevelopmental literature today.

We can, however, provide some general, plausible hypotheses. The timing (23rd week) adds to existing evidence that SPD is not a disorder of proliferation or migration. By the 23rd week of gestation, proliferation and migration to cortical and important subcortical areas are almost complete. At about this time, connections are forming between the cortex and subcortical layers. Axon growth is a central developmental focus. Of special interest are the connections and integration between deeper cortical layers and the thalamus and basal ganglia.[46,47] Thus, while we cannot be highly specific regarding brain systems at risk, we can say that our findings tend to:

1) Rule out disturbance of proliferation and migration as critical factors in the etiology of SPD
2) Support the study of deficits in axon growth between deeper cortical layers and the thalamus and basal ganglia.

MECHANISM OF ACTION IN PATHOGENESIS

Huttunen previously reported that rats subjected to prenatal stress evidenced disturbances in brain neurochemistry and behavior after their births.[48] More recent findings point to the key role that heat stress proteins play in regulating both the genetically and environmentally induced apoptosis of neuronal cells.[49] These proteins represent a central reaction of the body cells against all kinds of stress and their levels are increased in fever, stress, and so on. Their increase is known to distract the metabolism of fetal neurons from synaptic formation. This process may result in a failure of connection of the crucial neurons at a critical period (in the 23rd week) of the formation of connections.

McGlashan and Hoffman have proposed a model of schizophrenia as a disorder of developmentally reduced synaptic connectivity.[50] Early neurobiological lesions (neurodevelopmental deficits) are major determinants of childhood synaptic density and vulnerability to psychosis. Deterioration to full-blown schizophrenia results from the vulnerable-to-psychosis brain system being subjected to a normal or abnormal, developmentally-driven synaptic pruning process, which is accelerated during adolescence and young adulthood. Friston has posited an alternative mechanism.[51] He proposes that the pathophysiology of schizophrenia is marked by synaptic abnormalities and dysfunctional connectivity.

Thus, is schizophrenia a disorder of abnormal structural or functional/synaptic plasticity? Though these systems are commonly regarded as separate, they may represent two manifestations of a common, underlying process. The meaningful reconciliation of these two non-independent processes will undoubtedly advance our understanding of the etiology of schizophrenia spectrum disorders.

TYPE OF STRESSOR VS. TIMING OF STRESSOR

The bulk of the epidemiological studies supporting the neurodevelopmental hypothesis have shown the importance of exposure to prenatal influenza and later adult psychiatric outcomes.[1,32,52] Huttunen and Niskanen reported elevated rates of psychosis in the offspring of mothers who were informed during their second trimester of pregnancy that their husbands had been killed during the war.[53] Otake and Schull have noted that Hiroshima survivors who were second-trimester fetuses when the atomic bomb exploded later evidenced increased levels of cognitive disturbances (mainly mental retardation).[54] More recently, Selten and colleagues have reported that prenatal maternal exposure to severe stress (1953 Dutch flood) was associated with an increased risk for psychosis in the offspring.[55] Our recent findings reported above are the first to link exposure to an earthquake with a subsequent, young adult outcome. These findings, as a whole, tend to support the interpretation that the timing of the stressor during relevant and critical brain neurodevelopment is a more salient factor than the type of stressor.

REFERENCES

1. Bagalkote H, Pang D, Jones PB. Maternal influenza and schizophrenia in the offspring. In: *Risk Factors for Schizophrenia and Implications for Prevention–2, Int J Ment Health* (Bark N, guest ed) 2001; **29**(4): 3–21.
2. Kraepelin E. *Dementia Praecox and Paraphrenia*. New York: Robert E Krieger, 1919/1971.
3. Bleuler E. *Dementia Praecox or the Group of Schizophrenias*. New York: International Universities Press, 1911/1950.
4. Menninger KA. Influenza and schizophrenia. An analysis of post-influenzal 'dementia praecox' as of 1918 and five years later. *Am J Psychiatry* 1926; **5**: 469–529.

5. Crow TJ. Viral causes of psychiatric disease. *Postgrad Med J* 1978; **54**: 763–7.
6. Tramer M. Über die biologische Bedeutung des Geburtsmonates, insbesondere für die Psychoseerkrankung. *Schweitzer Archiv Neurologie Psychiatrie* 1929; **24**: 17–24.
7. Peterson WF. *The Patient and the Weather: Mental and Nervous Diseases*. Ann Harbor MI: Edwards Brothers, 1934.
8. Huntington E. *Season of Birth: Its Relation to Human Abilities*. New York: John Wiley & Sons, Inc, 1938.
9. Nolting WJJ de Sauvage. Het verband tusschen schizophrenie en aanverwante ziektebeelden en de geboortemaand. *Ned T Geneesk* 1934; **78**: 528–30.
10. Videbech T, Weeke A, Dupont A. Endogenous psychoses and season of birth. *Acta Psychiatr Scand* 1974; **50**: 202–18.
11. Dalén P. Month of birth and schizophrenia. *Acta Psychiatr Scand* 1968; **203**: 55–60.
12. Dalén P. *Season of Birth: A Study of Schizophrenia and Other Mental Disorders*. Amsterdam: North-Holland Publishing Co, 1975.
13. Odegaard O. Season of birth in the general population and inpatients with mental disorder in Norway. *Br J Psychiatry* 1974; **125**: 397–405.
14. Torrey EF, Torrey BB, Peterson MR. Seasonality of schizophrenic births in the United States. *Arch Gen Psychiatry* 1977; **34**: 1065–70.
15. Shimura M, Nakamura I, Miura T. Season of birth of schizophrenics in Tokyo, Japan. *Acta Psychiatr Scand* 1977; **55**: 225–32.
16. Dalén P, Roche SD. The South African sample. In: *Season of Birth: A Study of Schizophrenia and Other Mental Disorders* (Dalén P, ed). Amsterdam: North-Holland Publishing Co, 1975: 95–8.
17. Parker G, Neilson M. Mental disorder and season of birth: a southern hemisphere study. *Br J Psychiatry* 1976; **129**: 355–61.
18. Hakosalo JK, Saxén L. Influenza epidemic and congenital defects. *Lancet* 1971; **2**: 1346–7.
19. Coffey VP, Jessop WJE. Maternal influenza and congenital deformities. A follow-up study. *Lancet* 1963; **1**: 748.
20. Torrey EF, Peterson MR. The viral hypothesis of schizophrenia. *Schizophr Bull* 1976; **2**: 136–46.
21. Akbarian S, Bunney WE Jr, Potkin SG et al. Altered distribution of nicotinamide-adenine dinucleotide phosphate-diaphorase cells in frontal lobe of schizophrenics implies disturbances of cortical development. *Arch Gen Psychiatry* 1993; **50**: 169–77.
22. Akbarian S, Vinuela A, Kim JJ et al. Distorted distribution of nicotinamide-adenine dinucleotide phosphate-diaphorase neurons in temporal lobe of schizophrenics implies anomalous cortical development. *Arch Gen Psychiatry* 1993; **50**: 178–87.
23. Weinberger DR. Implications of normal brain development for the pathogenesis of schizophrenia. *Arch Gen Psychiatry* 1987; **44**: 660–9.
24. Mednick SA, Cannon TD, Barr CE, Lyon M (eds). *Fetal Neural Development and Adult Schizophrenia*. New York: Cambridge University Press, 1991.
25. Nowakowski RS. Basic processes in fetal neural development. In: *Fetal Neural Development and Adult Schizophrenia* (Mednick SA, Cannon TD, Barr CE, Lyon M, eds). New York: Cambridge University Press, 1991: 15–40.
26. Barr CE, Mednick SA, Munk-Jørgensen P. Exposure to influenza epidemics during gestation and adult schizophrenia: a 40-year study. *Arch Gen Psychiatry* 1990; **47**: 869–74.
27. Kendell RE, Kemp IW. Maternal influenza in the etiology of schizophrenia. *Arch Gen Psychiatry* 1989; **46**: 878–82.
28. Kunugi H, Nanko S, Takei N et al. Schizophrenia following in utero exposure to the 1957 influenza epidemics in Japan. *Am J Psychiatry* 1995; **152**: 450–2.
29. O'Callaghan E, Sham P, Takei N et al. Schizophrenia and influenza. *Lancet* 1991; **337**: 118–9.
30. Sham PC, O'Callaghan E, Takei N et al. Schizophrenia following prenatal exposure to influenza epidemics between 1939 and 1960. *Br J Psychiatry* 1992; **160**: 461–6.
31. Watson JB, Mednick SA, Huttunen MO, Wang X. Prenatal teratogens and the development of adult mental illness. *Dev Psychopathol* 1999; **11**: 457–66.
32. Machón RA, Mednick SA, Huttunen MO. Adult major affective disorder after prenatal exposure to an influenza epidemic. *Arch Gen Psychiatry* 1997; **54**: 322–8.
33. Machón RA, Huttunen MO, Mednick SA et al. Adult schizotypal personality characteristics and prenatal influenza in a Finnish birth cohort. *Schizophr Res* 2002; **54**: 7–16.
34. Rubin SA, Bautista JR, Moran TH et al. Viral teratogenesis: brain developmental damage associated with maturation state at time of infection. *Brain Res Dev Brain Res* 1999; **112**: 237–44.
35. Mednick SA, Hollister JM (eds). *Neural Development and Schizophrenia: Theory and Research*. NATO ASI Series. Series A, Life Sciences, **275**. New York: Plenum Press, 1995.
36. American Psychiatric Association. *Diagnostic and Statistical Manual of Mental Disorders* (4th ed). Washington DC: American Psychiatric Association, 1994.
37. Meehl P. Schizotaxia, schizotypy and schizophrenia. *Am Psychologist* 1962; **17**: 827–38.
38. Venables PH. Schizotypy and maternal exposure to influenza and to cold temperature: the Mauritius study. *J Abnormal Psychol* 1996; **105**: 53–60.
39. Siever LJ, Bernstein DP, Silverman JM. Schizotypal personality disorder. In: *The DSM-IV Personality Disorders* (Livesley WJ, ed). New York: Guilford Press, 1995: 71–90.
40. Raine A, Reynolds C, Lencz T et al. Cognitive-perceptual, interpersonal and disorganized features of individual differences in schizotypal personality in the general population. *Schizophr Bull* 1994; **21**: 191–201.
41. Raine A, Benishay D. The SPQ-B: a brief screening instrument for schizotypal personality disorder. *J Personality Disord* 1995; **9**: 346–55.
42. Chen WJ, Hsiao CK, Lin CCH. Schizotypy in community samples: the three-factor structure and correlation with sustained attention. *J Abnormal Psychol* 1997; **106**: 649–54.
43. Eagles JM. Are polioviruses a cause of schizophrenia? *Br J Psychiatry* 1992; **160**: 598–600.
44. Bruno RL, Cohen JM, Galski T, Frick NM. The neuroanatomy of post-polio fatigue. *Arch Phys Med Rehab* 1994; **75**: 498–504.
45. Suvisaari J, Haukka J, Tanskanen A et al. Association between prenatal exposure to poliovirus infection and adult schizophrenia. *Am J Psychiatry* 1999; **156**: 1100–2.
46. Hatten MB. Central nervous system neuronal migration. *Ann Rev Neuroscience* 1999; **22**: 511–40.
47. O'Leary DDM, Koester SE. Development of projection neuron types, axon pathways, and patterned connections of the mammalian cortex. *Neuron* 1993; **10**: 991–1006.
48. Huttunen MO. Persistent alternation of turnover of brain noradrenaline in the offspring of rats subjected to stress during pregnancy. *Nature* 1971; **35**: 53–5.
49. Srivastava P. Roles of heat-shock proteins in innate and adaptive immunity. *Nature Rev Immunol* 2002; **2**: 185–94.
50. McGlashan TH, Hoffman RE. Schizophrenia as a disorder of developmentally reduced synaptic connectivity. *Arch Gen Psychiatry* 2000; **57**: 637–48.
51. Friston KJ. Dysfunctional connectivity in schizophrenia. *World Psychiatry* 2002; **1**: 66–71.
52. Mednick SA, Machón RA, Huttunen MO, Bonett D. Adult schizophrenia following prenatal exposure to an influenza epidemic. *Arch Gen Psychiatry* 1998; **45**: 189–92.

53. Huttunen MO, Niskanen P. Prenatal loss of father and psychiatric disorders. *Arch Gen Psychiatry* 1978; **35**: 429–31.
54. Otake M, Schull WJ. In utero exposure to A-bomb radiation and mental retardation: a reassessment. *Br J Radiol* 1984; **57**: 409–14.
55. Selten JP, van Duursen R, van der Graaf C et al. Second-trimester exposure to maternal stress is a possible risk factor for psychotic illness in the child. *Schizophr Res* 1997; **24**: 258.

Index

5-HT *see* serotonin
23rd week of gestation   267–8

adaptive immunity *see* immunity, adaptive
adrenocorticotrophic hormone (ACTH)   254
   amino acid sequences in bacteria/viruses   256
   autoantibodies against   255–6
      in eating disorders   256–7
      origin of   257–8
   and puberty   258
affective disorders
   Borna disease virus in   129, 130
   stress as immunomodulator in   107–11
AIDS *see* HIV/AIDS
AIDS dementia complex (ADC)   55, 241–2
   cognitive manifestations   242
   Memorial Sloan Kettering Staging   242–3
AIDS lethargy   240
AIDS mania   113, 114
AIDS subacute encephalopathy   241
α-melanocyte-stimulating hormone (α-MSH)   253–4
   amino acid sequences in bacteria/viruses   256
   autoantibodies against   254–5
      in eating disorders   256–7
      origin of   257–8
   and puberty   258
Alzheimer's disease   229–30
   Chlamydia pneumoniae in   229–38
      presence in brain tissue   230–1
         studies   233–4
      viability in brain tissue   231
   glial inflammation mechanisms   248
   late-onset   229
      Chlamydia pneumoniae in   230–5
amenorrhea in eating disorders   257
American Academy of Neurology AIDS Task Force nomenclature   242
β-amyloid peptide   229
anandamide   24
animal models
   Borna disease virus (BDV)   113, 115, 125
   CB1 receptor knockout mice   24
   and cytokines   97, 99, 100–1
   developmental behavioral disorders   207

   eating disorders   253
   homologous modeling   207
   IL-1/LPS and sickness behavior   108
   influenza   71
   LPS model of infection   100–1
   Lyme borreliosis and sporadic schizophrenia   24
   maternal infection   92–4
      behavioral abnormalities   83–90
      inflammatory perinatal brain damage   218
   schizophrenia   48
   Semliki forest virus (SFV)   117
   toxoplasmosis   117
   viral, of neuropsychiatric diseases   213
anorexia nervosa   253
   antineuronal antibody assays   163
   autoimmune component   253–62
   genetic links   258
   and infections   258
   yellow palms   254
antenatal infections *see* prenatal infections
anti-basal ganglia antibodies   163
antibiotic prophylaxis
   PANDAS   149–50
   Sydenham chorea   159
antibodies
   anti-basal ganglia   163, 167
   anti-casein   182
   anti-CD26   180, 182
   anti-cerebellar   179
   anti-cerebellar, assay of   178–9
   anti-gliadin   179, 181, 182
   anti-neuronal   145–6, 157–8, 159
      assays for OCD/tic disorders   163
      removal   164
      and symptom recurrence   168
   anti-Purkinje cells   176, 178
   anti-streptokinase   182
   and autism   172–4, 201
   Borna disease virus detection   125–6, 129
   against CNS antigens   172–4
   gluten/casein/streptokinase   181
      simultaneous detection   181–2
   monoclonal antibody D8/17   146
   to neuron-specific antigens   174

antibodies *continued*
  to streptococcal antigens   137–8
  in stress   108
  viral, in schizophrenia   38, 96
antibody tests for syphilis   51–2
antidepressants and cytokines   115
antifungal medication in autism   193
antigens, cerebellar   176–9
antipsychotics and psychosis in syphilis/HIV   56
antiretroviral therapy   56, 239, 247
  and psychoses   240
antistreptolysin O   159
anxiety disorders in syphilis/HIV   56
APOE ε4   229, 234–5
appetite regulation   253
arcuate nucleus   256
ASD *see* autistic spectrum disorder (ASD)
astrocytes
  in Borna disease model   209
  Chlamydia pneumoniae in   232
  in HIV/AIDS   244–6
attention deficit hyperactivity disorder (ADHD)
  gastrointestinal symptoms   199
  and neurological soft signs   146
  in PANDAS   156
autism   198–203
  antibodies   172–4
  autoantibodies   180–1
    triggers   182–3
  autoimmunity pathogenesis/mechanism   183–5
  children at risk
    defining   203
    increase over time   204
  etiology   200
  gastrointestinal immunopathology   198–200
    immunohistochemistry   200, 202
  with gastrointestinal symptoms   199
    hypothesis   203
  gut–brain axis   202–3
  immunoglobulins   173–4
  mechanism of injury   183, 184
  mucosal pathology   199
  neuroimmune disorders   172–4
    mechanisms, possible   176
  season-of-birth effect   203
  and systemic immunity   200
  and viral infection   198
autistic enterocolitis   199–200, 201
  immunohistochemistry   202
autistic spectrum disorder (ASD)   187
  autoimmunity
    central nervous system   190–1
    systemic   191
  immunological issues   187–97
    abnormalities   188–9
    mechanisms, potential   190–5
      CNS autoimmunity   191
      dietary protein intolerance   193–5
      gut microflora disruption   193
      respiratory infections   191–3
  macrophages   194–5
  medical problems, associated   187
  opioid excess   203
autoantibodies   145–6
  anti-α-MSH   254–5, 256–8
  anti-ACTH   255–8
  anti-LHRH   257–8
  anti-myelin   171–2
  in appetite regulation   253
  in autism   172, 180–1
    triggers   182–3
  in bipolar disorder   116
  in different conditions   173
  in PANDAS   138, 168
autoimmune lymphoproliferative syndrome (ALPS)   191
autoimmune neurological disorders   171–2
autoimmunity
  and autism   183–5
  and autistic spectrum disorder   190–1
  in eating disorders   253–62
  pathogen-triggered   191–2
  systemic   191
autonomic nervous system
  and autistic spectrum disorder   190
  in eating disorders   253
AZT (zidovudine)   247

B cells
  in autistic spectrum disorder   191
  in depression   109
  in PANDAS/Sydenham's chorea   164, 168
bacterial amino acid sequences   256, 259
bacterial toxins binding to DPP IV (CD26)   183
basal ganglia, immune reactivity to   163, 192
Bcl-2 gene   68
behavioral abnormalities/changes
  in Borna disease   125
  in HIV/AIDS   241
    children   240
  maternal infection animal models   83–90
    bacterial infection   87
    double stranded DNA   87–8
    exploratory behavior   84, 87
    latent inhibition   88
    locomotor stimulation by amphetamine   88
    pup–mother attachment   86–7
    sensorimotor coordination   84
    sensorimotor gating   85–6, 87
    social behavior   86
    spontaneous activity   83–4
    viral infection   83–7
  in mumps   225
  regression in autism   199
  schizophrenia   70
benzathine penicillin therapy   56
β-amyloid peptide   229
β-caseomorphine   203
bipolar disorder   112–22
  diagnosis   112
    relevance for patient/research   113
  differential diagnoses   112
  factors, convergence of   119
  future research   119
  hypotheses   118
  and immunity   115, 116
  and infection   113–15
  medication   115, 119
  neurodevelopment and infection/immunity   117
  pathophysiology   115, 117–18
    neurotransmitters and infection/immunity   115, 117

signal transduction and infection/immunity 117–18
birth complications *see* pregnancy/birth complications (PBCs)
birthweight, low, in schizophrenia   3
blood–brain barrier
   Chlamydia pneumoniae crossing   232
   permeability in eating disorders   257
Borna disease   123
   symptoms   125
Borna disease virus (BDV)   123–4
   animal infections
      experimental   125
      natural   124–5
   and bipolar disorder   113, 114
   diagnosis
      antibody detection   125–6, 127, 129, 130
      antigen detection   126, 130
      marker detection in psychiatric disorders   131
      nucleic acid detection   126, 129, 130, 131
   genetics   123–4
   human infections   127–30
      incidence   127
      in psychiatric disorders   129–30, 131
         affective disorders   129, 130
         schizophrenia   127–9
   isolation from blood/brain tissue   126
   neonatal   207–15
   neonatal rat model   207–8
      appearance/growth of animal   208
      behavioral alterations
         cognitive abnormalities   211–12
         emotional disturbances   211
         sensorimotor deficits   211
         social behavior deficits   212
      brain pathology
         cerebellum   208
         cortex   209
         hippocampus   208–9
      direct effects of infection   210
      genetic background, effects of   212–13
      hormonal effects   211
      immune system, role of   209–10
      neurochemical changes   210–11
   neuronal death   38
   and neurotransmitters   115, 117
   replication   124
Borrelia spp.
   B. burgdorferi
      and bipolar disorder   113–14
      cytokine-mediated mutagenesis   20
      DNA recombination with human   21
      global distribution of vectors   22
      zooprophylaxis   23
   B. garinii   23
   see also Lyme borreliosis
brain abnormalities
   in schizophrenia   66
   see also white matter damage, perinatal
brain abscess   241
brain cell proliferation in influenza animal model   75
brain derived neurotrophic factor (BDNF)   99, 100–1
brain development
   and cytokines   97
   guidance by brain proteins   67–8
   human   66–7
   mice   67
   prenatal infections   97
brain infections, opportunistic, and AIDS   241
bulimia nervosa   253
   autoimmune component   253–62
   genetic links   258

Cajal–Rezius neurons   68, 72
calretinin   72
candida overgrowth in autism   193
cannabinoid receptor gene *see CB1* gene
cannabinoid system in schizophrenia   20
cannabis and schizophrenia   23, 24, 26
carbamazepine
   and immunity   115
   psychosis in syphilis/HIV   57
   in Sydenham chorea   159
casein
   antibodies   181
   binding to DPP IV (CD26)   179–80
β-caseomorphine   203
catatonias *see* periodic catatonia; systematic catatonia
CB1 gene
   anatomical distribution in brain   21
   B. burgdorferi/human recombination   20, 21
   and borrelia DNA   18
   receptor densities in brain   20, 21
   and schizophrenia   23
CB1 protein/receptors
   constraints on mechanism of action   25
   in schizophrenia   24–6
CB1 receptor knockout mice   24, 25
CD8+ lymphocytes in autism   200, 201
ceftriaxone   55
celiac disease   176, 178
   neurological manifestations   189
central nervous system
   antigens/antibodies   173
   autoimmunity and ASD   190–1
   development   66–7
   enteroviruses in   31–2
      coxsackievirus B5 (CBV-5)   34, 35
   HIV-related compromise   242
   HIV symptoms   53
   and innate immunity   189
   markers for CNS injury   145–6
   rheumatic disease   60–1
   spirochetes in   26, 28
   syphilis symptoms   53
   vasculitis   59
   see also specific organs/areas
cerebellar antigens   176–9
cerebellar damage   208
cerebral lesions and cytokines   98
cerebral palsy   98, 217
cerebroventricular enlargement   66
Chagas' disease   241
chemokines
   in Borna disease model   209–10
   in HIV/AIDS   245–7
   in inflammatory perinatal brain damage   218
Child Health and Development Plan (CHDP)   44
childhood infections
   enteroviruses   32
   and schizophrenia   34–5

childhood-onset schizophrenia 4
children
   autism, risk of
      defining 203
      increase over time 204
   HIV-infected 240, 241, 242
      CNS disease classification system 243
Chlamydia pneumoniae 175, 230, 232
   in Alzheimer's disease 229–38
      late-onset 230–5
   blood–brain barrier, crossing 232
   inflammatory response 230
   presence in brain tissue 230–1
      studies 233–4
choreiform movements in PANDAS 146
chorioamnionitis 216–17
chromosomal locus of schizophrenia 69
chronic catatonic schizophrenia 14
climate factors in schizophrenia 2
clozapine
   and prepulse inhibition 86
   psychosis in syphilis/HIV 56
CNS lymphoma 241
cognitive abnormalities
   AIDS dementia complex (ADC) 242
   Borna disease virus (BDV) 211–12
   HIV-1 associated dementia 242
   with *Treponema pallidum* 55
cognitive fragmentation 70
Collaborative Perinatal Study 97
complement system in eating disorders 257
conditioned responses in Borna disease model 212
corticotrophin releasing factor (CRH) 253, 254
cow's milk protein (CMP) intolerance 193–4
coxsackievirus B5 (CBV-5) 34, 35
CREB 117, 118
cryptitis 199, 200
α-B-crystallin 172
cyclic AMP responsive element binding *see* CREB
cycloid psychoses 11
   prenatal infections 14, 15–16
   season-of-birth effect 12
cystic spirochete structures in multiple sclerosis 26–7
cytokines 47
   in autistic spectrum disorder 188, 189–90
   and autoimmunity 184
   and brain development 97
   in cerebral palsy 98
   in depression 109–10
   HIV/AIDS 246–7
   as immunotransmitters 107
   in inflammatory perinatal brain damage 216, 217, 218
   in lipopolysaccharide model of infection 100–1
   and microglial cells 189–90
   and neuron development 98–9
   and neuronal death 38
   and neurotransmitters 38–9
   and neurotrophic factor expression 99, 100–1
   in periventricular leukomalacia 98
   and schizophrenia 47, 98
   serotonin, interaction with 39–40
   and sickness behavior 108
   in stress 107–8
   and susceptibility genes 38
   in Sydenham chorea 158

D8/17 *see* monoclonal antibody D8/17
Dana Consortium on Therapy for HIV Dementia 243
daylight/sunlight in schizophrenia 1–2, 3
deficit/non-deficit schizophrenia 4
delirium 52–3
dementia
   in HIV infection 55
   in syphilis 55
demyelinating diseases 171
   antibodies 173
demyelination, secondary 184
dentate gyrus in Borna disease model 208, 212
depression 109–10
   differential diagnosis 112
   in eating disorders 255
   in HIV/AIDS 240
developmental behavioral disorders 207
developmental regression in autism 199
diabetes and olanzapine therapy 56–7
dietary-derived opioid peptides 203
dietary proteins and neuroimmunity 176, 180, 183, 184
   in autistic spectrum disorder 193–5
differentiated psychopathology 11–12
   season-of-birth effect 12
disease resistance 59
DNA, *B. burgdorferi*/human infectious recombination of 21
DNA microarray studies of influenza 73, 75
dopamine
   in Borna disease model 210, 211
   in CNS autoimmune disorders 191
   in schizophrenia 39
   in Sydenham chorea 157
double stranded DNA 87–8
DPP IV (CD26)
   autoantibodies and autism 180–1
   binding 179–80, 183

earthquake and schizotypal personality 265–7
eating disorders 253–62
   autoantibodies 256–7
   neurotransmission 256
   role of peptides/monoamines 253
electroencephalogram (EEG) power measures 6
elimination diets in ASD 194
emotional disturbances
   in Borna disease model 211
   in HIV-infected children 240
   in Sydenham chorea 155
encephalitis 31, 35, 241
   HIV-1-related (HIVE) 243
   in mumps 225
encephalopathy, HIV-related 243
endotoxin in autistic spectrum disorder 194
enterocolitis 199–200, 201
enteroviruses 31
   persistence 32
   and schizophrenia
      childhood infections 34–5
      prenatal infections 32–4
      symptoms/diseases caused 31
epigenetic regulation 49
ethnicity and schizophrenia 4
exorphins 203

exploratory behavior and prenatal infections   84, 87, 93, 175–6

familial Mediterranean fever (FMF)   60
family history
    schizophrenia   3–4
    Sydenham chorea   159
FBRP virulence factor   20, 21

GABA *see* gamma aminobutyric acid (GABA)
GAD65/67 protein levels   73, 76
gamma aminobutyric acid (GABA) in Sydenham chorea   157
GAS *see* group A streptococcus (GAS)
gastrointestinal conditions and autistic spectrum disorder   189, 193
    autonomic nerve system   190
gastrointestinal immunopathology in autism   198–200
gene profile analysis   75, 77–9
genetics
    Borna disease virus   123–4
    as component of infectious disease   59, 60, 63
    and PANDAS   145
    schizophrenia   5
    Sydenham chorea   158–9
GFAP   68
    immunoreactivity   72–3
    protein levels   73, 75, 76
gliadin peptides   176–9
    antibody assays   178
    binding to DPP IV (CD26)   179–80
gliadmorphine   203
gliosis   66
    in Borna disease model   209
    marker   72
    in neurodegenerative disorders   248
glucocorticoids   107, 108
    in stress/depression   110
gluten antibodies   181
gluten ataxia   176
group A streptococcus (GAS)
    and autistic spectrum disorder   192
    diagnosis/treatment   149–50
    diseases caused   162
    M-proteins   158, 166–7
    neurological sequelae   146
    and PANDAS   157, 162–3
    pathogenesis   137–8
    persistent immune reaction   138
    prophage-encoded superantigens   165–6
    seasonality   144
    and Sydenham chorea   154, 157
    virulence factors   138, 164–5
    vulnerability   144–5

HAART   239, 247
hallucinations
    in psychosis/delirium   52–3
    in schizophrenia   24
haloperidol   56, 159
hapten carrier formation   183
heat shock proteins (HSPs)
    in multiple sclerosis   29
    in spirochetes   22, 27–8
    in stress response   268

heavy metals and neuroimmunity   174–5
    mercury   203, 204
herpes virus
    and autism   203
    and bipolar disorder   113, 114
    herpes simplex virus in Alzheimer's disease   230
highly active antiretroviral therapy (HAART)   239, 247
hippocampus in Borna disease model   208–9, 211–12
HIV-1 associated dementia
    cellular involvement and neurotoxicity   244–6
    cognitive manifestations   242
    glial inflammation mechanisms   248
    macrophages, infected   244
    neuroimaging   243–4
        techniques   244, 245
    neuropathology   243–4
    psychometric tests   242
HIV-1-associated encephalitis (HIVE)   243
HIV-1 encephalopathy   239
    chemokines   246
HIV/AIDS
    and α-MSH   258
    and bipolar disorder   113, 114
    CNS symptoms   53
    comorbid syphilis   52
        management recommendations   55–6
        psychosis treatment   56–7
    cytokines/chemokines   246–7
    dementia in   55
    incidence/transmission   52
    management recommendations   56
    neurological factors   240–2
    neuropsychological findings   242–3
    opportunistic brain infections   241
    prenatal/perinatal infections   239
    psychiatric disorders associated   239–40
    psychosis in   54–5
    transmission   239
    treatment   247–8
    viral proteins   244, 245, 246
    see also AIDS-related entries
HIV-related CNS compromise   242
HIV-related encephalopathy diagnosis   243
HLA haplotype   6
hydrocephalus   225
hypercortisolism   255
hypomania   112
hypothalamo–pituitary–adrenal (HPA) axis   255, 256
hypoxic brain damage in schizophrenia   23

imaging *see* neuroimaging
immune system
    in anorexia nervosa   254–5
    ASD, mechanisms underlying   190–5
        appropriate reactions, lack of   192
        dietary protein intolerance   193–5
        gut microflora disruption   193
        respiratory infections   191–3
    and bipolar disorder   112–22
    in depression   109, 110
    genetically-mediated response to infection   59
    gut   194
    and life events   109, 240

immune system *continued*
  multiple sclerosis   28
  neuroimmune disorders
    and dietary proteins   176
    and infections   175–6
    and xenobiotics/metals   174–5
  and obsessive–compulsive disorder   139–43
  and psychiatric disorder symptoms   107
  respiratory, and GI inflammatory conditions   189
  schizophrenia pathophysiology   37–42
  stress in affective disorders   107–11
  and tic disorders   139–43
immunity
  adaptive   188
  cell-mediated, in eating disorders   257
  innate
    aberrant   187
    and adaptive immunity   188
    and central nervous system   188
    and immune tolerance   188–9
  systemic, and autism   200
immunoglobulins   96
  antibodies   184
  IgA in autism   174, 179, 180, 181–2
    and systemic immunity   200
  IgG in autism   173–4, 179, 180, 181–2
    and systemic immunity   200
  IgM
    in autism   174, 179, 180, 181–2
    in bipolar disorder   116
  IVIG PANDAS trial   150, 163–4
immunopathogenesis of Sydenham chorea   157–8
infections
  and autoimmunity   182, 183, 184
  and bipolar disorder   112–22
  and neuroimmunity   175–6
  schizophrenia   3
  see also prenatal infections
infectious disease, genetic component of   59, 60, 63
inflammatory perinatal brain damage   216–21
  brain infection models   218
  experiments   217–18
  explanations   218–19
  fetal systemic infection models   218
  maternal infection animal models   218
  necrosis *vs* apoptosis   219
  observations   216–17
inflammatory response
  Chlamydia pneumoniae   230
  HIV/AIDS   246–7
  protective   246, 247
influenza   70
  maternal infection animal models *see under* influenza A/WS/33
  mouse infection studies   71
    DNA microarray studies   73, 75
    GFAP/GAD65/67 protein levels   73, 76
    GFAP immunoreactivity   72–3
    nNOS immunoreactivity   71
    pyramidal cell atrophy   73, 74
    Reelin-positive cells   72
    SNAP-25 immunoreactivity   71–2
  pathogenic mechanisms   47
  prenatal
    and cycloid psychoses   14

  and schizophrenia   3, 37, 43–4, 70, 96, 263
    serologic study   45
    and schizotypal personality   264–5
  transplacental passage   91, 92, 97
influenza A/WS/33   91–4
  maternal infection animal models
    offspring behavioral abnormalities   93–4
    offspring survival   92–3
    persistence of viral RNA   93
    transplacental passage   92
  postnatal infection animal model   93
innate immunity *see* immunity, innate
interleukins
  IL-1
    in HIV/AIDS   246
    in inflammatory cascade   107–8
    in LPS model of infection   97
    and neuron survival   99
    in schizophrenia   38, 39, 47, 98
    and sickness behavior   108
    transplacental passage   97
  IL-2
    in inflammatory perinatal brain damage   218
    in schizophrenia   39
  IL-6
    in HIV/AIDS   246
    in inflammatory cascade   108
    in LPS model of infection   97
    and neuron survival   99
    in schizophrenia   38, 39, 47
    transplacental passage   97
  IL-8 in schizophrenia   47–8
    factors causing increase   48
  IL-12 in bipolar disorder   115, 116
  see also soluble interleukin receptors (sIL-Rs)
intravenous immunoglobulin (IVIG) trial   163–4
Ixodes spp.
  animal reservoirs   21–3, 28
  global distribution   22
  I. holocyclus   23
  I. ovatus   23
  I. persulcatus   18, 19–20, 23
  I. ricinus   19, 20
  I. scapularis   18–19
  I. uriae   23
  see also Lyme borreliosis

Jones criteria   154

Kaiser Foundation Health Plan (KFHP)   44, 45
ketamine and prepulse inhibition   86
Kraepelinian schizophrenia   4
kyrenurate–quinolinate balance   40

latent inhibition   88
Leishmania major infection model   203
life events and immune system   109, 240
lipopolysaccharide (LPS)
  model of infection   100–1
  and sickness behavior   108
lithium
  in bipolar disorder   115, 118
  and immunity   115
  psychosis in syphilis/HIV   57
locomotor activity and prenatal infections   83, 88

LPS *see* lipopolysaccharide
luteinizing hormone releasing hormone (LHRH) 253, 254, 255
   amino acid sequences in bacteria/viruses 259
   autoantibodies against 257
      origin of 257–8
   and puberty 258
Lyme borreliosis and sporadic schizophrenia 18–30
   animal reservoirs 23
   genetic correlate 23
   geographical correlation 19, 20–3
   multiple sclerosis, correlation with 26–9
      biological plausibility 27–9
      etiological correlate 26–7
      season/locality as correlates 26, 28
   phenotypic correlate
      animal models 24
      pharmacological evidence 24–6
   prenatal transuterine transmission 20
   seasonal correlation 18–20
      biological plausibility 20
   zooprophylaxis 23
lymphatic choriomeningitis virus (LCMV) 37–8
lymphocytes in autism 200, 201
lymphocytic choriomeningitis virus (LCV) 115
lymphoid nodular hyperplasia (LNH) 199, 200, 201

macrophages in HIV/AIDS 244
magnetic resonance (MR) imaging
   in inflammatory perinatal brain damage 217
   in Sydenham chorea 157
mania 112
   and infection 113
markers for CNS injury 145–6
maternal gestational infection *see* prenatal infections
MCP-1 *see* monocyte chemoattractant protein (MCP-1)
measles
   and autism 198, 201, 203
   and schizophrenia 3
measles–mumps–rubella (MMR) vaccination 198
   in autism 193, 201, 204
melanin-concentrating hormone 254
melanocortin receptors in eating disorders 253
α-melanocyte-stimulating hormone (α-MSH) 253
memantine 247
Memorial Sloan Kettering Staging 242–3
meningoencephalitic syndrome 241
meningitis 31, 35, 241
   mumps meningitis 225
mental status examinations in HIV/AIDS 241
mercury 203, 204
metals and neuroimmunity 174–5
meteorological factors in schizophrenia 1–2, 3
microglial cells 39
   in autistic spectrum disorder 190
   in Borna disease model 209
   Chlamydia pneumoniae in 232
   and cytokines 189–90
   in HIV/AIDS 244, 248
   in neurodegenerative disorders 248
milk peptides, antibodies against 176
minocycline 247–8
MMR vaccination *see* measles–mumps–rubella (MMR) vaccination

molecular mimicry 157, 166
   triggering autoimmunity 189, 258
monoclonal antibody D8/17 146, 192
   in anorexia nervosa 258
   studies 147–8
monocyte chemoattractant protein (MCP-1) 245–7
mood disorders
   in HIV/AIDS 240
   in syphilis/HIV 56
mood stabilizers
   and cytokines 115
   and signal transduction 118
motor symptoms in HIV/AIDS 241
movement disorders in Sydenham chorea 155
multiple sclerosis 171
   autoimmunity in 191
   and sporadic schizophrenia/Lyme disease 26–9
      biological plausibility 27–9
      etiological correlate 26–7
      season/locality as correlates 26
mumps
   and autism 198
   history 222
   symptoms/complications 223
mumps encephalitis 225
mumps meningitis 225
mumps vaccination risks 224
mumps virus 222–8
   acoustic startle response 226
   in choroid plexus 224
   CNS disease/pathogenesis 224–5
   in ependymal lining of ventricle 224, 225
   epidemiology 223–4
   neurological deficits 225–7
   persistence 227
   rat brain, effect on 226
   replication 222–3
   structure 222
   transmission 223
myelin
   in influenza animal model 75
   see also demyelinating diseases; demyelination, secondary
myelopathy 241

NADPH-diaphorase 68, 71
nailfold capillary abnormalities 62
naloxone (Narcan) 24, 25
necrotizing vasculitis 241
nerve growth factor (NGF) 99, 100–1
neuroanatomical features in schizophrenia 4–5
neuroanatomy of Sydenham chorea 156–7
neurodevelopment
   23rd week 268
   23rd week of gestation 267–8
   and infection/immunity 117
   schizophrenia 37–8
   schizophrenia spectrum disorders 263–4
neurodevelopmental hypothesis of schizophrenia 43
neurofibrillary tangles 229
neurogenesis 67
neuroimaging
   HIV-1 associated dementia 243–4
   techniques 244, 245

neuroimaging *continued*
  in inflammatory perinatal brain damage   216–17
  Sydenham chorea   157
neuroimmune disorders   171–2
  in autism   172–4
    mechanisms, possible   176
    and dietary proteins   176
    and infections   175–6
    and xenobiotics/metals   174–5
neuron development and cytokines   98–9
neuronal adhesion molecule (N-CAM)   115, 116
neuronal migration   67
  abnormalities   68, 264
  marker   72
  in schizophrenia   23
neuropathology   157–8
  HIV-1 associated dementia   243–4
neurophysiological features of schizophrenia   5
neuropsychologic development in schizophrenia   66
neurosyphilis   18, 51
  AIDS-related   241
  case reports   54
  management recommendations   55
    with comorbid HIV   55–6
  neuroradiological findings   53
  symptoms   53
neurotoxicity   244–6
neurotoxins and neuroimmune disorders   174
neurotransmitters/neurotransmission
  from autonomic nerve fibers   190
  in bipolar disorder/infection   115, 117
  in CNS autoimmune disorders   191
  in eating disorders   256
  and peptide hormones   189
  in stress/depression   110
  in Sydenham chorea   157
neurotrophic factor expression   99, 100–1
neurotrophins
  in Borna disease model   210
  neurotrophin 3 (NT-3)   99
neuritic senile plaques (NSP)   229
nNOS   68, 72
  immunoreactivity   71
non-nucleoside reverse transcriptase inhibitors (NNRTIs)   56
norepinephrine   210
Northeast AIDS Dementia (NEAD) Consortium study   243
Northern Finland 1966 Birth Cohort study   34
nosology
  differentiated psychopathology   11–12
  and prenatal infections   11–17
novelty stress test   84–5
nucleoside reverse transcriptase inhibitors (NRTIs)   56

obsessive–compulsive disorder (OCD)   135–53
  age of onset   135
  antineuronal antibody assays   163
  case studies   149
  characteristics   137
  childhood onset *see* PANDAS
  diagnosis/treatment   149–50
  immune basis, evidence of   139–43
  marker   146
  and neurological soft signs   146
  in PANDAS   156

  in rheumatic fever   156
  and Sydenham chorea   136, 155–6
olanzapine   56–7
open field test   84
opioid excess   203
opportunistic brain infections and AIDS   241
PANDAS   135, 137, 162–4, 192
  and anorexia nervosa   258
  anti-basal ganglia antibodies   167
  and autism   204
  case studies   149
  characteristics   136–7
  diagnosis/treatment issues   149–50
  diagnostic criteria   136, 162
  future research   168
  GAS pathogenesis   137–8, 157
  genetic predisposition   145
  history   155
  immune/infection triggers, possible   144
  immune response   164–5
  intravenous immunoglobulin (IVIG) trial   150, 163–4
  neurological factors   146, 149
  neuropsychiatric manifestations   144
  onset   144
  plasmapheresis trial   150, 163–4
  seasonality   138
  streptococcal antibodies   138
  vulnerability   145
paraneoplastic cerebellar degeneration (PCD)   176, 178
paranoid/non-paranoid schizophrenia   3
parasitic infections and bipolar disorder   113, 114
parotitis   223–4
pathogen-associated molecular patterns (PAMPs)   188
  in autistic spectrum disorder   194
pattern recognition receptors (PRRs)   188
Pediatric AIDS Clinical Trials Late Outcomes Study   240
pediatric autoimmune neuropsychiatric disorders associated with streptococcus *see* PANDAS
penicillin therapy   55, 159
peptide hormones   189
peptides
  β-amyloid   229
  dietary-derived opioid   203
  in eating disorders   253
  gliadin   176–80
  milk   176
periodic catatonia   11–12
  demographic/environmental/genetic factors   15
  familial transmission   14, 15
  prenatal infections   14
peripheral blood mononuclear cells (PBMCs) in bipolar disorder   115, 116
peripheral neuritis   241
periventricular leukomalacia   98
pharyngitis, streptococcal   144
physical anomalies in schizophrenia   66
plasmapheresis   150, 163–4
polio virus/poliomyelitis   31
  and schizophrenia   3, 32–4, 96, 267
    environmental/geographic factors   32
    season-of-birth effect   32, 33
    vaccination   33–4

polymerase chain reaction (PCR)
  for *C. pneumoniae*   230–1
  RT/RT-nested for Borna disease virus   126–7, 129, 130
post-streptococcal reactive arthritis (PSRA)   137
post-streptococcal syndromes   60, 154–61, 192
  as autoimmune childhood diseases   154
  autoimmunity   157, 159
pregnancy/birth complications (PBCs) in schizophrenia   2–3
Prenatal Determinants of Schizophrenia (PDS) study   44, 45
prenatal infections
  and autism   175
  behavioral abnormalities   83–90
    bacterial infection   87
    double stranded DNA   87–8
    exploratory behavior   84, 87
    latent inhibition   88
    locomotor stimulation by amphetamine   88
    pup–mother attachment   86–7
    sensorimotor coordination   84
    sensorimotor gating   85–6, 87
    social behavior   86
    spontaneous activity   83–4
    viral infection   83–7
  brain damage, role in   218–19
  fetal inflammatory responses   216
  HIV/AIDS   239
  preterm birth, role in   218
  and schizophrenia   34–5, 43–50, 70, 96–7
    future research
      animal models   48
      gene–environment interaction   49
      neuroimaging   48–9
    history taking   12
    immunology   37–8
    infectious agents   44
    mechanisms, suggested   69
    obstetric complications   13, 16, 96
    pathogenic mechanisms   47–8
    prevention   48
    and psychiatric nosology   11, 12–17
    serology   45–7
    time of infection
      5th vs 6th month   264
      23rd week   267–8
      first trimester   14, 15, 46
      second trimester (midgestational)   13, 14, 15, 32, 33, 37, 44, 45
  transuterine transmission of borreliosis   20
prepulse inhibition (PPI) deficits   70, 85–6, 94
  and prenatal infections   175
Probenecid   55
procaine penicillin   55
progressive encephalopathy   242
progressive multifocal leukoencephalopathy   241, 244
prostaglandin E2 (PGE2) in stress/depression   108, 110
proteinase inhibitors (PI)   56
PSA-NCAM   68
psychiatric disorders, Borna disease virus in   127–30
psychometric tests   242
psychosis/psychoses
  in bipolar disorder   112
  classification   11
  cycloid   11
    prenatal infections   14, 15–16
    season-of-birth effect   12
  definition of   52–3
  in HIV/AIDS   54–5, 240
    prognostic value   54
  and rheumatic disease   59, 60, 61–2
  in syphilis   53–4
  treatment in comorbid syphilis/HIV   56–7
  vascular abnormalities   59–60
pup–mother attachment   86–7
Purkinje cells
  antibodies against   176, 178
  in Borna disease model   208
pyramidal cell atrophy   73, 74, 75

quetiapine   57
quinolinate–kyrenurate balance   40

radiculitis/radiculmyelitis   241
rainfall and schizophrenia   2
Reelin   68, 72
Reelin-positive cells   37, 47
respiratory immune system   189
respiratory infections   43–4
  and cycloid psychoses   14
  and schizophrenia   14–15, 44–5
retinitis   241
rheumatic disease
  neuropathology   60–1
  and psychoses   59, 60, 61–2
rheumatic fever (RF)
  and GAS   137
    M18 strains   166
  and PANDAS   135, 136
  predisposition   145
  Salt Lake City outbreaks   166
  and Sydenham chorea   154
risperidone   56
Rubella Birth Defects Evaluation Project (RBDEP)   45
  follow-up investigations   46
rubella, prenatal
  and partial autistic syndrome   198
  pathogenic mechanisms   47
  and schizophrenia   96
    serologic study   45–6

schizophrenia
  age of onset   3
  behavioral abnormalities   70
  birth excesses worldwide   22
  Borna disease virus in   127–9
  brain asymmetry   24
  cannabinoid system in   20
  chronic   13
  climate factors   2
  clinical symptoms   3
  cytokines   98
    viral infection induced   37–40
  daylight/sunlight   1–2, 3
  deficit/non-deficit   4
  differential diagnosis   112
  and enteroviruses   31–6

schizophrenia *continued*
  childhood infections 34–5
    prenatal infections 32–4
  environmental factors 69
  epidemiology
    enteroviruses 31–6
    and Lyme borreliosis 18–30
    prenatal infections 12–17
    season-of-birth effect 1–10, 12
  ethnicity 4
  familial nature 69
  family history 3–4
  gender 5
  genetics 5, 69
  heat shock proteins 268
  history 18
  infections 3
    influenza 263
      schizotypy scores 264–5
  infectious–inflammatory model 62
  Kraepelinian 4
  low birthweight 3
  mechanism of pathogenesis 268
  nailfold capillary abnormalities 62
  neuroanatomical features 4–5
  neurodegeneration 39–40
  neurodevelopment in 37–8
  neurodevelopmental hypothesis 43, 66, 67
  neuropathologic studies 68–9
  neurophysiological features 5
  neurotransmitters 39
  paranoid/non-paranoid 3
  'parental procreational habits' hypothesis 5
  place of birth
    city *vs* country 4, 43
    distance from equator 2
    latitude 1–2
  and polio virus 267
  pregnancy/birth complications (PBCs) 2–3
  premorbid antecedents 46
  prenatal infections 12–17, 34–5, 43–50, 70, 96–7
    future research
      animal models 48
      gene–environment interaction 49
      neuroimaging 48–9
    history taking 12
    immunology 37–8
    infectious agents 44
    mechanisms, suggested 69
    obstetric complications 13, 16, 96
    pathogenic mechanisms 47–8
    prevention 48
    and psychiatric nosology 11, 12–17
    serology 45–7
    time of infection
      5th *vs* 6th month 264
      23rd week 267–8
      first trimester 14, 15, 46
      second trimester (midgestational) 13, 14, 15, 32, 33, 37, 44, 45
    transuterine transmission of borreliosis 20
  prognosis and season of birth 3
  rainfall 2
  season-of-birth effect 1–10, 12, 43, 96
    differentiated psychopathology 12
    Lyme borreliosis, correlation with 18–20

    poliomyelitis 32, 33
    population attributable risk 1
    shifts over time 5
  skin conductance 1
  social class 4
  and stress 265–7
  susceptibility genes 38, 49
  timing of contributing factors 264, 267–8
  vitamin D seasonal variations 3
  winter temperatures 2
  see also schizophrenia subtypes
schizophrenia spectrum disorders 263–4
schizotypal personality 263–70
  and earthquake 265–7
  and influenza 264–5
schizotypy scores
  and influenza 264–5
  and stress 265–7
school difficulties
  with HIV/AIDS 242
  with PANDAS 155
season-of-birth effect *see under* schizophrenia
seizures 241
sensorimotor coordination 84
sensorimotor gating 85–6, 87
sensory overload 70
serotonin (5-HT)
  in Borna disease model 210–11
  depletion by cytokines 109–10
  in schizophrenia 39–40
shingles 241
signal transduction and infection/immunity 117–19
simian immunodeficiency virus study 246–7
skin conductance in schizophrenia 1
SNAP-25 68
  immunoreactivity 71–2
  in psychiatric disorders 117
social behavior
  Borna disease 212
  and prenatal infections 86, 176
social class and schizophrenia 4
soluble interleukin receptors (sIL-Rs)
  sIL-2R 115, 116
  sIL-6R 115, 116
SPECT imaging 157
spirochetes
  cystic structures 26–7
  heat shock proteins 22, 27–8
spontaneous activity 83–4
sporadic schizophrenia and Lyme borreliosis 18–30
  genetic correlate 23
  geographical correlation 19, 20–3
  multiple sclerosis, correlation with 26–9
    biological plausibility 27–9
    etiological correlate 26–7
    season/locality as correlates 26
  phenotypic correlate
    animal models 24
    pharmacological evidence 24–6
  prenatal transuterine transmission 20
  seasonal correlation 18–20
    biological plausibility 20
Streptococcus pyogenes see group A streptococcus (GAS)
streptococcal infections and psychiatric illness 60
streptococcal pharyngitis 144

streptokinase
  antibodies 181
  binding to DPP IV (CD26) 179–80
stress
  and cellular immunity 108–9
  coping strategies 109
  in HIV-infected children 240
  and life events 109
  physiological effects 108
  and schizotypal personality 265–7
  timing 267–8
  vs type of stressor 268
subcortical dementia 241–2
substance abuse 59
superantigens 138, 165–6
  and psychiatric disease 166–8
susceptibility genes for schizophrenia 38, 49
Sydenham chorea 60, 135, 154–61
  anti-basal ganglia antibodies 163, 167
  antineuronal antibody assays 163
  characteristics 137
  clinical features
    movement disorders 155
    multi-organ involvement 156
    neurological signs 155
    psychiatric disorders 155–6
  emotional lability 155
  GAS 137
    pathogenesis 157
  genetics 158–9
  history 154–5
  immune response 164–5
  implications for neuropsychiatric disorders 159
  neurological manifestations 137–8
  and obsessive–compulsive disorder 136
  pathogenesis
    immunopathogenesis 157–8
    neuroanatomy/neuropathology 156–7
    neurochemistry 157
    neuroimaging 157
  treatment 159
synaptophysins 117
  SNAP-25 68
    immunoreactivity 71–2
    psychiatric disorders 117
syphilis
  CNS symptoms 53
  comorbid HIV infection 52
    management recommendations 55–6
    psychosis treatment 56–7
  dementia in 55
  incidence 51
  psychosis in 53–4
  transmission 51–2
systematic catatonia 12
  demographic/environmental/genetic factors 15
  prenatal infections 14, 15
systematic schizophrenias
  prenatal infections 13
  season-of-birth effect 12
systemic immunity 200

T cells
  activated, in autoimmunity 171, 184

autoreactive
  in autistic spectrum disorder 191
  in neuroimmunity 183, 184
  in Borna disease 125
  in depression 109
  in PANDAS/Sydenham's chorea 164, 167
  regulatory 188
  and superantigens 165
T-helper cells 203
  Th1/Th2 balance 188
temporal cortex, *Chlamydia pneumoniae* in 233
tetrahydrocannabinol (THC) 24
thioridazine 56
tic disorders 135–53
  age of onset 135
  characteristics 137
  diagnosis/treatment 149–50
  immune basis, evidence of 139–43
  and neurological soft signs 146
  seasonality 144
tonsillopharyngitis 144
Tourette syndrome 135–53, 192
  anti-basal ganglia antibodies 163
  antineuronal antibodies 159
  antineuronal antibody assays 163
  characteristics 137
  marker 146
toxic gut–brain interactions 202–3
Toxoplasma gondii 114, 115
  in bipolar disorder 117
  and schizophrenia 113
Treponema pallidum 18, 28, 52, 53
  causing cognitive dysfunction 55
treponematoses 27, 28
  see also neurosyphilis; syphilis
tumor growth factor-β (TNF-β) 97
  in HIV/AIDS 246
tumor necrosis factor-alpha (TNF-α)
  in HIV/AIDS 246
  in inflammatory perinatal brain damage 216
  in LPS model of infection 97
  and neuron survival 99
  in schizophrenia 38, 47
  and schizophrenia 98
  transplacental passage 97

ultrasound 216–17
unsystematic schizophrenias 11
  season-of-birth effect 12

vaccination
  measles 198
  measles–mumps–rubella 193, 198, 201, 204
  mumps 224
  poliomyelitis 33–4
  rubella 48
vaccine adverse events reporting system (VAERS) 204
valproate
  in bipolar disorder 115, 118
  and immunity 115
  psychosis in syphilis/HIV 57
  in Sydenham chorea 159
vancomycin 193
vascular abnormalities
  in depression 60
  and psychoses 59–60

vascular disease, inflammatory 60, 62
vasculitis, CNS 59, 60
ventricle to brain ratio (VBR)
 in influenza animal model 73, 74
 schizophrenia 5–6
viral amino acid sequences 256, 259
viral animal models of neuropsychiatric diseases 213
viral infection and autism 198
viral persistence 91, 93
viral sequestration 239
vitamin D seasonal variations 3

white matter damage
 in HIV/AIDS 244
 perinatal 216–21
winter temperatures and schizophrenia 2
Wnt pathway 118

xenobiotics and neuroimmunity 174–5, 183

zidovudine (AZT) 247
ziprasidone 57
zooprophylaxis 23